Self Assessment & Re~~

Obstetrics

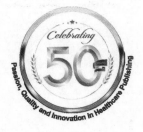

M000250065

Self Assessment & Review

Obstetrics

Thirteenth Edition

SAKSHI ARORA HANS

Faculty of Leading PG and FMGE Coachings
MBBS "Gold Medalist" (GSVM, Kanpur)
DGO (MLNMC, Allahabad)
India

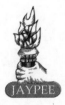

JAYPEE BROTHERS MEDICAL PUBLISHERS
The Health Sciences Publisher
New Delhi | London

Jaypee Brothers Medical Publishers (P) Ltd

Headquarters
Jaypee Brothers Medical Publishers (P) Ltd
4838/24, Ansari Road, Daryaganj
New Delhi 110 002, India
Phone: +91-11-43574357
Fax: +91-11-43574314
Email: jaypee@jaypeebrothers.com

Overseas Office
J.P. Medical Ltd
83 Victoria Street, London
SW1H 0HW (UK)
Phone: +44 20 3170 8910
Fax: +44 (0)20 3008 6180
Email: info@jpmedpub.com

Website: www.jaypeebrothers.com
Website: www.jaypeedigital.com

© 2020, Jaypee Brothers Medical Publishers

The views and opinions expressed in this book are solely those of the original contributor(s)/author(s) and do not necessarily represent those of editor(s) of the book.

All rights reserved. No part of this publication may be reproduced, stored or transmitted in any form or by any means, electronic, mechanical, photocopying, recording or otherwise, without the prior permission in writing of the publishers.

All brand names and product names used in this book are trade names, service marks, trademarks or registered trademarks of their respective owners. The publisher is not associated with any product or vendor mentioned in this book.

Medical knowledge and practice change constantly. This book is designed to provide accurate, authoritative information about the subject matter in question. However, readers are advised to check the most current information available on procedures included and check information from the manufacturer of each product to be administered, to verify the recommended dose, formula, method and duration of administration, adverse effects and contraindications. It is the responsibility of the practitioner to take all appropriate safety precautions. Neither the publisher nor the author(s)/editor(s) assume any liability for any injury and/ or damage to persons or property arising from or related to use of material in this book.

This book is sold on the understanding that the publisher is not engaged in providing professional medical services. If such advice or services are required, the services of a competent medical professional should be sought.

Every effort has been made where necessary to contact holders of copyright to obtain permission to reproduce copyright material. If any have been inadvertently overlooked, the publisher will be pleased to make the necessary arrangements at the first opportunity. The **CD/DVD-ROM** (if any) provided in the sealed envelope with this book is complimentary and free of cost. **Not meant for sale**.

Inquiries for bulk sales may be solicited at: jaypee@jaypeebrothers.com

Self Assessment & Review: Obstetrics

First Edition	:	2007
Second Edition	:	2009
Third Edition	:	2010
Fourth Edition	:	2011
Fifth Edition	:	2012
Sixth Edition	:	2013
Seventh Edition	:	2014
Eighth Edition	:	2015
Ninth Edition	:	2016
Tenth Edition	:	2017
Eleventh Edition	:	2018
Twelfth Edition	:	2019
Thirteenth Edition	:	**2020**

ISBN: 978-93-90020-52-2
Printed at: Sanat Printers

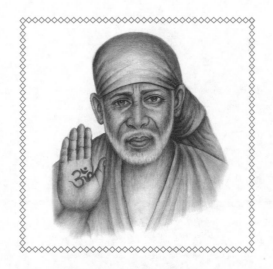

Dedicated to

SAI BABA

Just sitting here reflecting on where I am and where I started, I could not have done it without you Sai baba... I praise you and love you for all that you have given me... and thank you for another beautiful day... to be able to sing and praise you and glorify you... you are "*My Amazing God*".

'I met a man under a tree succumbed, unhappy and diseased. Howling in tears, hating his destiny. Unknowing reasons for his suffering and complexity. A disciple of god approched. Explaining his boundless and inevitable sufferings pointing karma for his hardship and obstacles and chanting god's name, the only way to fight the battle.

Making him understand about mystic law. His past karma is his only flaw.

Guiding him to courageously challenge his transitory life condition.

Earnestly praying gohonzon, manifesting his life mission.

Standing strong unshakable as mighty tree Concentrating power of mystic law to being happiness limitlessly, free. Expediting karmas for your own good. Virtues will then lead you to attain Buddahood.

Dear Students,

I extend my heartfelt thanks to all of you for giving so much love and acceptance to my books. It feels nostalgic to think that this is the 13th year of my books. This journey of 12 years wouldn't have been so wonderful without your support. I humbly accept that my books were not error-free but your acceptance had still made them to remain the best-selling books on the subjects. In the new edition (13/e) of my books, I have aspired to resolve all the queries and complaints.

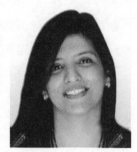

The 13/e includes:

○ Completely colored book
○ Theory before each chapter for the first time ever
○ USG'S & figures needed for exams.
○ Annexures for last minute revision
○ New guidelines of HIV in pregnancy
○ New diagnostic techniques
○ X-rays
○ AIIMS New Pattern Questions

I have put in my best effort in 13/e and I am sure this edition will mark the beginning of a new era. But I cannot achieve this alone. I request all of you to forward me the corrections and the mistakes that you encounter while reading the books. Together we can ensure that the books can remain the best-sellers for years to come and together we can pave the road of dreams of all the aspiring medicos. You can send your suggestions/corrections via the following routes:

Email: gsogclassesbydrsakshiarora@gmail.com
YouTube Channel — Dr Sakshi Arora Hans Obs and Gynae
Instagram Handle — Dr Sakshi Arora Hans
Telegram Group — obgbysakshiarorahans

I look forward to your support and cooperation.

Yours truly
Dr Sakshi Arora Hans

Acknowledgments

Everything what we are is the outcome of a series of factors and circumstances, in addition to ourselves.

It would not be fair, therefore, to ignore the people who have played an important part in making me known as 'Dr Sakshi Arora' and to whom I am deeply grateful.

My Teachers

Dr Manju Verma (Professor & Head, Department of Obstetrics and Gynecology, MLNMC, Allahabad) and Dr **Gauri Ganguli** (Professor & Ex-Head, Department of Obstetrics and Gynecology, MLNMC, Allahabad) for teaching me to focus on the basic concepts of any subject.

My Family

Dr Pankaj Hans, my better-half, who has always been a mountain of support and who is, to a large measure, responsible for what I am today. He has always encouraged me to deliver my best.

My Father: Shri HC Arora, who has overcome all odds with his discipline, hard work, and perfection.

My Mother: Smt. Sunita Arora, who has always believed in my abilities and supported me in all my ventures—be it authoring a book or teaching.

My in-laws (Hans family): For happily accepting my maiden surname 'Arora' and taking pride in all my achievements.

My Brothers: Mr Bhupesh Arora and Mr Sachit Arora, who encouraged me to write books and have always thought (wrong although) their sister is a perfectionist.

My Daughter: Shreya Hans (A priceless gift of god): For accepting my books and work as her siblings (who is now showing signs of intense sibling rivalry!!) and letting me use her share of my time. Thanks 'betu' for everything—your smile, your hugs, and tantrums!

My Colleagues: I am grateful to all my seniors, friends and colleagues of past and present for their moral support.

- Dr Manoj Rawal
- Dr Ruchi Aggrawal
- Dr Parminder Sehgal
- Dr Pooja Aggrawal
- Dr Shalini Tripathi
- Dr Amit Jain
- Dr Parul Aggrawal Jain
- Dr Kushant Gupta
- Dr Sonika Lamba Rawal

Directors of PG Entrance coaching, who helped me in realizing my potential as an academician:

- **Dr Vineet Gupta** (Director MIST Coaching)
- **Mr Parcha R Sundar Rao** (SIMS Academy)

Students

Dr Ahmed Savani—Surat, Gujarat

Dr Nazir Ahmad

Dr Sachin Paparikar

Dr Rakshit Chakravarty

Dr Linkan Verma, intern, Gandhi Medical College, Bhopal

Dr Asharam Panda, MKCG Medical College, Behrampur district, Odisha

Dr Hamik Patel

Dr Pankaj Zanwar

Dr Sreedhanya Sreedharan, Final year MBBS, Jubilee Mission Medical College, Thrissur

Dr Vinit Singh, Intern, RG Kar Medical College, Kolkata

Dr Junaid Shaikh, CU Shah Medical College, Dudhrej, Gujarat

Dr Niraj R Shah (Student of DIAMS) Academy, Smolensk State Medical Academy, Russia

Dr Aarti Dalwani, Baroda Medical College, Vadodara, Gujarat

Dr Rola Turki, King Abdulaziz University, Jeddah, Saudi Arabia
Dr Ronak Kadia, Baroda Medical College, Vadodara, Gujarat
Dr Anita Basoode, Raichur Institute of Medical Sciences, Raichur, Karnataka
Dr Neerja Barve, Bukovinian State Medical University, Ukraine
Dr Vinod Babu Veerapalli, Gandhi Medical College, Hyderabad

- Dr Indraneel Sharma
- Dr Vishal Sadana
- Dr Kumuda Gandikota
- Dr Shiraz Sheikh
- Dr Innie Sri
- Dr Ulhas Patil Medical College, Jalgaon, Maharashtra
- Dr Prasanna Lakshmi
- Dr Ankit Baswal

- Dr Ashutosh Singh
- Dr Azizul Hasan
- Dr Vaibhav Thakare
- Dr Gayatri Mittal
- Dr Chhavi Goel

- Dr Nelson Thomas
- **Dr S Jayasri Medhi**, Gauhati Medical College, Assam

- Dr Surender Morodia
- Dr Awanish Kant
- Dr Ramesh Ammati
- Dr Mariya Shabnam Sheikh
- Dr Jayesh Gosavi
- Dr Sandeepan Saha
- Dr Sana Ravon

My Publishers – Jaypee Brothers Medical Publishers (P) Ltd
Shri Jitendar P Vij (Group Chairman) for being my role model and a father-like figure. I will always remain indebted to him for all that he has done for me.
Mr Ankit Vij (Managing Director) for being so down-to-earth and always approachable.
Ms Chetna Malhotra Vohra (Associate Director—Content Strategy) for working hard with the team to **achieve the deadlines.**
The entire MCQs team for working laborious hours in designing and typesetting the book.

Last but not the least—

All the Students/Readers for sharing their invaluable, constructive criticism for the improvement of the book.

My sincere thanks to all FMGE/UG/PG students, present and past, for their tremendous support, words of appreciation (rather I should say e-mails of encouragement), which have helped me in the betterment of the book.

Dr Sakshi Arora Hans
delhisakshiarora@gmail.com

1. FOR PRE FINAL/FINAL YEAR STUDENTS:

Obstetrics and Gynaecology is a major subject not only for Final year but for all PG entrance examinations and supposedly for the Exit exam (if it comes). So you cannot take this subject lightly. I would suggest you all to start reading my book during your Third year MBBS to build your basics right from the beginning.

Sequence to Read Chapters

Now the sequence in which I want you read the chapters- (This will help you in understanding and building the concepts in a better way)

Entire Obstetrics should be read in 4 parts

Part 1–General Obstetrics

Part 2–Labor

Part 3–Complications Specific to Pregnancy

Part 4–Medical Complication in Pregnancy

Sequence to follow while reading each chapter

Read the theory of a chapter from this book and then read the textbook. You will be able to easily understand the textbook now.
Now read the theory of that chapter once again.
Now solve the MCQ from the book.
Follow this with another reading from the textbook.
- This completes your chapter with one reading and revision.
- While reading the book, either make notes or mark in the book itself for quick revision. Mark the difficult and important MCQ for further revision.
- Do this for all the chapters.
- After completing the syllabus, start revising.
- Remember minimum 4–5 readings are required before exams.

2. FOR INTERNS AND POST-INTERNS:

○ I do not recommend studying textbook now due to scarcity of time. However, textbook should be kept as a reference material

○ Do not confuse yourself by studying many books.

○ You should spend 10 days on both obs and gynae—6 for obs and 4 for gynae for first reading.

Read the theory of a chapter and solve MCQ of that chapter.
While solving MCQs, solve all questions at a stretch and only after this compare the answers.

↓

Re-read the theory of this chapter and now mark the important points for revision.
Remember, you should mark only that much so that the next reading of book can be finished in one third of the time. Similarly, encircle or mark the important MCQ for revision.
Just keep cutting those questions which you were able to solve at one go.

↓

Do same for all the chapters.

↓

During revision, study only marked portion with encircled MCQ only.
Second reading of entire obs and gynae should be finished in 4–5 days.

↓

Similarly third and fourth revision should be completed in 3 days each.

↓

Give one last revision just before exams in a day or two.

○ Remember, obs and gynae is a very important subject. You can answer nearly all questions asked in any exam on gynaecology from this book if you concentrate.

In the end test yourself by attempting the 102 questions question paper given of new pattern AIIMS exam and evaluate yourself.

I wish you all good luck for your exams and a very happy learning.

Dr Sakshi Arora Hans

Contents

SECTION 5—LATEST PAPERS

SECTION 6—MOST RECENT PAPERS

Most Important ★★★★★
Very Important ★★★★
Important ★★★

Symbols used in the book

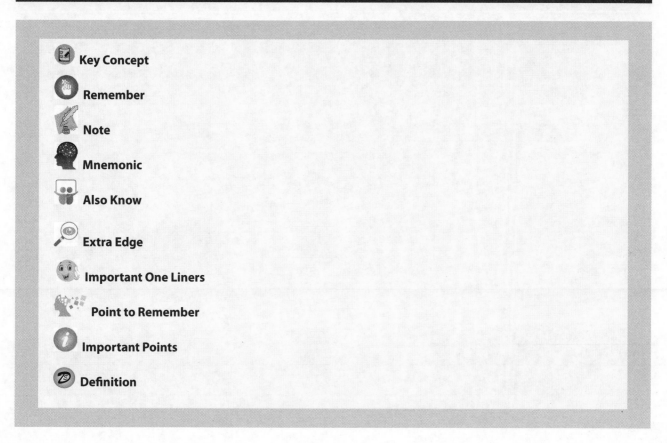

Key Concept

Remember

Note

Mnemonic

Also Know

Extra Edge

Important One Liners

Point to Remember

Important Points

Definition

Important Topic: **SLE in Pregnancy**

SLE IN PREGNANCY

It is due to immune system abnormalities including over-active B lymphocytes that are responsible for autoantibody production.

Antibodies formed in SLE with their clinical associations:

1. *Antinuclear (ANA)*:
   - Best screening test[Q]
   - A second negative test makes SLE unlikely.
2. *Anti ds DNA*:
   - High titres are specific for SLE
   - May correlate with disease activity—nephritis and vasculitis
3. *Anti sm (smith)*:
   - Specific for SLE[Q]
4. *Anti RNP*:
   - Associated with rheumatic syndromes
   - Not SLE specific
5. *Anti RO/SSA or SS-B*: Associated with:
   - Sicca syndrome
   - Predisposes to cutaneous lupus
   - Neonatal lupus with[Q] congenital heart block
   - Reduced risk of nephritis
6. *Anti histone*:
   - Common in drug induced lupus
7. Anti phospholipid
   - Lupus anticoagulant and anticardiolipin antibodies are associated with thrombosis, fetal loss, valvular heart disease
   - Chances of renal insufficiency are more.
8. Anti-erythrocyte
   - Direct Coombs test is negative
   - Hemolysis may develop

Important Parts

- 90% of SLE cases are in women
- 10 year survival rate = 70–90%
- Genetic influence → M/C in monozygotic twins than Dizygotic twins

- Familial inheritance seen (10%)
- Risk of disease increases if there is inheritance of "Autoimmunity gene" on chromosome 16.

Lupus and Pregnancy

- During pregnancy:
  - SLE improves in 1/3rd of women
  - Remains unchanged in 1/3rd of women
  - Worsens in 1/3rd of women
- Any newly diagnosed SLE during pregnancy tends to be severe
- In general pregnancy outcome is best in women in whom
  - Lupus activity has been quiescent for at least 6 months before conception
  - There is NO
    - Lupus nephritis
    - Antiphospholipid antibody syndrome
    - Super imposed pre-eclampsia

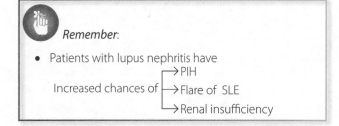

Remember:

- Patients with lupus nephritis have

  Increased chances of → PIH
  → Flare of SLE
  → Renal insufficiency

Management

- No permanent cure
- In mild cases → *symptomatic cure*
  - *For arthralgia/serositis*: NSAIDs

Note: Avoid chronic or large intermittent dosing due to related oligohydramnios or ductus arteriosus closure

- Low dose aspirin throughout pregnancy
- Severe disease is managed by Prednisolone (1 to 2 mg/kg/day) orally

Side Effect:

Corticosteroid can lead to gestational diabetes

- In case of lupus nephritis/SLE resistant to corticosteroid. Best drug is Azathioprine

Others:

- Cyclophosphamide in 2nd/3rd trimester
- Mycophenolate

Note: If before pregnancy, patient of SLE was on antimalarials then they should be continued in pregnancy

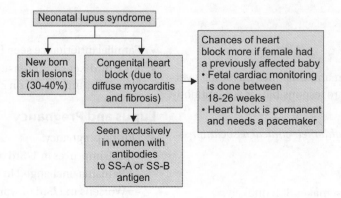

Annexures

Colour of amniotic fluid	Seen in condition
Colorless	Preterm
Straw coloured	Term
Green colour (meconium)	Fetal distress/breech or transverse lie/listeria infection
Golden yellow	Rh-incompatibility
Saffron	Postdated pregnancy
Tobacco juice	IUFD

ANNEXURE - 2

Causes of oligohydramnios:

- *Drugs*: PG synthetase inhibitor–Indomethacin
- Maternal conditions–High BP (Gestational HT/Preeclampsia/Eclampsia)
- Post-term pregnancy
- Premature rupture of membrane (PROM)
- Amnion nodosum
- Chromosomal anomaly–Triploidy
- Renal anomalies: Renal agenesis
- Posterior urethral valve.

ANNEXURE - 3

Causes of polyhydramnios:

- **Fetus produces more urine for example:**
  a. Twin/multifetal pregnancy (number of fetus is more: more of urine)
  b. Maternal hyperglycemia/diabetes
     Maternal hyperglycemia → Fetalhyperglycemia → Fetal polyuria → Increased amniotic fluid
  c. Twin-to-twin transfusion syndrome.
- **Besides producing amniotic fluid fetus also swallows amniotic fluid. The amount of amniotic fluid will increase if; fetal swallowing is impaired as in case of:**
  a. Cleft lip and cleft palate
  b. Esophageal atresia or stenosis
  c. Duodenal atresia or stenosis
  d. Bowel obstruction
  e. Anencephaly (swallowing is decreased + increased transudation of CSF into amniotic fluid due to absence of cranial vault).
- **Other important causes of polyhydraminos which need to mugged up are:**
  1. *Placental Causes:*
     a. Chorangioma of placenta and circumvallate placenta.
  2. *Fetal Causes:*
     a. Hydrops fetalis
     b. Rubella, syphilis, toxoplasma infection of fetus
     c. Trisomy (note—Triploidy leads to oligohydraminos)

d. Sacrococcygeal teratoma
e. Thallasemia of fetus.

ANNEXURE - 4

Types of pelvis and important points on them

Caldwell and Mohoy classification:

Gynaecoid	50%
Anthropoid	25%
Android	20%
Platypelloid	5%

Important points:

 Key Concept

Remember the following points on pelvi (most of the questions are asked on them):

- Normal female pelvis – Gynaecoid pelvis[Q].
- Male type pelvis – Android pelvis[Q].
- Most common type of pelvis – Gynaecoid pelvis[Q].
- Least common type pelvis – Platypelloid pelvis[Q].
- The only pelvis with AP diameter more than transverse diameter – Anthropoid pelvis[Q].
- Face to pubes delivery is most common in Anthropoid pelvis[Q].
- Direct occipitoposterior position is most common in Anthropoid pelvis[Q].
- Persistent occipitoposterior position is most common in Android pelvis[Q].
- Deep transverse arrest/ Nonrotation/Dystocia is most common in Android pelvis[Q].
- Broad flat pelvis – Platypelloid pelvis[Q].
- Transverse diameter is much more than AP diameter – Platypelloid pelvis[Q].
- Engagement by exaggerated posterior asynclitism occurs in platypelloid pelvis[Q].
- Super subparietal instead of biparietal diameter engages in platypelloid pelvis[Q].

ANNEXURE - 5

Definitive signs of early pregnancy:

Sign	Feature	Seen in
Jacquemier's/ Chadwick's sign	Dusky hue of the vestibule and anterior vaginal wall due to local vascular congestion	8th week of pregnancy
Osiander's sign	Increased pulsation felt through the lateral fornices	8th week of pregnancy
Goodell's sign	Softening of cervix (cervix feels like lip of mouth whereas in non pregnant state it feels like tip of nose)	6th week of pregnancy
Hegar's sign	On bimanual examination with 2 fingers in anterior fornix and fingers of other hand behind the uterus, the abdominal and vaginal fingers seem to appose below the body of uterus. It occurs because of softening of isthmus[Q]	6-10 weeks of pregnancy
Palmer's sign	Regular and rhythmic uterine contraction which can be felt on bimanual examination	6-8 weeks of pregnancy

- In the first trimester *uterus* enlarges to the size of hens egg at 6th week, cricket ball size at 8th week and size of fetal head by 12th week. It remains an intrapelvic organ.
- **Other signs seen in early pregnancy:**
  - Hartman sign—bleeding present at the time of implantation in few females.

ANNEXURE - 6

Best parameters for estimation of fetal age:

• 1st trimester	Crown Rump length (CRL)
• 2nd trimester	Biparietal diameter (BPD)
• 3rd trimester	Femur length
• Overall	Crown Rump length

- **BPD is measured in the trans thalamic view at the level of the thalami and cavum septum pellucidum. From outer table of skull to inner table.**

- Cephalic index = BPD divided by occipito frontal diameter (OFD).
- It head shape is flattened (dolichocephaly) or rounded (brachycephaly), then HC is more reliable than BPD. As BPD is affected by shape of head but not HC.

USG in pregnancy
- Best time to assess gestational age by USG is 9-12 weeks (by crown rump length).[Q]
- Best indicator of fetal growth – Abdominal circumference.[Q]
- So the best USG parameter to detect IUGR is Abdominal circumference.[Q]
- The best USG parameter to detect macrosomia is abdominal circumference.[Q]
- **AC is measured at the junction of left and right portal vein or liver and cystic duct.[Q]**
- Mean sac diameter (CMSD) is used to determine gestational age before CRL can be measured.
- MSD = Length + height + width/3.
- Normal MSD (in mm) + 30 = days of pregnancy.
- CRL (in mm) + 42 = gestation in days.
- The embryo should increase its CRL by 1 mm per day.
- Fetal anomaly which can be earliest detected by USG–Anencephaly.
- Lemon and Banana sign are seen in spina bifida on USG.
- The two best ultrasonographic markers of Down syndrome in first trimester:
  a. Absent or hypoplastic nasal bone
  b. Increased nuchal translucency.
- The diameter which in mm when measured between 14 and 24 weeks corresponds to the gestational age in weeks – Inter cerebellar diameter.[Q]
- If a single ultrasound examination is planned for the purpose of evaluating fetal anatomy, ACOG (2011) recommends it to be performed at 18–20 weeks.

ANNEXURE - 7

Safety of vaccines in pregnancy:

 Remember: A simple "FUNDA" (Proposed by CDC Society, 2002).
- Killed vaccine are safe in pregnancy.
- Live vaccines are best avoided in pregnancy.

Safety of Vaccines in Pregnancy:

Safe	Only in epidemics	To be given in case of travel to highly endemic area or exposed to contacts	Contraindicated
• H -Hepatitis A/B	• Tab-Typhoid • P-Pneumococcus • C-Cholera	• Yellow fever • Japenese encephalitis • Polio (IPV)	• Rubella • Measles • Varicella
• I-Influenza • T-Tetanus • Rabies-Rabies (mnemonic-HIT Rabies)	• M-Meningococcus (Tab PCM)		• BCG • Mumps • Small pox

ANNEXURE - 8

Important time table of events:

Important events	Following fertilization	
'0' hour	Fertilization	
4th day	16 cell stage	
	Morula enters uterine cavity	
5th day	Blastocyst	
7th day	Interstitial implantation occurs	
21st–22nd day	Placenta fully established/Fetal circulation established and heart formed	
8 weeks	Internal gonads formed	
10–12 weeks	Swallowing starts	
11 weeks	Fetal breathing movements	
12 weeks	External genitalia formed	
12 weeks	Urine formation occurs	
14 weeks	Gender can be identified on USG	

ANNEXURE - 9

Few named structures and their location:

Named structure	Seen in
• Nitabuch's layer	It is the zone of fibroid degeneration where trophoblast and decidua meet. Seen in basal plate of placenta
• Hoffbaeur cells	Phagocytic cell seen in connective tissue of chorionic villi of placenta
• Folds of Hobokon	Umbilical cord
• Whartons jelly	Connective tissue of umbilical cord
• Peg cells	Fallopian tube
• Langhans cells	Cytotrophoblast

ANNEXURE - 10

Recommended weight gain in pregnancy based on BMI in singleton pregnancy:

Weight - for - height		Recommended total weight gain		Weight gain/week
Category	BMI	kg	lb	In lb/week
Underweight	<18.5	12.5-18	28-40	1 (1-1.3)
Normal	18.5-24.9	11.5-14	25-35	1 (0.8-1)
Overweight	25-29.9	7-11.5	15-25	0.6 (0.5-0.7)
Obese	≥30	7	11-20	0.5 (0.4-0.6)

 Note: 1 lb = 0.454 kg
Recommended weight gain is 31–50 lb.
Recommended weight gain in twin pregnancy:
- Normal BMI = 37-54 lb
- Overweight = 31-50 lb
- Obese = 25-42 lb
- 1 lb = 0.454 kg

ANNEXURE - 11

Fetal heart rate traces as described by NICE (2015 guidelines):

Description	Feature baseline (bpm)	Baseline variability (bpm)	Deceleration
Reassuring/Normal	100-160	5 or more	None or early
Nonreassuring	161-180	Less than 5 for 30-90 minutes	Variable decelerations: • Dropping from baseline by 60 bpm or less and taking 60 seconds or less to recover • Present for over 90 minutes • Occurring with over 50% of contractions. OR Variable decelerations: • Dropping from baseline by more than 60 bpm or taking over 60 seconds to recover • Present for up to 30 minutes • Occurring with over 50% of contractions. OR Late deceleration: • Present for up to 30 minutes • Occurring with over 50% of contractions.
Abnormal	Above 180 or below 100	Less than 5 for over 90 minutes	Nonreassuring variable decelerations • Still observed 30 minutes after starting conservative measures • Occurring with over 50% of contractions. OR Late decelerations: • Present for over 30 minutes • Do not improve with conservative measures • Occurring with over 50% of contractions.

Description	Feature baseline (bpm)	Baseline variability (bpm)	Deceleration
			OR Bradycardia or a single prolonged Deceleration lasting 3 minutes or more

ANNEXURE - 12

Conditions in which alphafetoproteins are increased and decreased:

Elevated levels	Low levels

• Error in dates
• Multifetal pregnancy
• Severe oligohydramnios
• Neural tube defects
• Pilonidal cysts
• Esophageal or intestinal obstruction (and atresia)
• Liver necrosis
• Cystic hygroma
• Sacrococcygeal teratoma
• Fetal death
• Abdominal wall defects:
  – Omphalocele
  – Gastroschisis
• Urinary obstruction
• Renal anomalies:
  – Polycystic kidney
  – Absent kidneys
• Congenital nephrosis
• Osteogenesis imperfecta
• Congenital skin defects
• Cloacal exstrophy
• Chorioangioma of placenta
• Low birth weight
• Placental abruption
• Placenta accreta
• Preeclampsia
• Improper adjustment for low maternal weight
• Maternal hepatoma or teratoma
	• **G: G**estational trophoblastic diseases
	• **O²: O**verestimated gestational age, overweight mother
	• **A:** Spontaneous **a**bortion
	• **T: T**risomy (21 or 18)

ANNEXURE - 13

Conditions in which hCG levels are increased and decreased:

Increased	Decreased
M Multiple fetuses^Q	a. Ectopic pregnancy^Q
R Rh-incompatibility^Q	b. Impending spontaneous abortion^Q
D Down syndrome^Q	c. Other trisomies viz. 18, 13
C Choriocarcinoma^Q	
H Hydatidiform mole^Q	*Mnemonic:* **MR. DCH**

1. Hydraminos can be diagnosed by:
   1. **Single vertical pocket > 8 cm**
   2. **Single vertical pocket > 5 cm**
   3. **AFI > 24 cm**
   4. **AFI > 20cm**
   5. **Subjective assessment**

   a. 1, 4, 5   b. 1, 3, 5
   c. 2, 3, 5   d. 1, 4

   A 16 years old girl presents with episodes of right sided abdominal pain for 1 week. Her menstrual cycles are irregular, and she had normal period 32 days back. There is no history of any bladder or bowel symptoms. Her vitals are normal. Per abdominal examination shows vague mass in RIF with tenderness on it and restricted mobility. Per rectal examination revealed 6 cm cystic mass in right adnexal area with tenderness. Her Hb is 10 gm %, routine urine examination is normal.

2. The most likely diagnosis is:
   a. Ectopic pregnancy   b. Twisted ovarian cyst
   c. Appendicular abscess   d. Pelvic endometrioma

3. The most useful investigation in this case would be:
   a. Urine pregnancy test
   b. Total and differential leukocyte count
   c. Pelvic ultrasonography
   d. CT scan of abdomen

4. The most appropriate treatment would be:
   a. Administering antibiotics
   b. Danazol
   c. Laparotomy   d. Observation

5. Consider the following statements in respect of perinatal mortality (PNM):
   1. **The PNM rate is defined as the number of fetal deaths plus the deaths in the first week of life per 1000 total births.**
   2. **Anoxia/birth traumas are the leading causes of PNM.**
   3. **In about one-third of the cases, the cause is unknown.**

   Which of the above statements are correct?
   a. 1, 2 and 3   b. 1 and 2
   c. 2 and 3   d. 1 and 3

6. Which one of the following sets of agents/drugs can be used for ripening and dilatation of the cervix, prior to an MTP by suction evacuation of the uterus?
   a. Isabgol, mifepristone, and prostaglandins
   b. Isabgol and mifepristone
   c. Mifepristone and prostaglandins
   d. Isabgol and prostaglandins

7. In which of the following sets of conditions is methylergometrine contraindicated in the prophylactic management of third stage of labor?
   a. Suspected multiple pregnancy and organic cardiac disease
   b. Suspected multiple pregnancy and Rh-negative mother
   c. Organic cardiac disease and Rh-negative mother
   d. Suspected multiple pregnancy, organic cardiac disease, and Rh-negative mother

8. Assertion (A): Spontaneous correction of retroversion of uterus is unusual during pregnancy.
   Reason (R): Retroversion of uterus during pregnancy leads to stretching of urethra and retention of urine.
   a. Both A and R are correct and R is correct explanation of A
   b. Both A and R are correct and R is not correct explanation of A
   c. A is true, R is false
   d. A is false, R is true
   e. Both A and R are false

9. All of the following statements regarding perinatal transmission of hepatitis B in newborn are true except:
   a. HB vaccine can be delayed for newborn beyond 48 hours. If mother is HbsAg positive
   b. Maximum transmission of hepatitis B from mother to child occurs at the time of delivery
   c. HBeAg positivity in mother increases the risk of transmission
   d. 70% of newborns infected at birth can become chronic carriers

10. In a case of diabetes mellitus complicating pregnancy:
    a. Insulin requirement decreases as pregnancy advances
    b. Oral hypoglycemics are preferred to insulin therapy
    c. There is increased incidence of hydramnios and pre-eclampsia
    d. Congenital malformations are unrelated to diabetic control

11. Consider the following procedures:
    1. **A trial of labor in suspected CPD**
    2. **Prophylactic forceps delivery**
    3. **Prophylactic methergin at the birth of the anterior shoulder of the fetus**

    Which of these procedures are contraindicated in a case of heart disease complicating pregnancy?
    a. 1, 2 and 3   b. 1 and 2
    c. 2 and 3   d. 1 and 3

12. Consider the following statements:
    The expected date of delivery can be determined by:
    1. **Using the Naegele's formula**
    2. **Assessing uterine size during first trimester by pelvic examination**
    3. **Doing ultrasonography at 18 to 20 weeks**

Which of these statements are correct?
a. 1, 2 and 3   b. 1 and 2
c. 2 and 3   d. 1 and 3

13. A patient with hemoglobin 7 g% at 36 weeks' gestation is admitted in antenatal ward. If the anemia is hypochromic microcytic, the most appropriate management of the patient would be:
a. Induction of labor immediately so that further deterioration of anemia is prevented
b. Blood transfusion to raise the hemoglobin to 9 g%
c. Administration of intravenous Imferon so that anemia can get corrected more rapidly
d. Administration of intramuscular or intravenous Imferon depending upon her pulse rate

14. Consider the following complications:
1. Hydramnios
2. Placenta previa
3. Pregnancy-induced hypertension

Which of these complications occur more commonly in respect of monozygotic twins as compared with dizygotic twins?
a. 1, 2 and 3   b. 1 and 2
c. 2 and 3   d. 1 and 3

15. A young lady presents with history of amenorrhea of 12 weeks, pain in the lower abdomen, and bleeding per vaginam. On examination, uterus is of 12 weeks' size, both OS are closed, and bleeding per vaginam is present. The most likely clinical diagnosis is:
a. Threatened abortion   b. Missed abortion
c. Incomplete abortion   d. Complete abortion

16. Consider the following findings:
1. Increased vascularity of the chorionic villi
2. Edema of the mesoderm or stromal tissue
3. Proliferation of the syncytial and cytotrophoblastic epithelium

Those present in a hydatidiform mole would include:
a. 1, 2 and 3   b. 1 and 2 only
c. 2 and 3 only   d. 1 and 3 only

17. Which one of the following statements regarding palpation of ischial spines during labor is not true?
a. It determines the station of presenting part in the pelvis
b. It determines the transverse diameter of cavity
c. It selects the site to administer pudendal nerve block
d. It determines capacity of the pelvic brim

18. Consider the following features:
1. Fundal dominance
2. In between the contractions, the intrauterine amniotic pressure being 20 mmHg
3. Progressive retraction of the upper uterine segment

Which of the above features are typical of uterine contraction in normal labor?
a. 1, 2 and 3   b. 1 and 2
c. 2 and 3   d. 1 and 3

19. All of the following statements regarding placental separation in the third stage of labor are true except:

a. The separation starts during the latter part of the second stage of labor
b. Placental separation can occur by the Schultze mechanism or the Matthew-Duncan mechanism
c. The Schultze mechanism is the most common one
d. The plane of separation is through the spongy layer of the deciduas basalis

20. Abruptio placentae in labor should be treated by:
a. Cesarean section even if the fetal heart is absent
b. Rupture of membranes followed by oxytocin drip
c. Fibrinogen transfusion to prevent DIC
d. Heparin injection to prevent fibrinogen degradation

21. All of the following statements regarding vacuum extraction are correct except:
a. The cervix should be at least 6 cm dilated
b. The cup should be placed against the fetal head as near the occiput as possible
c. The maximum vacuum should not be more than 1.5 kg/cm²
d. Traction should be applied during uterine contractions

22. Consider the following statements:
Occipitoposterior position in labor is more disadvantageous than occipitoanterior position because:
1. It has to undergo a long rotation of 3/8th of the circle
2. The head is deflexed
3. The diameter of engagement is suboccipitofrontal or occipitofrontal

Which of the above statements are correct?
a. 1, 2 and 3   b. 1 and 2
c. 2 and 3   d. 1 and 3

23. A sixth gravida has postpartum hemorrhage immediately after a spontaneous vertex delivery. The placenta and membranes are expelled completely. The uterus is not very firm. The first-line of treatment would be:
a. Blood transfusion
b. Massaging the uterus and administering an oxytocic
c. Inspecting the vagina and cervix for laceration
d. Exploring the uterine cavity

24. Which one of the following drugs is used for suppression of lactation?
a. Progesterone   b. Pyridoxine
c. Metachlorpropamide
d. Chlorpromazine

25. Consider the following statements regarding puerperal sepsis:
1. It is essentially a wound infection
2. The uterus is the commonest site
3. The mode of infection by anaerobic Streptococcus is endogenous

Which of the above statements are correct?
a. 1, 2 and 3   b. 1 and 2
c. 2 and 3   d. 1 and 3

26. In which one of the following situations in amniocentesis not called for?

a. Mother's age is 35 years or more
b. Parents who are known to have chromosomal translocation
c. Raised α-fetoprotein in amniotic fluid during earlier pregnancy
d. An Rh-negative multipara mother aged 30 years with two live healthy boys

27. Amniocentesis to detect chromosomal abnormalities can be done as early as:
a. 14th week of gestation
b. 18th week of gestation
c. 22nd week of gestation
d. 26th week of gestation

28. Which one of the following endometrial histopathological findings is suggestive of an ectopic pregnancy?
a. Decidual reaction
b. Chorionic villi
c. Proliferative endometrium
d. Secretory endometrium

29. The following are the characteristics of caput succedaneum except:
a. It is present at birth
b. It does not cause jaundice in newborn
c. It is limited to individual bone
d. It disappears within a few hours of birth

30. The four cardinal movements (1) flexion, (2) internal rotation, (3) extension, (4) restitution and external rotation, constitute the normal mechanism of labor. The chronological order in which they occur is:
a. 1, 2, 3, 4   b. 2, 1, 3, 4
c. 1, 3, 4, 2   d. 2, 3, 4, 1

31. Match list I (feature) with list II (diagnosis) and select the correct answer using the codes given below the lists:

List I (Feature)	List II (Diagnosis)
A. Star gazing fetus	1. Transverse lie
B. Frog eye appearance	2. Breech with extended head
C. Buddha's position	3. Anencephaly
D. Partus conduplicato corpore	4. Hydrops fetalis

```
    A  B  C  D          A  B  C  D
    1  4  3  2          1  3  4  2
    2  4  3  1          2  3  4  1
```
a. A-1, B-4, C-3, D-2   b. A-1, B-3, C-4, D-2
c. A-2, B-4, C-3, D-1   d. A-2, B-3, C-4, D-1

32. With reference to abnormal labor, consider the following procedures:
1. Internal podalic version
2. Forceps application
3. Assisted breech delivery

In which of these, the cervix should be fully dilated?
a. 1, 2, and 3   b . 1 and 2
c. 2 and 3   d. 1 and 3

33. At which station of head is outlet forceps applied?
a. +2 station   b . +3 station
c. 0 station
d. After full engagement of head

34. In which one of the following combinations, ABO incompatibility is most common?
a. Mother's group 'A' and father's group 'O'
b. Mother's group 'A' and father's group 'B'
c. Mother's group 'O' and father's group 'A'
d. Mother's group 'B' and father's group 'AB'

35. The most important factor in hemostasis preventing PPH after placental separation is due to:
a. Uterine contraction and relaxation
b. Retraction of uterus
c. Thrombosis of blood vessels in myometrium
d. Retroplacental clot

36. Complete perineal tear is common in:
a. Face to pubes delivery
b. Breech delivery
c. Internal podalic version
d. Manual removal of placenta

37. Young women whose mothers took diethylstilbestrol during pregnancy are likely to develop one of the following genital malignancy:
a. Squamous cell carcinoma
b. Adenosquamous carcinoma
c. Papillary adenocarcinoma
d. Clear cell adenocarcinoma

38. Medical termination of Pregnancy Act was passed by the Parliament of India in:
a. 1950   b. 1965
c. 1971   d. 1981

39. A primipara with a cardiac lesion (MI) has come on the 40th day of delivery asking for contraception. The contraceptive of choice is:
a. Condom with spermicidal jelly
b. Oral contraceptive pill
c. Intrauterine contraceptive device
d. Laparoscopic sterilization

40. Which one of the following is not a contraindication to breastfeeding?
a. Infection of the breast
b. Psychiatric illness under treatment
c. Hepatitis B infection of the mother
d. Serve cleft palate with harelip

41. The engaging diameter of fetal head in right occipitoposterior position is:
a. Suboccipitobregmatic b. Occipitofrontal
c. Suboccipitovertical   d. Biparietal diameter

42. What dose of glucose has been recommended by WHO for oral glucose tolerance test during pregnancy?
a. 50 g   b. 75 g
c. 100 g   d. 150 g

43. With which one of the following fetal abnormalities is prolonged gestation associated?
a. Meningomyelocele   b. Spina bifida
c. Anencephaly   d. Omphalocele

44. Which one of the following is not cause of disseminated intravascular coagulopathy in pregnancy?
a. Abruptio placenta   b. Amniotic fluid embolism
c. Intrauterine death   d. Placenta previa

45. Match List I (sign) with List II (description) and select the correct answer using the code given below the lists:

List I (sign)	List II (description) (UPSC 2007 II question 28)
A. Palmer's sign	1. Bluish coloration of vagina in pregnancy
B. Braxton Hicks sign	2. Rhythmic painless uterine contractions felt per abdomen in second trimester
C. Goodell's sign	3. Softening of cervix in pregnancy
D. Chadwick sign	4. Rhythmic uterine contractions felt in first trimester

```
A B C D          A B C D
1 2 3 4          4 2 3 1
2 3 1 4          3 2 1 4
```
a. A-1, B-2, C-3, D-4   b. A-4, B-2, C-3, D-1
c. A-2, B-3, C-1, D-4   d. A-3, B-2, C-1, D-4

46. Consider the following:
   1. Fetal pulmonary hypoplasia
   2. Fetal chromosomal anomalies
   3. Prostaglandin synthetase inhibitors
   4. Amniotic fluid index of 15 cm

   Which of the above are associated with oligohydramnios?
   a. 1, 2 and 4   b. 2, 3 and 4
   c. 1, 3 and 4   d. 1, 2 and 3

47. A 32-year-old woman with two live children was brought to emergency with history of missed period for 15 days, spotting since 7 days and, pain abdomen since 8 hours. Her pulse was 120 per minute; pallor ++, systolic BP 80 mm Hg. There was fullness and tenderness on per abdomen examination, cervical movements were tender, uterus was anteverted, bulky and soft. There was fullness in pouch of Douglas. Most likely, she is suffering from:
   a. Pelvic inflammatory disease
   b. Missed abortion with infection
   c. Ruptured ectopic pregnancy
   d. Threatened abortion

48. A 20-year-old primigravida is admitted with full-term pregnancy and labour pains. At 4 am she goes into active phase of labour with 4 cm cervical dilatation. Membranes rupture during p/v examination showing clear liquor. A repeat p/v examination after 4 hours of good uterine contractions reveals a cervical dilatation of 5 cm. What should be the next step in management?
   a. Reassess after 4 hours
   b. Immediate caesarean section
   c. Oxytocin drip
   d. Reassess for occipitoposterior position and cephalopelvic disproportion

49. A G 2 P 1 A 0 presents with full term pregnancy with transverse lie in the first stage of labour. On examination, cervix is 5 cm dilated, membranes are intact and foetal heart sounds are regular. The appropriate management would be:
   a. Wait for spontaneous ovulation and expulsion
   b. External cephalic version
   c. Internal podalic version
   d. Caesarean section

50. Oxytocin is not responsible for:
   a. Milk production   b. Uterine involution
   c. After pains   d. Milk ejection

51. The causes for subinvolution of uterus are the following except:
   a. Multiple pregnancy   b. Pelvic infection
   c. Established breast feeding
   d. Retained placental fragments

52. Immediately after third stage of labour in a case of full term delivery, the fundus of the uterus is:
   a. At the level of xiphisternum
   b. At the level of umbilicus
   c. Below the level of umbilicus
   d. Just above the symphysis pubis

53. Arrange the following steps in which they occur form the entry of sperm into female Reproductive Tract and reptile fertilization(Sequential arrangement)
   a. Acrosomal reaction-capacitation-cortical reaction-zona Reaction
   b. Capacitation-acrosomal reaction-zona reaction-cortical reaction
   c. Capacitation-acrosomal reaction- cortical reaction-zona reaction
   d. Acrosomal-cortical reaction-capacitation-Zona reaction

54. Daily requirement of vitamin D in pregnancy and lactation is:
   a. 2.5 µg   b. 10 mcg
   c. 5 mcg   d 20 µg

55. The cells which surround the oocyte in Graafin follicle are called as:
   a. Disus proligerus   b. Cumulus oophorus
   c. Luteal cells   d. Villus cells

56. What is placental cotyledon
   a. Area drained by all branches from main stem villi
   b. Area drained supplied by one spiral arteriole
   c. Diameter of the placenta
   d. Area between 2 anchoring villi
   e. Area drained by on terminal villi

57. Median Umbilical Ligament is a remnant of:
   a. Umbilical artery   b. Umbilical Vein
   c. Urachus   d. Gubernaculum

58. The umbilical arteries near the insertion of cord to placenta are connected by:
   a. Funis anastomosis   b. Hyrtls anastomosis
   c. Hobner anastomosis   d. Hanis anastomosis

59. Following is essential to initiate labor:
   a. Fetal ACTH   b. Maternal ACTH
   c. HCG   d. Oxytocin

60. In Triple test all of the following are tested except:
   a. HCG   b. AFP
   c. Estradiol   d. Estriol

61. Chorionic villi sampling can detect all *except*:
    a. Phenylketonuria
    b. Thalassemia
    c. Anencephaly
    d. Trisomy 21

62. AG 1 female with previous H/0 Downs syndrome attends antenatal clinic at 10 weeks. She has monochorionic diamniotic twin pregnancy. What is the most appropriate method of excluding down syndrome in her
    a. CVS with sample from any one sac
    b. CVS with sample from both the sacs
    c. Triple test
    d. Perform cell free fetal DNA

63. All of the following are true about anencephaly *except*:
    a. Facial presentation
    b. Increased-alpha-fetoprotein
    c. Enlarged andrenal gland
    d. Polyhydramnios

64. The best marker for neural tube defect is:
    a. Acetylglucosaminidase
    b. Acetylcholinesterase
    c. Alpha-fetoprotein
    d. Chorionic gonadotropin

65. Cord Ph is:
    a. 7.1
    b. 7.2
    c. 6.1
    d. 6.2

66. All of the following are functions of amniotic fluid *except*:
    a. Maintenance of fetal temperature
    b. Allows for free movement of fetus
    c. Provides proteins to fetus
    d. Shock absorber

67. A primipara complains of lower abdomen pain at period of amenorrhea at 32 weeks. The fetus is in cephalic presentation.
    P/A = 1–2 contractions/10minutes
    FHR = 138 beats per minute
    O/E = Cx = 2 cm dilated 75% effaced membranes intact. What is the next step in management?
    a. Allows labor to progress normally
    b. Commence intramuscular corticosteroid and oral nifedipine
    c. Start intramuscular corticosteroid and I/V ritodrine
    d. Start I/V broad spectrum antibiotics

68. A primipara complains of sudden onset vaginal discharge at 32 weeks of pregnancy. P/A=No contractions
    Cephalic presentation
    Fetal heart sounds = Normal
    What is the first step in management?
    a. Start board spectrum antibiotics
    b. Start corticosteroid
    c. Perform sterile per speculum examination
    d. Perform sterile vaginal examination

69. A 35 years old female has twin pregnancy at 22 weeks. She has previous H/O of 2 abortions and has 5 years old child born at 38 weeks. Her gravida parity is:
    a. G4P 2 + 0 + 2 + 1
    b. G4P 1 + 0 + 2 + 1
    c. G4P 1 + 2 + 2 + 1
    d. G5P 1 + 0+ 2 + 1

70. Which of the following is best marker for gestational age:
    a. CRL@12 weeks
    b. BPD@16 weeks
    c. FL@32 weeks
    d. AC@20 weeks

71. Colostrum contains all in excess of milk *except*:
    a. Protein
    b. Fat
    c. Minerals
    d. Immunoglobulins

72. Which of the following test is the most sensitive for detection of iron depletion in pregnancy
    a. Serum iron
    b. Serum transferrin
    c. Serum erythroprotein
    d. Serum ferritin

73. Reticulocyte count reaches a peak after days of iron therapy:
    a. 3 days
    b. 5 days
    c. 10 days
    d. 1 month

74. A women with Mitral stenosis but no pulmonary HT is in labor at POG-39 weeks. She has dyspnea only on severe exertion. P/R-80bpm, No basal crepts in lungs. Fetus is in cephalic presentation. Cervix dilation 5cms. She is getting uterine contraction 2 in 10 minutes. Which of the following is best avoided in this patient?
    a. Active management of third stage of labor
    b. Use of epidural analgesia for pain relief
    c. Use of ergometrine in third stage of labor
    d. Ventouse delivery in second stage if delivery does not occur in half an hour

75. Caesarean section is mandatory in which cardiac disease?
    a. VSD
    b. Coarctation of aorta
    c. MVP
    d. MS

76. A 35-year-old second para with mitral stenosis has normal vaginal delivery at 40 weeks. The baby is healthy. Her first child is healthy and is 5 year old. Which of the following is the best method of contraception in this woman?
    a. Ligation and resection of fallopian tubes after 6 weeks
    b. Oral contraceptive pills
    c. Postpartum ligation and resection of fallopian tubes
    d. Subdermal progesterone implants

77. All of the following can be administered in acute hypertension during labor *except*:
    a. IV Labetalol
    b. IV nitroprusside
    c. IV hydralazine
    d. IV diazoxide

78. A primigravida who is admitted to the antenatal ward at 35 weeks is found to have a blood pressure of 160/100. Her urine does not contain albumin. Which one of the following drugs should not be used in her management?
    a. Furosemide
    b. Hydralazine
    c. Labetalol
    d. Methyldopa
    e. Nifedipine

79. What feature would be helpful in differentiating chronic HTN from PIH?

a. Episode of seizure
b. Hypertension nephropathy
c. Hypertensive retinopathy
d. HTN at 10 weeks of gestation

80. A 28 years old Eclamptic woman develop convulsions. The first measure to be done is:
a. Give MgSO$_4$
b. Sedation of patient
c. Immediate delivery
d. Care of Airway

81. A woman is admitted to the antenatal ward at 35 weeks. Her blood pressure is 170/110 and the urine contains albumin. She has a generalized seizure during examination. An oropharyngeal airway is inserted:

Which of the following would be the most appropriate next step in the management?
a. Admit to the intensive care unit
b. Give a 10 mg bolus intravenous injection of hydralazine
c. Give a 4 g bolus of magnesium sulphate by slow intravenous injection
d. Give oxygen inhalation
e. Insert an indwelling catheter

82. MgSO$_4$ is/are indicated in: (Multiple correct answers)
a. Severe pre eclampsia
b. Eclampsia
c. Pre term labour
d. Prevention of cerebral palsy

83. All are seen in gestational diabetes except:
a. Previous Macrosomic baby
b. Obesity
c. Malformations
d. Polyhydramnios

84. Best test for fetal maturity in a diabetic mother is:
a. L:S ratio
b. Lecithin—cephalin ratio
c. Phosphatidyl choline
d. Phosphatidyl glycerol

85. Which of the following is not used in DIC?
a. Heparin
b. Epsilon aminocaproic acid
c. Blood transfusion
d. Intravenous

86. A Primipara whose period of amenorrhoea is 39 weeks develops sudden onset of sharp continuous abdominal pain, shock and tender uterus without vaginal bleeding. She is not in labour. What is the most likely diagnosis:
a. Amniotic fluid embolism
b. Placental abruption
c. Red degeneration of fibroid
d. Rupture of the uterus

87. Partograph represents various stages of labor with respect to time. True about partograph is all except:
a. Each small square represents one hour
b. Alert and action lines are separated by a difference of 4 hours
c. Partograph recording should be started at a cervix dilation of 4 cm
d. Send the patient to first referral unit if the labor progression line crosses the alert line

88. A 38 weeks primigravida presented to the labor room with minimal labor pains and contraction. On examination, the cervix is 2 cm dilated and 50% effaced. The heart rate of the patient is 86/min and blood pressure is 126/76 mm hg> What should be done next?
a. Induce labor by artificial rupture of membranes
b. Give oxytocin to augment labor
c. Sedate the patient by and give Phenergan to decrease labor pains
d. Observe the patient and wait for increase in uterine contractions

89. A primigravida came with 6 cm cervical dilatation with contraction rate of 3/10 minutes which stage of labor is she in?
a. 1st stage
b. 2nd stage
c. 3rd stage
d. 4th stage

90. Vaginal delivery is allowed in all except:
a. Monochorionic monoamniotic twins
b. First twin cephalic and second breech
c. Extended breech
d. Mento anterior

91. A forceps rotation of 30° From left occiput anterior (LOA) to occiput anterior (OA) with extraction of the fetus from +2 Station is described as which type of forceps delivery?
a. High forcep
b. Mid forceps
c. Low forceps
d. Outlet forceps

92. In which one of the following conditions are the levels of maternal serum α-fetoprotein (AFP) not increased?
a. Down syndrome
b. Neural tube defects
c. Multiple pregnancy
d. Sacrococcygeal teratoma

93. Which one of the following is not a sign of separation of placenta?
a. Fundus of the uterus rises to the umbilicus
b. The uterine is well contracted and retracted
c. The cord "lengthens" when press the uterus down, but recedes on release
d. Exclusive vaginal bleeding

94. In deep transverse arrest, the head is arrested at the levels of:
a. Ischial tuberosity
b. Ischial spine
c. Inlet of pelvis
d. Perineum

95. Which one of the following is the most practiced regime of antenatal corticosteroid therapy for maturation of fetal:
a. Betamethasone 12 mg daily for 3 days
b. Betamethasone 12 mg 24 hourly × 2 dose
c. Dexamethasone 12 mg 12 hourly × 2 dose
d. Betamethasone 8 mg 8 hourly × 3 dose

96. A woman presents with abdominal pain and nausea with amenorrhea of 5-6 weeks. Ectopic pregnancy can be diagnosed if:
a. Serum progesterone > 25 ng/ml
b. Beta hCG > 1000 IU/L with endometrial thickness of 14 mm
c. Beta hCG > 2000 IU/L with no gestational sac in the uterus on transvaginal sonography
d. Beta hCG > 3000 IU/L with empty uterus on transvaginal sonography

97. A pregnant woman with 30 weeks gestation presents with BP 166/110 mm Hg with pulmonary edema with convulsions. the woman is given magnesium sulphate. The following drug should be avoided:
    a. Intravenous labetalol
    b. Sublingual Nifedipine
    c. Intravenous frusemide
    d. Intravenous hydralazine

98. Match the abnormal labor pattern with its definition:

List I	List II
A. Prolonged latest phase	1 > 14 hours in nulliparous
B. Prolonged third stage	2 > 20 hours in nulliparous
C. Active phase arrest	3 > 30 minutes
D. Prolonged second stage	4 > 45 minutes
	5 > 4 hours in in nulliparous
	6 > 2 hours in nulliparous

A	B	C	D		A	B	C	D
1	3	5	6		2	4	5	1
1	5	2	4		2	3	5	6

a. A-1, B-3, C-3, D-2   b. A-1, B-5, C-2, D-4
c. A-2, B-4, C-5, D-1   d. A-2, B-3, C-5, D-6

99. Assertion: Management of occupito posterior position in labor is wait and watch:
    Reason-Head of fetus is deflexed
    a. Both A & R are correct, and R is correct explanation of Assertion
    b. Both A & R are correct, and R is not correct explanation of A
    c. a is true, R is false
    d. R is true, A is false
    e. Both A and R are false

100. Assertion- Caesarean section should be done in all preterm breach:
    Reason-Caesarean section decreases the incidence of respiratory distress syndrome in breech

a. Both A & R are true, and R is correct explanation of A
b. Both A & B are true, R is not correct explanation of A
c. A is true, R is false
d. A is false, R is true
e. Both A & R are false

101. Match list I (Condition) with list II (treatment):

List I	List II
A Preterm breech	1 Classical caesarean section
B IUD	2 LSCS
C Transverse lie in 2nd twin	3 Induction of labor
D Shoulder dystocia	4 External cephalic version
	5 Internal podalic version
	6 MC Robert maneuver

A	B	C	D		A	B	C	D
2	3	5	6		4	2	1	6
4	3	5	6		2	3	5	1

a. A-2, B-3, C-5, D-6   b. A-4, B-2, C-1, D-6
c. A-4, B-3, C-5, D-6   d. A-2, B-3, C-5, D-1

102. Match List I (Procedure) with list II (Management of Complications):

List I	List II
A Burn Marshal technique	1. Delivery of placenta by controlled cord traction
B Andrews technique	2. To deliver extended leg in breech
C Prague Maneuver	3. To deliver dorso posterior breech
D Duhrssen incision	4. To deliver after coming head of breech
	5. To manage shoulder dystocia
	6. To deliver entrapped after coming head in breech

A	B	C	D		A	B	C	D
6	1	2	5		4	6	2	5
4	5	1	3		4	1	3	6

a. A-6, B-1, C-2, D-5   b. A-4, B-6, C-2, D-5
c. A-4, B-5, C-1, D-3   d. A-4, B-1, C-3, D-6

Answers with Explanations to New Pattern Questions

1. **Ans. is a, i.e. 1, 4, 5**

2. **Ans. is b, i.e. Twisted ovarian cyst**

Twisted ovarian cyst

Symptoms	Patient complains of sudden acute pain lower abdomen along with a lump
Clinical findings	• On examination—general condition remains unaffected except agony with pain • Abdominal examination—reveals a tense, tender cystic mass with restricted mobility situated in hypogastrium • Pelvic examination—mass separated from the uterus
Treatment	Laparotomy and ovariotomy (salpingo-oophorectomy)

3. **Ans. is c, i.e. Pelvic ultrasonography**

4. **Ans. is c, i.e. Laparotomy**

5. **Ans. is c, i.e. 2 and 3**

   Perinatal mortality rate: Late fetal and early neonatal death weighing more than 1000 g at birth expressed as a ratio per 1000 live births weighing more than 1000 g at birth.

   Important causes of perinatal mortality
   - Infections (sepsis, meningitis, pneumonia, neonatal tetanus, congenital syphilis)—33%
   - Birth asphyxia and trauma—28%
   - Preterm birth and/or low birth weight—24%
   - Congenital malformation and others—15%

6. **Ans. is c, i.e. Mifepristone and prostaglandins**

   Option "a" is for preparation of patient, whereas in question it has been asked about ripening of cervix.

7. **Ans. is d, i.e. Suspected multiple pregnancy, organic cardiac disease, and Rh-negative mother**

8. **Ans. is d, i.e. A is false but R is true**

   In majority cases of retroverted gravid uterus, spontaneous rectification occurs. In the minority, spontaneous rectification fails to occur between 12 and 16 weeks. The developing uterus gradually fills up the pelvic cavity and becomes incarcerated.

   Changes following incarceration

Organs	Changes
Uterus	• Cervix pointed upward and forward. • Anterior sacculation (rarely)—uterus continues to grow at the expense of the anterior wall while thick posterior wall lies in the sacral hollow.
Urethra and bladder	Retention of urine due to (i) mechanical compression of urethra by the cervix, (ii) elongation of urethra, and (iii) edema on bladder neck.

9. **Ans. is a, i.e. HB vaccine can be delayed for newborn beyond 48 hours. If mother is HbsAg positive**

10. **Ans. is c, i.e. There is increased incidence of hydramnios and pre-eclampsia**

11. **Ans. is d, i.e. 1 and 3**

12. **Ans. is a, i.e. 1, 2 and 3**

    Estimated due date (EDD)
    1. **Naegele's rule:** EDD = LMP—9 months + 7 days
       (a) EDD is early, if woman has shorter preovulatory phase
       (b) EDD is late, if woman has the longer preovulatory phase
    2. **Pelvic examination:** Bimanual examination of the pelvis and uterus. Because the uterus is usually in the pelvis until **12 week's gestation**, early pregnancy is the best time to correlate accurately uterine size and duration of gestation
    3. **Estimating weeks of gestation by abdominal examination:** Between 18 and 20 weeks, there is an excellent correlation between the size of the uterus and the gestation by weeks. The measurement in centimeters from the symphysis pubis

to the top of the fundus should approximate the weeks of gestation. At midpregnancy (20 weeks), the fundus of the uterus is at the level of umbilicus.

4. **Sonography:**
   (a) **First trimester:** Fetal gestational age is best determined by measuring the CRL between 7 and 12 weeks (variation ± 5 days).
   (b) **Second trimester:** By bronchopulmonary dysplasia (BPD), head circumference, abdominal circumference, abdominal circumference, femur length. It is most accurate when done between 12 and 20 weeks (± 8 days variation). BPD becomes more accurate after 12 weeks.
   (c) **Third trimester:** Least reliable (variation ± 16 days).

13. **Ans. is b, i.e. Blood transfusion to raise the hemoglobin to 9 gm%**

14. **Ans. is a, i.e. 1, 2 and 3**

All complications are more with monozygotic twins than dizygotic twins.

15. **Ans. is a, i.e. Threatened abortion**

Since size of uterus is equal to period of pregnancy and internal as is closed hence it is threatened abortion

16. **Ans. is c, i.e. 2 and 3 only**

Microscopic findings of hydatidiform mole

1. Marked proliferation of the syncytial and cytotrophoblastic epithelium
2. Marked thinning of the stromal tissue due to hydropic degeneration
3. **Absence of blood vessels in the villi,** which seems primary rather than due to pressure atrophy
4. The villus pattern is distinctly maintained

17. **Ans. is d, i.e. It determines capacity of the pelvic brim**

18. **Ans. is d, i.e. 1 and 3**

Physiology of normal labor
- There is good synchronization of the contraction waves of both halves of the uterus
- There is fundal dominance with gradual diminishing contraction wave through midzone down to lower segment which takes about 10–20 seconds
- The wave of contraction follows a regular pattern
- Intra-amniotic pressure rises beyond 20 mm Hg with the onset of true labor pain during contraction
- Good relaxation in between contraction brings down intra-amniotic pressure < 8 mm Hg
- During first stage, the tonus varies from 8–10 mm Hg (during pregnancy 2–3 mm Hg)
- During first stage, intrauterine pressure raised to 40–50 mm Hg and about 100–120 mm Hg in second and third stage of labor
- Retraction in upper segment, a gradual and progressive cervical dilation occurs with each contraction. Retraction in second stage results in expulsion of the baby and in the third stage causes separation of placenta and arrested bleeding.

19. **Ans. is c, i.e. The Schultze mechanism is the most common one**

Placental separation

Plane of separation—through deep spongy layer of deciduas basalis

Central separation (Schultze)	Marginal separation (Matthews-Duncan)
Separation starts at the center resulting in opening up of few uterine sinuses and accumulation of blood behind the placenta (retroplacental hematoma)	• More frequently • Separation starts at the margin • With progressive uterine contraction, more and more areas of the placenta get separated

20. **Ans. is b, i.e. Rupture of membranes followed by oxytocin drip**

Scheme of management of abruption placentae

1. Revealed type (most common)
   a. Patient is in labor: Low rupture of membrane + oxytocin
   b. Patient is not in labor:
      i. Pregnancy ≥ 37 weeks: Low rupture of membrane ± oxytocin; Indication of CS—fetal distress, failed amniotomy to controlled bleeding, and complication.
      ii. Pregnancy < 37 weeks:
         Bleeding (moderate to severe and continuing)—low rupture of membrane + oxytocin.
         Bleeding (slight or stopped)—on conservative treatment.
2. Mixed or concealed type: Correction of hypovolemia → ARM + oxytocin (if needed) → if no response, falling fibrinogen level, oliguria, fetal distress → CS → hysterectomy.

21. **Ans. is c, i.e. The maximum vacuum should not be more than 1.5 kg/cm²**

22. **Ans. a, i.e. 1, 2 and 3**

23. **Ans. b, i.e. Massaging the uterus and administering an oxytocic**

24. **Ans. is b, i.e. Pyridoxine**

25. **Ans. is a, i.e. 1, 2 and 3**

26. **Ans. is d, i.e. An Rh-negative multipara mother aged 30 years with two live healthy boys**
    Indications for amniocentesis
    - Advanced maternal age above 35 years
    - Abnormal serum triple marker test (α-fetoprotein, β-hCG, pregnancy-associated plasma protein A, or unconjugated estriol).
    - Family history of chromosomal abnormalities or Mendelian disorder amenable to genetic testing.

27. **Ans. is a, i.e. 14th week of gestation**

28. **Ans. is a, i.e. Decidual reaction**
    Finding of deciduous in endometrium sampling without chorionic villi is very much suggestive of ectopic pregnancy. Additional finding may be Arias-Stella reaction.

29. **Ans. is c, i.e. It is limited to individual bone**

30. **Ans. is a, i.e. 1, 2, 3, 4**

31. **Ans. is d, i.e. A-2, B-3, C-4, D-1**

32. **Ans. is a, i.e. 1, 2 and 3**

33. **Ans. is b, i.e. + 3 station**

34. **Ans. is c, i.e. Mother's group 'O' and father's group 'A'**

35. **Ans. is b, i.e. Retraction of uterus**

36. **Ans. is a, i.e. Face to pubes delivery**

37. **Ans. is d, i.e. Clear cell adenocarcinoma**

38. **Ans. is c, i.e. 1971**

39. **Ans. is a, i.e. Condom with spermicidal jelly**

40. **Ans. is c, i.e. Hepatitis B infection of the mother**
    - Contraindications of breastfeeding—markedly inverted nipple, mastitis, acute infection in mother if infant does not have same infection, septicemia, nephritis, eclampsia, hemorrhage, active tuberculosis, typhoid fever, breast cancer, malaria substance abuse, debility, severe neurosis, postpartum psychoses.
    - Mothers with the following conditions should be advised not to breastfeed—HIV infections, CMV, HTLV-I, HTLV-II, HSV-I, infants with galactosemia, drugs of abuse (amphetamines, cocaine, heroin, marijuana, phenocyclidine).
    - Conditions in which breastfeeding may be considered—hepatitis B, hepatitis C, rubell, varicella, infants with phenylketonuria, tobacco, and alcohol.

    Drugs contraindicated in breastfeeding women—antineoplastic agents, amphetamines, bromocriptine, clemastine cimetidine, chloramphenicol, cocaine, cyclophosphamide, cycloporine, diethylstilbestrol, doxorubicin, ergotamine, gold salts, heroin, immunosuppressants (azathioprine), iodides, Li, meprobamate, methimazole, methylamphetamine, nicotine, phencyclidine (PCP) phenindione, radiopharmaceuticals, tetracycline, thiouracil.

    Avoid or give with great caution—amiodarone, anthraquinones, aspirin (salicylates), atropine, birth control pill, bromides, calciferol, cascara, danthron, dihydrotachysterol estrogen, ethanol, metoclopramide, metronidazole, narcotics, phenobarbital, primidone, psychotropic drugs, reserpine, sulfasalazine.

41. **Ans. is b, i.e. Occipitofrontal**

42. **Ans. is b, i.e. 75 g**

43. **Ans. is c, i.e. Anencephaly**

44. **Ans. is d, i.e. Placenta previa**

45. **Ans. is b, i.e. A-4 B-2 C-3 D-1**

46. **Ans. is d, i.e. 1, 2 and 3**

47. **Ans. is c, i.e. Ruptured ectopic pregnancy**

48. **Ans. is c, i.e. Oxytocin drip**

49. **Ans. is d, i.e. Caesarean section**

50. **Ans. is a, i.e. Milk production**

51. **Ans. is c, i.e. Established breast feeding**

52. **Ans. is b, i.e. At the level of umbilicus**

53. **Ans. is c, i.e. Capacitation-acrosomal reaction- cortical reaction- zona reaction**

54. **Ans. is b, i.e. 10 mcg**
    Daily requirement of vitamin D:
    • Adult —2.5 µg (100 IU)
    • Infant and child—5.0 µg (200 IU)
    • Pregnancy and Laction—10.0 µg (400 IU)

55. **Ans. is b, i.e. Cumulus oophorus**

56. **Ans. is a, i.e. Area drained by All branches from main stem villi**

57. **Ans. is c, i.e. Urachus**

58. **Ans. is b i.e. Hyrtls anastomosis**

59. **Ans. is a, i.e. Fetal ACTH**

60. **Ans. is c, i.e. Estradiol**

61. **Ans. is c, i.e. Anencephaly**

62. **Ans. is a, i.e. CVS with sample from any one sac**
    The female has previous H/O Down syndrome, hence diagnostic test is used. Now since she is 10 weeks, it is chorionic villi sampling

63. **Ans. is c, i.e. Enlarged andrenal gland**

64. **Ans. is b, i.e. Acetylcholinesterase**

65. **Ans. is b, i.e. 7.2**

66. **Ans. is c, i.e. Provides proteins to fetus**

67. **Ans. is b, i.e. Commence intramuscular corticosteroid and oral nifedipine**

68. **Ans. is c, i.e. Perform sterile per speculum examination**

69. **Ans. is b, i.e. G4P 1 + 0 + 2 + 1**

70. **Ans. is b, i.e. BPD@16 weeks**
    The earlier the USG is done for gestational age, the better it is. Now @ 16 weeks, BPD is the best parameter, not CRL

71. **Ans. is b, i.e. Fat**

72. **Ans. is d, i.e. Serum ferritin**

73. **Ans. is c, i.e. 10 days**

74. **Ans. is c, i.e. Use of ergometrine in third stage of labor**

75. **Ans. is b, i.e. Coarctation of aorta**

76. **Ans. is a, i.e. Ligation and resection of fallopian tubes after 6 weeks**

77. **Ans. is d, i.e. IV** diazoxide

78. **Ans. is a, i.e. Furosemide**

79. Ans. is d, i.e. HTN at 10 weeks of gestation

80. Ans. is d, i.e. Care of Airway

81. Ans. is c, i.e. Give a 4 g bolus of magnesium sulphate by slow intravenous injection

82. Ans. is a, b, c and d, i.e. a. Severe pre eclampsia; b. Eclampsia; c. Pre term labour; d. Prevention of cerebral palsy

83. Ans. is c, i.e. Malformations

84. Ans. is d, i.e. Phosphatidyl glycerol

85. Ans. is b, i.e. Epsilon aminocaproic acid

86. Ans. is b, i.e. Placental abruption

87. Ans. is a, i.e. Each small square represents one hour

88. Ans. is d, i.e. Observe the patient and wait for increase in uterine contractions

89. Ans. is a, i.e. 1st stage

90. Ans. is a, i.e. Monochorionic monoamniotic twins

91. Ans. is c, i.e. Low forceps

92. Ans. is a, i.e. Down syndrome

93. Ans. is c, i.e. The cord "lengthens" when press the uterus down, but recedes on release

94. Ans. is b, i.e. Ischial spine

95. Ans. is b, i.e. Betamethasone 12 mg 24 hourly × 2 dose

96. Ans. is c, i.e. Beta hCG > 2000 IU/L with no gestational sac in the uterus on transvaginal sonography

97. Ans. is c, i.e. Intravenous frusemide

98. Ans. is d, i.e. A-2, B-3, C-5, D-6

99. Ans. is a, i.e. Both A & R are correct, and R is correct explanation of Assertion

100. Ans. is a, i.e. Both A & R are true, and R is correct explanation of A

101. Ans. is a, i.e. A-2, B-3, C-5, D-6

102. Ans. is a, i.e. A-6, B-1, C-2, D-5

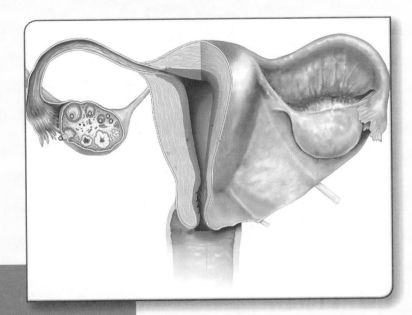

1

Section

General Obstetrics

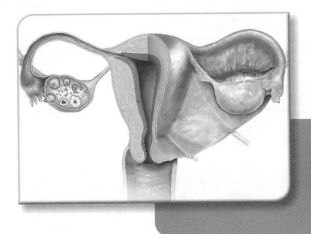

Basics of Reproduction

 Chapter at a Glance

➢ Germ Cell and its Differentiation
➢ Spermatogenesis
➢ Oogenesis

➢ Fertilization
➢ Implantation

GERM CELL AND ITS DIFFERENTIATION

GERM CELLS

- Germ cells are derived from **Epiblast (Best answer)** or **Ectoderm of yolk sac**[Q] (2nd best answer)
- If SRY gene (i.e. sex-determining region on Y chromosome, is present) the germ cells differentiate into spermatogonia (i.e. sex of baby is male) and if SRY gene is absent (i.e. Y chromosome is absent) the germ cells differentiate into oogonia. (i.e. sex of baby is female)

 Key Concept

Y chromosome determines the sex of baby
- If Y chromosome is present: Sex of baby is male
- If Y chromosome is absent sex of baby is female
- Best method of sex determination: **Karyotyping**

GERM CELL DIFFERENTIATION— SPERMATOGENESIS

- The process involved in the development of spermatids from the primordial germ cells and their differentiation into the spermatozoa (or sperms) is called **spermatogenesis.**
- Spermatogenesis begins at puberty in seminiferous tubules of male testis.
- The entire process is shown in Figure 1.1
- **Time taken for spermatogenesis is 72–74 days.**

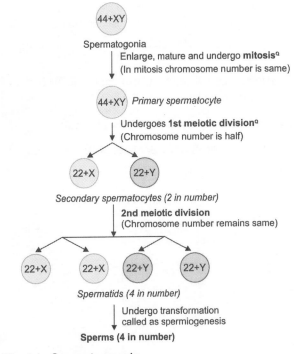

Fig. 1.1: Spermatogenesis

 Important One Liners

- Number of sperms formed by one primary spermatocyte: 4
- Number of primary spermatocytes formed from one spermatogonia: 16.

Contd…

Contd...

- Number of sperms formed by one spermatogonia (16 × 4): 64
- Spermatids attain maturity and motility: Caudal part of epididymis, i.e. tail of epididymis
- Ion responsible for motility of sperm: Calcium
- Gene responsible for motility = Catsper gene
- Size of sperms: 55 microns
- Fertilisable span of sperms: 48 hours.
- One spermatogonia gives rise to **16 primary spermatocytes**[Q].

Spermiogenesis

It is the process by which spherical spermatids transform into tailed spermatozoa without any change in the chromosomal number.

There is no mitosis or meiosis in spermio genesis. In this process following changes occur: (Table 1.1)

Table 1.1: Spermiogenesis

Part of spermatid	Part formed in sperm
Nuclear material	Head of sperm
Golgi body	Acrosomal cap
Mitochondria	Middle piece
Microtubules or Centrioles	Axial filament/Tail of sperm

Note: Sperms lack endoplasmic reticulum (especially Rough Endoplasmic reticulum).

- **Time taken for spermiogenesis = 14 days**

Hormonal Support of Spermatogenesis (Fig. 1.2)

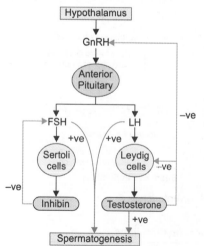

Fig. 1.2: Hormonal support of spernatogenesis.

Note: (Via GnRH), testosterone not only decreases LH but also FSH.

Key Concept

- Thus all 3 hormones—LH FSH, and testosterone—are needed for spermatogenesis. But the main hormone for spermatogenesis is testosterone.

Remember:

- Inhibin always has a negative feedback on FSH whether in males or females

Capacitation

- It is a biochemical change in the sperms enabling them to bind and fertilise the ovum.
- **Begins in female genital tract**[Q].
- It begins in the cervix but **major part takes place in fallopian tube**.
- Time taken for capacitation is 7 hours.
- **After capacitation sperms attain** full maturity and **hypermotility**.

Note:

- Sperms **become motile** in caudal end of epididymis.
- Sperms **become hypermotile** in Fallopian tube as major part of capacitation occurs in Fallopian tube.

OOGENESIS

The process involved in the development of mature ovum is called Oogenesis (Fig. 1.3).

- Oogenesis begins in the ovary in intrauterine life at *6–8 weeks of gestation.*[Q]

The primitive germ cells take their origin from yolk sac at about the end of 3rd week and migrate to the developing gonadal ridge, at about the end of 4th week.

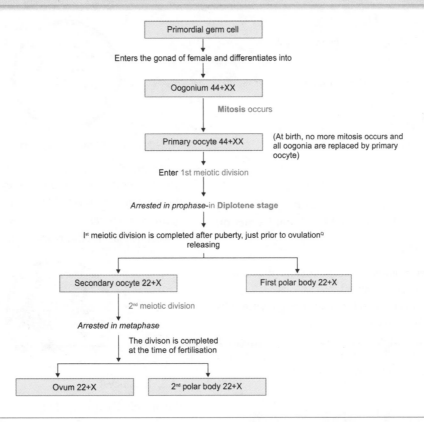

Fig. 1.3: Oogenesis.

 Important One Liners

- Maximum number of oocytes/oogonia are in the ovary at 5th month development[Q] (20 weeks of gestation number in patients 6–7 million)[Q].
- At birth no more mitotic division occurs, all oogonia are replaced by primary oocyte.[Q]
- At birth total content of both ovaries is 2 million primary oocytes.[Q]
- At puberty, number is further decreased and is ~300000–500000 of which only 500 are destined to mature during an individual's life time.[Q] and a 1000 undergo atresia every month
- All the primary oocytes in the ovary of a newborn are *arrested in the diplotene stage of prophase* (of meiosis).[Q]
- All the primary oocytes then remain arrested and the arrested stage is called as "**Dictyate stage**" till puberty.[Q]
- **Hence the stage which is absent in spermatogenesis is dictyate stage**. (as their is no arrested stage in Spermatogeneses)
- The primary oocyte gets surrounded by follicular cells in the ovary and this structure is now called as **Primordial follicle**. (Fig. 1.4)
- Hence ovary is a Reservoir of many such primary follicles. Thus in patients of infertility when we do test for ovarian reserve we are actually checking whether follicles are present in ovary or not.

- At puberty as a result of mid cycle preovulatory surge, meiosis is resumed and completed just prior to ovulation.[Q]
- Hence Meiosis I is hormone dependant — it depends on LH.
- Release of secondary oocyte from primary oocyte is called **ovulation**.
- First polar body is released at the time of ovulation.
- The **second division** starts immediately after it but gets *arrested in metaphase*.[Q]
- At the time of fertilization second division is completed which results in the release of ova and second polar body.
- *Therefore second polar body and ova/female pronucleus is released only at the time of fertilisation.*[Q]
- **Size of mature ovum:** 120–130 microns (It is the largest cell in the body).
- **Size of mature follicle:** 18–20 mm
- **Fertilisable span of ova:** 12–24 hours.

Time table of events	
Event	Time (In weeks)
• Germ cells reach genital ridge	@ 3 weeks
• Germ cells reach yolk sac	@ 6 weeks
• Oogonia formed	@ 9 weeks
• Primary Oocyte formed	@ 12 weeks
• Follicle formation begins by	@ 14 weeks
• It completed by	@ 22–24 weeks

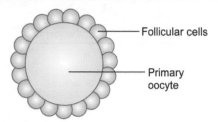

Fig. 1.4: Primordial follicle.

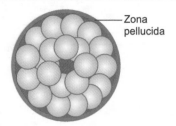

Fig. 1.5: Morula—Mulberry shaped

FERTILISATION

- For sperm to fuse with ova – First sperm should attach to secondary oocyte. This is called **Acrosomal Reaction**

Acrosomal Reaction

- It occurs after sperm binds to zona pellucida. (membrane surrounding secondary oocyte)
- Acrosomal reaction is due to the release of enzymes like Hyaluronidase, Acrosin etc.
- Zona pellucida has sperm receptors (zona proteins), namely ZP1, ZP2 and ZP3 which mediate the acrosomal reaction and binding. Main receptor is ZP3.

Fertilisation

- It is the fusion of female pronucleus and male pronucleus to form the zygote (conceptus).
- Fertilisation occurs in the **Ampulla of fallopian** tube.[Q]
- Gene responsible for fusion of male and female pronuclecus is **Fertilin**.
- The zygote undergoes cell division and becomes – 2 cell, 4 cell, 8 cells and 16 cell stage. **The 16 cell stage is called Morula**
- The zygote stays in fallopian tube **for 3 days after** fertilisation. At this time nutrition is provided to every zygote by secretory cells of Fallopian tube in the form of Pyruvate.
- **Morula enters the uterine cavity**, 4 days after fertilisation, i.e. on day 18 of the cycle.
- The zygote enters uterine cavity because of:
  i. Movement of cilia
  ii. Peristalsis is fallopian tube (Main)
Most important factor is: Peristalsis in tube. This is the reason why smooth muscle relaxation caused by Progesterone only Pills can lead to Ectopic pregnancy.
- Zygote enters the uterine cavity in the **form of Morula** (16 celled stage zygote) (Fig. 1.5).
- Morula like ova is surrounded by **zona pellucida** whose function is to prevent polyspermy.
- The zona pellucida is lost 5 days after fertilisation. This is **called as Zona Hatching**

- As the morula enters the uterine cavity, fluid enters it and morula gets converted to **Blastocyst (Fig 1.6).**
- The cells of blastocyst differentiate into:
  – Inner cell mass
  – Trophoblast (cells arranged in periphery)

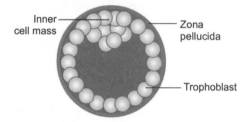

Fig. 1.6: Blastocyst

- The protein E cadherin helps in differentiation.

- The inner cell mass forms the **Embryo proper** in future
- The trophoblast forms Future Placenta and Fetal Membranes.

IMPLANTATION

- Implantation is the process by which the **blastocyst** penetrates the uterine mucosa to get implanted in the endometrium.
- **Implantation begins 6–7 days after fertilisation, i.e. 20-21st of regular menstrual cycle.**
- The process of implantation involves 3 stages:

Phase	Molecule
Apposition	Selectin
Adhesion	Integrin
Invasion	D/t Enzyme matrix metalloproteinases

Note: **Invasion**—The blastocyst implants by penetrating and invading the secretory endometrium completely. This is called **Interstitial implantation (Fig 1.7)** which is completed **by 10th–11th day after fertilisation.**

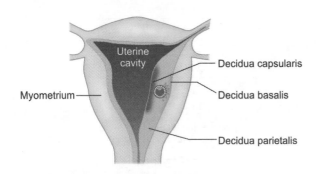

Fig. 1.7: Showing interstitial implantation

Site of Implantation

M/C (In 2/3)—Posterior surface of the upper uterine segment. (Don't say fundus of uterus)

In 1/3rd—Anterior surface of the upper uterine segment.

 Note: Implantation is eccentric i.e. on one side of uterus. D/t this, their is unequal growth of uterus is early pregnancy called as Piskacek's sign.

- In some females bleeding arceus at the time of implantation called as Hartman sign

Decidua

- After implantation, the endometrium is called as **Decidua**.
- Decidua becomes differentiated into:
  - **Decidua basalis**—Part of the decidua which lies between Embryo and myometrium. It forms the site of attachment of placenta and forms the maternal side of the placenta.
  - **Decidua capsularis**—This is the part of decidua which lies between Embryo and uterine cavity.
  - **Decidua parietalis**—This is the rest of decidua which lines the cavity of uterus.

 Note: As the embryo grows, Decidua capsularis and Decidua Parietalis fuse with each other and then together they are called as **Decidua vera** (Understand from Fig. 1.7). The happens by 14–16 weeks of pregnancy

In other words, obliteration of decidual space is complete by 14–16 weeks. Thus, **theoretically, twinning (superfetation) can occur uptil 16 weeks**.

- The decidua parietalis and basalis are composed of three layers—zona compacta, zona spongiosa (middle layer) and zona basalis.

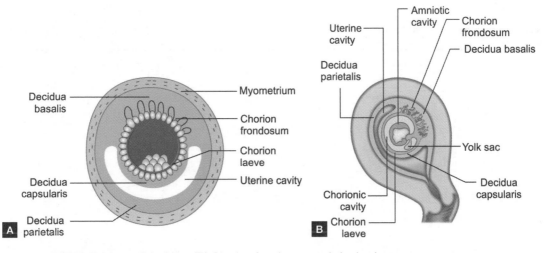

Figs. 1.8A and B: (A) Subdivisions of decidua; (B) Chorion frondosum and chorion laeve

Further Differentiation of Blastocyst

- **On 8th day after fertilisation[Q], the Trophoblast differentiates into two layers:**
  i. **Cytotrophoblast (Langhan's cell layer)**—Mononucleate cell layer
  ii. **Syncytiotrophoblast**—Outer, multilayered multinucleated zone without any distinct cell borders (See flowchart 1.1 for further discussions and functions of Trophoblast).

Flowchart 1.1: Differentiation of trophoblast

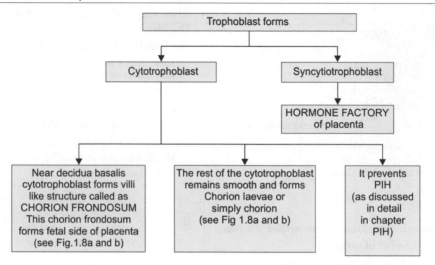

 Remember:

- The cytotrophoblast thus forms the fetal side of placenta and the fetal membrane chorion.
- The inner cell mass forms the entire embryo.
- First germ layer to be formed is Endoderm (by 7 days after fertilisation) and all 3 germ layers are formed by 21 days after fertilisation.

 Note: All the important events and the time related to embryogenesis have been summarised in the Appendix.

New Pattern Questions

N1. Figure F1 shows T:S of uterus with implanted zygote Identify structure A.

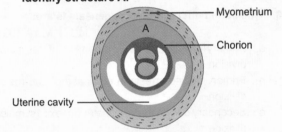

Myometrium

Chorion

Uterine cavity

Fig. F1

    a. Decidua basalis   b. Decidua capsularis
    c. Decidua parietalis   d. None of the above

N2. Maximum oogonia can be seen in ovaries at:
    a. 5th month of IUL   b. 7th month of IUL
    c. At birth   d. At puberty

N3. Zona hatching occurs:
    a. 4 days after fertilisation
    b. 5 days after fertilisation
    c. 6 days after fertilisation
    d. 8 days after fertilisation

N4. 1st meiotic division of oogenesis gets arrested at:
    a. Pachytene stage of prophase
    b. Diplotene stage of prophase
    c. Leptotene stage of prophase
    d. Metaphase stage of prophase

N5. Time taken for spermatogenesis is:
    a. 50–60 days   b. 60–70 days
    c. 70–80 days   d. 80–90 days

N6. Time taken for capacitation of sperms is:
    a. 2–4 hours   b. 4–6 hours
    c. 6–8 hours   d. 8–10 hours

N7. During spermiogenesis, middle piece of spermatid forms _____ of the sperm.
    a. Acrosomal cap   b. Middle piece
    c. Axial filament   d. Head of sperm

N8. Germ cells appear in yolk sac at:
    a. 3 weeks   b. 6 weeks
    c. 9 weeks   d. 5 weeks

N9. Formation of a follicle is completed by:
    a. 6 weeks   b. 9 weeks
    c. 14 weeks   d. 24 weeks

N10. Secondary sex ratio of female:male is:
    a. 100:160   b. 100:106
    c. 940:1000   d. 880:1000

N11. Obliteration of uterine cavity occurs by:
    a. 10–12 weeks   b. 8–10 weeks
    c. 12–16 weeks   d. 12–20 weeks

N12. True statement with regards to resumption of Meiosis I is:
    a. It is not hormone dependant
    b. Resumed due to LH
    c. Resumed due to FSH
    d. Resumed due to GnRH

N13. Size of resting follicle:
    a. 0.2 mm   b. 0.02 mm
    c. 2 mm   d. 20 mm

N14. Time taken by sperms to reach fallopian tube:
    a. 30 mins   b. 1 hr
    c. 2 hrs   d. 7 hrs

N15. Cells of embryo are totipotent uptil which cell state:
    a. 8 cell   b. 16 cell
    c. 20 cell   d. 24 cell

N16. Sperms attain maturity and motility in:
    a. Cranial end of epididymis
    b. Caudal end of epididymis
    c. Vas deferens
    d. Ejaculatory duct

N17. Langhans cells are seen in:
    a. Placenta   b. Fallopian tube
    c. Cytotrophoblast d. Syncytiotrophoblast

N18. Main source of prolactin in amniotic fluid is:
    a. Decidua   b. Syncytiotrophoblast
    c. Cytotrophoblast d. Yolk sac of fetus

N19. Primary oocyte is formed after:
    a. 1st meiotic division b. 2nd meiotic division
    c. Mitotic division   d. None of above

N20. 1 primary oocyte forms _____ number of ova:
    a. 1   b. 2
    c. 3   d. 4

N21. Fertilisation is said to be complete if:
    a. 1st polar body is formed
    b. 2nd polar body is formed
    c. Primary oocyte is formed
    d. Secondary oocyte is formed

N22. The first stimulus in intrauterine life for Leydig cells to produce testosterone:
    a. LH   b. FSH
    c. hCG   d. Progesterone

Previous Year Questions

1. **Fertilised ovum reaches uterine cavity by:**
   a. 4 to 5 days after implantation   [AIIMS Nov 13]
   b. 6 to 7 days after implantation
   c. 7 to 9 days after implantation
   d. 2 to 3 days after implantation

2. **After how many days of ovulation embryo implantation occurs?**   [AIIMS May 06]
   a. 3–5 days   b. 7–9 days
   c. 10–12 days   d. 13–15 days

3. **The thickness of endometrium at the time of implantation is:**   [PGI June 99]
   a. 3–4 mm   b. 20–30 mm
   c. 15–20 mm   d. 30–40 mm

4. **In which of the following transition meiosis occurs?**   [AIIMS Nov 07]
   a. Primary to secondary spermatocyte
   b. Second spermatocyte to globular spermatid
   c. Germ cells to spermatogonium
   d. Spermatogonium to primary spermatocyte

5. **Primary oocyte:**   [PGI June 02]
   a. Is formed after single meiotic division
   b. Maximum in number in 5 months of the fetus
   c. Is in prophase arrest
   d. Also called as blastocyst

6. **True statement regarding oogenesis is/are:**
   [PGI May 2010]
   a. Primary oocyte arrests in prophase of 1st meiotic division
   b. Primary oocyte arrests in prophase of 2nd meiotic division
   c. Secondary oocyte arrest in metaphase of 1st meiotic division
   d. Secondary oocyte arrest in metaphase of 2nd meiotic division
   e. 1st polar body is extruded during 1st meiotic division of primary oocytes

7. **In a young female of reproductive age with regular menstrual cycles of 28 days, ovulation occurs around 14th day of periods. When is the first polar body extruded?**   [AIIMS May 05]
   a. 24 hours prior to ovulation
   b. Accompanied by ovulation
   c. 48 hours after the ovulation
   d. At the time of fertilization

Answers with Explanations to New Pattern Questions

N1. Ans. is a, i.e. Decidua basalis *Ref. Dutta Obs 8/e, p 28*

When zygote implants in endometrium, the endometrium is called as Decidua. The part 'A' in the figure is that part of endometrium which is lying in between embryo and myometrium is called Decidua basalis.

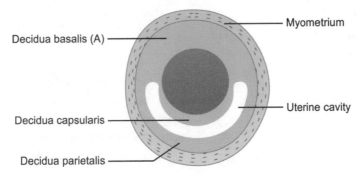

Fig. F1: Subdivisions of decidua

N2. Ans. is a, i.e. 5th month of IUL *Ref Dutta Obs 8/e, p 19*

Maximum number of oogonia are seen at 20 weeks (5th month), numbering 6–7 million.

At birth number is 2 million

At puberty = 3 to 5 lacs. Out of these 400–500 are destined to ovulate throughout life.

N3. Ans. is b, i.e. 5 days after fertilization

Zona hatching occurs just before implantation, i.e. 5 days after fertilization, i.e. D19 of the cycle.

N4. Ans. is b, i.e. Diplotene stage of prophase *Ref. Novaks Gynae 15/e, p 152*

Meiosis 1 is arrested in prophase.

Prophase is further divided into five stages—leptotene, zygotene, patchytene, diplotene and diakinesis.

The first meiotic division gets arrested in the embryonic life in the late diplotene stage of prophase.

The arrested stage is called Dictyate stage

The division is completed only after puberty just prior to ovulation.

N5. Ans. is c, i.e. 70–80 days *Ref. Novaks Gynae, 15/e*

Spermatogenesis on average takes 70–80 days (75 days).

N6. Ans. is d, i.e. 8–10 hours

Capacitation: The term capacitation refers to the changes which occurs in the sperm before it fertilizes the ova. It is the functional maturation of the spermatozoa.
- Average time required = 6–8 hours.
- Capacitation occurs in female reproductive tract.
- It begins in the cervix
- Majority part occurs in fallopian tube.

N7. Ans. is b, i.e. Middle piece

During spermiogenesis – spermatid transforms into the sperm.

Part of spermatid	Part of sperm which it forms
• Nuclear material	Head of sperm
• Golgi body	Acrosomal cap
• Mitochondrion	Middle piece of sperm
• Microtubules	Axial filament/Tail of sperm

 Note: Sperms lack endoplasmic reticulum.

N8. **Ans. is a, i.e. 3 weeks**

N9. **Ans. is d, i.e. 24 weeks**

3 weeks: Time table of events

At 6 weeks POG	Germ cells migrate to ovary
9 weeks	Form oogonia
12 weeks	Form primary oocyte
14 weeks	Follicle formation begins
24 weeks	Follicle completed

N10. **Ans. is b, i.e. 100:106**

You all have studied sex ratio in PSM—the number of females per 1000 males. Primary sex ratio is the sex ratio at fertilisation, i.e. 100:160, which means 100 female zygotes are produced as compared to 160 male zygotes due to higher mobility of Y chromosome.

Secondary sex ratio, i.e. sex ratio at birth is 100:106 i.e. 100 females are born against 106 males as miscarriage rate is higher in male fetuses, probably, due to higher metabolism.

N11. **Ans. is c, i.e. 12–16 weeks** *(Callen's usg in and Gynae pg 189)*

Obliteration of uterine cavity, i.e. decidual cavity occurs by 12–16 weeks.

N12. **Ans. is b, i.e. Resumed due to LH**

Resumption of Meiosis I is hormone, dependent. It resumes with LH surge, i.e. Meiosis I is completed 32–36 hrs before ovulation

Meiosis II is not hormone-dependent.

N13. **Ans. is b, i.e. 0.02 mm**

Size of resting follicle = 0.02 mm
Size of follicle just before ovulation = 20 mm
Size of ova = 120 microns (largest cell in body)
Size of sperm = 55 microns

N14. **Ans. is a, i.e. 30 mins.**

Time taken for sperms to reach the site of fertilisation = 30 mins.

N15. **Ans. is a, i.e. 8 cell**

The cells of embryo are totipotent uptil 8 cell stage.

N16. **Ans. is b, i.e. Caudal end of epididymis.**

Sperms attain maturity and motility in the caudal end of epididymis.

N17. **Ans. is c, i.e. Cytotrophoblast**

Name of cells	Seen in
Langhans cells	Cytotrophoblast
Hofbauer cells	Placenta
Peg cells	Fallopian tube

N18. Ans. is a, i.e. Decidua   *Ref. William Obs, 24 edition, p 88*

The decidua is the main source of prolactin that is present in amniotic fluid. Decidual prolactin is not to be confused with human placental lactogen (hPl), which is produced only by syncytiotrophoblast.

N19. Ans. is c, i.e. Mitotic division

N20. Ans. is a, i.e. 1

Primary oocyte is formed after mitotic division and from 1 primary oocyte only 1 ovum is formed

N21. Ans. is b, i.e. 2nd polar body is formed

See Fig. 1.3 for explanation.

N22. Ans. is c, i.e. hCG

The first stimulus for Leydig cells to produce testosterone in Intrauterine in hCG.

Remember:

- The main stimulus for Leydig cells to produce testosterone is LH
- The first stimulus for Leydig cells to produce testosterone is hCG

Answers with Explanations to Previous Year Questions

1. **Ans. is a, i.e. 4 to 5 days after implantation**   *Ref. JB Sharma Obs, pg 19*

   "The morula enters the uterine cavity on the 4th day"
   Questions on Morula

   > Zygote enters the uterine cavity in the form of Morula (16 celled stage).
   > Zygote enters the uterine cavity 4th day after fertilisation, i.e. Day 18 of the cycle.

2. **Ans. is b, i.e. 7–9 days**   *Ref. JB Sharma Obs, pg 20*

   Implantation is the process by which blastocyst penetrates the uterine mucosa to get implanted in the endometrium. It starts on the 6–7th day after ovulation i.e. 20–21st day of a regular menstrual cycle.   *Ref. JB Sharma Obs, pg 20*

3. **Ans. is b i.e. 20–30 mm (caller USG in obs and gynae.**

   At the time of implantation, endometrium is 8–10 mm thick)

4. **Ans. is a i.e. Primary to secondary spermatocyte**

 Key Concept

Cell division is of 2 types:
Mitosis—Here the number of chromosomes remains the same
Meiosis—Includes 2 divisions
Meiosis I—This is Reduction division. Here the number of chromosomes becomes half
Meiosis II—Here the number of chromosomes remains the same.

In spermatogenesis, meiosis occurs at 2 steps:

i. When primary spermatocyte changes to secondary spermatocyte.

ii. When secondary spermatolcyte changes to spermatid.

But reduction division, i.e. Meiosis I occurs in step (i). So, we are taking it as the correct answer.

5. **Ans. is b and c, i.e. Maximum number in 5 months of fetus and Is in prophase arrest.**

See the text for explanation.

6. **Ans. is a, d and e, i.e. Primary oocyte arrest in prophase of 1st meiotic division, Secondary oocyte arrests in metaphase of 2nd meiotic division and 1st polar body is extruded during 1st meiotic division of primary oocyte.**

See the text for explanation.

7. **Ans. is b, i.e. Accompanied by ovulation**   *Ref. Guyton 10/e, p 944; Ganong 21/e, p 438*

    • Most of the standard textbooks say the first polar body is expelled just before or shortly before ovulation approximately 10–12 hours before ovulation.

    • Which does not mean that it is released 24 hours before ovulation.

    • *"While still in the ovary, the ovum is in the primary oocyte stage. Shortly before it is released from ovarian follicle (i.e. shortly before ovulation), its nucleus divides by meiosis and a first polar body is expelled from the nucleus of the oocyte. The primary oocyte then becomes the secondary oocyte. In this process, each of the 23 unpaired chromosomes loses one of its partners which become the first polar body that is expelled. These leave 23 unpaired chromosomes in the secondary oocyte. It is at this time that the ovum still in the secondary oocyte stage is ovulated into the abdominal cavity."*   *—Guyton 10/e, p 944*

    So, first polar body is released at the time of ovulation, i.e. *Option "b"*

 Note:

• The secondary oocyte immediately begins the second meiotic division, but this division stops at metaphase and is completed only when sperm penetrates the oocyte.

• At this time second polar body is cast off. So, *second polar body is cast off at the time of fertilization.*

• Friends, this is an often repeated question and for those who find it difficult to remember this basic fact, I have a mnemonic:

 Mnemonic

• **PP1 and M2F**

• **PP1**, i.e. **1st** meiotic division is arrested in **prophase** and 1st polar body is released at puberty

• **M2F**, i.e. **2nd** meiotic division is arrested in **metaphase** and **2nd polar body** is released at the time of **fertilisation.**

Placenta, Fetal Membranes and Umbilical Cord

PLACENTA

The human placenta is **discoid**, because of its shape; **hemochorial**, because of direct contact of the chorion with the maternal blood and **deciduate**, because some maternal tissue is shed at parturition.

Extra Edge

The human hemochorial placenta can be subdivided into

a. **Hemodichorial:** Where there is a continuous inner layer of cytotrophoblast and outer layer of syncytiotrophoblast. This is seen in 1st trimester.

b. **Hemomonochorial:** Later in gestation, the inner layer of cytotrophoblast is no longer continuous, by term there are only scattered cells present. This is hemomonochorial.

DEVELOPMENT

The placenta is formed by 2 sources:

1. **Fetal surface:** Chorion frondosum

2. **Maternal surface:** Decidua basalis

• The chorion frondosum has many finger like projections called villi (Fig. 2.1). In between the villi, there are intervillous spaces.

• The syncytiotrophoblast and cytotrophoblast grows inside the Villi. Thus now the villi have trophoblastic

shell. This is called as **Primary Villi which is formed** before 12 days after fertilisation (Fig. 2.2). The maternal blood vessels open in the inter villous space at 15 days after fertilization.

• In the next step extra embryonic mesoderm grows into the villi. Thus now these villi have a mesodermal core. This is a **Secondary Villi** (Fig 2.3). It is formed between day 12 day – 16 day after fertilisation.

• **In the last step:** The fetal blood capillaries open in the villi and now the villi is called Tertiary Villi. Fetal circulation is established by D17 after fertilisation.

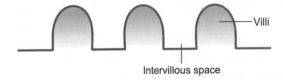

Fig. 2.1

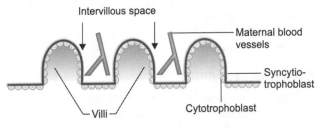

Fig. 2.2: Primary villi

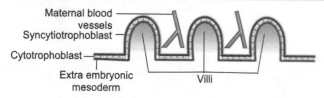

Fig. 2.3: Secondary villi

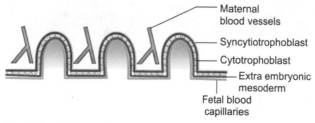

Fig. 2.4: Tertiary villi

 Also Know:

- When the maternal spiral arterioles open in the intervillous space, their lining is replaced by cytotrophoblast. This is called as **Trophoblastic Invasion**.
- Trophoblastic invasion occurs in 2 phases.
- Trophoblastic invasion converts high pressure/ (resistance) vessels into low pressure vessels (p ∝1/r) so more volume of blood goes to fetus. This prevents PIH also.
- If there is no trophoblastic/incomplete trophoblastic invasion, then resistance in maternal vessels remains high and female develops PIH.

- Thus from above discussion it is clear that villi has fetal blood and maternal blood is present in intervillous space
- So both maternal and fetal blood are present in placenta but they never mix with each other. They are separated by
  - Syncytiotrophoblast
  - Cytotrophoblast
  - Extraembryonic mesoderm
  - Endothelium of fetal capillaries

  Together called as **placental barrier** or **placental membrane**
- **Maternal arterial blood enters placental circulation by D15 after fertilization**
- **Tertiary villi (with fetal blood vessel) are seen 17 days after fertilisation**
- Thus feto placental circulation is established by **17 days after fertilisition.**

Structure of a Villi

- The villi are attached on the fetal side to the extra-embryonic mesoderm and on maternal side to the cytotrophoblastic shell.

- The villi are called anchoring villi or stem villi.
- Each anchoring villi consists of a stem-**(Trunchus chorii)**
- It divides into number of branches-**(ramus chorii)** which further divides into many small branches **(Ramuli chorii)**
- One such anchoring villi and its branches is called a cotyledon (which is the functional unit of placental) (see Fig. 2.5).
- Apart from anchoring villi, most villi are free within the intervillous space and are called Nutritive villi.

 Note: Blood vessels within the branching villi have no anastomosis with the neighbouring villi.

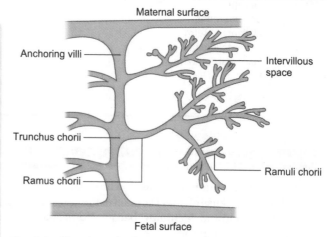

Fig. 2.5: Structure of villi

PLACENTA AT TERM

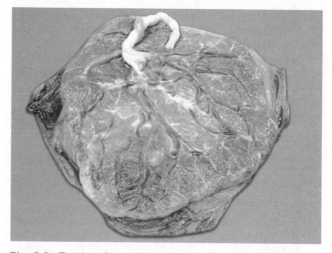

Fig. 2.6: Fetal surface of the placenta showing attachment of the umbilical cord

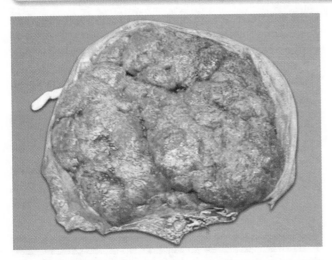

Fig. 2.7: Maternal surface of the placenta showing shaggy look with cotyledons limited by fissures

- The placenta, at term, is almost a circular disc with a diameter of 15–20 cm and thickness **of 3 cms** at its center.
- It weighs **500 gm.**[Q]
- The ratio of weight of placenta to the weight of the baby being roughly **1 : 6 at term.**[Q]
- **At 17 weeks of gestation the weight of the placenta and fetus are equal.**[Q]
- It occupies about 30% of the uterine wall and is attached to upper part of uterine wall either at posterior wall (2/3 cases) or at anterior wall (1/3 cases)
- **It has two surfaces, fetal surface and maternal surface.**

Fetal Surface

- **At term, four-fifth of the placenta is of fetal origin (Fig. 2.6).**
- But area-wise both fetal and maternal surface occupy same area on placenta
- Fetal side is formed by chorion frondosum

- The fetal surface is shiny, grey in color and covered with shining amnion.
- The umbilical cord is attached at or near its center.

Maternal Surface

- The maternal surface is dull red in color and rough.
- It has 10–38 convex polygonal areas called as **lobes**. The total number of placental lobes remains the same throughout gestation and individual lobes continue to grow. Some people refer to lobes as cotyledons. This is not correct.

- **A cotyledon** or lobule is the functional unit of placenta originating from a main (stem villus) as discussed in structure of villi.
- The maternal portion of the placenta is one-fifth of the total placenta.
- **Maternal side is formed by decidua basalis**
- **Separation: The line of separation of placenta is through the decidua spongiosum.** (Intermediate layer of the decidua basalis).
- **Nitabuch's membrane** is the fibrinoid deposition in the outer syncytiotrophoblast. It limits the further invasion of the decidua by the trophoblast. Absence of the membrane causes **Placenta Accreta, Increta and Percreta.**
- **FFN (fetal fibronectin)** has been called **trophoblast glue** to suggest a critical role for this protein in the migration and attachment of trophoblasts to maternal decidua. The presence of FFN in cervical or vaginal fluid can be used as a prognostic indicator for preterm labor or PROM.
- The stroma of placenta has fetal macrophages called as **Hoffbauer cells.**

 Also Know:
- Placenta formation begins by 6 weeks (on USG it can be seen as early as 10 weeks) and is completed by 14–15 weeks
- For placental localization—USG should be done in 3rd trimester[Q]
- At term placenta has following characteristic which enables efficient transport between placenta and fetus:
  - No cytotrophoblast
  - Syncytiotrophoblast thin
  - Stroma—decreases
  - Fetal capillaries increase and move towards periphery villi
  - Hoffbauer cells are present

PLACENTAL CIRCULATION

- As discussed above, placenta has villi and intervillous space.
- **The villi** carry fetal blood (Fig. 2.8).
- Volume = 350 mL.
- **Intervillous space**—which has maternal blood. Volume = 150 mL (Fig. 2.8)
- Thus volume of placenta is 500 mL (150 + 350 = 500)
- Also worth noting is, that although both maternal and fetal blood are present in placenta, they do not mix with each other
- So placental circulation consists of 2 independent circulations:

i. **Uteroplacental circulation**
ii. **Fetoplacental circulation**

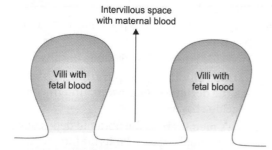

Fig. 2.8: Placental villi

Uteroplacental Circulation

- **It is concerned with the circulation of the maternal blood through the intervillous space.**
- It is established by D15 after fertilisation.
- The uteroplacental blood flow at term is 500–750 mL/min.

 Remember: If question says uterine blood flow at term it is 750 mL/minute

- The number of spiral arterioles opening in the intervillous space are 100–200 (≈120).

Table 2.1: Summary of intervillous hemodynamics

• Volume of blood in mature placenta	500 mL
• Volume of blood in intervillous space	150 mL
• Oxygen saturation	65–75%

Fetoplacental Circulation

- Established by D 17 after fertilisation
- Fetoplacental circulation is via umbilical veins and umbilical arteries.
- The umbilical vein carries oxygenated blood from placenta to fetus. (Fig. 2.9)

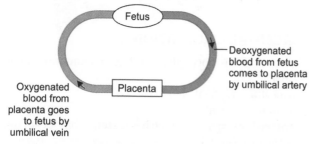

Fig. 2.9: Blood flow between placenta & fetus

- The two umbilical arteries carry the impure blood from the fetus to the placenta.
- These arteries branch repeatedly underneath the amnion to form the chorionic arteries which are end arteries. There branches are called as **truncal arteries**.

- Each truncal artery supplies one main stem villus and thus one cotyledon.
- The oxygenated blood then returns to the fetus via single umbilical vein.
- **The fetal blood flow through the placenta is about 400 mL/min.**

 Remember:
- If question say Fetal blood flow at term-125 mL/kg
- Rate of O_2 delivery to fetus - 8 mL/kg/min

Table 2.2: Summary of fetal hemodynamics

Umbilical vein	Umbilical artery
Carries oxygenated blood	Carries deoxygenated blood
O_2 Saturation 70 – 80%	50 – 60%
SPO_2 35 – 40 mm Hg	20–25 mm Hg
Pressure –10 mm	60 mm of Hg
Remnant in adult- Ligamentum teres	Medial umbilical ligament

 Points to Remember

- **The uteroplacental circulation** is established day 15 after fertilization.
- **Fetoplacental circulation** is established by17 days post fertilization.
- Uterine blood flow at term = 750 mL/min (In nonpregnant females: 50 mL/min)
- Uteroplacental blood flow at term = 400–600 mL/min
- Fetal blood volume at term = 125 mL/kg
- Fetoplacental blood flow = 400 mL/min

PLACENTAL PATHOLOGY

Placental Infarction

- These are the most common placental lesion. If they are numerous, placental insufficiency may develop. When they are thick, centrally located and randomly distributed, they may be associated with **preeclampsia** or **lupus anticoagulant. They can also lead to placental abruption.**

Placentomegaly

- During pregnancy, the normal placental increases its thickness at rate of approx 1 mm per week.
- If placental thickness is more than 40 mm at term, It is called as **placentomegaly.**

Thick placenta can be due to many causes. Based on the USG appearance it can be divided into:

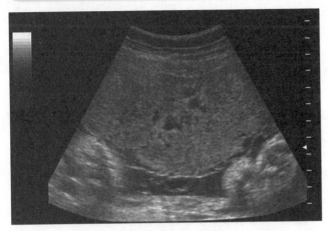

Fig. 2.10 Homogeneous thick placenta

Causes of homogeneous thickening (Fig. 2.10):

- Diabetes mellitus or Gestational diabetes
- Anemia
- Hydrops fetalis
- TORCH infection
- Rarely-aneuploidy

Causes of multiple cystic spaces seen within thick placenta (Fig. 2.11):

- Triploidy
- Placental hemorrhage
- Mesenchymal dysplasia
- Beckwith-Wiedemann syndrome

Causes of heterogeneous thickening: Intraplacental hemorrhage

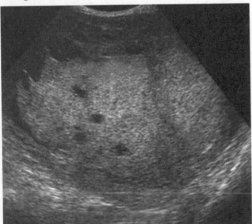

Fig. 2.11: Thick placenta with multiple cystic lesions

Small Placenta

- **Small placentas are seen in:**
  - Postdatism
  - IUGR
  - Placental infarcts

Abnormalities of Placenta

Placenta with a Small Lobe Detached (Figs. 2.12A to C)

A. **Succenturiate lobe:** Here a small part of placenta is separated from the rest of placenta. A leash of vessels connects the mass to the small lobe.

B. **Placenta bilobata:** When both the separated lobe and main lobe are of equal size, and are connected by blood vessels. It is called as placenta bilobata.

C. **Placenta spuria:** In this condition, a small part of placenta is separated from the rest of placenta, but there are no communicating blood vessels.

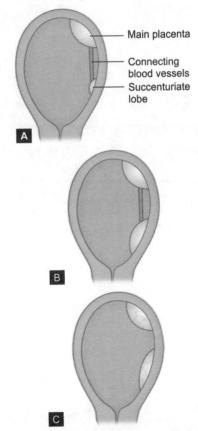

Figs. 2.12A to C: (A) Succenturiate lobe; (B) Placenta bilobata; (C) Placenta spuria

 Note: All these 3 can lead to PPH (postpartum hemorrhage)

Extrachorial Placenta

The chorionic plate normally extends to the periphery of the placenta and has a diameter similar to the basal plate.

In extrachorial placentation, the chorionic plate is smaller to the basal plate. This is of 2 varieties (Figs. 2.13 & 2.14):

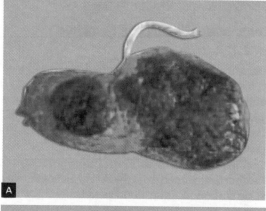

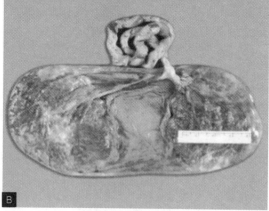

Figs. 2.13A and B: (A) Succenturiate lobe; (B) Placenta bilobata

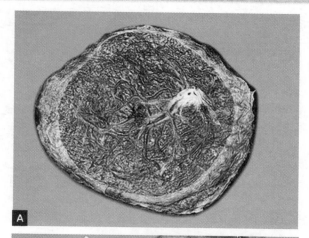

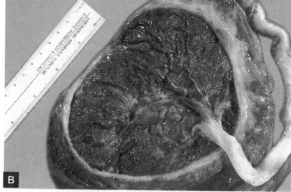

Figs. 2.14A and B: (A) Circummarginate placenta; (B) Circumvallate placenta

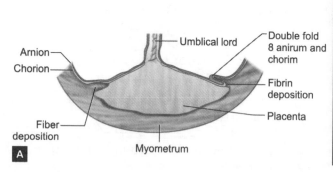

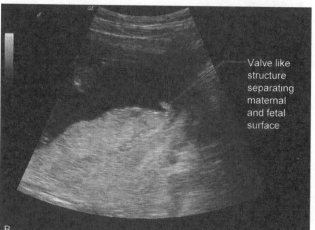

Figs. 2.15A and B: (A) Circumvallate placenta diagram; (B) Circumvallate placenta on USG

i. **Circummarginate placenta**

   Here the chorionic plate is covered by a single fold of amnion and chorion and there is fibrin and old hemorrhage between the placenta and overlying amnio-chorion. **Thus the transition between fetal surface and maternal surface is smooth.**

ii. **Circumvallate placenta**

Here chorionic plate is covered by a double fold of amnion and chorion so between maternal surface and fetal surface a valve like structure is seen. Sonographically this double fold appears as a thick linear band or shelf-like structure (see Figs. 2.14A and B).

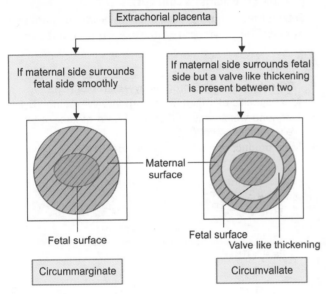

Both these conditions can lead to antepartum hemorrhage or IUGR in fetus.

Also Know:
- Battledore placenta (given in section on umbilical cord)

Placental Tumors

- M/C begin neoplasm of placenta is **chorangioma of the placenta** consisting of avascular mass arising from chronic tissue.
- Chorangioma is the M/C benign neoplasm of placenta (Figs. 2.16A and B)
- It consists of vascular mass arising from chorionic tissue
- Incidence = 1%
- Small chorangiomas are insignificant
- Large chorangiomas (>5 cm) can lead to:
  i. **Maternal complications**
     - Polyhydramnios
     - PIH
     - Preterm labor
     - ↑ AFP
  ii. **Fetal complications**
     - Hydrops fetalis
     - Fetal cardiomegaly
     - IVGR

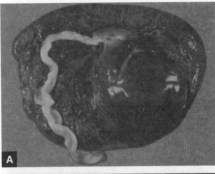
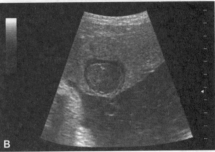
Figs. 2.16A and B: (A) Chorangioma of placenta appearing as a small, round mass on fetal surface of placenta; (B) Chorangioma of appearance on USG

- The feature which distinguishes this tumor from other placental tumors is prominent blood flow
- **Management:** In utero laser coagulation of the blood supply of the tumor.

- **The tumors which can metastasize to placenta** are melanoma, leukemia, lymphoma and breast cancer.
- Placental tumor which can metastasize to fetus also is **melanoma.**[Q]

FUNCTION OF PLACENTA

i. Transfer of gases, nutrients and waste products—i.e. respiratory, nutritive and excretory function.

Note: Oxygen delivery to the fetus is about 8 mL/kg of fetal weight/min which is achieved by placental blood flow of about 400 mL/min.

Glucose is the main source of energy for fetus. Fetus obtains its glucose from maternal blood by facilitated diffusion using GLUT-1 and GLUT-3.

- Lipids are transferred from mother to fetus in early pregnancy but are synthesized in fetus in late pregnancy **so fat has a dual origin in fetus.**

ii. Immunological function
iii. Endocrine function/hormonal function (details given below)
iv. Enzymatic functions
v. Barrier function

Hormonal Function of Placenta

- **Important hormones synthesized by placenta are:**
  - Progesterone
  - Estrogen
  - Human placental lactogen (HPL) most specific
  - Human chorionic gonadotropin (hCG)
- Others are:
  - Human chorionic thyrotropin
  - Pregnancy specific β, glycoprotein
  - Pregnancy associated plasma protein A (PAPP-A)
- Main site of hormonal synthesis is placenta—**syncytio-trophoblast**

Progesterone

- It is the Main hormone during pregnancy
- During initial 6–7 weeks, progesterone is synthesized by corpus luteum (17 alpha hydroxyprogesterone)
- At 8–10 weeks, placenta takes over the function of corpus luteum
- Progesteron is synthesized by placenta all by itself using **cholesterol/LDL from mother (Precursor of progesterone)**

Points on corpus luteum of pregnancy

- Hormone maintaining corpus luteum of pregnancy– hCG
- Life span of CL of pregnancy 10 to 12 weeks

Points on progesterone

- Progesterone is a smooth muscle relaxant
- Two reactions in pregnancy due to progesterone
  - **Decidual reaction:** i.e. conversion of endometrium to decidua
  - **Arias stella reaction:** (See ectopic pregnancy for details)

Table 2.3: Levels of progesterone

12 weeks	25 ng/mL
28 weeks	80 ng/mL
Term	300 ng/mL

Table 2.4: Abnormal levels of progesterone

Low levels	High levels
Ectopic pregnancy	Molar pregnancy
Abortion	Rh isoimmunization

Estrogen

- Estrogen cannot be synthesized by placenta alone as it cannot utilize C_{21} steroid due to lack of enzyme **17 alpha hydroxylase.** Hence conversion of C_{21} to C_{19} is not possible (**Diczfalusy's concept**).
- Fetal adrenal gland produce DHEA-S which is utilized by placental enzymes to synthesize estradiol and estriol.

 Important One Liners

- M/C estrogen during pregnancy—estradiol (E_2)
- Most specific estrogen during pregnancy—estriol (E_3)
- Hormone which was earlier used as a marker of fetal well- being—estriol (E_3)
- Main product of fetal adrenal gland—DHEA-S.

Key Concept

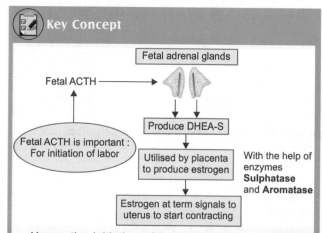

- Hence the initiation of labor depends on sufficient availability of estrogen, which in turn depends on fetal DHE AS - which depends on fetal ACTH.
- So if question says: Labor is initiated by: look for fetal ACTH/maternal estrogen in answer.
- This is the reason why **in anencephaly** where the adrenal glands are hypoplastic or absent, the complication is **Post Dated Pregnancy.**

Fetal Adrenal Gland

- Morphologically, functionally and physiologically, the fetal adrenal glands are a remarkable organ.
- At term fetal adrenal gland weighs almost the same as adult adrenal gland.
- More than 85% of gland is made up of unique fetal zone which has a great capacity for steroid synthesis.
- Daily steroid production of fetal adrenal gland is 100–200 mg/day (In adults = 40 mg/day).
- The fetal zone is lost in first year of life and is not present in adults.

- Growth of fetal adrenal gland depends not only on ACTH but also on factors secreted by placenta (that is why after delivery, rapid involution of fetal adrenal gland occurs).

Human Placental Lactogen

- Also called as **human chorionic somatotropin (hCS)**
- It is synthesized by syncytiotrophoblast
- Can be detected in maternal serum at 3 weeks of gestation
- Highest amount—34–36 weeks in maternal serum
- Half life = 10–30 minutes ($\approx$ 15 minutes)

Functions

- Main role is to conserve glucose so that it is utilised by the fetus
- It Promotes **maternal lipolysis** so maternal levels of free fatty acids are increased, which mother utilizes as a source of energy, sparing glucose for fetus.
- It increases **insulin resistance** hence again mother's glucose is high & it can be utilized by fetus.

Note: hPL has no role in lactation
- Functioning of placenta is determined by hPL
- Its production rate = 1 g/day at term, maximum for any hormone

Human Chorionic Gonadotropin

- It is a glycoprotein hormone[Q]
- **This hormone has highest carbohydrate content of any human hormone**[Q]
- It has 2 subunits:
  - α subunit—biologically similar in LH, FSH and TSH (i.e. non-specific)
  - β subunit—unique to hCG (specific)
- Structurally it is similar to LH, FSH, TSH but functionally it is similar to LH (i.e. luteotropic), i.e. helps in maintaining corpus luteum
- Half-life of hCG is 24–36 hours
- Doubling time = 2 days (1.4–2 days)
- It can be detected in maternal serum as early as 8 days following fertilization/day 22 of menstrual cycle/5–6 days before missed period (Fig. 2.17)

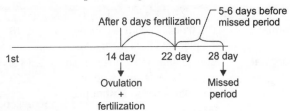
Fig. 2.17: Menstrual cycle

Order of Sensitivity of hCG Tests

Fluorescent Immunoassay (FIA) > Radioimmunoassay (RIA) > ELISA and Radioreceptor assay > Immunoradiometric assay (IRMA)

- At the time of missed period its level = 100 IU/L.
- It reaches maximum = 100,000 IU/L (MIU/mL) by 8–10 weeks (70 days)
- It then falls and minimum levels are seen at 16 weeks and remains at low level up to term (Fig. 2.18)
- hCG disappears from urine—48 hours after delivery

In Blood

hCG disappears after

Normal pregnancy	After 1-2 weeks
After abortion	In 2-4 weeks
After partial mole evacuation	In 7 weeks
After complete mole evacuation	In 9 weeks

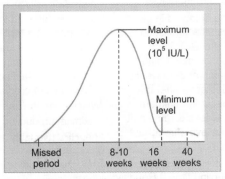
Fig. 2.18: hCG levels during pregnancy

Clinical implications of the measurement of hCG	
Increased hCG values	**Decreased hCG levels**
• Multifetal pregnancy • Gestational Trophoblastic disease • Down syndrome • Under estimated gestational age • Erythroblastosis fetalis as it is associated with fetal hemolytic anemia	• Abortion • Trisomy other than Down syndrome • Ectopic pregnancy

Critical titre of hCG:
- The titre of hCG at which gestational sac should be visible on TVS in case of intrauterine pregnancy = 1500 IU/L
- The titre of hCG at which gestational sac should be visible on TAS in case of intrauterine pregnancy = 6000 IU/L – 6500 IU/L

Functions of hCG

- Maintains corpus luteum of pregnancy (functionally similar to LH)
- It simulates LH and provides the first stimulus for release of testosterone from fetal testis
- It has immuno suppressive action and prevents rejection of fetus.
- It stimulates maternal thyroid gland.
- It is used for diagnostic test like triple test for down syndrome (See Table 2.5)

Table 2.5: hCG & hPL

hCG	hPL
• Glycoprotein hormone with 2 subunits α and β. β is the specific subunit It is the hormone with highest carbohydrate content	(also called hCS human carbonic somatotropin) • It has a single polypeptide chain
• Synthesised by syncytiotrophoblast	• Synthesised by syncytiotrophoblast
• Can be detected in blood 8 days after fertilisation (D22 of cycle). Then the levels increase, being maximum at 8-10 weeks and decrease after that and become minimum by 16 weeks & remain at this low level throughout pregnancy.	• Can be detected in blood 3 weeks after fertilisation. Then the levels keep on increasing steadily and maximum levels seen at 36 weeks of pregnancy (Which hormone has maximum production at term Ans. HPL (Roughly 1g/day)
– T1/2 = 24 - 48 hrs – Doubling time = Roughly 48 hours – (atleast by 48 hours in a viable pregnancy increase in hCG > 66%)	T1/2 - 10-30 min

FETAL MEMBRANES

- **Amnion**
  - Innermost fetal membrane.
  - It is avascular.
  - It provides almost all tensile strength of the fetal membranes.
  - It lacks smooth muscle cells, nerves, lymphatics and blood vessels.
  - It is now being considered as a derivative of fetal ectoderm.
  - The layer is formed between 10 and 11 days after fertilization.
- **Chorion**
  - Formed 8 days after fertilization.
  - Chorion frondosum forms placental villi while chorion leave or chorion gets merged with amnion

- **Yolk sac:** It is the first site of hematopoiesis
- **Allantois:** Diverticulum which arises from hindgut and grows into the connecting stalk.

UMBILICAL CORD

- Umbilical cord (or funis) extends from the fetal umbilicus to the fetal surface of the placenta or chorionic plate.
- It develops from the connecting stalk.[Q]
- In the early fetal life, cord has 2 arteries and 2 veins but later right umbilical vein disappears, leaving only the original left vein (**i.e. Left is left**)[Q]. *Thus at term umbilical cord has 2 arteries and 1 vein.*[Q]
- The two arteries are smaller in diameter than the veins.[Q]
- It is covered only by amnion not chorion.
- Normal cord pH = 7.2.

Structure and Function

- Anatomically umbilical cord can be regarded as a fetal membrane.[Q]
- Its length is ≈ 55 cm, Range is between 30 and 100 cm (If it is < 32 cm it is considered abnormally short).[Q]
- Folding and tortuosity of the vessels within the cord itself creates false knots (which are essentially varices).
- When fixed in their normally distended state, the umbilical arteries exhibit transverse **intimal folds of Hoboken**[Q] across their lumen.
- Number of coils/cm is called as **umbilical coiling index** which is seen on USG.
- Normal coiling index = 0.17 coils/cm
- Hypocoiling (< 0.07) is linked to IUD.
- Hypercoiling is linked to IUGR and fetal acidosis.
- The extracellular matrix, which is specialized connective tissue consists of Wharton's Jelly.[Q]

Short cord is associated with	Excessively long cord is associated with
• IUGR • Abnormal lie/presentation • Congenital malformations • Premature placental separation	• Cord entanglement • Cord around the neck of fetus • Fetal distress • Cord prolapse • Fetal anomalies

Abnormalities of the Cord Insertion

Abnormality	Features	Diagram
Normal	The umbilical cord is attached to the placenta near the centre	2.18
Marginal	Cord is attached to the margin of the placenta (this type of placenta is called **Battledore placenta**).	2.18 and 2.19

Contd...

Contd...

Abnormality	Features	Diagram
Furcate	Cord is attached to centre of placenta but just before insertion, it loses its Warton's jelly and is covered only by amnion Thus there are more chances of cord compression twisting and thrombosis	2.18

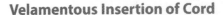

Figs. 2.19A to C: Abnormalities of cord insertion

Velamentous Insertion of Cord

Here the cord is attached to the center of placenta but the vessels split much before attaching to placenta and are attached to membranes first then they attach to placenta. This is called as **velamentous insertion of cord**.

Velamentous insertion of cord can give rise to serious fetal condition called as Vasa Previa (discussed in detail in chapter on APH)

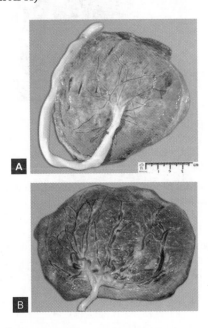

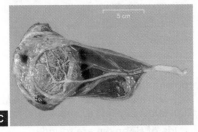

Figs. 2.20A to C: (A) Normal cord insertion; (B) Battledore placenta; (C) Velamentous insertion of cord

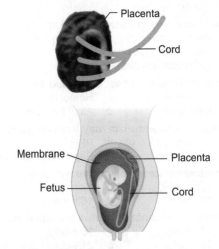

Fig. 2.21: Diagrammatic representation of velamentous insertion of cord

Single umbilical artery (SUA)

- It is the M/C vascular anomaly of the cord.
- It is seen in 0.7–0.8% cases of single pregnancy and 5% of twin pregnancy.
- More common in diabetic patients, black patients, with eclampsia, hydramnios and oligohydramnios, epilepsy patients and in APH.
- Finding of a single umbilical artery is not insignificant and is associated with:
  - **Congenital malformations of the fetus seen in 20–25% cases** amongst which cardiovascular anomalies and Renal anomalies are more common. If single umbilical artery is an isolated finding, chances of aneuploidy in fetus are not increased but if SUA is associated, with other major malformations—then chances of aneuploidy in the fetus are high and amniocentesis should be done.
  - M/c aneuploidy associated with SUA—Trisomy (Trisomy 18).
  - SUA also causes increased chances of abortion, prematurity, IUGR and perinatal mortality.

New Pattern Questions

N1. Uteroplacental blood flow at term is:
a. 300–500 mL/min   b. 500–700 mL/min
c. 700–900 mL/min   d. 900–1100 mL/min

N2. The folds of Hoboken are found in:
a. The amnion   b. The placenta
c. Uterus   d. Umbilical cord
e. Ductus venosus

N3. Fetal blood loss in abnormal cord insertion is seen in:
a. Vasa previa   b. Decidua basalis
c. Battle dore placenta
d. Succenturiate placenta

N4. Human placenta is best described as:
a. Discoidal   b. Hemochorial
c. Deciduate   d. All of the above

N5. Placenta succenturiata may have all except:
a. Preterm delivery   b. PPH
c. Missing lobe   d. Sepsis and subinvolution

N6. Decidual space is obliterated by:
a. 10th week   b. 12th week
c. 18th week   d. 16th week

N7. Weight of placenta and fetus are equal at:
a. 14 weeks   b. 15 weeks
c. 17 weeks   d. 21 weeks

N8. What is a placental cotyledon?
a. All branches from one stem villi
b. Area supplied by one spiral artery
c. Quarter of placenta
d. Area drained by one terminal villi

N9. Blood flow in intervillous space at term:
a. 150 mL   b. 250 mL
c. 300 mL   d. 500 mL

N10. Uterine blood flow at term:
a. 50 mL/min   b. 450 mL
c. 550 mL   d. 750 mL/min

N11. Which prostaglandin is present predominantly in fetal membranes:
a. PGE1   b. PGE2
c. PGF-2α d. PGI2

N12. Normal cord pH is:
a. 7.1   b. 7.2
c. 6.1   d. 6.2

N13. Whaton's jelly of umbilical cord is devided from:
a. Ectoderm   b. Mesoderm
c. Endoderm   d. Trophoblast

N14. Schwangershaft protein is the other name of:
a. hCG   b. Papp-1
c. Pregnancy specific beta 1 glycoprotein
d. Activin

N15. The role of human placental lactogen is:
a. Stimulate milk production
b. Fetal breast development
c. Growth of fetus   d. Endocrine regulation

N16. α and β subunits are not seen in:
a. FSH   b. hCG
c. Prolactin   d. Insulin

N17. Placental grading on ultrasound is based on:
a. Placental location   b. Placental deviations
c. Amniotic fluid and placental lactogen
d. Chorionic plate undulations

N18. Placentamegaly is diagnosed on USG if size of placenta is more near:
a. 25 mm   b. 30 mm
c. 35 mm   d. 40 mm

N19. Process of labor is initiated by:
a. Fetal ACTH   b. Maternal ACTH
c. Fetal progesterone d. Maternal progesterone

N20. Identify the placental abnormality shown in figure:

a. Succenturiate lobe b. Placenta bilobata
c. Velamentous insertion of cord
d. Battledore placenta

N21. Identify the placental abnormality shown in figure

a. Battledore placental
b. Velamentous insertion of cord
c. Circumvallate placental
d. Circummarginate placental

N22. Maternal blood enters intervillous space by _____ days after fertilisation:
a. 12   b. 15
c. 17   d. 21

N23. Fetoplacental circulation is established by _____ days are fertilisation:
a. 12   b. 15
c. 17   d. 21

Previous Year Questions

1. **Estrogen and progesterone in first two months of pregnancy are produced by:** [AIIMS Nov 2015]
   a. Fetal ovaries
   b. Fetal adrenal
   c. Placenta
   d. Corpus luteum

2. **Following hormones secreted by placenta exclusively:** [PGI June 03]
   a. hCG
   b. Estrogen
   c. HPL
   d. Prolactin

3. **hCG is secreted by:** [AIIMS May 06/PGI June 08]
   a. Trophoblast cells
   b. Amniotic membrane
   c. Fetal yolk sac
   d. Hypothalamus

4. **False statement regarding hCG is:** [AI 01]
   a. It is secreted by cytotrophoblast
   b. It acts on same receptor as LH
   c. It has luteotrophic acton
   d. It is a glycoprotein

5. **True about hCG:** [PGI Nov 10]
   a. α subunit identical to LH, FSH and TSH
   b. Causes involution of corpus luteum
   c. Doubles in 7–10 days
   d. Max. level seen at 60–70 days of gestation
   e. Detected in serum and urine 8–9 days after ovulation

6. **Best test for estimating hCG:** [AI 2011]
   a. Radioimmunoassay
   b. ELISA
   c. Radioreceptor assay
   d. Bioassay

7. **Hormone responsible for decidual reaction and Arias stella reaction in ectopic pregnancy is:** [AIIMS June 00]
   a. Oestrogen
   b. Progesterone
   c. hCG
   d. HPL

8. **High level of hCG found in:** [PGI Nov 2014]
   a. Twin
   b. Down syndrome
   c. Choriocarcinoma
   d. Ectopic pregnancy

9. **The foetal blood is separated from syncytiotrophoblast with all except:** [AI 08, UP 07]
   a. Fetal blood capillary membrane
   b. Mesenchyme of intervillous blood space
   c. Cytotrophoblast
   d. Decidua parietalis

10. **The uterine blood flow at term:** [AIIMS Nov 09]
    a. 50 mL/min
    b. 100–150 mL/min
    c. 350–375 mL/min
    d. 500–750 mL/min

11. **The finding of a single umbilical artery on examination of the umbilical cord after delivery is:**
    a. Insignificant [AIIMS Nov 09]
    b. Occurs in 10% of newborns
    c. An indicator of considerably increased incidence of major malformation of the fetus
    d. Equally common in newborn of diabetic and nondiabetic mothers

Answers with Explanations to New Pattern Questions

N1. **Ans. is b, i.e. 500–700 mL/min** *Ref. Williams Obs. 25/e, p 132*

"Using ultrasound to study the uterine arteries, utero placental blood flow has been measured to increase progressively during pregnancy from approximately 450 mL/min in mid trimester to nearly 500–750 mL/min at 36 weeks"

N2. **Ans. is d, i.e. Umbilical cord** *Ref. Williams Obs. 22/e, p 68, 69; 23/e, p 61, 62; 23/e, p 61, 62*

Here are few named structures frequently asked and the organ/structure where it is found.

Named structure	Seen in
• Nitabuch's layer	It is the zone of fibroid degeneration where trophoblast and decidua meet. Seen in basal plate of placenta.
• Hofbauer cells	Phagocytic cell seen in connective tissue of chorionic villi of placenta.
• Folds of Hoboken	Umbilical arteries
• Wharton's jelly	Connective tissue of umbilical cord
• Peg cells	Fallopian tube
• Langhans cells	Cytotrophoblast

N3. **Ans. is a, i.e. Vasa previa** *Ref. Dutta Obs. 9/e, p 36, 206*

Normally, the umbilical cord is inserted at the centre of the fetal surface of the placenta.
In velamentous insertion of cord

> **The blood vessels are attached to the amnion, where they ramify before reaching the placenta. Whenever patient goes into labour and cervix dilates, there are chances of umbilical cord being injured leading to fetal blood loss. This is called as vasa previa.**

N4. **Ans. is d, i.e. All of the above** *Ref: Dutta Obs 9/e, p 25*

• Human placenta is **discoid-disc like** in shape **hemochorial** because of direct contact of chorion with blood maternal **deciduate**, i.e. it is shed at the time of parturition.

N5. **Ans. is a, i.e. Preterm delivery** *Ref. Dutta Obs 9/e, p 205*

> Succenturiate lobe can lead to PPH, sub involution, uterine sepsis and polyp.

 Note: The accessory lobe in succenturiate placenta is developed from the activated villi on the chorionic laeva.

N6. **Ans. is d, i.e. 16th week** *Ref. Dutta Obs 9/e, p 22*

The decidual space (is the space between decidua capsularis and parietalis seen in early pregnancy because the gestational sac does not fill the uterine cavity. By 14–16 weeks gestational sac has enlarged to fill the uterine cavity completely by 4th month (16 weeks).

 Note: These 2 layers become atrophied at term whereas decidua basalis retains its characteristic appearance till term.

N7. **Ans. is c, i.e. 17 weeks** *Ref. Williams Obs 24/e, p 95*

"In the first trimester, placental growth is more rapid than that of the fetus. But by approximately 17 post menstrual weeks, placental and fetal weights are approximately equal" *Ref. Williams 24/e, p 95*

N8. **Ans is a, i.e. All branches from one stem villi** *Ref. Williams 24/e, p 94*

"Each of the truncal or main stem villi and their ramifications constitutes a placental lobule or cotyledon. Each lobule is supplied with a single truncal branch of the chorionic artery. And each lobule has a single vein so that lobules constitute functional units of placental architecture." —*Williams 24/e, p 94*

N9. **Ans is a, i.e. 150 mL** *Ref. Dutta Obs 9/e, p 29, Table 3.1*

A mature placenta has 500 mL blood out of which 150 mL is in the intervillous space and 350 mL in villi system.

N10. **Ans is d, i.e. 750 mL/min** *Ref. Dutta Obs 8/e, p 61*

"Uterine blood flow is increased from 50 mL/min in non pregnant state to about 750 mL near term".
Ref. Dutta Obs 8/e, p 61

N11. **Ans is b, i.e. PGE2** *Internet search*

N12. **Ans is b, i.e. 7.2** *Internet search*

N13. **Ans is b, i.e. Mesoderm**

N14. **Ans. is c, i.e. Pregnancy specific beta 1 glycoprotein** *Internet search*
Schwangershaft Protein:
- It is the other name for pregnancy specific B1 glycoprotein.
- Produced by trophoblast.
- Can be detected 18 days after ovulation.
- Its concentration rises steadily and reaches 200 mg/mL at term.
- Role-measure of placental function for fertility control.

N15. **Ans. is d, i.e. Endocrine regulation**
See the text for explanation

N16. **Ans. is c, i.e. Prolactin** *Ref. Dutta Obs. 7/e, p 58*

hCG (Human chorionic gonadotropic hormone) has alpha and beta subunits. Its alpha subunit is similar to that of LH (leutinizing hormone), FSH (Follicular stimulating hormone) and TSH (Thyroid stimulating hormone) whereas beta subunits is specific. We have also studied that insulin hormone has alpha and beta subunits.

Remember:

Hormones with alpha and beta subunits:
hCG[Q]   LH[Q]
FSH[Q]   TSH[Q]
Insulin[Q]

N17. **Ans. is d, i.e. Chorionic plate undulations**
Placental grading is done as follow:

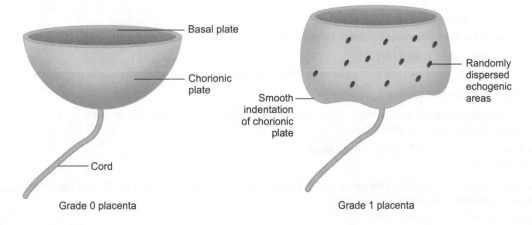

Grade 0 placenta   Grade 1 placenta

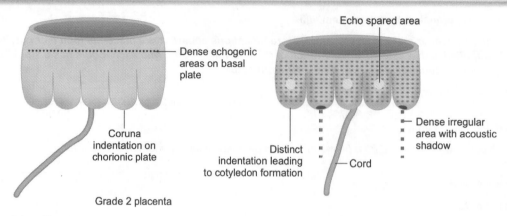

Grade 2 placenta

N18 Ans is d, i.e. 40 mm

Placental thickness increases by 1 mm/week. If placental thickness is more than 40 mm at term, it is called as placentomegaly

N19 Ans. is a, i.e. Fetal ACTH

Read the text for explanation

N20 Ans is c, i.e. Velamentous insertion of cord

The image shows cord is attached to membranes first and then to placenta

N21 Ans is c, i.e. Circumvallate placental

As seen in the image, the fetal side of placenta is smaller than maternal side & maternal side is secondary the fetal side in the maternal form of a ring, separated by a valve like thickening

N22 Ans is b, i.e. 15

See the text for explanation

N23 Ans is c, i.e. 17

Feto placental circulation is established by D17 after fertilisation

Answers with Explanations to Previous Year Questions

1. **Ans. is d, i.e. Corpus luteum**

   In the initial few weeks- the main source of estrogen and progesterone is corpus luteum.

2. **Ans. is a and c, i.e. hCG and HPL**

   Estrogen is not produced exclusively by placenta. For synthesizing estrogen, placenta needs precursors from fetus.

3. **Ans. is a, i.e. Trophoblast cells**   *Ref. Dutta Obs. 9/e, p 53*

   "Syncytiotrophoblasts are the principal site of protein and steroid hormones in pregnancy" *Ref. Dutta Obs. 9/e, p 53*
   hCG is synthesized by syncytiotrophoblast

4. **Ans. is a, i.e. It is secreted by cytotrophoblast**

   See the text for explanation.

5. **Ans. is a, d and e, i.e. α subunit identical to LH, FSH and TSH; Max level seen at 60–70 days of gestation; Detected in serum and urine 8–9 days after ovulation**

   All of us know hCG in detail now:

Let focus on false statements
- **Option b**: Causes involution of corpus luteum–false–rather hCG maintains corpus luteum
- **Option c**: Doubles in 7–10 days–false. Doubling time of hCG = 1.4 to 2 days.

6. **Ans. is a, i.e. Radioimmunoassay**   *Ref. JB Sharma Obs, p 65*

   Order of sensitivity test

FIA > RIA > ELISA = RRA > IRMA

7. **Ans. is b, i.e. Progesterone**   *Ref. Dutta Obs. 9/e, p 170*

   Arias stella reaction
   - Arias stella reaction is characterized by adenomatous change of the endometrial glands.
   - Cells loose their polarity, have hyperchromatic nucleus, vacuolated cytoplasm and occasional mitosis.
   - The reaction is seen in ectopic pregnancy *(in 10–15% cases)* and indicates blightening of conceptus be it intrauterine or extrauterine. (therfore it is not specific for ectopic pregnancy)
   - It occurs under the influence of progesterone.[Q]

   Decidual reaction: *Ref. Williams Obs. 23/e, p 44, 45*
   - Decidua is the specialised highly modified endometrium of pregnancy.
   - Decidual reaction/decidualisation is the conversion of secretory endometrium into decidua and is dependent on estrogen and progesterone.
   - Decidual reaction is completed only with blastocyst implantation.

   So, hormone which is common to both Arias stella reaction and decidual reaction is progesterone which is our answer of choice.

8. **Ans. is a, b and c, i.e. Twin, Down syndrome and Choriocarcinoma**

   See the text for explanation

9. **Ans. is d, i.e. Decidua parietalis**   *Ref. IB Singh, Embryology, p 66, 67*

The maternal blood in the lacuna is never in direct contact with fetal blood. They are separated by:	
• Syncytiotrophoblast • Cytotrophoblast • Basement membrane • Mesoderm • Endothelium of fetal capillaries	Together called as **placental barrier or membrane (0.025 mm)**

10. **Ans. is d, i.e. 500–750 mL/min**   *Ref: Williams 25/e*

    Uterine blood flow in nonpregnant females = 50 mL/min
    Uterine blood flow in pregnant females = 750 mL/min
    Uteroplacental flow at term = 500–750 mL/min
    Fetal volume at term = 125 mL/kg
    Placental volume at term = 500 mL
    Volume of blood in intervillous space = 150 mL
    Fetal blood flow through placenta at term = 400 mL/min

11. **Ans. is c, i.e. An indicator of considerably increased incidence of major malformation of the fetus**
    Ref: Williams Obs 23/e, p 582

 Single Umblical Artery
- It is seen in 0.7–0.8% cases of single pregnancy and 5% of twin pregnancy
- More common in diabetic patients and black patients.
- Finding of a single umbilical artery is not insignificant and is associated with:
  i. Congenital malformations of the fetus in 20–25% cases amongst which cardiovascular and genitourinary anomalies are common.
  ii. Increased chances of abortion, prematurity, IUGR and perinatal mortality.

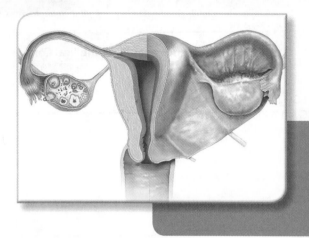

Chapter 3

Amniotic Fluid and its Abnormalities

Chapter at a Glance

AMNIOTIC FLUID

Important Facts

- Specific gravity of Amniotic fluid: 1.008 to 1.010.
- Osmolality: 250 mosm/L.
- It is completely replaced in 3 hours.
- Rate of amniotic fluid turn over is 500 cc/hr.
- Volume of Amniotic fluid maximum is between 32–34 weeks (1 litre) and then decreases such that at term it is roughly 800–900 mL.

Composition of Amniotic Fluid

- Water: 98–99%
- Solids: 1–2%-include, organic solids like proteins, glucose, lipid, urea, uric acid, creatinine and hormones like—Prolactin, insulin and renin
- Inorganic solids are Na, K and Cl

Origin of Amniotic Fluid

Amniotic fluid originates both from maternal and fetal sources:

- **In early pregnancy:** As an ultrafiltrate of maternal plasma.
- **By beginning of the second trimester:** It consists of extracellular fluid which diffuses through the fetal skin.
- **After 20 weeks:** Cornification of skin prevents this diffusion. The main contributors then are of fetal urine and fetal lungs.
- **Major contributor of amniotic fluid is fetal urine.**

Contributor	Approximate contribution daily (in mL)
• Fetal urine	1000
• Fetal lung	350

Fetal amniotic fluid volume production is kept in balance by 2 processes:
- Fetal swallowing = 750 mL/day.
- Intramembranous flow across fetal vessels on the placental surface = 400 mL/day

Colour of Amniotic Fluid

- *Early pregnancy* – Colourless
- *Near term* – Pale straw coloured due to presence of exfoliated lanugo hairs and epidermal cells from the fetal skin.

Abnormal colour of amniotic fluid

- *Green* (meconium stained)—fetal distress/Breech or transverse lie/Listeria infection
- *Golden yellow* - Rh incompatibility (Because bilirubin levels are increased in amniotic fluid in case of Rhincompatibility).
- *Greenish yellow saffron* - postmaturity.
- *Tobacco juice or prune juice on Dark brown* - in case of IUD due to presence of old HbA
- *Dark maroon* - concealed hemorrhage.

Function of Amniotic Fluid

- **Its main function is to protect the fetus.**
- It acts as a shock absorber and protects fetus from trauma
- Maintains temperature
- The fluid distends the amniotic sac and so gives space for growth of the fetus
- *It prevents adhesion formation between fetal parts and amniotic sac.*

 Remember: Amniotic fluid has no role in nutrition.

- The assessment of amniotic fluid is an integral part of antepartum fetal assessment.
- Techniques used for measurement of Amniotic fluid—ultrasonographically:

Amniotic fluid index (AFI) is calculated by dividing the uterus into four quadrants and measuring the largest vertical pocket of liquor in each of the four quadrants. The sum of the four measurements is the AFI in cm. The range of 5–24 cm is considered normal. **AFI less than 5 is considered oligohydramnios and 25 or more is polyhydramnios.**

Single deepest pocket (SDP) is the depth of a single cord free pocket of amniotic fluid. The normal range is 2–8 cm. Over 8 cm is considered polyhydramnios. Less than 2 cm is considered as oligohydramnios.

ABNORMALITIES OF AMNIOTIC FLUID

Oligohydramnios

Oligohydramnios is a condition where liquor amnii is deficient (< 200 mL at term).
Sonographically it is defined as:

- Absence of amniotic fluid pocket.[Q]
- Maximum vertical diameter of amniotic fluid pocket less than 2 cm.[Q]
- Amniotic fluid index less than 5 cm.[Q]

Causes of Oligohydramnios

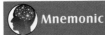 **Mnemonic**

Dil Mein Ppaar (read as pyaar)

D	•	Drug (Prostaglandin Synthetase inhibitors like indomethacin and ACE inhibitors).
I	•	IUGR
L	•	Leaking of fluid following amniocentesis or chorionic villus sampling.

Contd…

Contd…

Mein	•	**M**aternal conditions like hypertension and preeclampsia.
P	•	**P**ost-term pregnancy
P	•	**P**remature rupture of membrane
A	•	**A**bruptiochronic
A	•	**A**mnion Nodosum[Q] and chromosomal **a**nomaly like triploidy
R	•	**R**enal anomalies of fetus (leading to decreased urine production):
		– *Renal agenesis[Q]*
		– Urethral obstruction (posterior urethral valve)
		– Prune-Belly syndrome
		– Bilateral multicystic dysplastic kidneys.

 M/C cause of mild oligohydramnios—Idiopathic
M/C cause of severe oligohydramnios is Gross Congenital anomaly–Renal anomalies.

Complications of Oligohydramnios

1. Fetal complications

A. If oligohydramnios occurs early:

- It leads to fetal anomalies due to less space

  M/C = Pulmonary hypoplasia

  Other = Limb deformities like talipes,

  Potters face = Low set ears, epicanthic fold receding mandible and flattered nose.

- It can lead to IUGR

B. If oligohydramnios occur late in pregnancy-(by this time organogenesis is complete)

- It leads to cord compression and meconium aspiration syndrome.

2. Maternal complications

- Prolonged labor due to inertia
- Increased operative interference due to malpresentation. The sum effect may lead to increased maternal morbidity.

Treatment

- Isolated oligohydramnios in the third trimester with a normal fetus may be managed conservatively.
- Oral administration of water increases amniotic fluid volume.
- Amnioinfusion (prophylactic or therapeutic) for meconium liquor is found to improve neonatal outcome.

Key Concept

Amnioinfusion is the technique to increase the intrauterine fluid volume with normal saline (500 mL).
Indications are: —*Williams Obs. 22/e, p 462, 23/e, p 433*

- Treatment of variable or prolonged deceleration (i.e. fetal distress).
- Prophylaxis for cases of known oligohydramnios as with prolonged rupture of membrane.
- In an attempt to dilute or wash out thick meconium.

Besides the above mentioned therapeutic indications it can be used for diagnosis of:

i. Renal agenesis
ii. PROM (premature rupture of membrane)

 Note:

- Temperature at which saline is infused = 37°C.
- 250 mL of saline is infused in 30 minutes.

Intrauterine resting pressure should not be more than 25 mm of Hg at any time during infusion. —*Fernando Arias 3/e, p 94*

Polyhydramnios

- It is a condition where liquor amnii is in excessive amount, i.e. > 2 litres^Q. But since quantitative assessment of liquor amnii is impractical. Most common used definition is by ultrasound assessment, i.e. when amniotic fluid index (AFI) is $\geq$ 25 cm^Q or finding of a pocket of fluid measuring 8 cm^Q or more in vertical diameter.

Grades of Polyhydramnios^Q

- **Mild** defined as pockets measuring 8–11 cm in vertical dimension (seen in 80% cases).
- **Moderate** defined as pocket measuring 12–15 cm in vertical dimension (seen in 15% cases).
- **Severe** defined as free floating fetus found in pockets of fluid of 16 cm or more (seen in 5% cases).

Causes of Polyhydramnios

All of us know: The main contributor of amniotic fluid is fetal urine

Amount of amniotic fluid will be more (i.e. polyhydramnios) if:

- **Fetus produces more urine for example:**
  a. Twin/multifetal pregnancy (number of fetus is more: more of urine)
  b. Maternal hyperglycemia/diabetes
     Maternal hyperglycemia → Fetal hyperglycemia → Fetal polyuria → increased amniotic fluid.
  c. Twin to Twin transfusion syndrome

- **Besides producing Amniotic fluid fetus also swallows amniotic fluid. The amount of amniotic fluid will increase if; fetal swallowing is impaired as in case of:**
  a. Cleft lip and cleft palate
  b. Esophageal atresia or stenosis
  c. Duodenal atresia or stenosis
  d. Bowel obstruction
  e. Anencephaly (swallowing is decreased + increased transudation of CSF into amniotic fluid due to absence of cranial vault)

- **Other important causes of polyhydramnios which need to mugged up are:**
  1. Placental Causes
  a. Chorangioma of placenta and circumvallate placenta.

  2. Fetal Causes
  a. Hydropsfetalis
  b. Rubella, syphilis, Toxoplasma infection of fetus.
  c. Trisomy (note – Triploidy leads to oligohydramnios)
  d. Sacrococcygeal Teratoma
  e. Thalassemia of fetus.

M/C cause of mild polyhydramnios: Idiopathic
M/C cause of severe polyhydramnios: Gross congenital anomaly, i.e. GIT malformation > CNS malformation

Complications

Maternal

- Due to excessive fluid membranes are overstretched so it can lead to premature rupture of membranes (PROM) and preterm labour.
- Abruptio placenta
- PPH (due to overstretching, tone of uterus decreases)
- Subinvolution of uterus
- PIH (25% cases)
- Cord prolapse
- Malpresentation
- Unstable lie

In Fetus = Due to prematurity and congenital anomalies, there is increased perinatal mortality.

Management

- **Serial amniocentesis** is the TOC^Q if the patient is in distress (*Remember:* Amount of fluid removed is 500 mL/hr, maximum up to 1500–2000 mL).
- **Indomethacin therapy** is alternative management. It acts by decreasing fetal urinary output and by increasing reabsorption of fluid via lungs.
  Dose: 1.5–3 mg/kg/day.

Potential hazard of Indomethacin therapy – Premature closure of fetal ductus arteriosus.

So, the therapy should be stopped at 32 weeks.

New Pattern Questions

N1. Amount of liquor is maximum at:
- a. 32–34 weeks
- b. 36–38 weeks
- c. 34–36 weeks
- d. 38–40 weeks

N2. Golden colour amniotic fluid is seen in:
- a. Rh incompatibility
- b. Fetal death
- c. IUGR
- d. Fetal distress

N3. The major contribution of the amniotic fluid after 20 weeks of gestation:
- a. Ultrafiltrate and maternal plasma
- b. Fetal urine
- c. Fetal lung fluid
- d. Fetal skin

N4. Not a function of amniotic fluid:
- a. Maintain temperature
- b. Reduce trauma to fetus
- c. Provide nutrition in the form of fat and protein
- d. Prevent ascending infection to uterine cavity during labor

N5. Keratinization of fetal skin occurs at:
- a. 16–18 weeks
- b. 18–20 weeks
- c. 24–26 weeks
- d. 30–32 weeks

N6. Percentage of water in liquor amnia:
- a. 42%
- b. 64%
- c. 76%
- d. 99%

Previous Year Questions

1. True about amniotic fluid: **[PGI Nov 2014]**
- a. Same concentration of plasma throughout pregnancy
- b. Forms from transudation of plasma through fetus skin before 20 weeks of gestation
- c. Fetus swallows amniotic fluid
- d. Protects fetus from injury
- e. Main channel for gaseous exchange

2. Amniotic fluid is mainly produced by:
- a. Placenta
- b. Fetus **[AIIMS June 98]**
- c. Chorion
- d. Amnion

3. The pH of amniotic fluid is: **[AIIMS Nov 01]**
- a. 6.8 to 6.9
- b. 7.1 to 7.3
- c. 7.4 to 7.6
- d. 6.7 to 6.8

4. Surfactant appears in amniotic fluid at the gestational age of: **[AIIMS Nov 01]**
- a. 20 weeks
- b. 32 weeks
- c. 36 weeks
- d. 28 weeks

5. The amniotic fluid is in balance by: **[PGI Dec 01]**
- a. Excretion by fetal kidneys
- b. Maternal hemostasis
- c. Fetal intestinal absorption
- d. Fetal membrane absorption
- e. Fetal sweating

6. Oligohydramnios is seen in: **[AIIMS Nov 99]**
- a. Renal agenesis
- b. Oesophageal atresia
- c. Exomphalos
- d. Neural tube defect

7. Oligohydramnios is/are associated with:
[PGI May 2010]
- a. Neural tube defect
- b. Renal agenesis
- c. Postmature birth
- d. Premature birth

8. Renal agenesis is associated with: **[AIIMS Feb 97]**
- a. Hydramnios
- b. Anencephaly
- c. Tracheo-oesophageal fistula
- d. Oligohydramnios

9. Which of the following conditions is associated with polyhydramnios? **[AIIMS May 2010]**
- a. Posterior urethral valve
- b. Cleft palate
- c. Congenital diaphragmatic hernia
- d. Bladder exostrophy

10. A pregnant woman is found to have excessive accumulation of amniotic fluid. Such polyhydramnios is likely to be associated with all of the following conditions *except*: **[AIIMS Nov 03; Nov 07]**
- a. Twinning
- b. Microencephaly
- c. Oesophageal atresia
- d. Bilateral renal agenesis

11. Causes of polyhydraminos include: **[PGI Dec 01]**
- a. Diabetes mellitus
- b. Preeclampsia
- c. Esophageal atresia
- d. Renal agenesis
- e. Anencephaly

12. Causes of hydramnios: **[PGI June 04]**
- a. Anencephaly
- b. Oesophageal atresia
- c. Renal agenesis
- d. Posterior urethral valve
- e. Twins

13. All are associated with hydramnios *except*:
[PGI]
- a. Premature labour
- b. Gestational diabetes
- c. Renal agenesis
- d. Increased amniotic fluid

14. Indication of amnioinfusion is: **[PGI Dec 06]**
- a. Oligohydramnios
- b. Suspected renal anomalies
- c. To facilitate labour
- d. In case of fetal distress

15. A case of 35 week pregnancy with hydramnios and marked respiratory distress is best treated by:
- a. Intravenous frusemide **[AI 04]**
- b. Saline infusion
- c. Amniocentesis
- d. Artificial rupture of membranes

Answers with Explanations to New Pattern Questions

N1. **Ans. is a, 32–34 weeks**

This is a very controversial question. The volume of amniotic fluid varies at different gestation & different books have a different say on it. But most of the books agree at 32–34 weeks.

N2. **Ans is a, Rh incompatibility**

Golden color amniotic fluid is due to bilirubin in amniotic fluid because Rh incompatibility

N3. **Ans. is b, i.e. Fetal urine** *Ref. Williams Obs. 22/e, p 102*

Origin of amniotic fluid:

Gestation	Major contributor of amniotic fluid
Early week	Maternal plasma
2nd trimester	Fetal skin
Beyond 20 weeks	Fetal urine

N4. **Ans is c, i.e. Provide nutrition in the form of fat and protein**

As discussed in the text, amniotic fluid has a number of functions but it has no role in nutrition to the fetus.

N5. **Ans is c, i.e. 24–26 weeks** *(Callen's USG in Obs and Gynae, 5/e, p 758)*

"Fetal keratinization occurs at 24–26 weeks of gestation"

N6. **Ans is d. 99%** *Ref. Dutta Obs 9/e, p 34*

Water in amniotic fluid is 98–99%.

Answers with Explanations to Previous Year Questions

1. **Ans. is b, c and d, i.e. Forms from transudation of plasma through fetus skin before 20 weeks of gestation, Fetus swallows amniotic fluid and Protects fetus from injury**

   See the text for explanantion

2. **Ans. is b, i.e. Fetus** *Ref. Dutta Obs. 7/e, p 37; Williams Obs. 22/e, p 102, 23/e, p 88, 89*

   "The precise origin of the amniotic fluid remains is still not well understood. It is probably of mixed maternal and fetal origin."
   —*Dutta Obs. 9/e, p 34*

   But this cannot help us to solve this question.

   Let's see what *Williams Obs.* has to say on Origin of Amniotic fluid.

   "In early pregnancy, amniotic fluid is an ultrafiltrate of maternal plasma. By the beginning of second trimester, it consists largely of extracellular fluid which diffuses through the fetal skin, and thus reflects the composition of fetal plasma".

   After 20 weeks, however, the cornification of fetal skin prevents this diffusion and amniotic fluid is composed largely of fetal urine."
   —*Williams Obs. 23/e, p 88, 89*

   Reading the above text, it can be concluded that in early pregnancy - Mother is the main contributor whereas during rest of the pregnancy - Fetus is the main contributor.

3. **Ans. is b, i.e. 7.1 to 7.3** *Ref. COGDT 10/e, p 184*

"Amniotic fluid has a low specific gravity (1.008) and a pH of 7.2." *—COGDT 10/e, p 184*

"Amniotic fluid usually has a pH of 7.0 to 7.5." *—Fernando Arias 3/e, p 245*

Amongst the given options—7.1 to 7.3 seems to be the most appropriate option.

4. **Ans. is d, i.e. 28 weeks**

Friends, I had to search a lot for this answer but all in vain.
By concensus the following facts on surfactant need to be remembered.
Surfactant synthesis begins at 20 weeks.
Surfactant appear in amniotic fluid by 28 weeks.

5. **Ans. is a, b, c, d and e, i.e. Excretion by fetal kidneys; Maternal hemostasis; Fetal intestinal absorption; Fetal membrane absorption and Fetal sweating**

Ref. Dutta Obs. 9/e, p 34, 38; Williams Obs. 22/e, p 102; 23/e, p 88, 89; COGDT 10/e, p 184

Read the text for explanation.

6. **Ans. is a, i.e. Renal agenesis**

7. **Ans. is b and c, i.e. Renal agenesis and Postmature birth**

Ref. Dutta Obs. 9/e, p 203; Fernando Arias 2/e, p 321, 322; Williams Obs. 22/e, p 530, 532, 23/e, p 495

Causes of oligohydramnios:

> **Mnemonic**
>
> **Dil Mein Ppaar (read as pyaar)**
>
> | | | |
> |---|---|---|
> | **Dil** | • | **D**rug (Prostaglandin synthetase inhibitors and ACE inhibitors). |
> | | | **I**UGR |
> | | | **L**eaking of fluid following amniocentesis or chorionic villus sampling. |
> | **Mein** | • | **M**aternal conditions like hypertension and preeclampsia. |
> | **Ppaar** | • | **P**ostterm pregnancy |
> | | • | **P**remature rupture of membrane |
> | | • | **A**bruptio-chronic |
> | | • | **A**mnion Nodosum.[Q] and chromosomal **a**nomaly like triploidy |
> | | • | **R**enal anomalies of fetus(leading to decreased urine production): |
>
> - *Renal agenesis*[Q]
> - Urethral obstruction (Posterior urethral valve)
> - Prune-Belly syndrome
> - Bilateral multicystic dysplastic kidneys.

Note: Most common complication of oligohydramnios is *Pulmonary hypoplasia*[Q].

8. **Ans. is d, i.e. Oligohydramnios** *Ref. Dutta Obs. 7/e, p 215*

Fetal urine is the main contributor of Amniotic fluid beyond 20 weeks therefore. In case of Renal agenesis → decreased urine or/no urine → oligohydramnios.

9. **Ans. is b, i.e. Cleft palate**

10. **Ans. is d, i.e. Bilateral renal agenesis** *Ref. Dutta Obs. 7/e, p 215; Fernando Arias 2/e, p 3201; Williams Obs 23/e, p 495, 496, Ultrasound in Obs and Gynee by Merz 2004, 11/e, p 411*

Discussed in detail in preceding text.

11. **Ans. is a, c and e, i.e. Diabetes mellitus; Esophageal atresia; and Anencephaly** *Ref. Dutta Obs. 9/e, p 203, 212*

Friends, for a second - let's forget the lists of conditions leading to Oligohydramnios/Polyhydramnios (This happens quite often in exams).
Let's reason out each option one by one.

Option "a" Diabetes mellitus

We all know polyhydramnios is a complication of maternal diabetes.

Pathophysiology:

Maternal hyperglycemia
↓
Fetal hyperglycemia
↓
Polyuria (of fetus) and osmotic diuresis
↓
Polyhydramnios (*Option "a"* is correct)

Option "b" Preeclampsia

Preeclampsia (↑ BP)
↓
Decreased uteroplacental circulation (as Pressure and volume are inversely related)
↓
Decreased fetal renal blood flow
↓
Decrease urine production by fetus (↓ GFR)
↓
Oligohydramnios

Option "c" Esophageal atresia

We all know - Amniotic fluid is kept in balance with the rate of production, by fetal swallowing of amniotic fluid.

In case of esophageal atresia
↓
Decrease fetal swallowing
↓
i.e., Decrease absorption
↓
Polyhydramnios (*option "c"* is correct)

Same is the case with congenital diaphragmatic hernia/Facial clefts/Neck masses.

Option "d" Renal agenesis

Renal agenesis
↓
Decrease urine production
↓
Oligohydramnios (*Option "d"* is incorrect)

Same holds good for posterior urethral value in males.[Q]

Option "e" Anencephaly

In anencephaly (or meningomyelocele or spina bifida)
↓
Meninges are exposed
↓
Increase transudation of fluid from exposed meninges
↓
Polyhydramnios (*Option "e"* is correct)

So friends, it is not essential to mug up most of the causes of oligo/polyhydramnios.

Most of the causes can be understood logically except for a few which you need to mug up. You cannot in these cases reason out whether there will be oligohydraminos or polyhydramnios.

Some causes which need to mugged up are:

	Polyhydramnios	Oligohydramnios
Placental causes	• Placental chorioangioma[Q] • Circumvallate placenta[Q]	• Amnion Nodosum[Q]
Chromosomal anomalies	• Trisomy 13, 18 and 21 Down syndrome	• Triploidy
Fetal tumors	• Sacrococcygeal tumors	
Hematological disorders	• Rh isoimmunization • Alpha thalassemia	
Intrauterine infections	• Rubella • Syphilis and Toxoplasma	

12. **Ans. is a, b and e, i.e. Anencephaly; Oesophageal atresia; and Twins**   *Ref. Dutta Obs. 9/e, p 200*

13. **Ans. is c, i.e. Renal agenesis**   *Ref. Dutta Obs. 9/e, p 200*
    Already explained

14. **Ans. is a, b and d, i.e. Oligohydramnios; Suspected renal anomalies; In case of fetal distress**
    Ref. Dutta Obs. 7/e, p 614; Fernando Arias 3/e, p 94; Williams Obs. 22/e, p 462, 23/e, p 432 433

Amnioinfusion is the technique to increase the intrauterine fluid volume with normal saline (500 mL).

Indications are: *—Williams Obs. 22/e, p 462, 23/e, p 433*
- Treatment of variable or prolonged deceleration (i.e. fetal distress).
- Prophylaxis for cases of known oligohydramnios as with prolonged rupture of membrane.
- In an attempt to dilute or wash out thick meconium.

Besides the above mentioned therapeutic indications it can be used for diagnosis of:
   i.   Renal agenesis
   ii. PROM (Premature rupture of membrane)   *—Fernando Arias 3/e, p 94*

"Amnioinfusion in patients with oligohydramnios is not a simple procedure. The needle should be advanced slowly with continuous ultrasound visualization and when its tip has reached the interface between the fetus and the membranes warmed saline solution should be infused.

In majority of cases, 250–350 mL of saline solution will be necessary to achieve optimal ultrasound transmission and perform a careful level II examination. A normal fetus will swallow the infused fluid, and its bladder will be easily seen with ultrasound after 20 minutes. The bladder will not be seen in fetuses with renal agenesis.

Before ending the amnioinfusion, 1 mL of indigo carmine is injected inside the amniotic sac. The patient is instructed to wear a tampon for a few hours following the procedure and observe for evidence of blue discoloration. This finding will confirm the presence of PROM."   *—Fernando Arias 3/e, p 94*

Note:
- Temperature at which saline is infused = 37°C.
- 250 ml of saline is infused in 30 minutes.
- Intrauterine resting pressure should not be more than 25 mm of Hg at any time during infusion.

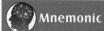

Mnemonic

Remember: Mnemonic for aminoinfusion:

P- Premature rupture of membranes
R- Renal agenesis (diagnostic purpose)
O- Oligohydramnios
M- to dilute or wash meconium in case of fetal distress

15. Ans. is c, i.e. Amniocentesis   *Ref. Dutta Obs. 9/e, p 203; Williams Obs. 22/e, p 529, 530, 23/e, p 494, 495*

The patient in the question has marked respiratory distress (i.e. it is a severe polyhydramnios and requires treatment) and gestational age is 35 weeks (i.e., fetal maturity is not yet achieved).
So our aim should be to relieve the distress of patient in hope of continuing the pregnancy till atleast 37 weeks.

This can be achieved by:
• Amniocentesis or
• Use of Indomethacin—but because gestational age is 35 weeks we should not use Indomethacin as it can lead to premature closure of ductus arteriosus.

4

Fetal Physiology

Chapter at a Glance

➢ Landmarks in Fetal Development
➢ Fetal Growth Period
➢ Haase's Rule

➢ Fetal Hemopoiesis
➢ Fetal Circulation

LANDMARKS IN FETAL DEVELOPMENT

Event	Time of occurrence
• Genital ridge is formed	5 weeks
• Gonads develop by:	
Testis	7 weeks
Ovary	8 weeks
• Internal genitalia develop by	10 weeks
• External genitalia	12 weeks
• Sex can be identified on USG by	14 weeks
• Gross body movement	8 weeks
• Fetal breathing movements	11 weeks
• Swallowing begins by	10–12 weeks
• Urine production begins by	12 weeks
• Meconium passage	16 weeks
• Snoring movements	24 weeks
• Fetus can hear by	24 weeks
• Light perception is by Endocrine	28 weeks
• Fetal Fibrinogen production	5 weeks
• ACTH synthesis	7 weeks
• Glucagon synthesis	8 weeks
• Post pituitary hormones synthesis	10–12 weeks
• Thyroxine synthesis	11 weeks
• Insulin synthesis and all clotting factors produced by	12 weeks
• Growth hormone and LH[Q]	13 weeks
• Rest all pituitary hormones	17 weeks

FETAL GROWTH PERIOD

There are 3 phases in the prenatal fetal development.

Period	Timing	Comment
Ovular period	From the day of fertilization to 2 weeks after that (i.e. 4 weeks of gestational age)	
Embryonic period	From 3rd week to 8th week after fertilization (i.e. 5–10 week of gestational age)	• This is the period of organogenesis • **It is the most[Q] teratogenic period** • Average Crown Rump length at this time = 4 mm
Fetal period	Beginning from 9th week after fertilization (i.e. 11 weeks of gestation age) till the end of pregnancy	

Concept: Pregnancy or period of gestation is calculated from the first day of last menstrual period.

Day 1	Day 14	Day 28
1st day of last menstrual period	Ovulation and fertilization 4 weeks	Missed period

↳ Pregnancy is calculated from here

This means when a female misses her period, her gestational age is 4 weeks.

Now all events related to pregnancy are calculated from the first day of last menstrual period and never from the day of fertilization.

Only in case of fetal growth period, it is calculated from the day of fertilization.

HAASE'S RULE

Upto 5th month: Fetal length is square of lunar months in centimeters.

From the 6th month: Fetal length is 5 times the number of month.

Weight of fetus: can be calculated:
• Clinically = by using **Johnson formula** • On Ultrasound = by using **Shephard formula** and **Hadlock formula**.

 Note: On USG: Only one parameter tells about fetal growth i.e. Abdominal circumference of fetus (AC)

$$\frac{\text{Femur length (FL)}}{\text{Abdominal circumference (AC)}} = 20–40\%$$

• If FL/AC ratio is increased: It indicates IUGR
• If FL/AC ratio is decreased: It indicates skeletal dysplasia (< 18%)

FETAL HEMOPOIESIS

Site	Time	Main hemoglobin
Yolk sac	1st site	Gower 1, Gower 2, Portland
Liver	6 weeks onwards	HbF ($\alpha_2\gamma_2$)
Bone marrow	24th week	HbA ($\alpha_2\beta_2$)

Fetal RBCs are bigger in size and have a shorter life span (90 days) as compared to adult RBC.[Q]

At birth:
Total Hb = 16–18 g/dl Fetal Hb = 70–80% Adult Hb (HbA) = 20% HbA$_2$ = 5–10% **Note:** 6–12 months after birth, HbF is 1–2% This change is mediated by glucocorticoids and is irreversible.

Differences between HbF and HbA

HbF	HbA
• Has higher affinity for oxygen due to less binding of 2, 3 diphoshoglycerate	• Has less afinity for oxygen due to higher binding of 2, 3 diphosphoglycerate
• Resistant to acid and alkali	• Sensitive to acid and alkali
• Less carbonic anhydrase enzyme	• More carbonic anhydrase enzyme

Clinical Correlation

Fetal hemoglobin (HbF) is resistant to acid and alkali forms the basis of two very important tests—**Singers Alkali**

Denaturation test (also called as **Apt-Downey test** or simply **Apt test**) and **Kleihauer-Betke test**.

In Singers Alkali denaturation test, reagent used is NaOH or KOH and is used for differentiating maternal blood from fetal blood:

i.   In case of vasa previa to differentiate it from placenta previa

ii. In newborns' having bloody vomitting, bloody stool or active bleeding from nasogastric tube to differentiate whether blood is of neonate origin or he/she has swallowed maternal blood during delivery.

In Kleihauer-Betke test, reagent is citric acid phosphate buffer. This test is used to quantitate the number of fetal cells present in maternal circulation in Rh-negative females. Once the amount of fetomaternal hemorrhage is determined, dose of Anti D can be calculated appropriately.

 Important One Liners

• **Qualitative test:** Singers Alkali Denaturation test (Apt test)
• **Quantitative test:** Kleihauer-Betke test
• **Test which differentiates fetal blood from maternal blood:** Singers Alkali Denaturation test
• **Test which differentiates fetal RBC from maternal RBC:** Kleihauer-Betke test.

FETAL CIRCULATION

• The embryo develops separate fetal circulation from 17th day after fertilization and fetus heart starts beating from 21st day of fertilization.
• Fetal cardiovascular system is of mesodermal origin.

Details of Fetal Circulation (Fig. 4.1)

The circulation in the fetus is essentially the same as in the adult except for the following:

• *The source of oxygenated blood is not the lung but the placenta.*[Q]
• Oxygenated blood from the **placenta** comes to the fetus through the umbilical vein[Q], which joins the left *branch of the portal vein*. A small portion of this blood passes through the substance of the liver to the *inferior vena cava*[Q], but the greater part passes directly to the inferior vena cava through the *ductus venosus*[Q]. A sphincter mechanism in the ductus venosus controls blood flow.
• *The inferior vena cava* carries the oxygen rich blood from the **liver to the right atrium**[Q].
• The oxygen rich blood reaching the **right atrium** through the inferior vena cava is directed by the valve of the inferior vena cava towards the foramen ovale. Here it is

divided into two portions by the lower edge of the septum secundum (crista dividens):

– Most of it passes through the *foramen ovale* into the **left atrium**.

– The rest of it gets mixed up with the blood returning to the right atrium through the *superior vena cava,* and passes into the **right ventricle.**

- From the right ventricle, the blood (mostly deoxygenated) enters the *pulmonary trunk.* Only a small portion of this blood reaches the **lungs** and passes through it to the **left atrium.** The greater part is short – circuited by the *ductus arteriosus into the aorta.*

- We have seen that the **left atrium receives:**

– Oxygenated blood from the *right atrium,* and

– A small amount of deoxygenated blood from the *lungs.*

The blood in this chamber is, therefore, fairly rich in oxygen. This blood passes into the left ventricle and then into the aorta. Some of this oxygen rich blood passes into the carotid and subclavian arteries to supply the brain, the head and neck and the upper extremities. The rest of it gets mixed up with poorly oxygenated blood from the ductus arteriosus. The parts of the body that are supplied by branches of the aorta arising distal to its junction with the ductus arteriosus, therefore, receive blood with only a moderate oxygen content.

- Much of the blood of the aorta is carried by the *umbilical arteries* to the **placenta** where it is again oxygenated[Q] and returned to the **heart**.

Changes in the Circulation at Birth

Soon after birth, several changes take place in the fetal blood vessels which lead to establishment of the adult type of circulation. The changes are as follows:

- The muscle in the wall of the *umbilical arteries contracts* immediately after birth, and occludes their lumen. This prevents loss of fetal blood into the placenta.

- The *lumen of the umbilical veins* and the ductus venosus is also occluded, but this takes place a few minutes after birth, so that all fetal blood that is in the placenta has time to drain back to the fetus.

- The ductus arteriosus is occluded, so that all blood from the right ventricle now goes to the lungs, where it is oxygenated.

- The pulmonary vessels increase in size and, consequently, a much larger volume of blood reaches the left atrium from the lungs. As a result, the pressure inside the left atrium is greatly increased. Simultaneously, the pressure in the right atrium is diminished because blood from the placenta no longer reaches it. The net result of these

pressure changes is that pressure in the left atrium now exceeds that in the right atrium causing the valve of the foramen ovale to close.

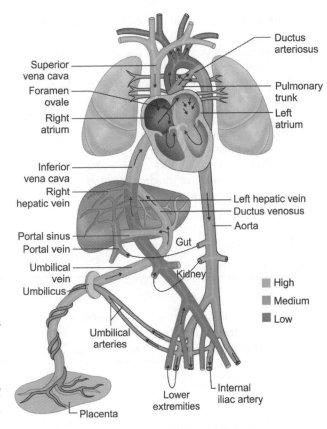

Fig. 4.1: Fetal circulation. (FO: Foramen ovale)

- The vessels that are occluded soon after birth are replaced by fibrous tissue and form the following ligaments:

Vessel	Remnant
a. Umbilical **Arteries**	**Medial Umbilical Ligaments**[Q]
b. Left umbilical vein	Ligamentum teres of the liver[Q]
c. Ductus venosus	Ligamentum venosum[Q]
d. Ductus arteriosus	Ligamentum arteriosum[Q]

 Mnemonic

- **Friends this table is easy to memorise, if you remember the mnemonic**
- **AMUL**-**A**rtery forms **M**edial **U**mblilical **L**igament

 Note: **Median umbilical ligament is a** remnant of urachus

- **Lateral umbilical ligament is a** remnant of inferior epigastric arteries.

New Pattern Questions

N1. The following are related to fetal erythropoiesis *except*:
a. In the embryonic phase, the erythropoiesis is first demonstrated in the primitive mesoderm
b. By 10th week, the liver becomes the major site
c. Near term, the bone marrow becomes the major site
d. At terms 75–80% of hemoglobin is fetal type (HbF)

N2. All are true regarding HbF *except*:
a. Higher affinity for oxygen
b. Binds less to 2, 3, DPG
c. More carbonic anhydrase
d. Resistant to acid

N3. Fetal sex can be detected by USG at:
a. 14 weeks
b. 16 weeks
c. 18 weeks
d. 20 weeks

N4. The percentage of HbF at birth is:
a. 20%
b. 50%
c. 70%
d. 90%

N5. Median umbilical ligament is a remnant of:
a. Umbilical artery
b. Umbilical vein
c. Gubernaculum
d. Urachus

N6. Urine production by fetus at term is:
a. 650 mL/hour
b. 65 mL/hour
c. 27 mL/hour
d. 50 mL/hour

N7. 1st stimulant for production of testosterone from fetal testis is:
a. LH
b. FSH
c. hCG
d. Steroids

N8. Insulin and Glucagon can be identified in fetal pancreas by:
a. Both at 11 weeks
b. Insulin at 12 weeks, glucagon at 8 weeks
c. Insulin at 9–10 weeks, glucagon at 8 weeks
d. Insulin at 12 weeks, glucagon at 14 weeks

N9. Hormone responsible for fetal growth:
a. Growth hormone
b. Insulin
c. Parathyroid hormone
d. Thyroxine

N10. What is the main product of fetal adrenal gland?
a. Cortisol
b. DHEA-S
c. Testosterone
d. Progesterone

Previous Year Questions

1. Fetal kidneys start producing urine by:
a. 3 months
b. 4 months
c. 5 months
d. 6 months

2. Fetal stage starts at: [JIPMER 04]
a. 9 weeks
b. 3 weeks
c. 6 weeks
d. 12 weeks

3. Lifespan of the fetal RBC approximates:
a. 60 days
b. 80 days
c. 100 days
d. 120 days

4. Which test differentiates maternal and fetal blood cell? [AIIMS May 2013]
a. APT test
b. Kleihauer-Betke test
c. Bubble test
d. Lilly's test

5. Ligamentum teres is formed after: [COMED 06]
a. Obliteration of the umbilical vein
b. Obliteration of the ductus venous
c. Obliteration of the ductus arteriosus
d. Obliteration of the hypogastric artery

Answers with Explanations to New Pattern Questions

N1. Ans. is a, i.e. In the embryonic phase, the erythropoiesis is first demonstrated on the primitive mesoderm
For details see the text.

N2. Ans. is c, i.e. More carbonic anhydrase
See the text for explanation.

N3. Ans. is a, i.e. 14 weeks *Ref. William's 23/e, p 79*

> *"Gender can be determined by experienced observers by inspection of the external genitalia by 14 weeks".*
> *Ref. Williams Obs 23/e, p 79*

N4. Ans. is c, i.e. 70% *Ref. Nelson*
During Intrauterine life HbF = 90%
At birth HbF = 70%
At 6 months after birth HbF = 1–2%
In Adults (HbF) is in traces.

N5. Ans. is d, i.e. Urachus

> **Median** umbilical ligament is a remnant of urachus
> **Medial** umbilical ligament is a remnant of umbilical arteries.

N6. Ans. is c, i.e. 27 mL/hour
See the text for explanation.

N7. Ans. is c, i.e. hCG *Ref. William's 24/e, p 148*
The initial/First stimulus for fetal testis to secrete testosterone is hCG and later it is fetal pituitary LH.

N8. Ans. is c, i.e. Insulin at 9–10 weeks and glucagon at 8 weeks *Ref. William's 24/e, p 141*

 Remember:

- Insulin containing granules can be identified is fetal pancreas by 9–10 weeks but insulin secretion (i.e. insulin can be identified in fetal plasma) by 12 weeks
- Glucagon can be identified in fetal pancreas by 8 weeks but is secreted only after birth.

N9. Ans. is b, i.e. Insulin
Hormone responsible for fetal growth is Insulin or Insulin like growth factors.

N10. Ans. is b, i.e. DHEA-S
Main product of fetal adrenal gland is DHEA-S which it synthesises using cholesterol.
The fetal DHEA-S is then used by placenta to synthesize estrogen (E_3 and E_2)

 Extra Edge

- At term, fetal adrenal glands weigh the same as those of adults.
- More than 80% of fetal gland is composed of unique fetal zone which has a great capacity for steroid synthesis.
- Daily steroid production of fetal adrenal gland is 100–200 mg/day as compared to adults 30–40 mg/day.
- Fetal zone is lost in the first year of life and is not present in adults.
- In anencephaly, fetal adrenal gland is absent or hypoplastic.

Answers with Explanations to Previous Year Questions

1. **Ans. is a, i.e. 3 months**   *Ref. Williams Obs. 24/e, p 142*

   Fetal kidneys start producing urine at 12 weeks = 3 months.
   Initial rate of production of urine = 7–14 ml/day.
   At term it is = 27 ml/hr or 650 ml/day.

2. **Ans. is a, i.e. 9 weeks**

   Fetal age starts at 9 weeks after fertilisation or 11 weeks of gestation or 11 weeks of pregnancy.

3. **Ans. is b, i.e. 80 days**   *Ref. Dutta Obs 9/e, p 38*

   The life span of the fetal RBC is about two-thirds of the adult RBC, i.e. about 90 days. The activities of all glycolytic enzymes in fetal erythrocytes except phosphofructokinase and 6-phosphogluconate dehydrogenase are higher than those of adults or term or premature infants.

4. **Ans. is b, i.e. Kleihauer-Betke test**

   Fetal blood cells can be differentiated from maternal blood cells using Kleihauer-Betke test
   Fetal blood can be differentiated from maternal blood using Singers Alkali Denaturation test (Apt test)

5. **Ans. is a, i.e. Obliteration of the umbilical vein**

Vessel	Remnant
Umbilical artery	Medial umbilical ligament
Left umbilical vein	Ligamentum teres of the liver

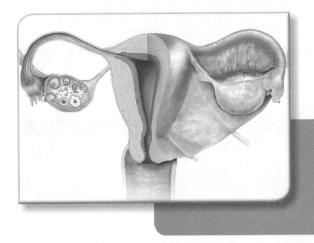

Chapter 5

Maternal Adaptations in Pregnancy

Chapter at a Glance

➢ Maternal Adaptation in Pregnancy
➢ General Considerations
➢ Systemic Changes in Pregnancy
  • Changes in Hematological System
  • Changes in Cardiovascular System
  • Changes in Respiratory System
  • Changes in Renal System
  • Changes in Endocrinological System

➢ Some other Changes in Pregnancy
➢ Diagnosis of Pregnancy
➢ Signs of Pregnancy
➢ Antenatal Care
➢ Vaccination during Pregnancy

MATERNAL ADAPTATIONS IN PREGNANCY

GENERAL CONSIDERATIONS

• BMR increases by 10–20% during pregnancy.
• Total amount of water retained during pregnancy is 6.5 litres
• There is Na⁺ and K⁺ retention during pregnancy but values of serum K⁺ and serum Na⁺ are less as water retained is more during pregnancy.
• Osmolality decreases during pregnancy as there is water retention during pregnancy.
• Extra caloric requirement during pregnancy = 350 kcal/day

Weight Gained during Pregnancy

• Total weight gained during pregnancy = 11–12 kg
• Net weight gained during pregnancy = 6 kg

Table 5.1: BMI and recommended weight gain

BMI	Recommended weight gain
Underweight BMI = < 18.5 kg/m²	12.5–18 kg
Normal weight (BMI 18.5–24.9 kg/m²)	11.5–14 kg
Overweight (BMI ≥ 25)	7–11.5 kg
Obese (BMI ≥ 30 kg/m²)	< 7 kg

Factors which Affect Maternal Weight Gain during Pregnancy

a. *Prepregnancy weight:* If the prepregnancy weight is more than normal (obese), there is a tendency to gain excessive weight during pregnancy.

b. *Race and ethnicity:* American women tend to put on more weight during pregnancy as compared to Asians and Africans.

c. *Socioeconomic status:* Women from higher socio-economic group have more weight gain as compared to women from lower socio economic group. This is because malnutrition prevents optimum weight gain.

d. *Associated conditions* like women with gestational/over diabetes mellitus, twins and polyhydramnios have higher weight gain during pregnancy

e. *Parity:* Multigravida females tend to gain less weigh than primigravida.

 Remember: Smoking does not affect maternal weight gain during pregnancy. Smoking affects fetal weight gain and is one of the causes of IUGR.

SYSTEMIC CHANGES IN PREGNANCY
Hematological System

Parameters which increase in pregnancy	Parameters which decrease in pregnancy
• Blood volume – (40%) starts to increase at 10 weeks • Average increase in blood volume is 30–60% • In twin pregnancy 40–80% • Maximum increase seen at 34 weeks. In PIH increase is less • Plasma volume – (40–50%) →Leads to	• ↓ in hematocrit • ↓ in Packed Cell Volume • ↓ in viscosity of blood
• Red blood cell volume – (20–30% starts at 8 weeks) Since the increase in RBC volume is less in comparison to plasma volume → there is hemodilution during pregnancy.	
• Hb mass (in gms) (as RBC volume increases) • O_2 carrying capacity of blood	• Hb conc (i.e. g/dl) as increase in plasma volume is more
• WBC count (Neutrophilic leucocytosis) may increase uptil 15000 cells. At delivery 25000 cells • Humoral Immunity $$TH_2 \Rightarrow IL – 4, IL–6 \uparrow \Rightarrow$$ This is the reason why SLE flares up during pregnancy. *Note:* Thus in normal pregnancy there is a shift from TH1 to TH–2. This shift is not seen in pregnant females who develop PIH in pregnancy.	• **Platelet count** (Benign gestational) thrombocytopenia • Cell mediated immunity TH 1 decreases $$\Downarrow$$ IL–2 and TNf–β decreases $$\Downarrow$$ This is the reason why rheumatoid arthritis, Hashimotto Thyroiditis, Sarcoidosis are suppressed during pregnancy

• Plasma protein mass (gm)
• Serum globulin (G) conc (Sex hormone binding globulin, Thyroxine building globulin)
 	
   • Normally = A: G = 1.7:1
   • In pregnancy: A: G = 1:1
	• Plasma protein concentration
	• Serum albumin (A)
	• Clotting factor 11, 13
	• Fibrinolytic activity
	
	Note: Plasminogen $\xrightarrow[\text{Converted to}]{\text{Help of: TPA}}$ Plasmin
	
	TPA: Tissue plasminogen activator
	• There is a TPA–I– Tissue plasminogen activator inhibitor which inhibits it
	• During pregnancy TPA–I increases, so TPA decreases and thus Fibrinolytic activity decreases
	• Anticoagulant activity
	• Protein C
	• Protein S

• All clotting factors: hence pregnancy is a hypercoagulable state
• Serum fibrinogen clotting factor 1.
• All markers of inflammation increase:
  – ESR
  – C reactive protein
  – C_3, C4, Leukocyte alkaline phosphatase	

Remember: Clotting time and bleeding time and Anti Thrombin levels remain unaffected in pregnancy.

Cardiovascular System

Parameters which increase in pregnancy	Parameters which decrease in pregnancy
• Cardiac output = Stroke volume x HR (↑ by 20%) All these cardiac output, stroke volume and heart rate increase in pregnancy.	• Peripheral vascular resistances (as progesterone has a smooth muscle relaxant effect)
• **Remember:** Cardiac output increase by 40% during pregnancy, 50% during each uterine contraction in labor and 80% immediately postpartum	• Pulmonary vascular resistance.

Contd...

Contd...

Parameters which increase in pregnancy	Parameters which decrease in pregnancy
∴ Maximum risk of cardiac failure in pregnancy → is in immediate postpartum period[Q] > second stage > Late first stage > 28–32 weeks of pregnancy[Q].	• Arteriovenous O_2 gradient (venous blood causes more O_2)
The increases in cardiac output begins at 5 weeks of pregnancy	• Blood pressure decreases • Systolic BP • Diastolic BP • Arterial Pressure
During pregnancy, Gravid uterus presses on inferior Vena cava so there is pooling of blood in lower limb. Hence femoral venous pressure increases in pregnancy from 8 mm of Hg to 20 mm of Hg. Hence in pregnancy their is: • Pedal edema • Haemorrhoids • Varicose vein	Maximum decrease in BP is seen in: • Second Trimester • In Diastolic BP • In supine position
• BMR increases (10–20%) • O_2 Consumption increases	• A–V oxygen gradient decreases

Parameters which are unaffected:
1. JVP or central venous pressure
2. Pulmonary capillary wedge pressure

Cardiac Output

- Cardiac output begins to increase in early pregnancy (5 weeks) reaching a peak of 40–50% at 28–32 weeks.
- **Maximum cardiac output during pregnancy is seen @ 28–32 weeks and then it decreases at term.[Q]**
- Overall maximum cardiac output is seen immediately after delivery > 2nd stage of labor > late 1st stage of labor > 28–32 weeks > early 1st stage of labor (*See* Fig. 5.1).
- Cardiac output is maximum in left lateral or right or knee chest position and least in supine position
- Cardiac output returns to normal 2 weeks after delivery.

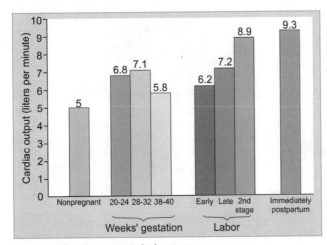

Fig. 5.1: Cardiac output during pregnancy

Clinical Findings Related to Cardiovascular Changes Occurring during Pregnancy

- *Heart rate (resting) increases by about 10–15 bpm.[Q]*
- *Apex beat shifts to the 4th intercoastal space, 2.5 cm outside the midclavicular line (as heart is pushed upwards, outward, with slight rotation to left).[Q]*
- Slightly enlarged cardiac silhouette.[Q] due to displacement 7 heart (5.4) (marked enlarged cardiac silhouette is not normal in pregnancy)
- Exaggerated splitting of the first heart sound (both components loud).[Q]
- Second heart sound: Normal[Q]
- Third heart sound: Loud and easily auscultated.[Q]
- *Murmurs:*
  - *In 80% cases Grade II systolic ejection murmur is audible in aortic or pulmonary area at about 10–12 weeks due to expanded intravenous volume. It disappears in the beginning of postpartum period.*
  - In 20% cases a soft diastolic murmur is transiently noted and a continuous murmur called as **Mammary murmur** arising from breast is heard in 10% cases.
- ECHO
  - Shows increased left atrial and ventricular diameters.[Q]
- *ECG*
  - *Shows left axis deviation.[Q]* (in 15% cases)
- Some women may have deep Q waves and low voltage complexes in ECG
- Chest X-ray - Straightening of left heart border.

 Note: None of the arrhythmias are normal during pregnancy, rather their presence indicates heart disease during pregnancy.

Plasma Proteins

Increase	Decrease
Total proteins (measured in g) (+ 20 to 30%) Globulin (+5%)	Plasma proteins concentration (measured in gm%) (−10%) Albumin (−30%) [Albumin/globulin ratio in-pregnancy − 1:1] In nonpregnant females− 1.7:1

Respiratory System

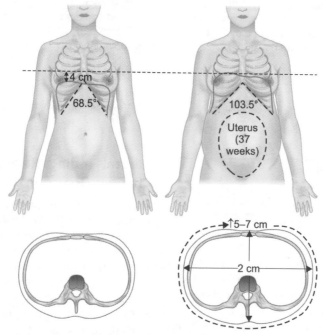

Fig. 5.2: Chest wall measurements in nonpregnant (left) and pregnant women (right). The subcostal angle increases, as does the anteroposterior and transverse diameters of the chest wall and chest wall circumference. These changes compensate for the 4-cm elevation of the diaphragm so that total lung capacity is not significantly reduced.

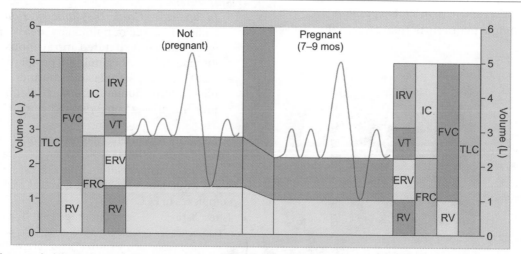

Fig. 5.3: Changes in lung volumes with pregnancy. The most significant changes are reduction in functional residual capacity (FRC) and its subcomponents, expiratory reserve volume (ERV) and residual volume (RV), as well as increases in inspiratory capacity (IC) and tidal volume (VT).

Changes in Respiratory System during Pregnancy

- The diaphragm is pushed up by 4 cm during pregnancy
- The subcostal angle increases from 68° to 103°
- The transverse diameter of the thoracic cage lengthens approximately by 2 cms
- The thoracic circumference increases by 6 cms

Implications

- As diaphragm is pushed up: Residual volume decreases and Expiratory Reserve volume decreases (significant reduction are observed by sixth months)
- As Transverse diameter of chest increases So, Tidal volume and minute ventilation increase.

Functional residual capacity (FRC)	Expiratory reserve volume	TV = ↑ IRV = Remains discharged ⎤ IC ↑
	Tidal volume	
Inspiratory Capacity (IC)	Inspiratory Reserve volume	Now In pregnancy: RV = ↓
	Residual volume	ERV = ↓ ⎤ FRC ↓

Total lung capacity is addition of IC and FRC, so it remains normal or is slightly decreased in pregnancy

Parameters which remain unchanged during pregnancy
1. Respiratory rate
2. Inspiratory reserve volume
3. Maximum breathing capacity
4. Vital capacity

- There is respiratory alkalosis during pregnancy.
- To compensate for this plasma bicarbonate levels drop from 26 to 22 mmol/L
- Their is a slight increase in blood pH & oxygen dissociation curve shift to left.

Renal System

Anatomical changes in renal system during pregnancy

- Kidney size enlarges by 1–1.5 cms during pregnancy
- There is renal pelvis-calyceal dilatation. This is more (15 mm) on right side and 5 mm on left side.
- The ureters become atonic and dilated due to mechanical compression by gravid uterus and due to smooth muscle relaxing effect of progesterone.
- This can lead to hydroureter and hydronephrosis, (which is M/C on right side due to dextro rotation of uterus).

- There is bladder congestion, hence bladder capacity decreases. To prevent stress urinary incontinence (SUI), bladder pressure and intraurethral pressure increases.
- During 1st trimester and 3rd trimester there is increased frequency of urine.

Increase	Decrease
Renal blood flow (+50%) GFR (+50%) Creatinine clearance Glucosuria	Plasma osmolality S. creatinine S. Urea S Uric acid S. Ka,⁺ Na⁺ S. Cl⁻

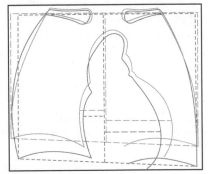

Fig. 5.4: Change in cardiac radiographic outline that occurs in pregnancy. The blue lines represent the relations between the heart and thorax in the nonpregnant woman, and the blue lines represent the conditions existing in pregnancy.

Changes in Iron Metabolism During Pregnancy

Marker	Change
• Serum iron concentration	Decreases
• Serum ferritin (reflecting Iron stores)	Decreases
• Serum total iron binding capacity	Increases
• Percentage saturation (Serum ferritin/TIBC)	Decreases
• Serum transferrin	Increases

 Remember: The two Ts i.e. Transferrin and TIBC increase during pregnancy, rest all parameters of iron metabolism decrease during pregnancy.

CHANGES IN GENITAL ORGAN DURING PREGNANCY

Vagina

- Vagina becomes edematous, more vascular and will have a bluish hue called as **Jacquemier sign/Chadwick sign**

- Doderlein bacteria increase during pregnancy so more of glycogen is converted to lactic acid hence vaginal pH decreases during pregnancy and becomes 3.5–6
- Main hormone during pregnancy is progesterone so there is increase in intermediate/navicular cells in vaginal cytology.
- There is Hobnailed appearance of vagina due to hypertrophy of the papillae of vaginal mucosa.

Uterus

- **Weight of nonpregnant uterus-70 g.**
- **Weight of pregnant uterus-1000 gms (Recent edition of Williams 25/e ....1100 grms)**
- **Length of nonpregnant uterus–7.5 cms.**
- **Length of pregnant uterus–35 cms**
- **Capacity of nonpregnant uterus–10 mL.**
- **Capacity of pregnant–5000 mL (but may be 20 L or more)**
- Shape of nonpregnant uterus is pyriform and pregnant uterus– globular (8-12 weeks), pyriform (12–36 weeks), and spherical at 36 weeks onwards.
- Uterine enlargement is mainly due to hypertrophy of muscle cells.
- Uterine hypertrophy is due to estrogen and perhaps progesterone. Thus similar changes are observed in ectopic pregnancy
- Within the uterus, enlargement is most marked in fundus
- The muscle layer of uterus during pregnancy is arranged in 3 layers:
  - **Outer: Longitudinal layer**
  - **Middle spiral layer:** The muscle fibres in this layer are arranged in figure of 8 pattern with blood vessels in between so on contraction they act as **living ligatures** by occluding the blood vessels running through them.
  - **Inner: Circular layer.**
- **Uteroplacental blood flow:** Uterine blood flow is increased from **10 mL/min in non-pregnant state to about 450 mL/min in mid trimester and nearly 500 to 750 mL/min at 36 weeks**. Out of the total blood flow to the uterus, 80% goes to placenta while 20% goes to myometrium.
- **Position of the uterus** in nonpregnant state- anteverted anteflexed. During pregnancy, as the uterus enlarges to occupy the abdominal cavity, it usually rotates on its long axis to the right (dextrorotation). This is due to the occupation of the rectosigmoid in the left posterior quadrant of the pelvis. The cervix, as a result, is deviated to the left side (levorotation) bringing it closer to the ureter.
- **Braxton Hicks Contractions:** From 2nd trimester onwards-Braxton **Hicks contractions are** felt. These are nonrhythmic, sporadic, painless contractions with

pressure-5–25 mm Hg. They do not lead to dilatation of cervix. Initially they are infrequent but later on towards end of pregnancy, frequency increase and in a few females it can lead to discomfort or false labor pains. Note- Braxton Hicks Contractions are absent in abdominal pregnancy.

> - **Fergusons reflex:** In labor, the nerve supply to the cervix causes stimulation of uterine contraction when pressure is put on cervix.
> - Utero placental Blood flow regulation: (Recent update William 25/e pg 50–51)

The increase in utero placental blood flow is due to:

1. Trophoblastic invastion–replacing the maternal spinal arteries wall. Leading to vasodilation by converting them into low resistance vessels.
2. As the diameter or radius of arteries increases, peripheral vascular resistance decreases & so blood flow increases. Blood flow is proportional to radius $(r)^4$
Hence All those factors which bring about angiogenesis: Also increase blood flow for e.g.
   - VEGF
   - Placental growth factor (PIGF)
   - Nitric oxide
   - Estrogen ⎤
   - Progesterone ⎬ Increase nitric oxide
   - Activin ⎦
3. Normal pregnancy is characterized by vascular refractoriness to pressor effect of angiotensin II
4. Adipocytokines which increase NO:
   - Chemerin (Produced by placenta)
   - VISFATIN (Produced by amnion)
4. Micro RNA species mediate vascular remodelling, e.g. MIR 17–92, MIR –34.

 Note: VEGF & PIGF actions are Mediated by Soluble FMS like tyrokinase 1 But if levels of S fit–1 is increased it inactivates & lowers the levels of VEGF & PIGF. This is what happens in patients of PIH.

Isthmus

- Forms the **lower uterine segment (LUS)** during pregnancy
- LUS begins to form in the second trimester. At term LUS is formed by isthmus–70% and cervix–30%.
- In nonpregnant females isthmus is 0.5 cms in length and extends from anatomical internal os to histological internal os.
- Taking up of cervix in the LUS is **effacement**
- Length of LUS at term-5 cm. It becomes 10 cm at the time of labor due to taking up of cervix.

Cervix

- There is marked softening of the cervix **(Goodell's sign)** which is evident as early as 6 weeks.
- There is marked proliferation of the endocervical mucosa with downward extension beyond the squamocolumnar junction.
- The cervical gland secretion is copious and tenacious-physiological leucorrhea of pregnancy. This is due to the effect of progesterone. The mucus not only fills up the glands but forms a thick mucus plug sealing the cervical canal. At the time of true labor, dilatation of cervix releases this mucus plug mixed with blood called as **Show.**
- On drying the mucus gives a **beaded appearance.**

Ovary

- Ovulation remains suspended throughout pregnancy
- Corpus luteum functions maximally until first 6–7 weeks.

 Important One Liners

- Corpus luteum of pregnancy is rescued from degeneration by hormone- hCG
- Corpus luteum of pregnancy synthesises progesterone exclusively till 6–7 weeks
- Placenta takes over the function of corpus luteum by- 8–10 weeks
- Life span of Corpus luteum of pregnancy is–10–12 weeks.

- **Theca Lutein cysts:** B/l ovarian cysts found whenever levels of hCG are high e.g. Trophoblastic diseases, large placenta-diabetes, anti-d alloimmunization, multiple pregnancy, chronic renal failure, hyperthyroidism. Occasionally they may be seen in normal pregnancy.
   Normally they are asymptomatic but because hCG is similar to LH and LH releases androgen from theca cells, so they can lead to maternal virilization.

Breast

- Increased size of the breasts becomes evident even in early weeks. This is due to marked hypertrophy and proliferation of the ducts (estrogen) and the alveoli (both estrogen and progesterone).
- The nipples become larger, erectile and deeply pigmented. Variable number of sebaceous glands (5–15) become hypertrophied and are called **Montgomery's tubercles.** Those are placed surrounding the nipples. An outer zone of less marked and irregular pigmented area appears in second trimester and is called secondary areola.
- **Colostrum:** can be squeezed out of the breast at about 12th week which at first becomes sticky. Later on, by 16th week, it becomes thick and yellowish.

 Remember: **Comparison between breast milk and colostrum:**
- Colostrum is yellow in color, alkaline in reaction and on microscopic examination consists of fat globules, watery fluid and colostrum corpuscles. Colostrum has high amount of immunoglobulins and everything more than breast milk except:
- K-: Potassium-**K**
- F: **F**at
- C: **C**arbohydrates (sugar), **c**esin.

Note: Ig A and other host resistant factors like IgM, IgG and lactoferrin are also seen in colostrum. Ig A protects the newborn against enteric infections. It also has laxative action.

Skin Changes in Pregnancy

Chloasma gravidarum or pregnancy mask: It is an extreme form of pigmentation around the cheek, forehead and around the eyes. It may be patchy or diffuse; disappears spontaneously after delivery (Fig. 5.5).

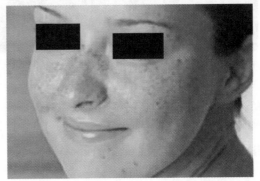

Fig. 5.5: Chloasma gravidarum

Linea nigra (Fig. 5.6): It is a brownish black pigmented area in the midline stretching from the xiphisternum to the symphysis pubis the pigmentary changes are due to melanocyte stimulating hormone from the anterior pituitary. Similar changes are observed in women taking oral contraceptives. The pigmentation disappears after delivery.

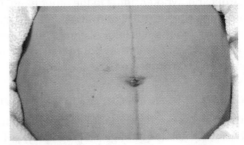

Fig. 5.6: Linea nigra

Striae gravidarum: These are linear marks with varying length and breadth found predominantly in the abdominal wall below the umbilicus, sometimes over the thighs and breasts. These stretch marks represent the scar tissues in the deeper layer of the cutis. Initially, these are pinkish but after the delivery, the scar tissues contract and they become glistening white in appearance and are called **striae albicans (Fig. 5.7).** These are due to mechanical stretching of the skin and increase in aldosterone production during pregnancy.

Apart from pregnancy, it may form in cases of generalized edema, marked obesity or in Cushing's syndrome.

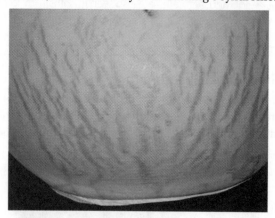

Fig. 5.7: Striae gravidarum

SOME OTHER IMPORTANT CHANGES DURING PREGNANCY

Supine Hypotension Syndrome— Mengerts Syndrome

During late pregnancy, the gravid uterus produces a compression effect on the inferior vena cava when the patient is in supine position. This, however, results in opening up of the collateral circulation by means of paravertebral and azygos veins. In some cases (10%), when the collateral circulation fails to open up, the venous return of the heart decreases, co-cardiac output of mother decreases, therefore she experiences tachycardia and hypotension. On the other hand, due to decrease in mothers cardiac output, the fetal blood flow also decreases, so there is fetal distress. **That is why all pregnant females are advised not to lie supine in late second and third trimester.**

Carbohydrate Metabolism during Pregnancy

- Transfer of increased amount of glucose from mother to the fetus is needed throughout pregnancy, as fetus is dependent on mother entirely for glucose.

- Insulin secretion is increased in response to glucose and amino acids. i.e. there is hyperinsulinemia in pregnancy
- There is hyperplasia and hypertrophy of beta cells of pancreas.
- Although insulin secretion increases during pregnancy, there is **insulin resistance during pregnancy** mediated by progesterone, estrogen, HPL, (main hormone responsible for insulin resistance) cortisol and free fatty acids. This results in postprandial hyperglycemia.
- Maximum insulin resistance is seen between 24–28 weeks.

 Key Concept

- Because of insulin resistance, pregnancy is a diabetogenic state.
- Best time to test for gestational diabetes during pregnancy is 24–28 weeks when the insulin resistance is maximum.

- During maternal fasting, there is hypoglycemia. (as glucose of mother is used by fetus)
- There is post-prandial hyperglycemia due to increase insulin resistance.
- Glycosuria maybe seen in 50% of normal pregnant females.
- There is no change in plasma glucagon levels during pregnancy.

Changes in GIT during Pregnancy

- Gastric emptying time does not change during pregnancy but increases in labor
- Reflux esophagitis is common as progesterone relaxes lower esophageal sphincter
- Splenic area increases by 50%.

Liver

- There is no change in the size of liver.
- With the exception of alkaline phosphatase (because of heat stable alkaline phosphatase produced by placenta), other liver enzymes (serum levels of bilirubin, AST, ALT, CPK, LDH) are slightly decreased.
- Alkaline phosphatase increase in pregnancy
- There is mild cholestasis (estrogen effect).
- There is marked atonicity of the gallbladder (progesterone effect). This, together with high blood cholesterol level during pregnancy, favor stone formation.

Changes in CNS during Pregnancy

- **Pituitary gland enlarges by 135% during pregnancy due to estrogen stimulation**

- Prolactin levels increase during pregnancy but incidence of prolactinomas does not increase.

  Changes in Regional Blood Flow during pregnancy
  - Uteroplacental blood flow increases during pregnancy and becomes roughly 450–650 ml/minute at term
  - Their is vascular refractoriness to angiotensin II, endothelin.
  - Skin perfusion increases.

Changes in Hormones in pregnancy	
Increase	**Decrease**
• All adrenal Hormones increase during pregnancy including cortisol and aldosterone	• Except DHEA–Sulphate

• All Pituitary hormones increase like
  – GH
  – ACTH
• Prolactin (150 ng/mL at term which is 10 times its 'N' value) non-pregnant female Paradoxically prolactin levels decrease after delivery even in females who are breastfeeding
	• Except LH and FSH (Due to negative feedback by Estrogen & Progesterone)

• Size of Pituitary Gland increases by 135% (Mainly the anterior lobe explaining why necrosis of anterior lobe of pituitary happens in Sheehan's syndrome) • The increase in size is due to estrogen stimulated hypertrophy and hyperplasia of lactotrophs. (This is the reason of increase in Prolactin during pregnancy)	

DIAGNOSIS OF PREGNANCY

Duration of pregnancy: The duration of pregnancy is 10 lunar months or 9 calendar months and 7 days or 280 days or 40 weeks, calculated from the first day of the last menstrual period. This is called **menstrual or gestational age.**

Calculation of EDD: Can be done by **Naegele's formula:** To the LMP i.e (First day of the last menstrual period) 7 days (6 days for a leap year) and count forwards and add 9 months or count backwards and substract 3 months.

 Important One Liners

- Only 4–6% of the females deliver on their exact EDD as calculated by Naegles formula.
- 50% females deliver either one week before or one week after their EDD.
- Hence whenever a female comes with postdated pregnancy–first step is to review her menstrual history.

Important Terminology

Early term pregnancy	37 to 38 weeks + 6 days
Term pregnancy	39 to 40 weeks + 6 days
Late term pregnancy	41 to 41 weeks + 6 days
Post term pregnancy	> 42 weeks
Preterm pregnancy	< 37 weeks

The entire duration of pregnancy is divided in three trimesters:
- First trimester: first 12 weeks
- Second trimester: 13–28 weeks
- Third trimester: 29–40 weeks.

First Trimester

Symptoms

- **'U'**—increased **u**rinary frequency
- **Are**—**a**menorrhea
- **My**—**m**orning sickness due to hCG
- **Best**—**b**reast discomfort
- **Friend**—**f**atigue

Sign	Feature	Seen in
Jacquemier's/Chadwick's sign	Dusky hue of the vestibule and anterior vaginal wall due to local vascular congestion	8th week of pregnancy and in pelvic tumors like fibroid
Osiander's sign	Increased pulsation felt through the lateral fornices	8th week of pregnancy and in acute PID
Goodell's sign	Softening of cervix (cervix feels like lip of mouth whereas in nonpregnant state it feels like tip of nose)	6th week of pregnancy and in OC pill users

Contd...

Contd...

Sign	Feature	Seen in
Hegar's sign	On Bimanual examination with 2 fingers in anterior fornix and fingers of other hand behind the uterus, the abdominal and vaginal fingers seem to appose below the body of uterus. It occurs because of softening of isthmus[Q]	6–10 weeks of pregnancy
Palmer's sign	Regular and rhythmic uterine contraction which can be felt on bimanual	4–8 weeks of pregnancy

 Also Know:

Size of uterus in 1st trimester: In the first trimester uterus enlarges to the size of hen egg at 6th week, cricket ball size at 8th week and size of fetal head by 12th week.

Position of uterus in 1st trimester: It remains an intrapelvic organ.

A few females may experience bleeding at the time of implantation. This is placental sign/Hant-man sign

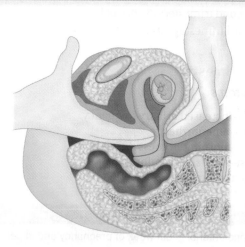

Fig. 5.8: Elicitation of Hegar's sign

Second Trimester of Pregnancy (13–28 Weeks) can be Diagnosed by

Symptoms

- *Quickening:* Perception of active fetal movements felt by 18 weeks of pregnancy in primipara and 2 weeks earlier in multiparae.

- *Progressive enlargement:* Of the lower abdomen by the growing uterus.

Signs

Sign	Feature
Chloasma	Pigmentation over forehead and cheeks
Breast changes	Appearance of secondary areola
	Secretion of colostrum
	Thickening of colostrum

Third Trimester

Symptoms

- Amenorrhea persists
- Enlargement of the abdomen is progressive which produces some mechanical discomfort to the patient such as palpitation or dyspnea following exertion
- **Lightening** — After 36 th week, specially in primigravidae, a sense of relief of the pressure symptoms is obtained due to engagement of the presenting part
- Frequency of micturition reappears
- Fetal movements are more pronounced

Signs of Pregnancy

Presumptive Symptoms and Signs (Subjective)

- **A**-Amenorrhea
- **N**—Nausea, vomiting
- **M**—frequency of **m**icturition
- **Q**uickly—**q**uickening
- **B**ring—**b**reast discomfort
- **F**emale (for)—**f**atigue
- **S**urgery—**s**kin changes

Uterine Changes in 2nd Trimester

Size	Increases with increasing gestational age and uterus feels soft and elastic. Uterus becomes an abdominal organ	
Braxton hick contractions	Irregular[Q], infrequent[Q] spasmodic and painless contractions without any effect on dilatation of the cervix. (Intrauterine pressure is <8 mm of Hg)	Begin in early pregnancy and continue till term
Palpation of fetal parts and active fetal movement	They are positive signs of pregnancy	Elicited by 20 weeks[Q]
Ballottement of uterus	Ballottement of uterus on bimanual examination gives the impression of a floating object inside the uterus. It may also be seen in case of uterine fibroid, ascites or ovarian cyst	Elicited between 16–20[Q] weeks of pregnancy
Auscultation of fetal heart sound	Most conclusive sign of pregnancy[Q]	Heard by stethoscope between 18–20 weeks of pregnancy[Q] Fetal cardiac motion can be detected by doppler by 10 weeks

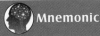

Mnemonic

ANM Quickly bring Females (for) Surgery

Positive or Absolute Signs of Pregnancy
- **Palpation of fetal parts and** perception of fetal movements by examiner, at about 20 weeks.
- **Auscultation of fetal heart sounds**.
- **USG evidence of embryo** (at 6th week) and later[Q] on of the fetus.
- **Radiological demonstration of fetal skeleton at 16 weeks and onwards**.

Note: Now all the signs which are objective which I have discussed above like for e.g., softening of cervix, abdominal enlargement, Braxton hicks contractions are included under **probable signs of pregnancy.**

PSEUDOCYESIS: PHANTOM PREGNANCY/ SPURIOUS PREGNANCY/FALSE PREGNANCY

Definition: *It is a psychological disorder where the women has a false but firm belief that she is pregnant, although no pregnancy exists. Patient is often infertile and has an intense desire to have a baby.*

Patient presents with:
- Cessation of menstruation.
- Enlargement of abdomen (due to deposition of fat).
- Secretions from breasts.
- Fetal movement (actually intestinal movement).

On examination: No positive signs of pregnancy are found, i.e. fetal heart sound is not heard, no fetal movement felt and no fetal parts palpable by the examiner.

USG and X-ray do not reveal any signs of pregnancy.

ANTENATAL CARE

Ideally the Schedule for Antenatal Visits Should be

- Monthly visits upto 28 weeks.
- Two weekly visit between 28 and 36 weeks.
- Weekly visit from 36 weeks onwards

This means a total of 12–15 visits.   *Ref. Dutta Obs 6/e, p 99*

WHO Recommends At Least 4 Visits

1st at	–	16 weeks
2nd at	–	24–28 weeks
3rd at	–	32 weeks
4th at	–	36 weeks

As per Indian Scenario-Minimum 3 Visits are Essential

1st at	–	20 weeks (or as soon as pregnancy is known)
2nd	–	32 weeks
3rd	–	36 weeks

- The first visit that a woman makes to a health care facility is called the **booking visit.**
- A **booked case** is one that has at least 3 antenatal visits with at least two in the last trimester.

Folic Acid Supplementation during Pregnancy

- Folic acid supplementation during pregnancy prevents neural tube defects.
- Dose of folic acid given to all pregnant females-**400** µg
- **When to initiate folic acid**—It should be given ideally 3 months before conception or at least 1 month before

conception and continued for 3 months after pregnancy. This dose is called as **prophylactic dose of folic acid.**

- Govt of India supplies Iron and Folic acid tablets free of cost- these tablets have 100 mg of Fe and 500 mcg of folic acid- so **RDA of folic acid during pregnancy is- 500** μg.
- In high-risk patients like
  i. Females with history of previous NTD babies
  ii. Diabetic females
  iii. Females with sickle cell anemia and
  iv. Females on antiepileptic drugs like valproic acid— dose of folic acid needed to prevent NTD is **-4 mg:** This is called as **Therapeutic dose of folic acid.**

> **Also Know:** Dose of folic acid to treat megaloblastic anemia during pregnancy—1 mg/day

Supplementary Iron Therapy during Pregnancy
Iron Requirements during Pregnancy

Total amount of iron required during pregnancy **is 1000 mg,** i.e. 4–6 mg/day which can be calculated as:

- **Fetus and placenta require** – **300 mg**
- Growing RBC of the mother require – 500 mg
- Lost through sweat, urine and faeces – 200 mg
- Lost at the time of delivery – 200 mg
- Amount of iron saved d/t amenorrhea – 300 mg

So approximately (1200–300 =) 900–1000 mg is required during pregnancy.

- No matter in what form iron is being taken–only 10%

of it is absorbed, which means in order to fulfill the requirement of 4–6 mg/day, approximately 40–60 mg of iron should be taken in diet daily during pregnancy. Which is not possible, this is the reason why Iron supplementation is absolutely necessary in pregnancy.

> **Other important points:**
> - RDA of calcium during preganacy–1200 mg/day
> - RDA of iodine during pregnancy–250 μg/day
> - Extra calory requirement = + 350 Kcal/day
> - Extra calory in lactation = +600 Kcal/day
> - Exta protein requirement in pregnancy = + 23 g/day
> - For moderate women total calories in pregnancy = 2230 + 350 = 2580 Kcal/day

VACCINATION DURING PREGNANCY

Tetanus

- Immunization against tetanus not only protects the mother but also the neonates. In unprotected women, 0.5 mL tetanus toxoid is given intramuscularly at 6 weeks interval for 2 such, the first one to be given between 16–20 weeks and second dose at 20–24 weeks.
- Women who are immunized in the past, a booster dose of 0.5 mL IM is given preferably 4 weeks before EDD.

Other Vaccines in Pregnancy

> **Remember:** A simple "FUNDA" - (Proposed by CDC Society - 2002).
>
> - Killed vaccine are safe in pregnancy.
> - Live vaccines are best avoided in pregnancy.

Safety of Vaccines in Pregnancy

(Table Based on table 9-9 p 185, Williams 24/e)

Safe	Only in epidemics	To be given in case of travel to highly endemic area or exposed to contacts	Contraindicated
• H-Hepatitis A/B	• **Tab**-Typhoid • **P**-Pneumococcus • **C**-Cholera	• Yellow fever • Japanese encephalitis • Polio (IPV)	• Rubella • Measles • Mumps
• I-Influenza • T-Tetanus • Rabies-Rabies (mnemonic-HIT Rabies)	• **M**-Meningococcus (Tab PCM)		• BCG • Smallpox • Chickenpox

GRAVIDA AND PARITY

It is a very important concept.

Gravida: Denotes pregnant state both present and past irrespective of the period of gestation.

The term gravida should only be used if the female is presently pregnant.

Parity: Denotes previous pregnancies which have reached beyond the period of viability. There are various ways in which Gravida and parity can be denoted:

1. G_aP_b **method:** It is the simplest method. Here Gravida and Parity are written as discussed above. For example,

   Case 1: If a female is 10 weeks pregnant now and has a

child of 4 years. She will be G_2P_1 (G_2 because this is the 2nd time she is pregnant and P_1 because she had a previous pregnancy which went beyond period of viability).

Case 2: If the same female did not have a 4 year child but had H/o abortion @ 12 weeks then she would be G_2P_0 (P_0 because none of her pregnancy went beyond the period of viability).

 Note: Gravida and parity refer to the number of pregnancies **but not babies**.

Case 3: A 12 weeks pregnant female with previous history of twin delivery @ 38 weeks is G_2P_1 (G_2 because this is the 2nd time she has become pregnant P_1 because her 1st pregnancy went beyond the period of viability. It will counted as 1 only, irrespective of the number of children delivered).

2. **G_aP_{b+c} method:** In clinical practice, it is mandatory to express parity by 2 digits, the first one (b) represents number of viable pregnancies and second one (c) relates with number of abortions. Gravida remains same as explained earlier, e.g.

Case 4: If a pregnant female has H/o one child of 4 years and 2 abortions, one @ 10 weeks and one @ 14 weeks. Her obstetric history will be:

$$G_4 \, P_{1+2}$$
↓

G4 = She is becoming pregnant for 4th time.

P1 = 1 pregnancy went beyond the period of viability as she has a child of 4 years

+2 = Number of abortions which are 2.

3. **$G_aP_{b+c+d+e}$ method:** In some centers parity is denoted by 4 numbers.

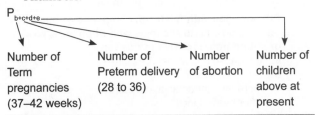

$P_{b+c+d+e}$

| Number of Term pregnancies (37–42 weeks) | Number of Preterm delivery (28 to 36) | Number of abortion | Number of children above at present |

That is why this is also called $GP_{T+P+A+L}$ method

 Also Know:

- A female who has her first pregnancy at the age of 30 or more is called Elderly primigravida
- A pregnant woman with previous history of four births or more is called Grand multipara.

ANEMIA MUKT BHARAT

As per Government of India

In all pregnant females:

60 mg elemental iron + 500 mcg of Folic acid is to be given daily, starting from 4th month of POG & continued throughout pregnancy, minimum for 180 days & to be continued for 180 days, partum

New Pattern Questions

N1. A 28-year-old primgravida had prepregnancy BMI of 30 kg/m². What is the recommended weight gain for her during pregnancy:
a. 5–7 kg
b. 8–11 kg
c. 10–13 kg
d. 14–16 kg

N2. Primigravida with full term, complains of faintness on lying down and she feels well when turns to side or sitting position. This is due to:
a. Increased abdominal pressure
b. IVC compression
c. Increased intracranial pressure
d. After heavy lunch

N3. The clotting factor which is not increased in pregnancy:
a. Factor 2
b. Factor 7
c. Factor 10
d. Factor 11

N4. A prosthetic valve patient switches to heparin at what time during pregnancy:
a. 28 weeks
b. 32 weeks
c. 36 weeks
d. Postpartum

N5. Schwangerschaft protein is the other name of:
a. hCG
b. Papp-1
c. Pregnancy specific beta1 glycoprotein
d. Activin

N6. All of the following are true about regional blood flow in pregnancy *except*:
a. Uterine blood flow at term is 750 ml/min
b. Blood flow through skin decreases
c. Renal blood flow increases by 50%
d. Pulmonary blood flow increase

N7. Prolactin levels:
a. Lowest in pregnancy and increases after delivery
b. Highest during pregnancy and fall during lactation
c. Unaffected by pregnancy and lactation
d. Variable in every pregnancy

N8. Intermediate cell predominance on a vaginal cytology is seen in:
a. Pregnancy
b. Menstruation
c. Postovulatory
d. Premenstrual

N9. The term "placental sign" denotes:
a. Alteration of FHR on pressing the head into the pelvis
b. Spotting on the expected date of period in early months of pregnancy
c. Permanent lengthening of the cord in 3rd stage of labour
d. Slight gush of bleeding in third stage of labour

N10. The following changes occur in urinary system in pregnancy *except*:
a. Increased GFR
b. Increased RBF
c. Hypertrophy of bladder musculature
d. Increased activity of ureters

N11. The subcostal angle during pregnancy is:
a. 85°
b. 95°
c. 105°
d. 75°

N12. A G_2P_1 female carrying twin fetuses has BMI of 26. What is the ideal weight gain in for this female?
a. 16.8 to 24.5 kg
b. 14.1 to 22.7 kg
c. 11.4–19.1 kg
d. None of the above

N13. The following are related to uterine souffle *except*:
a. It is a soft blowing systolic murmur heard on the sides of pregnant uterus
b. The sound is synchronous with the maternal pulse
c. It is due to increased in blood flow through the compressed umbilical arteries
d. It can be heard even in a big fibroid

N14. The following are related to fetal souffle *except*:
a. It is soft blowing murmur synchronous with the fetal heart sounds
b. It is due to rush of blood through the compressed umbilical arteries
c. It is heard in about 15% cases
d. When present is diagnostic of pregnancy

N15. Ideal number of antenatal visits:
a. 12–14
b. 6–8
c. 7–9
d. 10–11

N16. Daily caloric needs in pregnancy is about........ kilo cal:
a. 1000
b. 1500
c. 2500
d. 3500

N17. Which is not a feature of pseudocyesis?
a. Amenorrhea
b. Abdominal distension
c. Fetal heart sounds are audible
d. None of the above

N18. All of the following statements are true for parity *except*:
a. Parity refers to number of pregnancies reaching viability
b. In twin pregnancy, parity remains same
c. If a female has still birth her parity decreases
d. Parity is to affected by number of fetuses delivered

N19. An 18-year-old woman complains of lower abdominal pain and vaginal spotting for several days. She denies sexually transmitted disease although she is sexually active with her boyfriend; they use condoms for protection. Her last menstrual period was 6 weeks ago. Her blood pressure is 124/80 mm Hg, pulse is 90/min, and temperature is 37.2°C (99.0°F). Abdominal examination demonstrates vague left lower quadrant tenderness without rebound or guarding. Pelvic examination shows a

normal vagina and cervix without cervical motion tenderness. No adnexal masses are appreciated. Results of a complete blood cell count and metabolic panel are within normal limits. Which of the following is the next best step in mgt?
a. Transvaginal USG
b. Follow up after 3 months
c. Quantitative β-hCG measurement
d. Rapid urine β-hCG measurement
e. Methotrexate injection.

N20. What is approx fetal weight, if height of uterus is above pubic symphysis is 35 cm and station of head –2?
a. 2.5 kg   b. 3 kg
c. 3.5 kg   d. 4 kg

N21. Appropriate treatment of women having edema in pregnancy includes:
a. Salt restriction   b. Fluid restriction
c. Diuretics   d. Bed rest

N22. Teenage pregnancy is associated with all *except*:

a. Caesarean section is more common
b. Eclampsia more common
c. Postdated pregnancy
d. ↑ maternal mortality rate

N23. Term delivery implies that the gestational age of the foetus calculated from the time of onset of last menstrual period is:
a. 40 weeks   b. 42 weeks
c. 38 weeks   d. 260 days

N24. Use of one of the following vaccinations is absolutely contraindicated in pregnancy:
a. Hepatitis-B   b. Cholera
c. Rabies   d. Yellow fever

N25. Chadwick sign is seen in:
a. Cervix   b. Vagina
c. Uterus   d. Ovary

N26. Theca lutein cyst is not seen in:
a. Twin pregnancy   b. Molar pregnancy
c. Chronic renal failure during pregnancy
d. Hypothyroidism during pregnancy

Previous Year Questions

1. Weight gain in pregnancy is related to all *except*:
     a. Ethnicity   [AI 2011/AIIMS May 2010]
b. Smoking
c. Socioeconomic status
d. Preconceptional weight

2. Which of the following is the least likely physiological change in pregnancy?   [AIIMS Nov 06]
a. Increase in intravascular volume
b. Increase in cardiac output
c. Increase in stroke volume
d. Increase in peripheral vascular resistance

3. What are maternal physiological changes in pregnancy?
a. ↑ed cardiac output   b. ↑ed tidal volume
c. ↑ed vital capacity   d. ↓ed fibrinogen
e. ↓ed plasma protein concentration   [PGI June 03]

4. Physiological changes in pregnancy:
a. ↓residual volume   b. ↓GFR   [PGI June 09]
c. ↓cardiac output   d. ↓Hematocrit

5. Which of the following cardiovascular change is abnormal in pregnancy?   [PGI Dec 00]
a. Enlarged cardiac silhouette
b. Increased S1 split
c. Right axis deviation on ECG
d. Early diastolic murmur
e. HR increased by 10 to 15 per minute

6. Which cardiovascular change is physiological in last trimester of pregnancy?   [AIIMS Nov 01]

a. Mid-diastolic murmur
b. Occasional atrial fibrillation
c. Shift of apical impulse laterally and upwards in left 4th intercostal space
d. Cardiomegaly

7. All of the following changes are seen in pregnancy *except*:   [AIIMS Nov 2011]
a. Increased stroke volume
b. Increased cardiac output
c. Increased Intravascular volume
d. Increased peripheral vascular resistance

8. All of the following may be observed in a normal pregnancy *except*:   [AI 03]
a. Fall in serum iron concentration
b. Increase in serum iron binding capacity
c. Increase in blood viscosity
d. Increase in blood oxygen carrying capacity

9. Which of the following is increased in pregnancy?
a. Globulin   b. Fibrinogen   [PGI Dec 01]
c. Uric acid   d. Leukocytes
e. Transferrin

10. True about various changes in pregnancy is/are:
a. Fibrinogen levels are increased   [PGI Dec 00]
b. Uric acid levels are increased
c. Sr. potassium is decreased
d. Sodium retention

11. **Physiological changes of pregnancy include:**
    a. Insulin levels increase   [PGI June 02]
    b. Increased BMR
    c. Hypothyroidism   d. GH decreases
    e. Blood volume decreases

12. **Insulin resistance in pregnancy is because of:**
    a. Human placental lactogen   [PGI Dec 01]
    b. Thyroid hormone   c. Progesterone
    d. hCG   e. Estrogen

13. **Most common cause of platelet ↓ in pregnancy:**
    a. Immune   b. Incidental   [PGI June 00]
    c. Idiopathic   d. Infection
    e. Benign gestational

14. **During foetal life maximum growth is caused by:**
    a. Growth hormone   b. Insulin   [AI 99]
    c. Cortisol   d. Thyroxin

15. **In normal pregnancy character of vagina is:**
    a. ↑ed pH   [AI 02]
    b. ↑ed number of lactobacilli
    c. ↑ed glycogen content
    d. ↑ed number of pathogenic bacteria

16. **All of the following statements are true except:**   [AI 01]
    a. Oxytocin sensitivity is increased during delivery
    b. Prostaglandins may be given for inducing abortion during IIIrd trimester
    c. In lactating women genital stimulation enhances oxytocin release
    d. Oxytocin is used for inducing abortion in 1st trimester

17. **True regarding changes during pregnancy:**
    a. Hyperplasia of parathyroid   [PGI May 2010]
    b. Hyperplasia of thyroid
    c. Increased pigmentation
    d. Decreased BMR   e. Increased insulin

18. **Estrogen and progesterone is first two months of pregnancy are produced by:**   [AIIMS Nov 2015]
    a. Fetal ovaries   b. Fetal adrenal
    c. Placenta   d. Corpus luteum

19. **Signs positive in early pregnancy are:** [PGI Dec 00]
    a. Hegar's sign   b. Palmer's sign
    c. Goodell's sign   d. Osiander's sign

20. **Hegar's sign of pregnancy is:**   [PGI June 97]
    a. Uterine contraction
    b. Bluish discoloration of vagina
    c. Softening of isthmus
    d. Quickening

21. **Changes that are found in 2nd trimester of pregnancy:**
    a. Braxton-Hicks contraction   [PGI Dec 03]
    b. Show   c. Lightening
    d. Quickening   e. Broad ligament pain

22. **Pregnancy is confirmed by:**   [PGI 04]
    a. Morning sickness   b. Amenorrhea
    c. Fetal heart activity
    d. Fetal movement by examiner
    e. Fetal sac in USG

23. **An expectant mother feels quickening at:**
    a. 12–18 weeks   b. 16–20 weeks [PGI Dec 09]
    c. 26 weeks   d. 24–28 weeks
    e. 28–32 weeks

24. **Periconceptional use of the following agent leads to reduced incidence of neural tube defects:**
                              [AIIMS May 03, UP 08]
    a. Folic acid   b. Iron
    c. Calcium   d. Vitamin A

25. **Folic acid supplementation reduces the risk of:**
                              [PGI June 03]
    a. Neural tube defect b. Toxemia of pregnancy
    c. Down's syndrome   d. Placenta previa

26. **Use of folic acid to prevent congenital malformation should be best initiated:**   [AIIMS Nov 03]
    a. During 1st trimester of pregnancy
    b. During 2nd trimester of pregnancy
    c. During 3rd trimester of pregnancy
    d. Before conception

27. **Kegels exercise should begin:**   [AIPG 2012]
    a. Immediately after delivery
    b. 24 hours after delivery
    c. 3 weeks after delivery
    d. 6 weeks after delivery

28. **All of the following increase at full term in pregnancy except:**   [AIIMS May 2016]
    a. Minute volume   b. GFR
    c. Blood volume   d. Cardiac output

29. **Consider the following hemodynamic changes during pregnancy:**   [UPSC–2018]
    1. Cardiac output ↑   2. Stroke volume ↑
    3. ↑ In oncolytic pressure
    4. ↑ pulse rate
    Which of the following statements are correct
    a. 1, 3 and 4   b. 1, 2 and 4
    c. 1, 2 and 3   d. 2, 3 and 4

30. **A patient presented at 20 weeks of gestation. The patient's LMP was 9th January. What will be the estimated date of delivery?**   [AIIMS Nov 2017]
    a. 9th January   b. 16th September
    c. 16th October   d. 9th October

31. **Which of the following Leopold's grip is shown in the image?**   [AIIMS Nov 2017]

    a. Pawlick's grip   b. Pelvic
    c. Fundal   d. Abdominal

Answers with Explanations to New Pattern Questions

N1. **Ans. is a, i.e. 5–7 kg** *Ref. Williams 24/e, p 117*

Recommended Ranges of Total Gain for Pregnant Women by Prepregnancy Body Mass Index (BMI) for Singleton gestation.

Weight – for – Height		Recommended Total Weight Gain		Weight gain/week
Category	BMI	kg	lb	In lb/week
Underweight	<18.5	12.5–18	28–40	1 (1–1.3)
Normal	18.5–24.9	11.5–14	25–35	1 (0.8–1)
Overweight	25–29.9	7–11.5	15–25	0.6 (0.5–0.7)
Obese	≥30	7	11–20	0.5 (0.4–0.6)

Note: 1 lb = 0.454 kg.

N2. **Ans. is b, i.e. IVC compression** *Ref. Dutta Obs 9/e, p 49*

SUPINE HYPOTENSION SYNDROME (POSTURAL HYPOTENSION): During late pregnancy, the gravid uterus produces a compression effect on the inferior vena cava when the patient is in supine position. In 90% cases this, however, results in opening up of the collateral circulation by means of paravertebral and azygos veins. In some cases (10%), when the collateral circulation fails to open up, the venous return of the heart may be seriously curtailed. This results in production of hypotension, tachycardia and syncope called as supine hypotensive syndrome. The normal blood pressure is quickly restored by turning the patient to lateral position. That is why pregnant females are advised to lie in lateral positions best being left lateral.

N3. **Ans. is d, i.e. Factor 11** *Ref: Dutta Obs 9/e, p 48*

Pregnancy is a hypercoaguable state, all clotting factors increase in pregnancy except factor 11 and 13. Another frequently asked question is what happens to fibrinogen levels during pregnancy-since fibrinogen is clotting factor number 1 therefore it also increase in pregnancy.

N4. **Ans. is c, i.e. 36 weeks**

Anticoagulants in Pregnancy

2 main anticoagulants are:

	Warfarin	Heparin
Advantage	It is highly effective anticoagulant	Cannot cross placenta and so does not lead to fetal defects
Disadvantage	Can cross placenta and Lead to-short stature, Stippled epiphysis, Nasal hypoplasia, Saddle nose and frontal Bossing if used in 1st Trimester.	It is not as effective as warfarin and pregnancy is a hypercoagulable state. During pregnancy unfractionated heparin is used. LMWH can be used during pregnancy but should not be used in pregnant patients with valves replaced.

Keeping these things in mind, during pregnancy anticoagulants are used.

Period of gestation	Anticoagulant used
Uptil 12 weeks	Unfractionated heparin
12–36 weeks	Warfarin
36 weeks onwards and uptil 6 hours before delivery	IV heparin (since if warfarin is continued, there can be PPH after delivery)
From 6 hours after vaginal delivery and 24 hours after cesarean	Restart anticoagulants

N5. **Ans. is c, i.e. Pregnancy specific beta 1 glycoprotein.** *Ref. JB Sharma TB of Obs, p 58*
Schwangerchaft Protein:
- It is the other name for pregnancy specific B1 glycoprotein.
- Produced by syncytiotrophoblast.
- It appears in serum as early as 6 days after conception.
- Its concentration rises steadily and reaches 200 mg/mL at term.
- It is a potent immunosuppressor of lymphocyte proliferation and prevents rejection of the concepters.

N6. **Ans. is b, i.e. Blood flow through skin decreases** *Ref. Dutta Obs 9/e, p 49*
REGIONAL DISTRIBUTION OF BLOOD FLOW DURING PREGNANCY: Uterine blood flow is increased from 50 ml/min in non-pregnant state to about 750 ml near term. The increase is due to the combined effect of uteroplacental and fetoplacental vasodilatation. **Pulmonary blood flow** (normal 6000 ml/min) is increased by 2500 ml/min (i.e. 40% increase). **Renal blood flow** (normal 800 ml) increases by 400 ml/min (i.e. 50% increase) at 16th week and remains at this level till term. **The blood flow through the skin and mucous** membranes reaches a maximum of 500 mL/min by 36th week. **Heat sensation, sweating or stuffy nose complained by the pregnant women can be explained by the increased blood flow.**

N7. **Ans. is b, i.e. Highest during pregnancy and fall during lactation** *Ref. Williams Obs 25/e pg 69; Williams Obs. 23/e, p 126, 127*
"Maternal plasma levels of prolactin increase markedly during the course of normal pregnancy, serum concentration levels are usually 10-fold greater at term (about 150 ng/ml) compared with normal non pregnant women. Paradoxically, after delivery, the plasma prolactin concentration decreases even in women who are breast feeding. During early lactation, there are pulsatile bursts of prolation secretion in response to sucking." *Ref. Williams Obs. 23/e, p 126, 127*

N8. **Ans. is a, i.e. Pregnancy** *Ref. Dutta Gynae. 4/e, p 105*
This question has been explained in detail in 'Self Assessment and Review in Gynaecology' by the same author. In brief **Vaginal epithelium is stratified squamous epithelium and has the following layers:**

Layer	Cells seen	Characteristic
Basal and parabasal	Small, round and basophilic cells	This layer is dominant when there is *lack of any hormonal activity* as in **childhood[Q] uptil puberty[Q], postpartum[Q] and after menopause[Q].**
Intermediate cells	Transparent and basophilic cells	This layer is dominant under the influence of *Progesterone[Q], Androgen, Corticosteroid or, if patient is on OCP's.* It is the predominant layer **at birth[Q]**; during **pregnancy** or can be seen also at **menopause**.
Superficial cells	Large cells with pyknotic nucleus, Acidophilic on staining[Q]	This layer is dominant under the influence of *oestrogen[Q]* and is **predominant layer in reproductive period** and during **preovulatory phase**

N9. **Ans. is b, i.e. Spotting on the expected date of period in early months of pregnancy** *Ref. Dutta Obs 9/e, p 60*
All pregnant females have amenorrhea. In a few pregnant females however, cyclic bleeding may occur upto 12 weeks of pregnancy, i.e. until the decidual space is obliterated by the fusion of decidua vera with decidua capsularis. Such bleeding is usually scanty, lasting for a shorter duration than her usual cycle and roughly corresponds with the date of the expected period. This is termed as **placental sign**.

N10. **Ans. is d, i.e. Increased activity of ureters**
As discussed previously, during pregnancy – Glomerular filtration rate and renal blood flow increases i.e. option a and b are correct. Amongst option c and d; option d i.e. increased activity of ureters cannot be correct as the main hormone during pregnancy is progesterone which leads to relaxation of the smooth muscles of ureter. Therefore activity of ureters decreases and leads to urinary stasis.
Anatomical changes in renal system during pregnancy.
- Both kidneys enlarge in pregnancy 1 cm.
- Hydroureter and hydronephrosis occurs due to relaxant effect progesterone (These changes are M/c on right side).
- Congestion of bladder leading to decreased bladder capacity.
- To compensate bladder pressure increases and intraurethral pressure increases.

N11. **Ans is c, i.e. 105°** *Ref. Dutta Obs 9/e, p 50*
Anatomic changes in respiratory system:
1. Elevation of diaphragm by 4 cm
2. Transverse diameter of chest increases by 2 cm

3. Subcostal angle increases from 68–103°
4. Chest circumference increases by 5–7 cm

N12. **Ans is b, i.e. 14.1 to 22.7 kg**

BMI = 26 = overweight female

BMI	Category
<19	Underweight
19.1–24.9	Normal
25–29.9	Overweight
>30	Obese

Recommended weight gain in twin pregnancy
Normal BMI = 37–54 lb = 16.8 to 24.5 kg
Overweight = 31–50 lb = 14.1 to 22.7 kg
Obese = 25–42 lb = 11.4 to 19.1 kg
1 lb = 0.454 kg

N13. **Ans. is c, i.e. It is due to increase in blood flow through the compressed umbilical arteries.**   *Ref. Dutta 9/e, p 64*

Uterine souffle is a soft blowing and systolic murmur heard low down at the sides of the uterus, best on the left side. The sound is synchronous with the maternal pulse and is due to increase in blood flow through the dilated uterine vessels. It can be heard in big uterine fibroid.

N14. **Ans. is b, i.e. It is due to rush of blood through the compressed umbilical arteries**   *Ref. Dutta 9/e, p 64*

Funic or fetal souffle is due to rush of blood through the umbilical arteries. It is a soft, blowing murmur synchronous with the fetal heart sounds.

N15. **Ans. is a, i.e. 12–14**   *Ref. Dutta Obs. 7/e, p 99; SPM Park 19/e, p 417, 20/e, p 450*

Ideally the schedule for antenatal visits should be:

- Monthly visits upto 28 weeks.
- Two weekly visit between 28 and 36 weeks.
- Weekly visit from 36 weeks onwards

This means a total of 12–15 visits.   *Ref. Dutta Obs 9/e, p 99*

WHO recommends atleast 4 visits:

1st at   –   16 weeks
2nd at   –   24–28 weeks
3rd at   –   32 weeks
4th at   –   36 weeks

As per Indian scenario - minimum 3 visits are essential;

1st at   –   20 weeks (or as soon as pregnancy is known)
2nd   –   32 weeks
3rd   –   36 weeks

- The first visit that a woman makes to a health care facility is called the **booking visit.**
- A **booked case** is one that has atleast 3 antenatal visits with at least two in the last trimester.

N16. **Ans. is c, i.e. 2500 kcal**   *Ref. Park 21/e, p 588; Dutta Obs. 7/e, p 101*

Recommended daily allowance: in pregnancy and lactation   *Ref. Park 21/e, p 588*

Nutrient	RDA in nonpregnant female	RDA in pregnancy	RDA in lactation
Kilo calories (moderate work)	2200	2200 + 350	2200 + 600
Proteins	55 gm	78	74

Contd...

Contd...

Nutrient	RDA in nonpregnant female	RDA in pregnancy	RDA in lactation
Fat	20 gm	30 gm	30 g
Calcium	600 mg	1200 mg	1200
Iron	21 mg	35 mg	25 mg

So, it is clear in pregnant females extra 350 kcal should be added i.e. 2200 + 350 = 2550 kcal/day

N17. Ans. is c, i.e. Fetal heart sounds are audible *Ref. Dutta Obs. 7/e, p 72*

Pseudocyesis: Phantom pregnancy/Spurious pregnancy/False pregnancy.

Definition: *It is a psychological disorder where the women has a false but firm belief that she is pregnant, although no pregnancy exists. Patient is often infertile and has an intense desire to have a baby.*

Patient presents with:
- Cessation of menstruation.
- Enlargement of abdomen (due to deposition of fat).
- Secretions from breasts.
- Fetal movement (actually intestinal movement).

On examination: No positive signs of pregnancy are found, i.e. fetal heart sound is not heard, no fetal movement felt and no fetal parts palpable by the examiner.

USG and X-ray do not reveal any signs of pregnancy.

N18. Ans. is c, i.e. If a female has still birth her parity decreases

As discussed in the text option a, b and d are correct.

Option c i.e. if a female has stillbirth, her parity decreases is incorrect as stillbirth means pregnancy went beyond the period of viability.

N19. Ans. is d, i.e. Rapid urine β-hCG measurement *Ref. Read below.*

In the question patient is presenting with amenorrhea of 6 weeks and she has history of being sexually active. Now all of you know the most common cause of secondary amenorrhea is pregnancy, so first rule it out by doing a rapid urine hCG test, i.e urine pregnancy test and then do USG to see whether the pregnancy is intrauterine or extrauterine (the question specifically asks which is the next step in management).

N20. Ans. is c, i.e. 3.5 kg *Ref. Dutta Obs. 9/e, p 68*

Estimation of fetal weight can be done using Johnson formula:
- **If station of head below ischial spine**
  [Height of uterus above pubic symphysis (in cm) – 11] × 155
- **If fetal head is at or above ischial spine–**
  [Height of uterus above pubic symphysis (in cm) – 12] × 155
  Here fetal head is at – 2, i.e. above ischial spine, so it will be
  (35 – 12) × 155 = 3.5 kg.

 Also Know:

USG measurement of fetal weight =

Shephard formula = Log_{10} EFW (gm) =
1.2508 + [(0.166 × BPD) + 0.46 × AC] – (0.002646 × AC × BPD)

Hadlock formula = Log_{10} EFW (gm) = 1.3596 – 0.00386 (AC × FL) + 0.0064 (HC) + 0.00061 (BPD × AC) + 0.0425 (AC) + 0.0174 (FL)

N21. **Ans. is d, i.e. Bed rest** *Ref. Dutta Obs. 9/e, p 103*

- Femoral venous pressure is markedly raised in pregnancy especially in later months.
- *The pressure exerted by gravid uterus on the common iliac veins (more on right side due to dextrorotation of the uterus). causes pedal edema in pregnant women called as physiological edema of pregnancy.*
- **No treatment is required for physiological edema or orthostatic edema. It subsides on rest alone.**
- Diuretics should not be prescribed in case of physiological edema.

N22. **Ans. is c, i.e. Postdated pregnancy** *Ref. Textbook of Obstetrics Shiela Balakrishnan 1/e, p 407*

Friends-Teenage pregnancy is not only a new topic for PGME exams but has envolved as an emerging problem in our daily OPD'S

Hence I am giving it details about

TEENAGE PREGNANCY

Definition: Teenage pregnancy is defined as pregnancy occurring in a girl below the age of 19.
Incidence: Teenage pregnancy accounts for about 10–12% of all births.

Complications Maternal

In general, maternal mortality and morbidity are more among teenage pregnancies especially in the below 15 group and the unwed mothers because there is lack of antenatal care and a tendency to conceal the pregnancy in many cases.

   i. *Criminal and septic abortions* are more in these girls in spite of abortion being liberalized in India.

   ii. **Antepartum complications** like anaemia, malnutrition and pre-eclampsia are also much more in teenage pregnancy.

   iii. **Obstetric complications** are also increased like, preterm labour, fetal prematurity and IUGR. Cephalopelvic disproportion may be a problem in the very young teenagers, as they may not have attained complete skeletal maturity. Therefore, the incidence of caesarean section may be more in this group. Other labour complications are also increased if they present for the first time in labour, without proper antenatal care.

Long-Term consequences

   1. *Physical*. Induced abortions may increase the risk of recurrent miscarriage, preterm labour and low birth weight babies in the subsequent pregnancy. There is also a higher chance of infertility later on due to infection and blocked tubes. Early age of onset of sexual intercourse and first pregnancy increases the risk of cancer cervix and preinvasive lesions of the cervix. There is also an increased chance of sexually transmitted diseases in unmarried mothers.

   2. *Psychological, Social and educational problems*/–High suicide rates and depressive illness are common. Guilt feelings about a previous abortion or having given the baby for adoption, may occur, sometimes even years later. The girl may have to face social ostracim which would definitely affect her life.

     Problems of child –These mothers our not emotionally equipped to handle the responsibilities of motherhood. Hence there is poor maternal –child relationship, baby battering and behavioural disturbances in children of such mothers.

N23. **Ans. is a, i.e. 40 weeks** *Ref. Dutta Obs 7/e, p 64*

DURATION OF PREGNANCY: The duration of pregnancy has traditionally been calculated by the clinicians in terms of 10 lunar months or 9 calendar months and 7 days or 280 days or 40 weeks, calculated from the first day of the last menstrual period. This is called menstrual or gestational age.

But, fertilization usually occurs 14 days prior to the expected missed period and in a previously normal cycle of 28 days duration, it is about 14 days after the first day of the period. Thus, the true gestation period is to be calculated by subtracting 14 days from 280 days, i.e. 266 days. This is called fertilization or ovulatory age and is widely used by the embryologist.

N24. **Ans. is d, i.e. Yellow fever** *Ref. Williams Obs. 25/e, p 185-186 Table 8-10; Sheila Balakrishnan, p 696, 697*

Vaccines in pregnancy

Amongst the options given—hepatitis B and Rabies are absolutely safe. Cholera vaccine can be given during epidermis

- Yellow fever vaccine is an attenuated live virus vaccine and is contraindicated in pregnancy. The latest edition of Williams says that if the woman is travelling through an endemic area and cannot postpone her travel it may have to be given.[Q] But still the answer to this question is yellow fever.

N25. **Ans is b, i.e. Vagina**
Ref. Williams Obs 25/e, pg 52

During pregnancy, due to increased vascularity and hyperemia there is bluish discoloration of vagina. **This is called as Chadwick sign (Jacquemier sign).**

N26. **Ans is d, i.e. Hypothyroidism during pregnancy**
Ref. Williams Obs 25/e, p 52

Theca lutein cysts are bilateral cysts seen in ovary associated with markedly elevated levels of hCG.

Conditions of pregnancy where theca lutein cysts are seen:
- Molar pregnancy – ↑'ed level of hCG
- Diabetes
- Anti. D alloimmunization ⎤→ large placenta
- Multifetal gestation ⎦
- Chronic renal failure – decreased clearance of hCG
- Hyperthyroidism (hCG and TSH–anatomically similar)

Answers with Explanations to Previous Year Questions

1. **Ans. is b, i.e. Smoking**
Ref. Williams 22/e, p 213, 1012, Maternal Nutrition Kamini Rao, p 21-23; Handbook of Obesity: Eitology and Pathophysiology after 2/e, p 968

As discussed in text:
Smoking does not affect maternal weight gain during pregnancy, Smoking affects fetal weight gain and is one of the causes of IUGR.

"Studies have, indicated a lack of relationship between smoking and maternal weight gain while demonstrating a direct relationship between smoking and fetal grown rate." —Health Consequences of Smoking for Women (1985), p 237, 238

Remember: Rapid weight gain, i.e. more than 0.5 kg a week[Q] or 2 kg per month[Q] is an early manifestation of preeclampsia.[Q]
- Stationary or falling weight suggests IUGR or IUD[Q].
- In pregnancy – the amount of water retained is 6.5 L at term.[Q]

2. **Ans. is d, i.e. Increase in peripheral vascular resistance** *Ref. Dutta Obs. 7/e, p 52, 53; Fernando Arias 3/e, p 508, 509*

3. **Ans. is a, b, and e, i.e. ↑ed cardiac output; ↑ed tidal volume; and ↓ed plasma protein concentration**
Ref. Dutta Obs. 7/e, p 51, 53;

4. **Ans. is a and d, i.e. ↓ residual volume and ↓ hematocrit.**
Ref. Dutta Obs. 7/e, p 51, 53; Williams Obs. 23/e, p 121, 122 (see Pulmonary Function)
See the text explanation

5. **Ans. is c and d, i.e. Right axis deviation on ECG and Early diastolic murmur**

6. **Ans. is c, i.e. Shift of apical impulse laterally and upwards in the left 4th intercostal space**
Ref. Dutta Obs. 7/e, p 52; Williams Obs. 25/e, p 60–62, 119, 960

Clinical findings related to cardiovascular changes occuring during pregnancy:
- *Heart rate (resting) increases by about 10–15 bpm.[Q]*

- *Apex beat shifts to the 4th intercoastal space, 2.5 cm outside the mid clavicular line (as heart is pushed upwards, outward, with slight rotation to left).*[Q]
- Slightly enlarged cardiac silhouette.[Q] (marked enlarged cardiac silhouette is not normal in pregnancy)
- Exaggerated splitting of the first heart sound (both components loud).[Q]
- Second heart sound : Normal[Q]
- Third heart sound : Loud and easily auscultated.[Q]
- **Murmurs :**   – *Grade II systolic ejection murmur is* audible in aortic or pulmonary area at about 10–12 weeks due to expanded intravenous volume. It diappears in the beginning of postpartum period.
  - *Continuous hissing murmur*[Q] audible over tricuspid area in left 2nd and 3rd intercoastal spaces known as *Mammary murmur.*
- ECHO   – Shows increased left atrial and ventricular diameters.[Q]
- *ECG*   – *Shows left axis deviation.*[Q]
- Chest X-ray   – Straightening of left heart border.

 Note: None of the arrhythmia are normal during pregnancy, rather their presence indicates heart disease during pregnancy.

7. **Ans. is d, i.e. Increased peripheral vascular resistance**   *Ref: Dutta Obs. 7/e, p 51-53*

   As discussed in detail:
   - Blood volume increases during pregnancy
   - Cardiac output = Stroke volume × Heart rate

     All these three parameters increase during pregnancy
   - In pregnancy since the main hormone is progesterone, which has a smooth muscle relaxant effect so peripheral vascular resistance **decreases during pregnancy** (and not increases).

8. **Ans. is c, i.e. Increase in blood viscosity**   *Ref. Dutta Obs. 7/e, p 52, 263; Williams Obs. 25/e, p 54*

   In normal pregnancy – Since plasma volume increases more in comparison to Red cell volume so viscosity of blood decreases (not increases) i.e. *option "c"* is incorrect.[Q]
   - Since total hemoglobin mass increases during pregnancy. Therefore, oxygen carrying capacity of blood also increases (*William 23/e, p 115*). Therefore, *option "d"* is correct. **BEWARE** - *In pregnancy hemoglobin mass increases (to the extent of 18–20%) but hemoglobin concentration decreases due to hemodilution.*
   - Now let's have a look at **Iron metabolism in pregnancy.**
     - During pregnancy there is marked demand of extra iron especially in the second half.
     - Even an adequate diet cannot provide the extra demand of iron.

   Thus pregnancy is always a state of physiological iron deficiency.

   Changes in Iron Metabolism during Pregnancy:

Marker	Change
• Serum iron concentration	Decreases
• Serum ferritin (reflecting Iron stores)	Decreases
• Serum total iron binding capacity	Increases
• Percentage saturation (Serum ferritin/TIBC)	Decreases
• Serum transferrin	Increases

 Remember: The two Ts i.e. Transferrin and TIBC increase during pregnancy, rest all parameters of iron metabolism decrease during pregnancy.

9. **Ans. is a, b, d and e, i.e. Globulin; Fibrinogen; Leukocytes; and Transferrin**   *Ref. Dutta Obs. 7/e, p 52, 55, 263*

Increase during pregnancy	Decrease during pregnancy
• Hemoglobin[Q] mass	• Hemoglobin concentration
• Total plasma protein[Q]	• Factor XI and XIII

Contd...

• **Globulin**[Q]	• All parameters of iron metabolism except TIBC and transferrin
• **Leucocytes** (neutrophilic leucocytosis)	
• Fibrinogen[Q]	• Serum Urea[Q] ⟍ As their
• Factors II, VII, VIII, IX, X	• **Serum uric acid**[Q] ⟶ clearance
• Insulin[Q]	• Serum creatinine[Q] increases (normal in pregnancy is 0.7–0.9 mg/dL)
• Lipids, lipoproteins (LDL and HDL) and apolipoproteins	• Serum blood urea nitrogen[Q]
	• Serum Na/K/Ca/Mg/I_2
• **Serum Transferrin**[Q] **and TIBC.**	• Albumin
• C-reactive protein[Q]	• Platelets
• Placenta phosphatase[Q]	
• Total alkaline phosphatase[Q]	

10. **Ans. is a, c and d, i.e. Fibrinogen levels are increased, Sr. potassium is decreased and Sodium retention**

Ref. Dutta Obs. 7/e, p 52, 55, 57; William Obs. 25/e, p 57; Fernando Arias 3/e, p 490

- Pregnancy is a hyper coagulable state, all clotting factors are increased so serum fibrinogen levels are raised by 50% from 200–400 mg% in non pregnant to 300–600 mg% in pregnancy (i.e. *option "a"* is correct).
- Glomerular filtration rate is increased by 50% which means filtering capacity of the kidney is increased. So there is a decrease in maternal plasma levels of creatinine, blood urea nitrogen and uric acid (ruling out *option "b"*).
- In pregnancy there is active retention of Na[+], K[+] and water due to increased estrogen, progesterone, aldosterone and renin angiotensin activity (i.e. *option "d"* is correct).

And although there are increased total accumulation of sodium and potassium, their serum concentrations are decreased slightly because of expanded plasma volume... —*Williams Obs 25/e, p 57*

This fact is further strengthened by —*Fernando Arias 3/e, p 490*

"The average plasma sodium concentration during pregnancy is 136 mEq/L. This slight decrease in plasma sodium concentration during pregnancy is a result of the increased amount of filtered sodium caused by the increased GFR.

In fact during pregnancy the amount of sodium presented to the tubules for reabsorption is approximately 30240 mEq/L per day, whereas the nonpregnant woman filters only about 26160 mEq/L per day.

Although the efficiency of tubular sodium reabsorption during pregnancy is remarkable, the serum sodium equilibrates at slightly lower level than it does in nonpregnant status."

So though sodium retention and potassium retention occur in pregnant states, the serum concentrations are ultimately less than their non-pregnant status, i.e. *option "c"* and *"d"* both are correct.

11. **Ans. is a and b, i.e. Insulin levels increase; and Increased BMR**

Ref. Dutta Obs. 7/e, p 54, 62, 63

Hormones during pregnancy

Increased	Decreased	Unchanged
Growth hormone	LH	TSH
ACTH	FSH	ADH
Prolactin	S. iodine	
Thyroxine binding globulin	DHEA-S	
Total T3, T4		
Aldosterone		
Testosterone, androstenedione and cortisol		
Basal metabolic rate		
Insulin resistance		

Note: In pregnancy there is hyperinsulinemia but there is insulin resistance.

- In general plasma insulin level is increased, so as to ensure continuous supply of glucose to fetus.

To be specific: The overall effect of pregnancy is such that there is maternal fasting hypoglycemia (due to fetal consumption), whereas postprandial hyperglycemia and hyperinsulinemia.

12. **Ans. is a, c and e, i.e. Human placental lactogen; Progesterone; and Estrogen** *Ref. Dutta Obs. 7/e, p 54*

During pregnancy insulin levels are increased because of increased insulin secretion as well as increase in insulin resistance due to a number of contra insulin factors.

These are:
- *Estrogen*
- *Progesterone*
- *Human placental lactogen (HPL)*
- Cortisol
- Prolactin

Note:
- The main hormone responsible for insulin resistance is HPL
- Insulin resistance is maximum between 24–28 weeks of pregnancy.

13. **Ans. is e, i.e. Benign gestational** *Ref. Fernando Arias 3/e, p 475, Williams Obs, 23/e, p 1093*

Gestational thrombocytopenia/Benign Gestational Thrombocytopenia

It is the most common cause of thrombocytopenia accounting for 80–90% of all cases of thrombocytopenia occuring during pregnancy.
- Exact cause is not known (may be due to hemodilution and increased platelet consumption)
- Platelet count is rarely <70,000/mm³.
- Women are asymptomatic and there is no H/O bleeding.
- Condition is benign and has no risk to mother or infant.
- The only problem associated with it is - that anaesthesiologists are reluctant to give epidural or spinal anaesthesia if platelet count is < 1 lakh/mm³.
- Treatment with steroids and IgG or platelet transfusion before delivery is sometimes necessary.

14. **Ans. is b, i.e. Insulin** *Ref. Ghai 6/e, p 2, Dutta obs 7/e, p 42*

Fetal growth is predominantly controlled by:
1. IGF-1
2. Insulin
3. Other growth factors

Growth hormone is required for postnatal growth of fetus.

15. **Ans. is b, i.e. ↑ed number of lactobacilli** *Ref. Williams Obs. 23/e, p 111*

Changes in vagina during pregnancy:
- Increased vascularity and hyperemia (causes – violet colour characteristic of Chadwick sign).
- **Vaginal pH:** decreases i.e. becomes acidic and varies from 3.5 to 6.
- *Increase in number of lactobacillus acidophilus*[Q] *(which act on glycogen and cause increased production of lactic acid therefore, pH becomes more acidic).*
- As pH of vagina becomes acidic – it inhibits the growth of pathogenic bacteria.
- Histopathology:
- Early in pregnancy, the vaginal epithelial cells are similar to those seen in the luteal phase.
- **As pregnancy advances:**
  - Small intermediate cells known as **Navicular cells** are seen in abundance in small clusters.
  - Vesicular nuclei without cytoplasm or so called **Naked nuclei,** are also seen along with abundant Lactobacillus.

16. **Ans. is d, i.e. Oxytocin is used for inducing abortion in Ist trimester** *Ref. Dutta Obs. 7/e, p 177; Ganong 20/e, p 238*

Lets see each option one by one
- Oxytocin causes contraction of smooth muscles of uterus. The sensitivity of uterine musculature to oxytocin is enhanced by estrogen and inhibited by progesterone. The sensitivity of uterus to oxytocin becomes very much increased in late pregnancy. Oxytocin levels reach maximum at the time of birth (i.e. *option "a"* is correct).

- In lactating women genital stimulation enhances oxytocin release (*option "c"* is correct).
- Prostaglandins are used in Ist and IInd trimester for induction of abortion.

I can not understand what the examiner wants to say by *"IIIrd trimester abortion"* as beyond 28 weeks fetus is viable therefore, term abortion is never used. It may be a printing mistake.

As far as *option "d"* is concerned – It is absolutely incorrect as oxytocin is never used for Ist trimester abortions.

Friends don't get upset, if you don't remember *"methods used of inducing abortion"* right now, as we have dealt with it in detail in chapter *"Abortion & MTP"*.

17. **Ans. is a, b, c and e, i.e. Hyperplasia of parathyroid, Hyperplasia of thyroid, Increased pigmentation and Increased insulin**   *Ref: Dutta Obs 9/e, p 56 to 58; Williams, Obs 23/e, p 128 for a, 127 for b, 111 for c and 113 for e*

- In pregnancy- there is hyperplasia of the Thyroid, Parathyroid, Pituitary and Adrenal Cortex
- Although the size of thyroid gland increases, patient remains euthyroid.
- Basal metabolic rate increases (i.e. **option 'd'** is incorrect)
- There is hyperinsulinemia during pregnancy (due to insulin resistance) so as to ensure continuous supply of glucose to fetus.

Skin changes during pregnancy

During pregnancy, skin undergoes varying degrees of pigmentation, which varies among individuals. The dark line running centrally below the umbilicus is **called the linea nigra.**

Chloasma: It is hyperpigmentation of the skin around the cheeks, forehead and eyes. The pigmentation is thought to be due to increased levels of endorphins and melanocyte stimulating hormone and disappears spontaneously after delivery.

18. **Ans. is d, i.e Corpus luteum**   *Ref. Read below*

In the initial few weeks—the main source of estrogen and progesterone during pregnancy is corpus luteum

19. **Ans. is a, b, c and d, i.e. Hegar's sign; Palmer's sign; Goodell's sign; and Osiander's sign**

Ref. Dutta Obs. 9/e, p 61

See the text for explanation

20. **Ans. is c, i.e. Softening of isthmus**   *Ref. Dutta Obs. 9/e, p 61*

- Hegar's sign is present in 2/3rd cases and is demonstrated between 6–10 weeks.
- The sign is based on the fact that - upper part of the body is enlarged by the growing fetus whereas lower part of the body of the uterus, i.e. isthmus is empty and soft and cervix is comparatively firm. Because of these variations in consistency- on bimanual examination, the abdominal and vaginal fingers seem to appose below body of the uterus.

21. **Ans. is a and d, i.e. Braxton Hicks contraction; and Quickening**   *Ref. Dutta Obs. 9/e, p 63, 64*

Second trimester of pregnancy (13–28 weeks) can be diagnosed by:

Quickening and Braxton hicks contractions are seen in 2nd trimester. Lightening is seem in 3rd trimester show is seen during initiation of labor.

22. **Ans. is c, d and e, i.e. Fetal heart activity; Fetal movement by examiner; and Fetal sac in USG**

Ref. Dutta Obs. 9/e, p 68

Positive or absolute signs of pregnancy:

- **Palpation of fetal parts and perception of fetal movements by examiner, at about 20 weeks.**
- **Auscultation of fetal heart sounds.**
- USG evidence of embryo (at **6th week**) and later[Q] on of the fetus.
- Radiological demonstration of fetal skeleton at 16 **weeks and onwards.**

Friends there is no need to mug up the presumptive/probable signs of pregnancy. Generally it is not asked in exams.

Also remember: These positive or absolute signs of pregnancy are never seen in pseudocyesis or phantom pregnancy.

23. **Ans. is b, i.e. 16–20 weeks**   *Ref. Dutta Obs 9/e, p 63: Reddy 27/e, p 434*

"Quickening (feeling of life) denotes the perception of active fetal movements by the women. It is usually felt about the 18th week[Q], 2 weeks earlier in multiparae. Its appearance is a useful guide to calculate the expected date of delivery with reasonable accuracy"   *Ref. Dutta Obs, 9/e, p 63*

"Quickening is felt between 16th to 20th week[Q]"   —*Reddy 27/e, p 343*

Phenomenon	Time
Palpation of fetal part	20 weeks
Active fetal movement felt by placing a hand on abdomen	20 weeks
External ballottement	20 weeks
Internal ballottement	16–28 weeks
FHS audible by Stethoscope	18–20 weeks
Fetal movement can be detected by Doppler	10 weeks
Lightening	38 weeks

24. Ans. is a, i.e. Folic acid *Ref. Dutta Obs. 9/e, p 383; COGDT 10/e, p 197*

25. Ans. is a, i.e. Neural tube defect *Ref. Dutta Obs. 9/e, p 383; COGDT 10/e, p 197*

26. Ans. is d, i.e. Before conception *Ref. Dutta Obs. 9/e, p 383; COGDT 10/e, p 197*

"Folic acid has been shown to effectively reduce the risk of neural tube defects (NTD's). A daily 4 mg dose is recommended for patients who have had a previous pregnancy affected by neural tube defects. It should be started atleast 1 month (ideally 3 months) prior to pregnancy and continued through the first 6–12 weeks of pregnancy."

Ref. COGDT 10/e, p 197

Remember: Folic acid is used to reduce the risk of neural tube defect.

- More than half of NTDs could be prevented with daily intake of 400 µg of folic acid throughout the periconceptional period.
- *Thus dose* of folic acid which is given to all pregnant females = 0.4 mg, i.e. 400 mcg (also called as prophylactic dose).
- A woman with a prior pregnancy complicated by a neural tube defect can reduce the 23% recurrence risk by more than 70% if she takes 4 mg of folic acid for the month before conception and for the first trimester of pregnancy. This called a therapeutic dose of folic acid.
- *Therapeutic* dose of folic acid (to be given in females with previous history of baby with NTD)—4 mg.
- **Duration:** It should be started 1 month before conception and continued till first 6–12 weeks of pregnancy.
- **Dose of folic acid** given to pregnant women with megaloblastic anemia = 1 mg day.

27. Ans. b, i.e. 24 hours after delivery *Ref. Jeffcoates 7/e, p 286*

Kiegels exercise are pelvic floor exercises which consists of contracting and relaxing the muscles that form part of the pelvic floor.

The aim of Kegel exercises is to improve muscle tone by strengthening the pubococcygeus muscles of the pelvic floor.

Kegel exercises are good for treating vaginal prolapse, preventing uterine prolapse and to aid with child birth in females and for treating prostate pain and swelling resulting from benign prostatic hyperplasia (BPH) and prostatitis in males. These exercises reduce premature ejaculatory occurrences in men as well as increase the size and intensity of erections.

Kegel exercises may be beneficial in treating urinary incontinence in both men and women (The treatment effect might be greater in middle aged women in their 40s and 50s with stress urinary incontinence alone...".)

Kegels exercises - Time for initiating kegels exercise:

- Pregnancy-1st trimester
- After vaginal delivery-after 24 hours
- After cesarean section-after 24 hours.

28. Ans. d, i.e. Cardiac output *Ref: Dutta 7/e p 51-53; Williams 24/e p 59*

All the four options given in the question increase during pregnancy. Even cardiac output at term is more as compared to a non-pregnant female, but it is lesser than first and second trimester, mainly due to IVC compression (see Fig. 5.1). Hence, cardiac output is option of choice here.

29. Ans. is a, i.e. 1, 3 and 4

As discussed is text, options

1, 3, 4 dont need further explanation

Lets see how blood volume changes in accrue pregnancy

"Maternal blood volume begin to accure during the first trimester, By 12 weeks plasma volume expands by approximately 15% compared with that prior to pregnancy. Maternal blood volume grows most rapidly during the third trimester. and reaches a plateau during the last several weeks of pregnancy. The well known hypervolemia associated with pregnancy averages 40–45% above non pregnant blood volume after 32–34 weeks gestation." *Williams obs 25/e p 57*

Thus from above lines it is clear that option 1 is correct

Now as far as cardiac output is concerned it reaches maximum i.e. about 40–50% by 28–32 weeks (not 20%) hence it is incorrect.

30. **Ans. is c, i.e. 16th October**

EDD can be calculated by Naegele's formula

EDD= LMP + 9 months and 7 days

So to January add 9 months= October

To 9 add 7=16

Hence LMP of the female becomes- 16th october

31. **Ans. is a, i.e. Pawlick's grip.**

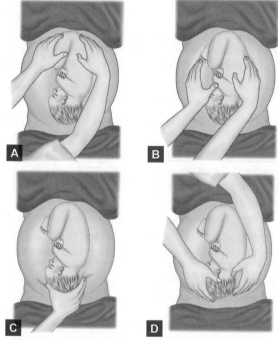

Obstetric grips (Leopold maneuvers)

(i) 1st leopold maneuver/Fundal grip: The palpation is done facing the patient's face. The whole of the fundal area is palpated using both hands laid flat on it to find out which pole of the fetus is lying in the fundus: (a) broad, soft and irregular mass suggestive of breech, or (b) smooth, hard and globular mass suggestive of head. In transverse lie, neither of the fetal poles are palpated in the fundal area.

(ii) Second leopold maneuver/Lateral or umbilical grip: The palpation is done facing the patient's face. The hands are to be placed flat on either side of the umbilicus to palpate one after the other, the sides and front of the uterus to find out the **position of the back, limbs and the anterior shoulder.** The back is suggested by smooth curved and resistant feel.

(iii) Pawlick's grip/Pelvic grip 2 (Third Leopold): The examination is done facing towards the patient's face. The overstretched thumb and four fingers of the right hand are placed over the lower pole of the uterus keeping the ulnar border of the palm on the upper border of the symphysis pubis. When the fingers and the thumb are approximated, the presenting part is grasped distinctly (if not engaged) and also the mobility from side to side is tested. In transverse lie, Pawlick's grip is empty.

(iv) Pelvic grip 1 (Fourth Leopold): The examination is done facing the patient's feet. Four fingers **of both the hands** are placed on either side of the midline in the lower pole of the uterus and parallel to the inguinal ligament. The fingers are pressed downwards and backwards in a manner of approximation of finger tips to palpate the part occupying the lower pole of the uterus (presentation). If it is head, the characteristics to note are: (1) precise presenting area (2) attitude and (3) engagement.

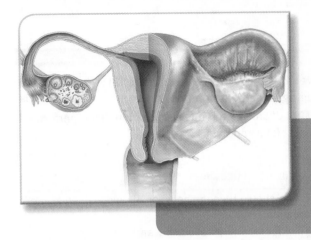

6

Diagnosis in Obstetrics and Fetal Monitoring

Chapter at a Glance

USG IN OBSTETRICS

BASICS ABOUT ULTRASOUND

- *Ultrasound* refers to sound waves traveling at a frequency above 20,000 hertz (cycles per second).
- Higher frequency transducers yield better image resolution, whereas lower frequencies penetrate tissue more effectively.
- Transducers use wide-bandwidth technology to perform within a range of frequencies. In early pregnancy, a 5- to 10-megahertz (MHz) transvaginal transducer usually provides excellent resolution because the early fetus is close to the transducer.
- And, in the first and second trimesters, a 4- to 6 MHz transabdominal transducer is similarly close enough to the fetus to yield precise image.
- By the third trimester, a lower frequency 2- to 5-MHz transducer may be needed for tissue penetration—particularly in obese patients.

FETAL SAFETY

- Sonography should be performed only for a valid medical indication, using the lowest possible exposure setting to gain necessary information—the *ALARA* principle— *a*s *l*ow *a*s *r*easonably *a*chievable.

- The International Society of Ultrasound in Obstetrics and Gynecology (2016) further concludes that there is no scientifically proven association between ultrasound exposure in the first to second trimesters and autism spectrum disorder or its severity.

- All sonography machines are required to display two indices: the *thermal index* and the *mechanical index*. The **thermal index** is a measure of the relative probability that the examination may raise the temperature, potentially high enough to induce injury. Fetal damage resulting from commercially available ultrasound equipment in routine practice is extremely unlikely. The potential for temperature elevation is higher with longer examination time and is greater near bone than in soft tissue. Theoretical risks are higher during organogenesis than later in gestation. The thermal index is higher with pulsed Doppler applications than with routine B-mode scanning.

- In the first trimester, if pulsed Doppler is clinically indicated, the thermal index should be ≤ 0.7, and the exposure time should be as brief as possible (American Institute of Ultrasound in Medicine, 2016). To document the embryonic or fetal heart rate, motion-mode (M-mode) imaging is used instead of pulsed Doppler imaging.

- The ***mechanical index*** is a measure of the likelihood of adverse effects related to rare factional pressure, such as cavitation—which is relevant only in tissues that contain air.

> *Note:* In mammalian tissues that do not contain gas bodies, no adverse effects have been reported over the range of diagnostically relevant exposures. Because foetuses cannot contain gas bodies, they are not considered at risk.

REASONS OF USG DURING PREGNANCY

USG during pregnancy is done for a number of reasons

1. Estimation of gestational age
2. Evaluation of fetal growth in single or multifetal growth
3. Vaginal bleeding of undetermined etiology in pregnancy
4. Determination of fetal presentation when the presenting part cannot be adequately assessed in labor
5. Suspected multiple gestation
6. Adjunct to amniocentesis/CVS
7. Significant uterine size/clinical dates discrepancy
8. Pelvis mass detected clinically
9. Suspected hydatidiform mole
10. Adjunct to cervical cerclage
11. Suspected ectopic pregnancy
12. Suspected fetal death
13. IUCD localization
14. Ovarian follicle development and surveillance
15. Biophysical profile for fetal well-being (after 28 weeks gestation)
16. Observation of intrapartum events (e.g. version/manual removal of placenta)
17. Suspected polyhydramnios or oligohydramnios
18. Suspected abruptio placenta
19. Adjunct to external version from breech to vertex presentation
20. Estimation of fetal weight and/or presentation in PROM or premature labor
21. Abnormal alpha fetoprotein
22. H/O previous congenital anomaly

Ultrasound Terminology

Level 1: Examination (**Routine/Basic examination**)

This is routine examination done during pregnancy to detect pregnancy for dating, number of fetus, for amniotic fluid, localization of placenta, etc.

Level 2: (**Targeted examination/TIFFA: Targeted imaging for fetal anomalies**)

It is a detailed anatomic examination that is performed to detect fetal anomalies.

 Important One Liners

- TIFFA should be done between 18 and 20 weeks in all pregnant females
- Time for routine ultrasound scan:
  - At the booking visit in first trimester
  - 18–22 weeks
  - In third trimester
- If throughout pregnancy only one ultrasound has to be done—best time to that ultrasound is 18–20 weeks
- Best time to do USG to localize placenta: 3rd trimester
- Best time to do USG to detect chorionicity in twins: 11 to 14 weeks
- Wavelength of USG used in obstetrics
  - TAS (transabdominal scan): 3 to 5 Hz
  - TVS (transvaginal scan): 5 to 10 Hz

THE FIRST TRIMESTER ULTRASOUND EXAMINATION

For Diagnosis of Pregnancy

Feature	TVS	TAS
Gestational sac	4 week 1 day–4 week 3 days	5 weeks
Yolk sac	5 weeks definitely by 5.5	6–7 weeks
Cardiac activity	6 weeks	7–8 weeks

Note: Fetal heart starts pulsating by 36–37 days

 Note: The embryo should be visible transvaginally once the mean sac diameter has reached 25 min —otherwise the gestation is **anembryonic**. Cardiac motion is usually visible with transvaginal imaging when the embryo length reaches 5 mm.

In embryos < 7 mm without cardiac activity, subsequent examination may be needed to determine viability (American College of Obstetricians and Gynecologists, 2016). (See Fig. 6.1A and B)

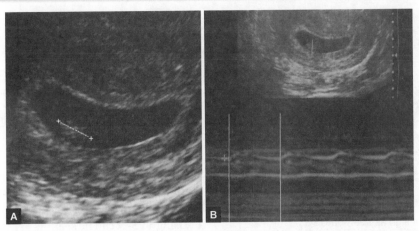

Figs. 6.1A and B: (A) The measured crown-rump length is approximately 7 mm in this 6 weeks embryo; (B) M-mode demonstrates embryonic cardiac activity and a heart rate of 124 beats per minute.

Gestational Sac

- The first sign of pregnancy on USG **is appearance of gestational sac.**
- At sonography, the earliest appearance of a gestational sac is a small round fluid collection surrounded completely by a hyperechogenic rim of tissue (Fig. 6.2).

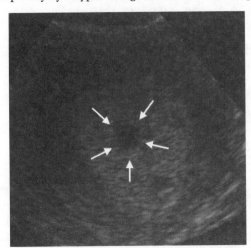

Fig. 6.2: An early gestational sac, measuring 4 mm in diameter, is visible as a small fluid-filled structure (the chorionic cavity) surrounded by an echogenic rim of tissue (chorionic villi and adjacent decidual tissue)

- The size of gestational sac must be determined by calculating the mean sac diameter (MSD).
- This value is obtained by adding the three orthogonal dimensions of chronic cavity and dividing by 3 (Fig. 6.3).
- The position of normal gestational sac is mid to upper uterus.
- As the sac implants into the decidualized endometrium, it lies adjacent to the linear central cavity echo

complex, without initially displacing or deforming the hyperechogenic anatomic landmark (**This is called intradecidual sign**) (Figs. 6.4 and 6.5).

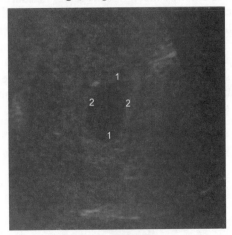

Fig. 6.3: Measurement of MSD

- Intradecidual sign is positive in intrauterine pregnancy. But it is very difficult to differentiate between ectopic and intrauterine pregnancy on the basis of this sign.

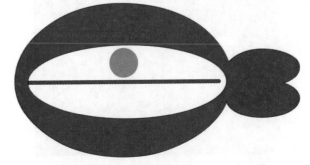

Fig. 6.4: The sac (black dot) implanting in the endometrium (white) without displacing the central cavity echo complex

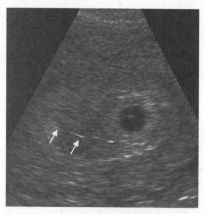

Fig. 6.5: Intradecidual sign as seen on USG

- As the sac enlarges, it gradually impresses and deforms the central cavity echo complex giving rise to a characteristic sonographic appearance called **Double decidual sac sign** (Figs. 6.6 and 6.7)
- The sign is present when MSD is ≥ 10 mm.
- It consists of two concentric echogenic lines, surrounding a part of the gestational sac.

  The line closest to the sac represents combined smooth chorion-decidua capsularis, whereas the one which is peripherally located represents decidua parietalis.
- This sign is seen on USG (TAS) between 5 to 6 weeks can confirm the presence of intrauterine pregnancy before a yolk sac is visualized.

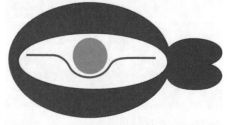

Fig. 6.6: The sac impressing on the central cavity echo complex

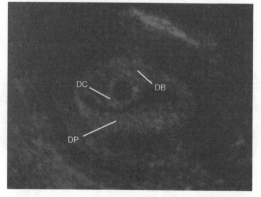

Fig. 6.7: The double decidual sac sign. The first sac is formed by decidua capsularis (DC) and second by decidua parietalis (DP)

Blood Flow in Early Pregnancy

- The characteristic first trimester uterine artery waveform consists of high resistance flow with a prominent diastolic notch.
- The diastolic notch typically disappears during second trimester (in some cases by 13 weeks). If diastolic notch persists, it indicates in future this female can have PIH or placental abnormalities.

Yolk Sac

- Yolk sac is the first anatomic structure seen with in gestational sac
- Using TVS- it can be seen:
  - As early as 5th week (MSD = 5 mm)
  - Definitely by 5.5 weeks (MSD = 8 mm)
- By TAS definitely it is seen by 7 weeks (MSD = 20 mm).
- Presence of yolk sac in the gestational sac is 100% confirmatory of intrauterine pregnancy.

Identification of Embryo and Cardiac Activity

- Cardiac contraction begin by 36-37 days gestational age
- Cardiac activity should be visible by:
  6 weeks on TVS (MSD = 13–18 mm)
  8 Weeks on TAS (MSD = 25 mm)
- During first trimester, cardiac rate should be recorded using M-mode.

 Remember: Distinctly appearing human embryo with hand and feet and no tail is seen by 10 weeks.

For Determination of Gestational Age

Remember: The earlier that sonography is performed, the more accurate the gestational age assessment. The only exception to revising the gestational age based on early sonography is if the pregnancy resulted from assisted reproductive technology, in which case accuracy of gestational age assessment is presumed.

- Sonographic measurement of the crown-rump length (CRL) is the most accurate method to establish or confirm gestational age.

Mean Sac Diameter

- Mean sac diameter (MSD) is a sonographic measurement of the gestational sac.
- Mean sac diameter measurement is used to determine gestational age before Crown Rump length can be clearly measured

- MSD = (length + height + width)/3
- Normal MSD (in mm) + 30 = days of pregnancy, i.e. MSD = 5 mm then gestational age = 35 days or 7 weeks.

Crown Rump Length

- Longest straight line measurement of the embryo from the outer margin of cephalic pole to rump midsagittal plane with fetus in neutral, non fixed position (Fig. 6.8).
- Best seen on TVS
- The measurement should include neither yolksac nor limb bud.

Overall best USG parameter to assess fetal age

- Ideal time to measure CRL is 7–10 weeks (error = /– 3 days)
- It is used as a marker for assessment of fetal age up to 14 weeks or till CRL is 84 mm.
- Smallest CRL at which embryo is visible on TVS-3–4 mm.

Until 13 weeks gestation, CRL is accurate to within 5 to 7 days (AOG 2017B).

A CRL of ≥7 mm with no cardiac activity seen or MSD ≥ 25 mm with no yolk sac indicates missed abortion.

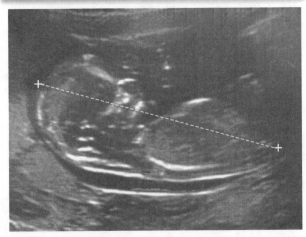

Fig. 6.8: The measured crown-rump length in this 12-week 3-day fetus approximates 6 cm.

 Key Concept

- Overall best parameter to determine fetal age: Crown Rump Length
- Best time to do USG to determine fetal age: 1st trimester
- Best USG parameter to determine gestational age in first trimester: CRL

Diagnosis of Fetal Anomalies (Excluding Nuchal Translucency)

By 10 weeks of gestational age, the fetal cranium, brain, neck, trunk and extremities can be visualized and gross anomalies can be detected in first trimester.

Anencephaly

- Earliest anomaly to be detected on USG: Anencephaly
- Anencephaly can be detected earliest by: 10 weeks
- For best diagnosis of anencephaly, USG should be done at 14 weeks
- Signs of Anencephaly on USG:
  - Fetal head has an irregular contour and no bone
  - No calcified cranium (Fig. 6.9)
  - Face shows-**Mickey mouse sign** (Fig. 6.9)
  - Eyes of fetus are big-**Frog eye sign** (Fig. 6.10)

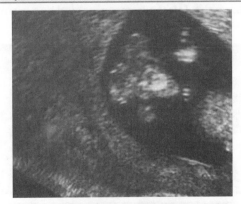

Fig. 6.9: Mickey mouse sign in anencephaly on USG.

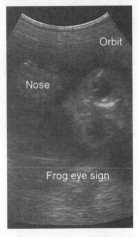

Fig. 6.10: Frog eye sign seen on **USG** in anencephaly.

Other Defects Detected in 1st Trimester

- The presence of large cystic spaces behind the fetal head, neck and trunk, like thickening of the nuchal translucency are called **cystic hygromas or lymphangiectasia.** These are associated with abnormal chromosomes, particularly trisomy 13, 18, 21 and Turner syndrome.

- **Large ventral wall defects, such as omphalocele** and **gastroschisis, can be differentiated from physiologic** bowel herniation based on the size of the protruding anterior abdominal mass and persistence of mass beyond 12 weeks GA.

  If the size of the mass before 12 weeks GA is more the 7 mm, a ventral wall defect should be suspected and follow up sonography should be performed after 12 weeks GA to confirm the diagnosis.

- **The protruding mass of an omphalocele typically has a smooth and rounded contour (Fig. 6.11A) because the extruded abdominal contents are contained by a peritoneal membrane. The contour of gastroschisis is typically irregular, because bowel looks protruding through the defect are not contained by a membrane (Fig. 6.11B).**

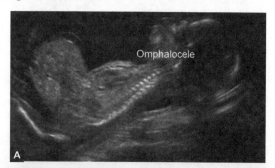

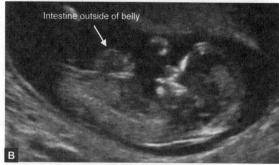

Figs. 6.11A and B: (A) Omphalocele with smooth contour; (B) Gastroschisis with irregular contour on USG

Twin Pregnancy

- The best time to detect chorionicity in twin pregnancy is 1st trimester
- In dichorionic twins on USG: Twin peak sign is seen (details given in Chapter 17)
- Twin peak sign is seen due to presence of chorion
- Best seen between 11–14 weeks

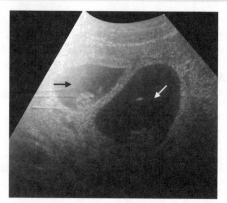

Fig. 6.12: USG of dichorionic twin showing twin peak sign

 Note: The placental tissue coming in between the two twins.

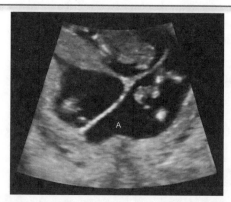

Fig. 6.13: USG of trichorionic twins showing 'Ipsilon zone'

- In triplet pregnancy a variation of twin peak sign is seen. In trichorionic twins the junction of the three interfetal membranes is seen called 'ipsilon zone'.

SECOND TRIMESTER USG EXAMINATION

Fetal Biometry

Biparietal Diameter

Prerequisites for measuring BPD:
- Fetal head should be perpendicular to ultrasound beam
- Fetal head should appear oval, symmetrical
- Third ventricle and thalamus should be seen called as bithalamic view
- Cavum septum pellucidum should be visible
- Cerebellum and orbit should not be seen
- BPD is measured from outer aspect of skull on one side to inner aspect of skull on other side

- HC is measured in the same plane as BPD
- It is measured by measuring the circumference in the outer aspect of the skull.

Significance: BPD is the best parameter for fetal age after 14 weeks and until 20 weeks.

 Note: Head circumference is more reliable than BPD-for fetal age when there is alteration in shape like dolichocephaly and brachycephaly.

 Note: Until 13 6/7 weeks gestation, the CRL is accurate to within 5 to 7 days (American College of Obstetricians and Gynecologists, 2017b).

- Starting at 14 0/7 weeks, equipment software formulas calculate estimated gestational age and fetal weight from measurements of the biparietal diameter, head and abdominal circumference, and femur length. The estimates are most accurate when multiple parameters are used but may over- or underestimate fetal weight by up to 20 percent (American College of Obstetricians and Gynecologists, 2016).

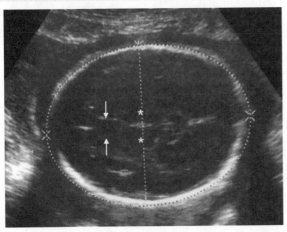

Fig. 6.14: Fetal biometry. Transthalamic view. A transverse (axial) image of the head is obtained at the level of the cavum septum pellucidum (arrows) and thalami (asterisks). The biparietal diameter is measured perpendicular to the sagittal midline, from the outer edge of the skull in the near field to the inner edge of the skull in the far field. By conversion, the near field is that which is closer to the sonographic transducer. The head circumference is measured circumferentially around the outer border of the skull.

Femur Length

- Full length of the femur should be visible
- Femur should be perpendicular to ultrasound beam
- Calipers should be placed at the junction of bone and cartilage. Femoral head should not be measured and epiphysis should be excluded.
  Clinical significance: It is the best parameter for gestational age in 3rd trimester.
- Femur can be visualized by 10 weeks GA.

- Gestational age estimation, it has a variation of 7 to 11 days in the second trimester.
- A femur measurement that is < 2.5th percentile for gestational age or that is shortened to < 90 percent of that expected based on the measured BPD is a minor marker for Down syndrome.
- The normal range for the FL to abdominal circumference (AC) ratio is generally 20 to 24 percent.
- A dramatically foreshortened FL or a FL-to-AC ratio below 18 percent prompts evaluation for a skeletal dysplasia.

 Also Know:
- Pregnancies not imaged prior to 22 weeks to confirm or revise gestational age are considered suboptimally dated (American College of Obstetricians and Gynecologists, 2017).

Abdominal Circumference

- It is the parameter affected most by fetal growth
- It is the best parameter for fetal growth, be it IUGR or macrosomia.

- In the plane for measuring abdominal circumference (AC)—Following landmarks should be visible (Fig. 6.15A and B):
  1. Felt stomach
  2. Umbilical vein
  3. Portal sinus
  Following should not be visible:
  1. Kidneys
  2. Umbilical cord insertion

- This is the plane at which liver is seen in maximum diameter.
- **Significance:** AC is the single best USG parameter for fetal growth.
- AC ≥ 35 cms means macrosomia.

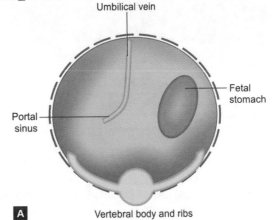

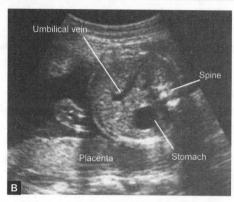

Figs. 6.15A and B: Plane for measuring abdominal circumference. (A) Diagrammatic representation; (B) USG view

Detection of Congenital Anomalies

Spina Bifida

- Spina bifida can be reliably diagnosed with second trimester sonography.

Ultrasonographic signs indicating Spina bifida...
Williams Obs. 25/e, p 193

- Small biparietal diameter.
- Ventriculomegaly.
- Frontal bone scalloping (**the so-called lemon sign**).[Q]
- Elongation and downward displacement of the cerebellum (**the so-called banana sign**) Figs. 6.16A and B.[Q]
- Effacement or obliteration of the cisterna magna.

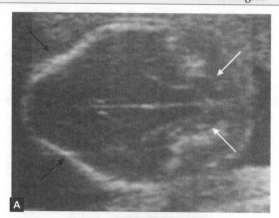

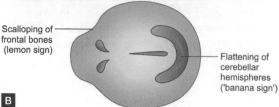

Figs. 6.16A and B: (A) Lemon sign-black arrows and banana sign-white arrows on USG; (B) Diagrammatic representation

Scalloping of frontal bones (lemon sign)

Flattening of cerebellar hemispheres ('banana sign')

Remember:

It is recommended that sonography be routinely offered to all pregnant women between 18 and 22 weeks gestation (American College of Obstetricians and Gynecologists, 2016). This time interval permits accurate assessment of gestational age, fetal anatomy, placental location, and cervical length.

FETAL MALFORMATIONS

NEURAL TUBE DEFECTS

- These result from incomplete closure of the neural tube by the embryonic age of 26 to 28 days. They are the second most common class of malformations after cardiac anomalies.
- **Anencephaly** is characterized by absence of the cranium and telencephalic structures, with the skull base and orbits covered only by angiomatous stroma. **Acrania** is absence of the cranium, with protrusion of disorganized brain tissue. Both are generally grouped together, and anencephaly is considered to be the final stage of acrania.
- **Cephalocele**—herniation of meninges through a cranial defect. When brain tissue herniates through the skull defect, the anomaly is termed an **encephalocele**.
- Cephalocele is an important feature of the autosomal recessive **Meckel-Gruber syndrome**.
- **Spina bifida** is a defect in the vertebrae, typically the dorsal arch, with exposure of the meninges and spinal cord.

Risk Factors for Neural Tube Defect

1. Diabetes—hyperglycemia
2. Medications—valproic acid, carbamazepine, coumadin, thalidomide, efavirenz
3. Family history—multifactorial inheritance
4. Syndromes with autosomal recessive inheritance—Meckel-Gruber, Roberts
5. Aneuploidy—trisomy 13 and 18, triploidy.

Recurrence

The recurrence risk of NTDs is:
- If H/O one affected child = 5%
- If H/O two affected children = 13%.

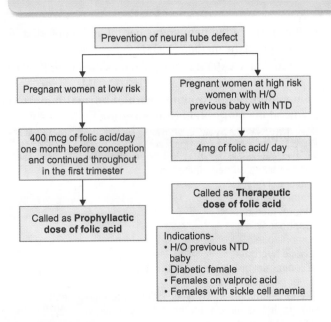

Anencephaly

Anencephaly is characterized by absence of the cranium and telencephalic structures above the level of the skull base and orbits. *Acrania* is absence of the cranium with protrusion of disorganized brain tissue. Both are uniformly lethal and are generally considered together, with anencephaly as the final stage of acrania.

Pathological Features

- Forebrain and midbrain are absent
- Cerebellum and hindbrain are less involved or completely spared
- Base of skull and facial bones are not affected
- Pituitary gland is either absent or hypoplastic.[Q]
- As a result: Adrenal gland is diminished in size.[Q]
- Such fetuses have *bulging eyes, short neck* and a *large tongue.*
- 70% cases are female.

Complications

Caused by Anencephaly during Pregnancy:

- **Polyhydramnios:** seen in 35% cases.[Q]
  Causes:
  - Diminished fetal swallowing[Q]
  - Secretion of CSF directly into the amniotic cavity[Q]
  - Excessive micturition.[Q]
- **Preterm labor:** due to associated polyhydramnios
- **Malpresentation:** face presentation (most common)[Q] and breech presentation

- **Most common fetal anomaly responsible for face presentation is anencephaly.**

- Tendency for **postmaturity.**[Q]
  Cause: Insufficient production of DHEA from fetal adrenals leading to diminished estriol.

Complications during Labor

- **Shoulder dystocia**[Q]**:** Most common complication of anencephaly during labor. This is **pseudo shoulder dystocia**.
- Obstructed labor.[Q]

Risk of recurrence is 5% after one affected child and 13% after two affected children.[Q]

Diagnosis

Screening Methods

- **Most common screening method to detect anencephaly is elevated levels of maternal serum alpha-fetoproteins.**[Q]
- **All pregnant women are offered screening for fetal open neural-tube defects in the second trimester, either with MSAFP screening or with sonography (American College of Obstetricians and Gynecologists, 2016c). Measurement of the MSAFP concentration between 15 and 20 weeks gestation has been offered as part of routine prenatal care for more than 30 years.**
- **Most specific marker for diagnosis of anencephaly—** acetylcholinesterase.
- **IOC is ultrasound:** These anomalies are often diagnosed in the late first trimester, and with adequate visualization, virtually all cases may be diagnosed in the second trimester. Inability to image the BPD raises suspicion. The face often appears triangular, and sagittal images readily demonstrate absence of the ossified cranium. Hydramnios from impaired fetal swallowing is common in the third trimester.

Management

Termination of pregnancy irrespective of gestational age.

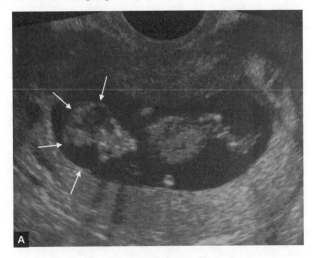

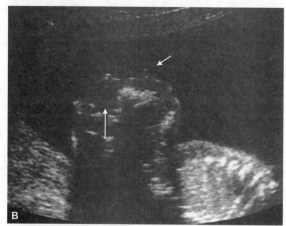

Figs. 6.17A and B: Anencephaly/acrania. (A) Acrania. This 11-week fetus has absence of the cranium, with protrusion of a disorganized mass of brain tissue that resembles a "shower cap" (*arrows*) and a characteristic triangular facial appearance; (B) Anencephaly. This sagittal image shows the absence of forebrain and cranium above the skull base and orbit. The long white arrow points to the fetal orbit, and the short white arrow indicates the nose

ALPHA FETOPROTEIN

- It is a glycoprotein[Q] synthesized by the fetal yolk sac[Q] in the early weeks of gestation and by the gastrointestinal tract[Q] and liver[Q] later.
- It is the most abundant protein in the fetal serum.
- It circulates in fetal serum and passes into fetal urine and amniotic fluid.
- Concentration of AFP increases steadily in fetal serum till 13 weeks[Q], (3 mg/mL) after which the level rapidly decreases throughout the rest of pregnancy.
- AFP level in fetal serum declines following birth and by one year of age, its concentration is 1 ng/mL which persists throughout life.
- AFP passes from the fetus to amniotic fluid when fetus passes urine.
- It passes into the maternal serum by diffusion across the placental membranes and via placental circulation and is found in steadily increasing quantities in maternal serum after 12 weeks. In maternal serum it continues to increase uptil 28–32 weeks of pregnancy.

  These are the usual ways of entry of serum alfa fetoprotein in maternal serum but serum alfa fetoprotein can find its way in maternal serum in other ways too.

- Open fetal body wall defects uncovered by integument permit allows additional AFP to leak into the amniotic fluid and thus maternal serum AFP are increased. **This is the reason for increase in serum alpha fetoprotein in neural tube defects and ventral wall defects.**
- Maternal screening is done between 15-20 weeks.

- It is measured in nanograms per ml and reported as a multiple of the median (MOM).
- MSAFP of 2.5 MOM is considered as the upper limit of normal (for twin pregnancy it is 3.5 MOM).

Some condition associated with abnormal maternal serum alpha fetoprotein concentration.

Conditions Associated with an Elevated MSAFP Concentration
Underestimated gestational age
Multifetal gestation
Fetal death
Neural-tube defect
Gastroschisis
Omphalocele
Cystic hygroma
Esophageal or intestinal obstruction
Liver necrosis
Renal anomalies—polycystic kidneys, renal agenesis, congenital nephrosis, urinary tract obstruction
Cloacal exstrophy
Osteogenesis imperfecta
Sacrococcygeal teratoma
Congenital skin abnormality
Pilonidal cyst
Chorioangioma of placenta
Placenta intervillous thrombosis
Placental abruption
Oligohydramnios
Preeclampsia
Fetal-growth restriction
Maternal hepatoma or teratoma

MSAFP = Maternal serum alpha-fetoprotein.

PRENATAL DIAGNOSIS

- Chromosomal abnormalities occur in approximately 0.9% of newborn and it is estimated that at least 10 to 15% of conceptions are chromosomally abnormal.

Indications of prenatal screening:

- Singleton pregnancy and maternal age 35 years or above.
- Twin pregnancy at age over 31 years of pregnancy.
- Previous chromosomally abnormal child.
- Family history of chromosome anomaly.
- Three or more spontaneous abortions.
- Patient or husband with chromosome anomaly.
- Possible female carrier of X-linked disease.
- Metabolic disease risk (because of previous experience or family history).
- NTD risk (because of previous experience or family history).
- Positive second-trimester maternal serum screen or major fetal structural defect identified by USG.

PRENATAL DIAGNOSTIC TECHNIQUES (FIG. 6.18)

1. Chorionic villi sampling
2. Amniocentesis
3. Cordocentesis
4. Fetal tissue biopsy (not done)

Chorionic villi sampling	Amniocentesis

• Study material
  – Chorionic villi
	• Study material
	  – Amniocytes, Fibroblast of amniotic fluid

• Time ≥ 10 weeks	• Time ≥ 15 weeks
• M/C done = 11–13 weeks	• M/C done 16–18 weeks
• Never be done before 9 weeks as it leads to fetal limb defects	
• Fetal loss = 1–2%	**Fetal loss:**0.1 to 0.3% In severe obesity = Rate double (BMI > 40 kg/m²) In twins = 1.8%

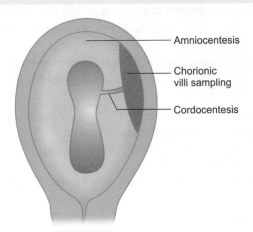

Fig. 6.18: Techniques of prenatal diagnosis

Chorionic Villi Sampling

Study material: Chorionic villi from which trophoblastic cells are used for study.

Time: Between 10–13 weeks.

Indications:

- To detect chromosomal anomalies
- For DNA analysis as in hemoglobinopathies, mallasenua, sickle cell anemia.
- To detect inborn errors of metabolism line phenylketonuria
- Appropriate for first trimester diagnosis of Down syndrome

Note: **It is not suitable to detect structural defects like of neural tube defects.**

Contd…

Contd…

Routes:

- Transabdominal (done using spinal needle)
- Transcervical (done using specially designed catheter)

Advantages over amniocentesis:

- The main advantage of CVS is that, results are available earlier in pregnancy, which allows earlier and safer methods of pregnancy termination when results are abnormal.
- Results can be obtained from direct analysis as well as culture in contrast to amino centers where diagnosis requires cultured cells.
- Preferred procedure for diagnosis needing DNA analysis as villi are a good source of DNA.
- CVS yields a larger amount of tissue and is therefore the method of choice when larger amount of DNA is needed for diagnosis.

Risks:

- Chances of fetal loss/abortion 1–2% (more than amniocentesis).
- If performed earlier than 9 weeks (typically around 7 weeks), increased chances of oromandibular limb hypogenesis and limb reduction defects.
- It can cause rupture of membranes, leakage of amniotic fluid and infection.
- Rh isoimmunization can occur in Rh-negative females.

Contraindications:

- Vaginal bleeding
- Active genital tract infection
- Extreme ante- or retroflexion of uterus.
- For transcervical route—cervical stenosis

Amniocentesis

Amniocentesis is the deliberate puncture of amniotic fluid sac per abdomen, used to diagnose fetal aneuploidy and other genetic conditions:

- Amniocentesis can be done anytime between 15-20 weeks.

Indications:

Diagnostic:

- *Early months (14-16 weeks):*

  Antenatal diagnosis of chromosomal and genetic disorder:

  i. Sex-linked disorders
  ii. Karyotyping
  iii. Inborn errors of metabolism
  iv. Neural tube defects as level of alpha fetoprotein is raised in amniotic fluid in NTD's.

Contd…

Contd...

- **Later months:**
  - Fetal lung maturity by measuring ratio of Lecithin and sphingomyelin.
  - Degree of fetal hemolysis in Rh-sensitised mother
  - Spectrophotometric analysis of amniotic fluid and deviation bulge of the optical density at 450 nm is obtained.
  - Meconium staining of liquor is an evidence of fetal distress.
  - Amniography or fetography following instillation of radio-opaque dye in the amniotic fluid cavity.

Therapeutic:
- **First half:**
  - Induction of abortion by instillation of chemicals such as hypertonic saline, urea or prostaglandins.
  - Repeated decompression of the uterus in acute hydramnios.
- **Second half:**
  - Decompression of uterus in unresponsive cases of chronic hydramnios producing distress or to stabilize the lie prior to induction.
  - To give intrauterine fetal transfusion in severe hemolysis following Rh-isoimmunization.
  - Amnioinfusion in oligohydramnios.

Procedure:
Amniocentesis is performed under sonographic guidance using a **20–22 gauze spinal needle** about 9 cm in length (About 30 ml of fluid is collected in a test tube for diagnostic purposes).

Precautions:
- Prior sonographic localization of placenta is desirable to prevent bloody tap and fetomaternal bleeding. Earlier methylene blue dye was used for the purpose but now it is contraindicated as it has been associated with jejunal atresia and neonatal methemoglobinemia.
- Prophylactic administration of 100 μg of anti-D immunoglobulin in Rh-negative nonimmunised mother.

Complications of Amniocentesis:
Maternal complications:
- Chorioamnionitis
- Hemorrhage (placental or uterine injury)
- Premature rupture of the membranes and premature labor
- Maternal isoimmunization in Rh-negative cases.

Fetal complications:
- Abortion (0.3–0.5%) (now even less = 1 in 300–in 500 pregnancies). The loss rate is doubled in twin pregnancy and obese women with BMI $\geq$ 40 kg/m²

Contd...

Contd...

- Trauma
- Fetomaternal hemorrhage
- Oligohydramnios due to leakage of amniotic fluid which may lead to:
  - Fetal lung hypoplasia
  - Respiratory distress
  - Talipes.

Cordocentesis

(Perumblical blood sampling-PUBS)

- Although there are theoretically, many indications for assessing the fetal circulation directly, advances in molecular genetic technology have greatly decreased the need for PUBS as well as for performing biopsy of fetal muscle, skin or liver.
- PUBS is done at ≥ 20 weeks gestational age
- Blood sample is taken from umbilical vein at the site where cord attaches to placenta
- Fetal loss rate is 1.5 to 2%. This is the reason why PUBS is not preferred
- The M/C indication of PUBS is evaluation and treatment of fetal isoimmunization, when a need for in utero transfusion is suspected.

> The sample collected by CVS, amniocentesis or cordocentesis is then subjected to either:
> i. Karyotyping (time taken 7–10 days)
> ii. FISH (24–48 hours)
> iii. CMA-chromosomal micro array analysis (3–5 days)

Karyotyping (Fig. 6.19)

- For karyotyping viable cells are needed. These are obtained either by chorionic villi sampling/amniocentesis.
- In amniocentesis, the specimen is centrifuged to obtain cells. In chorionic villus sampling (CVS) cells are obtained directly.
- The cells are cultured until enough cells in mitosis are obtained to make a cytogenetic diagnosis.
- It takes 2–3 weeks, 1–2 weeks and 24–48 hours for culturing of cells obtained by amniocentesis, CVS and cordocentesis respectively.
- These viable fetal cells obtained either by CVS/amniocentesis or cordocentesis are subjected to Giemsa staining, which produces a specific banding pattern called **G banding**.
- For karyotyping cells are arrested in metaphase using colchicine.

- Each chromosome stains in a characteristic pattern of light and dark bands.

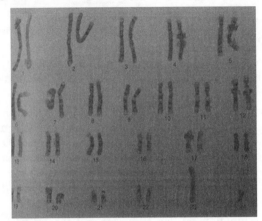

Fig. 6.19: Normal Karyotyping

- The light and dark bands on each chromosome are numbered. This numbering allows the location of any particular band and its involvement in any chromosomal abnormality.
- The results of karyotyping are obtained in 7–14 days.

FISH (Fig. 6.20)

Fluorescence In Situ Hybridization

- FISH is a technique that allows visualization of a small chromosomal region, generally too small to be seen with karyotyping.
- The results obtained by FISH are much faster than karyotyping = 6–8 hours.
- **FISH can be performed on interphase cells and therefore culturing is not required for analysis hence quick results are obtained.**
- FISH is carried out by using a small fragment of DNA (called a DNA probe) with the same nucleotide sequence as the stretch of chromosomal DNA of interest.

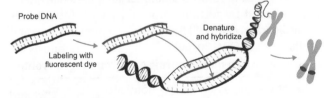

Fig. 6.20: FISH

Noninvasive Method of Prenatal Diagnosis

Cell Free Fetal DNA

Fetal cells can be isolated from maternal blood and used for diagnostic purpose.

- **Advantage:** Noninvasive, Gives rapid result.
- **Disadvantage:**
  - It is a screening test (Not diagnostic test)
  - Very expensive

The American College of Obstetricians and Gynecologists (2012 b) currently recommends that the test may be offered to the following groups:
- Women 35 years or older at delivery.
- Those with sonographic findings indicating increased risk for fetal aneuploidy.
- Those with a prior pregnancy complicated by trisomy 21, 18, or 13.
- Patient or partner carries a balanced robertsonian translocation indicating increased risk for fetal trisomy 21 or 13.
- The College does not recommend offering the test to women with low-risk pregnancies or multifetal gestations (American College of Obstetricians and Gynecologists, 2012 b).

ANEUPLOIDY SCREENING

Aneuploidy is the presence of one or more extra chromosomes, usually resulting in trisomy, or loss of a chromosome—monostomy.

Aneuploidy accounts for more than 50 percent of first-trimester abortions, about 20 percent of second-trimester losses, and 6 to 8 percent of stillbirths and early-childhood deaths. Of recognized pregnancies with chromosomal abnormalities, trisomy 21 composes approximately half of cases, trisomy 18 accounts for 15 percent; trisomy 13, for 5 percent; and the sex chromosomal abnormalities—45, X, 47, XXX, 47, XXY, and 47,XYY—for approximately 12 percent.

The risk for fetal trisomy increases with maternal age, particularly after age 35 except Monosomy X and Triploidy.

Broadly speaking, there are two types of aneuploidy screening tests, those that are traditional or analyte-based and those that are cell free DNA-based. All pregnant women should be offered aneuploidy screening or diagnostic testing early in pregnancy (American College of Obstetricians and Gynecologists, 2016c).

Note: Whenever a patient elects an aneuploidy screening test that does not include second-trimester serum analytes, screening for neural-tube defects should be performed separately, either with MSAFP assessment or with sonography (American College of Obstetricians and Gynecologists, 2016c).

DOWN SYNDROME

Introduction

- Down syndrome is Trisomy 21.
- Trisomy 21 due to nondisjunction of chromosomes is the etiology of 95% of Down syndrome cases, whereas 3 or 4% is due to a robertsonian translocation and 1–2% due to Mosaicism.
- The nondysjunction that results in trisomy 21 occurs during meiosis 1 in almost 75% of cases. The remaining events occur during meiosis II.
- Down syndrome is the most common nonlethal trisomy. Its prevalence is approximately 1 per 1000 pregnancies.
- As age of mother increases, risk of Down syndrome increases.

Maternal age	Risk of Down syndrome
30 years	1 in 1000
35 years	1 in 300
40 years	1 in 100
45 years	1 in 30

Clinical Findings

- It is estimated that 25 to 30% of second-trimester fetuses with Down syndrome will have a major malformation that can be identified sonographically.
- Approximately 40% of liveborn infants with Down syndrome are found to have cardiac defects, particularly endocardial cushion defects and ventricular septal defects. Gastrointestinal abnormalities develop in 7% and include duodenal atresia, esophageal atresia, and Hirschsprung disease.
- Typical findings in Down syndrome include brachycephaly; epicanthal folds and upslanting palpebral fissures: Brushfield spots, which are grayish spots on the periphery of the iris; a flat nasal bridge; and hypotonia. Infants often have loose skin at the nape of the neck, short fingers, a single palmar crease, hypoplasia of the middle phalanx of the fifth finger, and a prominent space or 'sandal-toe gap' between the first and second toes. Some of these findings are sonographic markers for Down syndrome.
- Health problems more common in children with Down syndrome include hearing loss in 75%, refractive errors in 50%, cataracts in 15%, thyroid disease in 15%, and an increased incidence of leukemia. Degree of mental impairment is usually mild to moderate, with an average intelligence quotient (IQ) score of 35 to 70.
- Recent data suggest that approximately 95% of liveborn infants with Down syndrome survive the first year. The 10-year survival rate is at least 90% overall and is 99%, if major malformations are absent.

Screening Tests for Down Syndrome/Aneuploidy Screening

Before we go to the screening test for Down syndrome, remember screening for Down is Universal and should be done in all pregnant females irrespective of age.

- **First-trimester screening** at 11 to 14 weeks' gestation, using the fetal nuchal translucency measurement together with serum analytes, has achieved Down syndrome detection rates comparable to those for second-trimester screening in women younger than 35 years (American College of Obstetricians and Gynecologists, 2013c).
- Combinations of first-trimester and second-trimester screening yield Down syndrome detection rates as high as 90 to 95%.
- Maternal serum cell-free fetal DNA testing for trisomy 21, 18 and 13 has become available as a screening test for high-risk pregnancies, with a 98% detection rate and a false-positive rate of 0.5% (American college).

First Trimester Screening

The most commonly used protocol involves measurement of sonographic nuchal translucency and biochemical test.

Nuchal Translucency (Figs. 6.21 and 6.22)

- Nuchal Translucency (NT) is a sonographic marker of Down syndrome/aneuploidy in 1st trimester.
- It is the most powerful marker.
- It is the maximum thickness of the subcutaneous translucent area between the skin and soft tissue that overlies the fetal spine in sagittal plane.
- **It is measured between 11–13 weeks**
- Nuchal translucency up to 3 mm = Normal
- If NT > 3 mm: Abnormal and all such patients should be offered targetted sonography with fetal echocardiography and cell free DNA screening and prenatal diagnosis (ACOG 2016c)
- Best Approach for measuring NT – Transvaginal route

 Note: Increased nuchal translucency is not a fetal abnormality, but rather a marker or soft sign that confers increased risk of fetal abnormality.

Causes of increased nuchal translucency	
• Down syndrome (Trisomy 21)	• Klinefelter syndrome
• Trisomy 18	• Triploidy
• Trisomy 13	• Congenital heart disease
• Turner syndrome	

Note:
- NT should be measured when Crown Rump Length is between 38–84 mm
- It should be measured in midsagittal plane
- Measuring calipers should be placed on the inner border of the echolucent space and should be perpendicular to long axis of fetus
- MIC cause of increased nuchal translucency is Down syndrome > Turner syndrome > cardiac anomalies

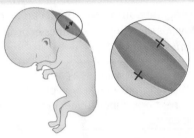

Fig. 6.21: Correct method of measurement of nuchal translucency

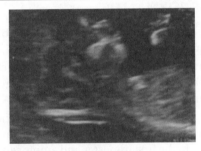

Fig. 6.22: Increased nuchal translucency

Other sonographic markers in 1st trimester of Down syndrome:
1. Absence of nasal bone.
2. Reversed 'a' wave in ductus venosus
3. Tricuspid regurgitation.

Biochemical Tests

- Two serum analytes used for first-trimester aneuploidy screening are human chorionic gonadotropin-either intact of free β-hCG—and pregnancy-associated plasma protein A (PAPP-A).
- In cases of fetal Down syndrome, the first-trimester serum free β-hCG level is higher (h for hCG and h for high) approximately 2.0 MoM and the PAPP-A level is lower, approximately 0.5 MoM.
- With trisomy 18 and trisomy 13, levels of both analytes are lower.

- If gestational age is correct, the use of these serum markers—without NT measurement—results in detection rates for fetal Down syndrome up to 67%.
- Aneuploidy detection is significantly greater, if these first-trimester analytes are either: (1) Combined with the sonographic NT measurement or (2) Combined with second-trimester analytes, which is termed serum integrated screening (p 291).

Note: In twin pregnancies, serum free β-hCG and PAPP-A levels are approximately doubled as compared to singleton values.

- β–hCG levels in Down syndrome are increased from the end of 1st trimester and throughout the second trimester, making it a useful marker in both 1st and 2nd trimester, whereas 'PAPP-1' levels are decreased only in 1st trimester, later there values start approaching normal, hence it is a useful marker only in 1st trimester.

Combined First Trimester Screening

The most commonly used screening protocol does PAPP at 9 weeks, NT measurement at 11 weeks and serum hCG at 12 weeks and. Using this protocol, 95% Down syndrome detection rates are as high as.

Maternal age does affect the performance of first-trimester aneuploidy screening tests.

Second Trimester Screening

(A) Biochemical Test

Triple Test
- It is a screening test for Down syndrome
- Done between 16 and 18 weeks of gestation
- It involves estimation of 3 hormones: hCG, AFP, and unconjugated estriol (UE3).

Interpretation

	hCG	AFP	UE3
Down's syndrome (T21)	↑	↓	↓
Edward syndrome (T18)	↓	↓	↓

To the triple test, if the level of a fourth-marker-dimeric **inhibin** alpha are added, the test is called as **Quad test or quadruple test**. Levels of inhibin A are elevated in Down syndrome.

Note:
- Free estriol is a breakdown product of DHEA-S produced by fetal adrenal gland in placenta.
- Inhibin A is produced by placenta during pregnancy and by corpus luteum in nonpregnant females.

The quad test is the most commonly used second-trimester serum screening test for aneuploidy

Screening Test	Detection of Down's Syndrome (%)
Double test (βhCG + PAPP) (done in first trimester)	60
Triple test	70
Quadruple test (hCG, AFP, UE3, + Inhibin A)	75
Serial integrated test (hCG, AFP, UE3, Inhibin A, PAPPA)	85

Integrated Screening

Combines results of first- and second-trimester tests. This includes a combined measurement of fetal NT and serum analyte levels at 11 to 14 weeks gestation plus quadruple markers at 15 to 20 weeks.

(B) USG in Second Trimester

Any 2 of the soft tissue markers listed below should be positive to diagnose Down Syndrome.

Sonographic Marker for Down in 2nd Trimester
Brachycephaly or shortened frontal lobe
Clinodactyly (hypoplasia of the 5th digit middle phalanx)
Hyperechogenic bowel
Echogenic intracardiac focus
Nasal bone absence or hypoplasia
Nuchal fold thickening
Aberrant right subclavian artery
'Sandal gap' between first and second toes
Shortened ear length
Single umbilical artery
Short femur
Short humerus
Mild hydronephrosis ventriculomegaly.

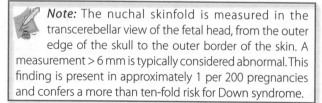

Note: The nuchal skinfold is measured in the transcerebellar view of the fetal head, from the outer edge of the skull to the outer border of the skin. A measurement > 6 mm is typically considered abnormal. This finding is present in approximately 1 per 200 pregnancies and confers a more than ten-fold risk for Down syndrome.

Cell-Free Fetal DNA Screening

- Using massively parallel sequencing or chromosome selective sequencing to isolate cell-free fetal DNA from maternal plasma, fetal Down syndrome and other autosomal trisomes may be detected as early as 10 weeks' gestation.
- Recent trials of these techniques in high-risk pregnancies have yielded detection rates for trisomies 21, 18, and 13 of approximately 98%.
- This novel technology has recently become clinically available as a screening test, but it is not considered a replacement diagnostic test.

Confirmatory Test

- The only 100% confirmatory test for Down syndrome is **karyotyping**, the sample for which can be obtained by chorionic villus sampling in 1st trimester or amniocentesis in 2nd trimester.

Note: In a patient who has a past history of fetus with Down syndrome, fetal karyotyping has to be done in the next pregnancy (screening test are not done in this case).

SCREENING OF TWINS FOR FETAL ABNORMALITIES

- Biochemical screening tests are unreliable in twin pregnancy, as the values tend to be elevated.
- Ultrasound scanning for nuchal translucency between 11 and 13 weeks can be performed as a screening test for trisomies.
- Occurrence of a trisomy and other genetic and chromosomal diseases are confirmed by chorionic villous sampling in the first trimester and amniocentesis in the second trimester.
- Monochorionic twins are monozygotic and only one sample is needed for karyotyping, as chromosomal and genetic defects will affect both fetuses.
- In dichorionic twins, both fetuses should be sampled.
- Maternal serum biochemistry is not reliable because of the contribution by each twin and is not used for second trimester screening. Amniocentesis will have to be done if a trisomy is suspected.
- The optimal method of diagnosing structural abnormalities is ultrasound scanning of each twin at 20 weeks. Structural abnormalities can affect either one or both twins in both monochorionic and dichorionic twins.

SCREENING AND DIAGNOSIS OF CYSTIC FIBROSIS

- Preconception diagnosis is preferred, but if not done, prenatal diagnosis is offered if a previous child is affected, or if there is a strong family history.

- DNA analysis of 23 most common CFTR mutations is carried out in one parent.
- If one parent is positive, the other parent is tested.
- If both parents are positive, there is 25% risk that the baby may be affected.
- If only one parent is positive, the baby will not develop the disease, because it is an autosomal recessive disorder.
- Confirmed by chorionic villous sampling at 10 weeks, or amniocentesis at 15 weeks and DNA probe testing on harvested cells if both parents are carriers.

PRENATAL DIAGNOSIS OF THALASSEMIA

Both parents have to be carriers for the fetus to be affected because it is an autosomal recessive disease.

The methods used in the prenatal diagnosis

- Preconception screening of parents should be done.
- Routine antenatal screening for carrier status of high risk mothers with a positive family history.
- Testing the father if the mother is a carrier.
- Testing the fetus if both parents are carriers.

Testing for Carrier Status

- **Red cell indices**
  - Low MCV (< 77 fl) and MCH (< 27 pg). However, low indices are not confirmatory as false positive results can occur in the presence of iron deficiency anemia.
- **Naked Eye Single Tube Red Cell Osmotic Fragility Test (NESTROFT)**
  - NESTROFT and red cell indices increase the negative predictive value to almost 100%. However, false positive results can occur in the presence of iron deficiency.
- **Hemoglobin A_2 Estimation**
  - Raised hemoglobin A_2 level is the gold standard for diagnosis of thalassemic trait.
  - Thalassemia carrier status is confirmed by HbA_2 measurement by hemoglobin electrophoresis, in couples found to be positive in preliminary screening, by red cell indices and NESTROFT.
- If the mother is found to be a carrier, the next step is to test the father for carrier status.
- If both parents are carriers, the next step is to perform DNA analysis of the fetus, by CVS in the first trimester or amniocentesis at 15 weeks.

DOPPLER STUDY DURING PREGNANCY

- Doppler ultrasound is used to assess the uterine, placental and fetal arterial and venous system.
- It is especially relevant in IUGR.

Ratios measured by Doppler:

- S/D — Systolic-diastolic ratio or S/D ratio *(most commonly)*
- S-D/S — Resistance index
- S-D/Mean — Pulsatility index

UMBILICAL ARTERY VESSELS

- Blood flow across the umbilical arteries provides a comprehensive overview of the - fetal blood supply and helps in detecting fetal circulatory compromise.
- The systolic component of blood flow reflects the cardiac pump and the diastolic component the distal vascular bed.
- In this case the distal vascular bed is the placental villous tree and hence umbilical artery Doppler is actually a placental and not a fetal Doppler.
- The umbilical artery is characterised by **forward^Q low resistance** flow.
- As gestation increases, there is gradual fall in all the resistance indices so the amount of forward diastolic flow increases. (As gestation increases peripheral vascular resistance decreases so diastolic flow increases as pregnancy advances).
- Systolic/diastolic ratio decreases as period of gestation increases.

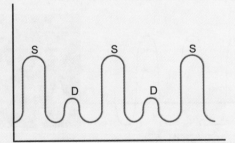

Fig. 6.23: Normal S/D ratio

- **There are three abnormal flow patterns; reduced EDF, absent EDF and finally reversal of flow.**

(i) *Reduced EDF:* (End diastolic flow)

SD ratio increases: It indicates uteroplacental insufficiency.

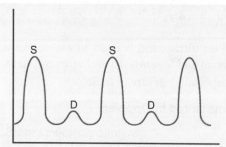

Fig. 6.24: Increased S/D ratio in PIH

- A normal Doppler is reassuring for at least a week and need only be repeated weekly to detect compromise.
- It the umbilical artery flow is abnormal, then further monitoring is with NST or BPP to decide on the time of delivery.

(ii) Absent end diastolic flow (AEDF):

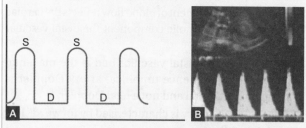

Figs. 6.25A and B: Absent end diastolic flow in umbilical artery

- These fetuses have a poorer outcome than those with only reduction in EDF, with the majority being delivered by cesarean section.
- The aim should be to deliver before reversal of flow.
- It is indication of termination of pregnancy, if pregnancy ≥ 34 weeks by cesarean section.

(iii) Reversed end diastolic flow (REDF)

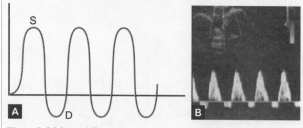

Figs. 6.26A and B: Reversed end diastolic flow

- Once reversal occurs the fetus usually dies within 1–2 days.
- It is an indication of termination of pregnancy irrespective of gestational age.

Umbilical artery velocimetry provides a useful adjunct in management of high risk pregnancy. They are however not recommended for screening low risk pregnancies.

— Williams Obs. 22/e, p 401

MIDDLE CEREBRAL ARTERY (MCA)

- Generally flow in MCA has a high resistance flow hence its diastolic component is lower than umbilical arteries at any age.
- Doppler measurement of middle cerebral artery velocimetry has been studied and employed clinically for detection of fetal anemia.
- With fetal anemia, **the peak systolic velocity is increased** (≥ 1.5 MoM) due to increased cardiac output and decreased blood viscosity. This has permitted the rhesus group alloimmunization (Figs. 6.27A and B).

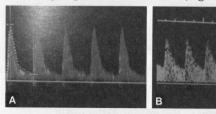

Figs. 6.27A and B: Peak systolic velocity in middle cerebral artery. (A) In anemia - PSV increased; (B) S/D ratio decreased in IUGR

- MCA Doppler has also been studied as an adjunct to the evaluation of fetal-growth restriction. In IUGR, there is brain sparing effect because of which the resistance in middle cerebral arteries decreases. Therefore S/D ratio decreases in middle cerebral artery in IUGR.

> *Note:* The last blood vessel to show changes in IUGR is ductus venosus (terminal event).
> In case of IUGR due to fetal hypoxia, there is redistribution of blood to middle cerebral artery (brain-sparing event) ultimately pressure in ductus venosus rises due to afterload in right side of fetal heart. This is a terminal event.

Doppler of Uterine Artery

- The uterine artery waveform consists of high resistance flow. A **diastolic notch** is seen in uterine artery Doppler waveform is early pregnancy.

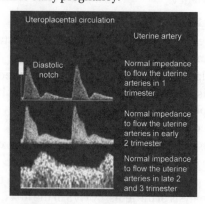

Fig. 6.28: Doppler of uterine artery

- This **diastolic notch** typically disappears during second trimester by 22 weeks. If the diastolic notch persists beyond 22 weeks, it is a predictor of preeclampsia.

ANTEPARTUM FETAL MONITORING

FETAL HEART RATE

Characteristics

Baseline fetal heart rate = 110–160 bpm (according to NICE criteria).

Bradycardia:

- Rate < 110 bpm
- Due to mild head compression in the second stage of labor
- Congenital heart block
- Indicates serious fetal compromise.

Tachycardia:

- Rate > 160 bpm
- Maternal fever due to *'amnionitis'* is the most common cause
- Cardiac arrhythmias
- Maternal parasympathomimetics (atropine) or sympathomimetics (terbutaline)
- May indicate fetal compromise.

Beat to beat variability:

- A baseline variability of 5–25 bpm is a sign of fetal well-being

Causes of decreased beat to beat variability:
- Fetal hypoxia **(it is the single most reliable sign of fetal compromise)**[Q]/Fetal acidemia[Q]
- Sleep phase[Q]
- Drugs (Sedatives, Analgesics, MgSO$_4$, Antihypertensives) given to mother[Q]
- Maternal acidemia.[Q]

Sinusoidal heart rate:
- It is a stable baseline FHR with fixed baseline variability without any acceleration
- Seen in cases of severe fetal anemia as in
  - Rh-isoimmunization[Q]
  - Ruptured vasa previa[Q]
  - Twin to twin transfusion.[Q]
- Also seen in fetal intracranial hemorrhage with severe fetal asphyxia.

Accelerations:

- Accelerations are increase in FHR by 15 bpm or more lasting for at least 15 sec.
- Accelerations denote an intact neurohormonal and cardiovascular activity and therefore denotes a healthy fetus at >32 weeks.
- At period < 32 weeks, acceleration is increase in FHR by 10 bpm or more lasting for at least 10 secs.

Decelerations:

Decrease in fetal heart 15 beats per minute for 15 secs with uterine contraction.

Three basic patterns of deceleration are observed, each of which has a diagnostic significance:

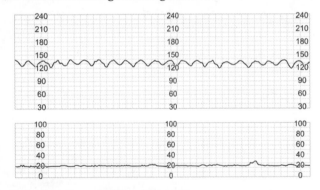

Fig. 6.29: Sinusoidal heart rate pattern

FHR pattern	Feature	Seen in	Diagram
Early deceleration	Deceleration coincidences with uterine contraction. Uniform onset, i.e. gradual takes > 30 sec and recovery. Magnitude rarely > 40 bpm	Head compression. Not associated with fetal hypoxia. It is physiological	A
Late deceleration	The dip in FHR occurs at or after the contraction peak and continues well after the end of uterine contraction. Uniform onset, i.e. gradual takes ≥ 30 secs and recovery. May be of low magnitude 10–20 bpm	Most ominous finding. Indicates uteroplacental insufficiency	B

Self Assessment & Review: Obstetrics

FHR pattern	Feature	Seen in	Diagram
Variable deceleration	Variable relationship to contraction Ragged waveform. Abrupt in onset < 30 sec Variable magnitude	Umbilical cord compression	C

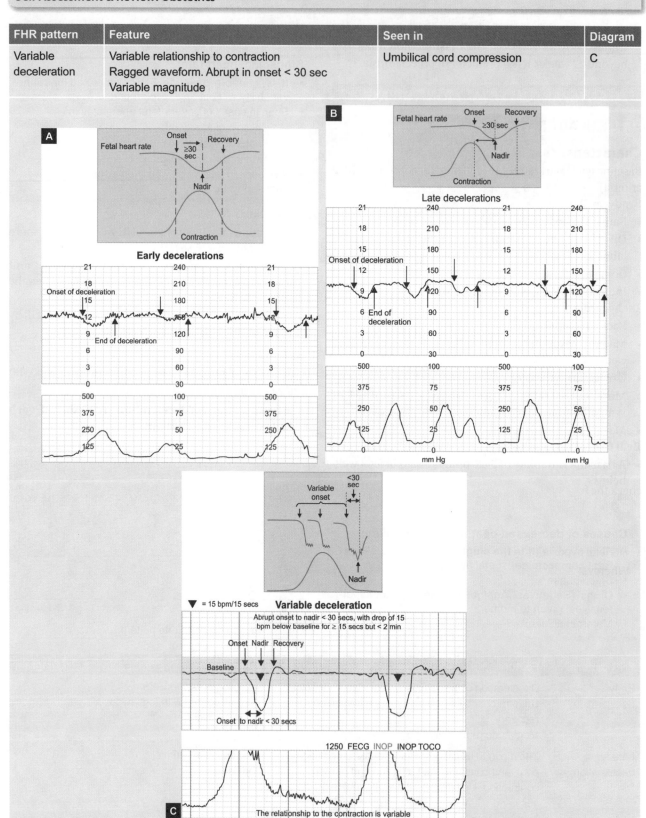

Figs. 6.30A to C: Fetal HR deceleration.

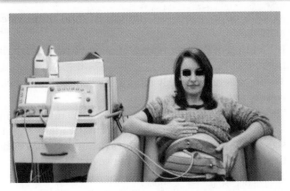

Fig. 6.31: Non-stress Test

- **The worst type of deceleration is—late deceleration**

  The most ominous picture is
  - Shallow late decelerations
  - Loss of baseline variability
  - Tachycardia

- **Management for late deceleration**
  - Check fetal pH
  - Immediate delivery

- **Management for variable deceleration**
  - Turn the patient on her side (as this will relieve pressure on the cord)
  - Maintain hydration
  - Stop oxytocics
  - Give oxygen by face mask

  If it is persistent variable deceleration—(3 in 20 minutes) check the fetal pH and deliver.

ANTEPARTUM FETAL MONITORING

Daily Fetal Movement Count: A pregnant female should have at least 10 movements in 2 hours, period of rest.

Whenever a pregnant female complains of decreased fetal movement, next step to do Modified Biophysical Score (which includes NST and Amniotic fluid index) or just non-stress test (these are screening tests).

Non-Stress Test (Fig. 6.31)

It is the most commonly used screening test for antepartum evaluation of the fetal status.

Principle: The test looks for the presence of temporary accelarations of fetal heart rate (FHR) associated with fetal movement. Presence of spontaneous fetal heart rate acceleration associated with fetal movements is an indicator of fetal well-being, likewise the absence of fetal reaction suggests the possibility of fetal hypoxia.

Method:
- Place patient in the semi-Fowler's position (Fig. 6.31).
- Apply the tococardiographic equipment to the maternal abdomen, and observe the uterine activity and FHR for 20 minutes. Instruct the patient to push the calibration button of the uterine contraction tracing every time she feels fetal movement.

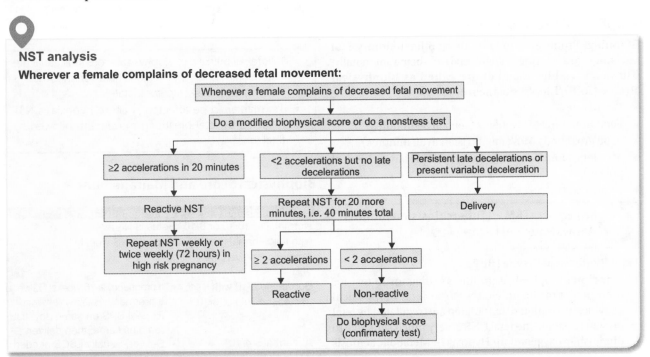

NST analysis

Wherever a female complains of decreased fetal movement:

Time for performing these test:[Q]

- Testing should begin by 32 to 34 weeks.
- In pregnancies with severe complications, begin at 26–28 weeks.

Note: In case test is being performed before 32 weeks, accelerations are defined as having 10 bpm or more above baseline for 10 seconds or longer:

- **Interval between NST testing**
  - Ideally – repeated weekly (a reactive NST means that fetus is not in danger for atleast 7 days)
  - In high risk pregnancies like diabetes mellitus, IUGR and Gestational hypertension, twice weekly
  - In severe preeclampsia remote from term – done daily
- The positive and negative predictive value of a NST is typically less than 50% and more than 90% which means a reactive NST is more reliable in excluding fetal hypoxia than a nonreactive test in predicting fetal compromise.

False normal stress test: Though a normal stress test means that fetus is not in danger for at least 7 days, but NST is inadequate to preclude an acute asphyxial insult.

Causes of death within a week of normal NST:

- Meconium aspiration associated with umbilical cord abnormalities
- IUGR
- Oligohydramnios
- Placental abruption
- Abnormal cord position.

Biophysical Score/Manning Score

Manning: Proposed a method using 5 fetal **biophysical variables**[Q] to assess the status of fetal well-being antenatally. **These 5 variables together are called as Biophysical Profile (BPP)/Biophysical score**

- Fetal **T**one
- Fetal **B**reathing Movements (seen in 30 minutes)
- Fetal gross body **M**ovements (seen in 30 minutes)
- Amniotic Fluid Volume (as seen by single largest vertical pocket)
- **N**on stress test

 Remember: **TBM - (Tuberculosis meningitis) Always Notorious** for these variables.

Fetal Biophysical Profile (BPP)

- **Principle:** Biophysical profile is a diagnostic test for uteroplacental insufficiency.[Q] The fetal biophysical activities are initiated, modulated and regulated by fetal nervous system. The fetal CNS is very much sensitive to diminished oxygenation/ Hypoxia → Metabolic acidosis

→ CNS depression → Changes in fetal biophysical activity.

- **Indication of BPP scoring:** Nonreactive NST[Q], high risk pregnancy[Q].
- **Test frequency:** Weekly after a normal NST, and twice weekly after an abnormal test.
- The variables are observed for at least 30 minutes[Q] and assigned a score of 2 each[Q] to normal variables and a score of 0[Q] to abnormal variables (all or none law either the score is 2 or 0, nothing in between).
- Thus the highest score possible for a normal fetus is 10.[Q]
- A score of 8 to 10 is normal, 6 is equivocal and 5 or less is abnormal.

Components and Their scores for the Biophysical profile:

Component	Score 2	Score 0
Non-stress test	≥ 2 accelerations of > 15 beats/min for > 15 sec in 2–40 min	0 or 1 acceleration in 2–40 minutes
Fetal breathing	≥ 1 episode of rhythmic breathing lasting > 30 second within 30 minutes	< 30 second of breathing in 30 min
Fetal movement	≥ 3 discrete body or limb movements within 30 minutes	< 3 discrete movements
Fetal tone	≥ 1 episode of extension of fetal extremity with return to flexion, or opening or closing of hand within 30 minute	No movements or no extension/ flexion
Amniotic fluid volume	Single vertical pocket ≥ 2 cm	Largest single vertical pocket < 2 cm

 Note: All markers of Biophysical score indicate acute state of fetus except Amniotic fluid volume which is a long-term marker (chronic state).

- 1st marker to be affected is acute hypoxia is NST followed by fetal breathing movement followed by fetal tone.

Biophysical Score and Management

Biophysical score	Management
Normal, i.e. 10/10 or 8/10 with fluid normal (i.e. Amniotic fluid volume 2/2)	Fetus is Normal. Repeat BPS weekly
Borderline 8/10 with decreased fluid or 6/10	• If pregnancy ≥ 36 weeks: Deliver • If pregnancy < 36 weeks: Repeat BPS on same day. If it remains same, then deliver.
Abnormal ≤ 4/10	• Deliver: Usually LSCS needed

Modified Biophysical Score

- To avoid the disadvantages of biophysical profile and to simplify monitoring, **Clark and co-authors (1989) developed** modified **biophysical profile**.
- The modified biophysical profile combines **the non-stress test with the amniotic fluid index (AFI)** as an indicator of long-term function of the placenta and takes only about 10 minutes to perform.

 Note: Modified BPS is not a confirmatory test. It is a screening test.

Interpretation

1. The modified biophysical profile is considered normal if the non-stress test is reactive and the amniotic fluid index is more than 5 cm. It is then repeated once a week or earlier if clinically indicated.
2. It is abnormal if the non-stress test is non-reactive or the amniotic fluid index is 5 cm or less. In such a situation a full biophysical profile is performed.
3. Negative results are repeated every 3–4 days.

INTRAPARTUM FETAL MONITORING

1. **Continuous CTG or Intermittent auscultation of FHS. CTG is done as discussed in antepartum monitoring**

FHS auscultation	Low Risk	High Risk
1st stage	30 mins	15 mins
2nd stage	15 mins	5 mins

2. **Fetal scalp pH monitoring**

7.25 – 7.35 = N
7.20 – 7.25 – Borderline pH
↓
Repeat in 30 mins
< 7.20 – Cesarean/delivery

 Note: Fetal scalp pH monitoring should not be done in HIV +ve females
- Avoid vacuum till 1 hr after doing fetal scalp pH.

New Pattern Questions

N1. Wavelength of USG used in obstetrics:
- a. 1–2 MHz
- b. 5–7.5 MHz
- c. 3.5–5 MHz
- d. 7.5–10 MHz

N2. During USG, fetal abdominal circumference is measured at the level of:
- a. Stomach and umbilical vein, perpendicular to spine
- b. Kidneys
- c. Stomach parallel to spine
- d. Liver and spleen

N3. At 9 weeks, approximate CRL in mm of a fetus would be:
- a. 8 mm
- b. 2.5 mm
- c. 9 mm
- d. 5 mm

N4. Which of the following is not an indication of amniocentesis for chromosomal anomaly detection?
- a. Gestation diabetes
- b. Previous Down's child
- c. Maternal age more than 35
- d. Parents with chromosomal anomaly

N5. Fetal anemia is detected on Doppler of:
- a. Uterine artery
- b. Umbilical artery
- c. Middle cerebral artery
- d. Any of the above

N6. On Doppler the most omnious sign indicating fetal compromise is:
- a. ↑ pulsatility index in umbilical art
- b. ↑ S/D blood flow ratio
- c. ↑ cerebral artery flow
- d. Absent diastolic flow

N7. Increased acidosis and hypoxaemia is associated with:
- a. Normal Doppler waveform
- b. Increased fetal diastolic flow in the middle cerebral artery with absent diastolic flow in the aorta
- c. Presence of the 'notch' in the uterine artery
- d. Absent umbilical artery

N8. A G2P1 woman at 35 weeks pregnancy complains of decreased fetal movement. Next step in Mgt is:
- a. Observation
- b. Do NST
- c. Do CST
- d. Do BPS
- e. Induction reliably of labor

N9. Which most significant finding in cardiotocography for detection of fetal hypoxia?
- a. Late deceleration
- b. Variable deceleration
- c. Sinusoidal deceleration
- d. Early deceleration

N10. Sinusoidal heart rate pattern is seen in:
- a. Placenta previa
- b. Vasa previa
- c. Battledore placenta
- d. Succenturiate placenta

N11. Which of the following explanations is not an explanation for decreased variability of the fetal heart tracing?
- a. Fetal 'sleep state'
- b. Prematurity
- c. Barbiturate ingestion
- d. Fetal stimulation

N12. Consider the following:
1. Reactive NST
2. Absence of deceleration
3. Sinusoidal pattern

Which of the above findings in an antepartum CTG indicate fetal well-being:
- a. 1 and 2 only
- b. 2 and 3 only
- c. 1 and 3 only
- d. 1, 2, 3

N13. A 17-year-old comes to an adolescent clinic with complain of nausea and vomiting. She did a home urine pregnancy test which was positive. She does not remember her date of last menstrual period. USG shows a viable pregnancy of 8 weeks gestation. Which of the following statements regarding first trimester ultrasound is correct?
- a. A gestational sac can be first seen 2 weeks after LMP
- b. The accuracy of determining gestational age using ultrasound begins to decrease after first trimester
- c. Yolk sac is the first sign of pregnancy on USG
- d. USG can be used to determine the sex of the baby

N14. A patient present for her first initial OB visit after performing a home pregnancy test and gives a last menstrual period of about 8 weeks ago. She says she is not entirely sure of her dates, however because she has a long history of irregular menses. Which of the following is the most accurate of way of dating the pregnancy?
- a. Determination of uterine size on pelvic examination
- b. Quantitative serum hCG levels
- c. Crown rump length on abdominal or vaginal examination
- d. Determination of progesterone level along with serum hCG level

N15. A 28 years female G2P1 presents to antenatal clinic at 24 weeks for routine check up. USG shows a normal for gestational age fetus at 24 weeks of gestation in frank breech position, with no other abnormalities. What is the most appropriate next step in mgt?
- a. Glucose challenge test with 50 gm of glucose

b. Culture for *Neisseria gonorrhoeae* and *Chlamydia trachomatis* (normally done at initial visit and in certain high-risk GRPs at 32-36 weeks along with GRP B streptococcal screening)

c. ECV

d. Immediate LSCS

e. Immediate induction and vaginal delivery

N16. In pregnancy with increased MSAFP which of the following should be done?

a. Repeat measurement of MSAFP at later date

b. USG

c. Amniocentesis

d. Termination of pregnancy

N17. During 1st stage of labor, FHR should be auscultated in low risk pregnancy after every:

a. 10 mins   b. 15 mins

c. 30 mins   d. 45 mins

N18. Parameter not used to determine fetal age in midtrimester USG:

a. BPD

b. Femur length

c. HC

d. CRL

N19. An HIV positive, 36 years old female on ART needs counseling. Which of the following 1st trimester markers of Down syndrome would be affected by HIV:

a. β–hCG

b. PAPP-A

c. NT

d. All of the above

N20. MIC hazard of chorionic villous biopsy is:

a. Limb abnormality   b. Spina bifida

c. Down's syndrome   d. Abortion

Previous Year Questions

PRENATAL DIAGNOSIS

1. **Appropriate material for antenatal diagnosis of genetic disorders includes all of the following *except*:** [AIIMS May 06]

   a. Fetal blood   b. Amniotic fluid

   c. Chorionic villi   d. Maternal urine

2. **Karyotyping of fetus can be done through all of the following invasive methods *except*:**

   a. Amniocentesis   [AIIMS Nov 11]

   b. Cordocentesis

   c. Chorionic villous sampling

   d. Fetal skin biopsy

ALPHA FETOPROTEIN

3. **In which of the following conditions would maternal serum alpha fetoprotein values be the highest?** [AIIMS Nov 05]

   a. Down's syndrome   b. Omphalocele

   c. Gastroschisis   d. Spina bifida occulta

4. **Screening by using maternal serum alpha feto-proteins helps to detect all of the following *except*:** [AI 04]

   a. Neural tube defects

   b. Congenital nephrosis

   c. Talipes equinovarus

   d. Omphalocele

5. **Increased AFP level is seen in:** [AIIMS Nov 07]

   a. Down syndrome

   b. Molar pregnancy

   c. Overestimated gestational age

   d. Congenital nephrotic syndrome

6. **Alpha fetoprotein concentration in serum is elevated in:** [PGI Dec 08]

   a. Hepatoma

   b. Hepatoblastoma

   c. Endodermal sinus tumor

   d. Cirrhosis

   e. Chromosomal trisomy

7. **AFP is raised in all *except*:** [PGI Dec 99]

   a. Polycystic kidney

   b. Trisomy

   c. IUD

   d. Esophageal atresia

8. **Maximum level of alpha fetoprotein is seen in:**

   a. Fetal serum   [AIIMS June 98]

   b. Placenta

   c. Amniotic fluid

   d. Maternal serum

9. **About AFP all are true *except*:** [PGI June 08]

   a. MSAFP detected 16-18 weeks of gestation

   b. Diabetic patients have increased AFP level

   c. MSAFP is unrelated to period of gestation

   d. Highest fetal level is seen around 13 weeks of gestation

   e. Increased in Down syndrome

10. **Regarding alpha fetoprotein true statement is:**
    [AIIMS May 08]
    a. Major source in fetal life is yolk sac
    b. Commonly increased in Wilm's tumor
    c. Maximum level at 20th week
    d. Half-life 5-7 days

11. **↓ed maternal serum α-FP is seen in:**
    a. Multiple pregnancy   [PGI June 03; Dec 97]
    b. Trisomy 21
    c. Open neural tube defect
    d. IUD

hCG

12. **↓ hCG level seen in:**   [PGI 04]
    a. Down syndrome   b. DM
    c. Multiple pregnancy d. Ectopic pregnancy
    e. Esophageal atresia

13. **Raised beta-hCG levels are seen in:**   [PGI June 01]
    a. DM   b. Preeclampsia
    c. Ectopic pregnancy d. Rh-incompatibility
    e. Down syndrome

14. **Monitoring of β-hCG is useful in management of:**
    [PGI Dec 08]
    a. H. mole   b. Choriocarcinoma
    c. Ectopic pregnancy d. Endodermal sinus tumor

AMNIOCENTESIS AND CVS

15. **Amniotic fluid contains acetylcholinesterase enzyme. What is the diagnosis?**
    a. Open spina bifida   [AIIMS May 07, Nov 06]
    b. Gastroschisis
    c. Omphalocele
    d. Osteogenesis imperfecta

16. **Which of the following tests on maternal serum is most useful in distinguishing between open neural tube defects and ventral wall defects in a fetus?**
    [AI 04]
    a. Carcinoembryogenic antigen
    b. Sphingomyelin
    c. Alpha-fetoprotein
    d. Pseudocholinesterase

17. **The best time to do chorionic villous sampling is:**
    [AIIMS May 05, 09]
    a. Between 6-8 weeks
    b. Between 7-9 weeks
    c. Between 9-11 weeks
    d. Between 11-13 weeks

18. **Chorionic villous sampling done before 10 weeks may result in:**   [AIIMS May 02, Dec 97]
    a. Fetal loss
    b. Fetomaternal hemorrhage
    c. Oromandibular limb defects
    d. Sufficient material not obtained

19. **DNA analysis of chorionic villus/amniocentesis is not likely to detect:**   [AI 01]
    a. Tay-Sach's disease
    b. Hemophilia A
    c. Sickle cell disease
    d. Duchenne muscular dystrophy

20. **Chorionic villous sampling is done in all except:**
    a. Phenylketonuria   [AIIMS Dec 97, AI 08]
    b. Down's syndrome
    c. Neural tube defect
    d. Thalassemia/sickle cell anemia

21. **True about chorionic villi biopsy:**   [PGI June 08]
    a. Strongly associated with faciomandibular defects
    b. Done in 10-12 weeks
    c. Rh immunoglobulin prophylaxis is not necessary
    d. Done to diagnose genetic disorders

22. **About amniocentesis following are true except:**
    a. It carries risk of miscarriage   [PGI June 00]
    b. Always done as a blind procedure
    c. Done between 10-18 weeks
    d. Chromosomal abnormality can be detected

23. **Amniocentesis done at:**   [PGI Dec 09]
    a. 14-18 weeks   b. 16-20 weeks
    c. 20-24 weeks   d. 24-28 weeks
    e. >34 weeks

FETAL IMAGING

24. **At what level of β-hCG is it that normal pregnancy can be earliest detected by TVS (transvaginal USG)?**
    [PGI Dec 06]
    a. 500 IU/mL   b. 1000 IU/mL
    c. 1500 IU/mL   d. 2000 IU/mL
    e. 2500 IU/mL

25. **Earliest of fetal heart can be detected at:**
    a. 6.0-6.5 weeks   [PGI June 06]
    b. 6.5-7 weeks
    c. 7.1-7.5 weeks
    d. 8 weeks

26. **What is the finding seen earliest in USG?**
    [PGI Dec 05]
    a. Yolk sac   b. Fetal heart
    c. Chorion   d. Placenta
    e. Embryo

27. **Best confirmation for pregnancy at six weeks?**
    a. USG for cardiac activity   [AIIMS Nov 13]
    b. Doppler
    c. Estimation of serum beta-hCG in urine
    d. Bimanual palpation

28. **Pseudogestational sac seen in ultrasonography of:**
    [PGI Dec 05]
    a. Missed abortion   b. Ectopic gestation
    c. Complete abortion d. Hematometra

29. Which one of the following congenital malformation of the fetus can be diagnosed in first trimester by ultrasound? [AI 06]
    a. Anencephaly
    b. Inencephaly
    c. Microcephaly
    d. Holoprosencephaly

30. Best marker of gestational age in 2nd trimester is: [AI 04]
    a. Biparietal diameter
    b. Head circumference
    c. CRL
    d. Femur length

31. Doppler ultrasound in pregnancy detect:
    a. Cardiovascular malformation [AI 98]
    b. Neural tube defect
    c. Abdominal masses
    d. IUGR

ANTENATAL FETAL ASSESSMENT

32. Late deceleration indicates: [AI 98]
    a. Head compression
    b. Cord compression
    c. Fetal hypoxia
    d. Breech presentation

33. A drop in fetal heart rate that typically last less than 2 minutes and usually associated with umbilical cord compression is called: [AIIMS May 03]
    a. Early deceleration
    b. Late deceleration
    c. Variable deceleration
    d. Prolonged deceleration

34. Early deceleration denotes: [PGI June 97]
    a. Head compression
    b. Cord compression
    c. Placental insufficiency
    d. Fetal distress

35. With reference to fetal heart rate, a nonstress test is considered reactive when: [AIIMS Nov 03]
    a. Two fetal heart rate accelerations are noted in 20 minutes
    b. One fetal heart rate acceleration is noted in 20 minutes
    c. Two fetal heart rate accelerations are noted in 10 minutes
    d. Three fetal heart rate accelerations are noted in 30 minutes

36. 35 weeks pregnant diabetic female with NST non-reactive. What should be done next?
    a. Induction of labor [AIIMS May 11]
    b. CS
    c. Do NST after 1 hour
    d. Proceed to biophysical profile

37. In a nondiabetic high-risk pregnancy the ideal time for non-stress test monitoring is: [AIIMS May 01]
    a. 48 hours
    b. 72 hours
    c. 96 hours
    d. 24 hours

38. All of the following are components of manning score/Biophysical score except: [AIIMS May 06, Nov 00; AI 97]
    a. Non-stress test
    b. Oxytocin challenge test
    c. Fetal body movement
    d. Respiratory activity of child

39. Manning score/Biophysical score includes: [PGI Dec 09, Dec 01]
    a. Fetal movements
    b. Respiratory movements
    c. Placental localization
    d. Uterine artery waveform
    e. Fetal heart rate accelerations

40. Following represents fetal hypoxia except:
    a. Excessive fetal movements [AI 98, 96]
    b. Meconium in vertex presentation
    c. Fetal scalp blood pH > 7.3
    d. Heart rate < 100

MIXED BAG

41. Modified BPS consists of: [AIIMS Nov 2015]
    a. NST with AFI
    b. NST with fetal breathing
    c. NST with fetal movement
    d. NST with fetal tone

42. Banana and lemon sign is seen in which fetal anomalies? [PGI June 05]
    a. Neural tube defect
    b. Hydrops fetalis
    c. Twins
    d. IUD
    e. Down syndrome

43. A G3P2, pregnant comes to your clinic at 18 weeks of gestation for genetic counseling. She has a history of two kids born with thalassemia major. Which test would you recommend now? [AIIMS Nov 2015]
    a. Amniocentesis
    b. Chorionic villus sampling
    c. Cordocentesis
    d. Noninvasive prenatal testing

44. A mother comes with history of antenatal fetal death due to neural tube defect in first child. What is the amount of folic acid you will prescribe during preconceptional counseling (in micrograms/day)? [AIIMS May 2015]
    a. 4
    b. 40
    c. 400
    d. 4000

45. Earliest diagnosis of pregnancy can be established safely by: [AIIMS May 2015]
    a. USG for fetal cardiac activity
    b. Fetal cardiac Doppler study
    c. hCG levels
    d. MRI pelvis

46. **Cause(s) of stillbirth:** [PGI Nov 2014]
    a. Prematurity
    b. Syphilis
    c. Abruptio placentae
    d. Diabetes

47. **High level of hCG found in:** [PGI Nov 2014]
    a. Twin
    b. Down syndrome
    c. Choriocarcinoma
    d. Ectopic pregnancy

DOWN SYNDROME

48. **Kamlesh, a 2-year-old girl, has Down's syndrome. Her karyotype is 21/21 translocation. What is the risk of recurrence in subsequent pregnancies, if the father is a balanced translocation carrier:**
    [AI 02; AIIMS June 00]
    a. 100%
    b. 50%
    c. 25%
    d. 0%

49. **Screening for Down's syndrome should be done in the age group in pregnancy:** [AIIMS 94]
    a. 30
    b. 35
    c. All in the reproductive age group
    d. None of the above

50. **Aneuploid in 1st trimester is detected by:**
    a. Nuchal translucency [PGI May 2015]
    b. MSAFP level
    c. PAPP-A
    d. Unconjugated estriol
    e. β-hCG

51. **All of the following are biochemical markers included for triple test *except*:** [AIIMS May 05, 03]
    a. Alfa-fetoprotein (AFP)
    b. Human chorionic gonadotropin (hCG)
    c. Human placental lactogen (HPL)
    d. Unconjugated estriol

52. **Which of the following is done for screening of Down's syndrome in first trimester?** [AIIMS Nov 16]
    a. Beta hCG and PAPP-A
    b. Unconjugated estradiol and PAPPA
    c. AFP and Inhibin A
    d. AFP and beta hCG

53. **Increased nuchal translucency at 14 weeks is suggestive of:** [AI 07]
    a. Down's syndrome
    b. Esophageal atresia
    c. Trisomy 18
    d. Foregut duplication cyst

54. **The best way of diagnosing Trisomy 21 during second trimester of pregnancy is:** [AI 06]
    a. Triple marker estimation
    b. Nuchal skin fold thickness measurement
    c. Chorionic villus sampling
    d. Amniocentesis

55. **Diagnosis of Down syndrome at 11 weeks is best assessed by:** [AI 98]
    a. Ultrasonography
    b. Amniocentesis
    c. Chorionic villous biopsy
    d. Doppler ultrasound

56. **Mr. and Mrs. Annadural have a 2-month-old baby suffering with Down's syndrome. Karyotype of Mrs. Annadural shows translocation variety of Down syndrome. Which of the following investigation will you advise to the parents before the next pregnancy?**
    a. Triple test [AI 04]
    b. α-fetoprotein
    c. Karyotyping
    d. β-human chorionic gonadotropin (hCG)

57. **Which of the following is the investigation of choice in a pregnant lady at 18 weeks of pregnancy with past history of delivering a baby with Down's syndrome?**
    a. Triple screen test [AI 04]
    b. Amniocentesis
    c. Chorionic villous biopsy
    d. Ultrasonography

58. **A pregnant female, 38-year-old, had a child with Down's syndrome. How do you assess the risk of Down's syndrome in the present pregnancy?**
    [AIIM May 01, June 00]
    a. Material alpha-fetoprotein
    b. Material hCG
    c. USG
    d. Chorionic villous biopsy

59. **A 32-year-old woman is 9 weeks pregnant and has a 10-year-old Down's syndrome child. What test would you recommend for the mother, so that she can know about her chances of getting a Down's syndrome baby is this present pregnancy. How will you assure the mother about the chances of Down's syndrome in the present pregnancy?** [AIIMS Nov 10]
    a. Blood test
    b. USG
    c. Chorionic villus sampling
    d. Assure her there is no chance since she is less than 35 years of age

60. **Which of the following feature on second-trimester ultrasound is not a marker of Down's syndrome?**
    a. Single umbilical artery [AI 03]
    b. Choroid plexus cyst
    c. Diaphragmatic hernia
    d. Duodenal atresia

RECENT QUESTIONS

61. A routine ultrasound done at 20 weeks period of gestation done in a 31 years old gravida 1 para 0 revealed an anomaly. The patient comes to you with the following ultrasound film for a second opinion. What congenital anomaly would you explain to the couple? **[AIIMS May 2016]**

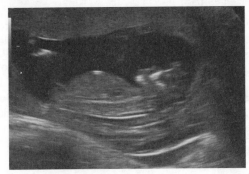

a. Omphalocele
b. Encephalocele
c. Cystic hygroma
d. Anencephaly

62. Double bleb signs in USG are depictive of:
[AIIMS May 2016]
a. Intrauterine two gestations sac
b. Amniotic sac and yolk sac

c. Ectopic pregnancy
d. Heterotopic pregnancy

63. Which of the following abnormalities can be diagnosed in the 1st trimester of pregnancy?
[AIIMS May 2017]
a. Anencephaly   b. Meningocele
c. Encephalocele   d. Microcephaly

64. True about significant variable decelerations is:
[AIIMS May 2017]
a. Drop in fetal heart rate to less than 90 bpm for 60 seconds
b. Drop in fetal heart rate to less than 100 bpm for 60 seconds
c. Drop in fetal heart rate to less than 80 bpm for 60 seconds
d. Drop in fetal heart rate to less than 70 bpm for 60 seconds

65. Screening test used to detect aneuploidy in 1st trimester includes: **[PGI May 2017]**
a. Estimation of PAAP-A and estradiol
b. Estimation of PAAP-A and βhCG
c. Estimation of PAAP-A and MSAFP
d. Estimation of βhCG and Inhibin
e. Estimation of MSAFP and βhCG

66. Pregnancy aggravates which of the following condition(s)? **[PGI May 2017]**
a. Hypertension   b. Anaemia
c. Rheumatoid arthritisd. Acne

Answers with Explanations to New Pattern Questions

N1. **Ans. is c, i.e. 3.5–5 MHz**

Whenever in questions, it does not specify TVS or TAS, always take it as TAS.

N2. **Ans. is a, i.e Stomach and umbilical vein, perpendicular to the spine** *Ref. Williams 24/e, p 198*

The abdominal circumference is measured at a transverse plane (i.e. plane perpendicular to fetal spine) at the level of stomach and conference of the umbilical vein with the portal sinus.

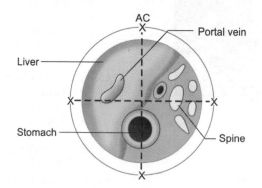

It is an indicator of fetal growth, hence is an indicator of IUGR/macrosomia in fetus.

Note: Biparietal diameter:- is measured in transthalamic view at the level of thalamic and cavut septum pellucidum (CSP), from the outer edge of the skull to inner edge of the distal skull.

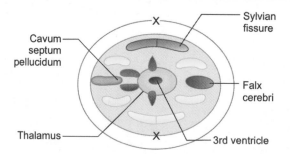

N3. **Ans. is b, i.e 2.5 mm**

Remember:

CRL (in mm) + 6.5 = No. of weeks of gestation
At 9 weeks, hence CRL would be 9–6.5 = 2.5 mm approximately.

Also Know:
- CRL (in mm) + 42 = gestational age in days
- MSD (in mm) + 30 = gestational age in days   MSD = mean sac diameter.

N4. **Ans. is a, i.e. Gestation diabetes**

Ref. Dutta Obs. 7/e, p 647; Fernando Arias 3/e, p 46, 47; COGDT 10/e, p 107, Williams Obs. 23/e, p 299, 300

- **Amniocentesis or chorionic villi sampling should be offered to the following class of patients:**
  - Singleton pregnancy and maternal age 35 years or above.
  - Twin pregnancy at age over 31 years of pregnancy.
  - Previous chromosomally abnormal child.
  - Three or more spontaneous abortions.
  - Patient or husband with chromosome anomaly.
  - Family history of chromosome anomaly.
  - Possible female carrier of X-linked disease.
  - Metabolic disease risk (because of previous experience or family history).
  - NTD risk (because of previous experience or family history).
  - Positive second-trimester maternal serum screen or major fetal structural defect identified by USG.

N5. **Ans. is c, i.e. Middle cerebral artery**

Ref. Williams 23/e, p 362, 363

As discussed in the text:

Doppler of Middle cerebral artery is used to detect.

(i) Fetal anemia as in Rh isoimmunization, vasa previa and TTTS

(ii) IUGR

N6. **Ans. is d, i.e. Absent diastolic flow**

Ref. Williams 23/e, p 645

See the text for explanation.

N7. **Ans. is b, i.e. Increased fetal diastolic flow in the middle cerebral artery with absent diastolic flow in the aorta**

Ref. Williams Obs. 23/e, p 363, 364; Dutta Obs. 7/e, p 645

Doppler Study of Middle Cerebral Vessels:

- Normally the middle cerebral vessels have high resistance flow and are characterized by little diastolic flow.
- In case of IUGR a brain-sparing effect is seen with a reduction in the resistance indices in the middle cerebral vessels (i.e. increased flow) due to the shunting of blood to the brain in IUGR. Whereas in other areas (as aorta in the options) show decreased flow.
- *"Increased fetal diastolic flow in middle cerebral artery with absent diastolic flow in aorta implies fetal acidemia."*
  —*Dutta Obs. 7/e, p 648*

As far as persistence of diastolic notch in uterine artery is concerned, it signifies pregnancies destined to develop preeclampsia.

N8. **Ans. is b, i.e. Do NST**

 Remember: **Whenever a pregnant female complains of decreased fetal movement**

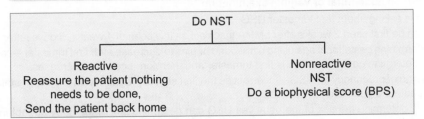

- A nonreactive NST earlier was being followed by a CST (contraction stress test) to confirm the diagnosis of hypoxia but CST is associated with risk of initiating labor and hence these days a nonreactive NST is being followed by a biophysical score (Manning score).

N9. **Ans. is a, i.e. Late deceleration** *Ref. Williams Obs. 23/e, p 420; COGDT 10/e, p 255, 257*

"Late decelerations are smooth falls in the FHR beginning after the contractions has started and ending after the contractions has ended. They are associated with fetal hypoxemia and potential for perinatal morbidity and mortality. Variable decelerations are abrupt in onset and return to baseline, vary in timing with the contractions, and usually represents cord compression."

As far as sinusoidal pattern is concerned - *Williams Obs. 23/e, p 420* says *"Intrapartum sinusoidal fetal heart patterns were not generally associated with fetal compromise".*

N10. **Ans. is b, i.e. Vasa previa**
Sinusoidal Pattern:
- Stable baseline heart rate of 120 to 160 beats/min with regular oscillations.
- Amplitude of 5 to 15 beats/min (rarely greater).
- Long-term variability frequency of 2 to 5 cycles per minute.
- Fixed or flat short-term variability.
- Oscillation of the sinusoidal waveform above or below a baseline.
- Absence of accelerations.

Causes of Sinusoidal Pattern:
- Serious fetal anemia due to Rh-isoimmunisation/rupture vasa previa/fetomaternal hemorrhage/twin-to-twin transfusion.
- Drugs — Meperidine, morphine, alphaprodine and butorphanol.
- Amnionitis.
- Fetal distress (+/–).
- Umbilical cord occlusion.

N11. **Ans. is d, i.e. Fetal stimulation** *—Williams 25/e, p 479*
Baseline variability on CTG is the oscillation of baseline FHR excluding acceleration and deceleration.
A variability of 5-25 BPM is a sign of fetal well-being.
Decreased variability is an omnious sign indicating seriously compromised fetus.
1. Fetal hypoxia and acidemia
2. Maternal acidemia
3. $MgSO_4$
4. Drugs given to mother such as analgesics during labor like narcotics, barbiturates, general anesthetics, etc.
5. Sleep phase
According to *Williams* increasing gestational age leads to increased baseline variability, so it can be taken prematurity will have decreased variability (i.e. **option 'b'** can be considered correct).

N12. **Ans. is a, i.e. 1 and 2 only** *Ref. Dutta Obs. 7/e, p 110, for 1, 612 for 2 and for 3; Williams 23/e, p 420*
Reactive NST, i.e. acceleration with fetal movements indicates a healthy fetus.
"Absence of deceleration in the NST is reassuring. Absence of accelerations in the NST may be a sign of fetal compromise."
—Fernando Arias 3/e, p 19
"Sinusoidal pattern is observed with serious fetal anemia, whether from D isoimmunization, ruptured vasa previa, fetomaternal hemorrhage or twin-to-twin transfusion."
—Williams 25/e, p 482

N13. **Ans. is b, i.e. The accuracy of determining gestational age using ultrasound begins to decrease after first trimester.**

N14. **Ans. is c, i.e. Crown rump length on abdominal or vaginal examination**
Coming to Q N13: The question is asking about first trimester USG.
Option a.	A gestational sac can be first seen 2 weeks after LMP – incorrect as it is seen at 4 weeks, 5 days after LMP
Option b.	The accuracy of determining gestational age using ultrasound begins to decrease after first trimester—correct as the best time to determine gestational age is first trimester and therefore accuracy decreases.
Option c.	Yolk sac is the first sign of pregnancy on USG—Incorrect as the first sign of pregnancy on USG is gestational sac, first sign of intrauterine pregnancy is yolk sac.
Option d.	USG can be used to determine the sex of the baby yes USG can determine sex of the baby but not in first trimester Sex of the baby can be determined positively on USG at 14 weeks.

N15. **Ans. is a, i.e. Glucose challenge test with 50 gm of glucose** *Ref. Read below*
Points worthnoting here are:

Patient is presenting to antenatal clinic at 24 weeks for routine check up and a coincidental finding on USG is fetus in frank breech position, with no other abnormalities.

- Now friends at 24 weeks, breech should not worry you as most of the times it spontaneously rotates and becomes cephalic by 32 weeks of pregnancy. Thus options '**c**' i.e. ECV and '**d**' i.e. immediate LSCS and '**e**' i.e. immediate induction and vaginal delivery are ruled out.
- Culture for *Neisseria gonorrhoeae* and *Chlamydia trachomatis*—It is normally done at initial visit and in certain high risk groups at 32-36 weeks along with group B streptococcal screening, so it is also ruled out.
- 24 weeks gestational age is the correct time for screening for gestational diabetes therefore we will do glucose challenge test with 50 gm of glucose.

Friends, mentioning about breech presentation was just given to confuse you, actually examiner wants to know whether you know the correct time for different screening tests or not.

N16. Ans. is b, i.e. USG   *Ref. Fernando Arias 2/e, p 35, 36; 3/e, p 54, Dutta Obs. 7/e, p 106*

MSAFP is a screening test. If it is raised, it should be followed by a diagnostic test, Level 2 USG. In earlier days, diagnostic test was amniocentesis or USG. But nowadays it is only USG.

N17. Ans. is c, i.e. 30 minutes

Auscultation of fetal heart sounds is a very good way of intrapartum fetal monitoring. Fetal heart sounds should be auscultated as here.

	1st stage	2nd stage
Low risk	every 30 mins	every 15 mins
High risk	every 15 mins	every 5 mins

N18. Ans. is d, i.e. CRL

CRL is used as a parameter to determine fetal age in 1st trimester and not midtrimester.

N19. Ans. is a, i.e. β-hCG   *Ref. Fernando Arias 4/e, p 4*

In women with HIV:

β-hCG levels in women who are HIV positive and are on treatment have been shown to have a lower value than women without HIV and those with HIV not receiving treatment. In contrast PAPP- A levels and NT are not affected by HIV status.

N20. Ans. is d, i.e. Abortion   *Ref. Williams Obs. 23/e, p 300; Dutta Obs. 7/e, p 107*

It must be quite surprising for some you that why I have not marked *option "a"* i.e. Limb abnormality as the answer.

This is because *Williams Obs. 23/e, p 300* says—

"Early reports of an association between CVS and limb reduction defects, oromandibular defects and cavernous hemangiomas have been disproved.

When CVS is performed after 9 weeks, Kuliev and Colleagues (1996) reported the incidence of limb-reduction defects to be 6 per 10,000 - the same as the background incidence.

The frequency of oromandibular limb hypogenesis however was increased after CVS when the procedure was performed before 9 weeks."

Therefore, It can be concluded—*M/C complication caused by CVS, if performed before 9 weeks is **oromandibular and limb defects** otherwise M/C complication of is CVS is **increased chances of fetal loss (abortion)**.*

Answers with Explanations to Previous Year Questions

1. **Ans. is d, i.e. Maternal urine**   *Ref. Dutta Obs. 9/e, p 103*

   Prenatal genetic diagnosis can be made by:
   - Chorion villi sampling
   - Amniocentesis: Amniotic fluid
   - Cordocentesis:
   - Fetal blood tests like Triple test/Maternal serum alpha fetoprotein done on maternal blood.

2. **Ans. None > Fetal skin biopsy**   *Ref. Williams 23/e, p 299-301*

   Currently there are 3 techniques available for obtaining fetal tissue for fetal karyotyping:
   i.   **Chorionic villi sampling**
   ii. **Amniocentesis**
   iii. **Percutaneous umbilical blood sampling (PUBS/Cordocentesis)**
   As far a **skin biopsy** is concerned obviously it can detect any chromosomal anomaly but is not used for this purpose.
   It is done between 17 and 20 weeks to detect serious skin disorders like epidermolysis bullosa, oculocutaneous albinism, etc.

3. **Ans. is c, i.e. Gastroschisis**

   Ref. Williams Obs. 25/e, p 284-285; Fernando Arias 3/e, p 83, 84; USG in Obs and Gynae by Callen 4/e, p 28

   Friends, many questions are asked on serum alpha fetoprotein, therefore basic knowledge of this protein is quite vital.

   Alpha Fetoprotein:

   Now after having this basic knowledge lets have a look at the question.
   In the question alpha fetoprotein will be increased in the following conditions.
   - Gastroschisis   – Ventral wall defect
   - Omphalocele   – Ventral wall defect
   - Spina bifida occulta   – Neural tube defect

   In Down's syndrome - AFP levels are decreased.
   Spina bifida occulta:
   Spina bifida occulta is usually a small, clinically asymptomatic defect, covered by skin, so there are less chances of mixing of fetal serum and maternal serum. Therefore the maternal serum alpha fetoprotein level usually does not increase in spina bifida occulta.
   "In the fetus with a defect such as anencephaly or spina bifida, AFP enters the amniotic fluid in increased amounts, leading to higher levels in the maternal serum as well. Levels of AFP are elevated in amniotic fluid and maternal serum only when such lesions are "open," i.e., when the neural tissue is exposed or covered by only a thin membrane. When NTDs are skin-covered, AFP does not escape from the fetal circulation, and such defects are generally not detected by maternal serum AFP (MSAFP) screening".   *Ref. USG in Obs. and Gynae by Callen 4/e, p 25*
   Omphalocele: *Ref. Fernando Arias 3/e, p 84*
   It is a midline defect of the anterior abdominal wall characterized by herniation of the abdominal viscera into the base of the umbilical cord.
   The protruding organs are typically covered by a thin aminoperitoneal membrane.
   Omphalocele has a strong association with high levels of maternal serum alpha-fetoprotein because the ventral wall defect allows mixing of fetal and maternal circulation.
   Gastroschisis: *Ref. Fernando Arias 2/e, p 83*
   Gastroschisis is a paraumbilical defect of the anterior abdominal wall, through which abdominal viscera herniates. The defect is usually located on the right side of the cord insertion and compromises the full thickness of the abdominal wall.
   There is no sac or membrane covering the herniated organs.
   This defect is associated with high alpha fetoprotein titre.
   Both gastroschisis and omphalocele are ventral wall defects containing abdominal organs and both are associated with high alphafetoprotein level in maternal serum.

But it is likely that alpha fetoprotein level will be higher in patients with gastroschisis as there is no sac or membrane which covers the herniated organs in this defect. So there is more possibility of fetoprotein leak into the maternal serum or amniotic fluid in Gastroschisis. The answer is further supported by the following graph from

Ref. USG in Obs. and Gynae by Callen 5/e, p 43

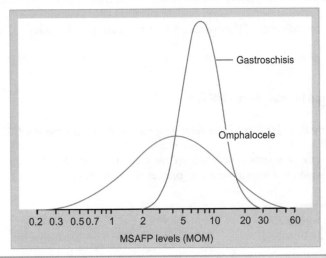

NdSAFP levels (MOM)

 Also Know:

Neural tube defects and abdominal wall defects can be differentiated by:
  i. USG
  ii. Amniotic fluid acetyl cholinesterase levels which are raised in open NTD but low in abdominal wall NTD
  iii. Pseudocholinesterase levels which are low in NTD but high in abdominal wall defects.
Gastroschisis and omphalocele can be differentiated by USG.

---

4. **Ans. is c, i.e. Talipes equinovarus**   *Ref. Callen USG in Obs. & Gynae 5/e, p 45; Fernando Arias 3/e, p54*

5. **Ans. is d, i.e. Congenital nephrotic syndrome**

6. **Ans. is a, c and d, i.e. Hepatoma, Endodermal sinus tumor, Cirrhosis**
   All the causes of increased AFP have been discussed. In Williams endodermal sinus tumor has not been mentioned as a cause of raised AFP but in Shaw 14/e, p 380 it has been given.

7. **Ans. is b, i.e. Trisomy**   *Ref. Williams Obs. 23/e, p 291, Shaw 14/e, p 380*
   As discussed in Ans. 4.
   Low levels of alpha fetoprotein are seen in:
   • **Devils:** Diabetes mellitus
   • **G:** Gestational trophoblastic tumor
   • **O:** Overestimated gestational age/obesity
   • **A:** Abortion
   • **T:** Trisomy 21 or 18

8. **Ans. is a, i.e. Fetal serum**   *Ref. COGDT 10/e, p 185; Callen USG in Obs & Gynae 5/e, p 42.*
   • Alpha fetoprotein is the most abundant protein in the fetal serum throughout fetal development.
   • It is transferred from fetus to amniotic fluid when fetus passes urine.
   • The concentration of AFP in amniotic fluid is approximately 100 folds less than in fetal serum, peaks at 13-14 weeks and then decreases in the second trimester (by 10% per week).
   • AFP reaches the maternal serum by diffusion across the amniotic membranes and via the placenta.
   • The level of AFP in maternal serum is less than fetal serum as is suggested by:
   "Fetal serum contains AFP in a concentration 150 times that of maternal serum".   *Ref. COGDT 10/e, p 185*
   "When the fetal serum level is 2 million U/L, the corresponding amniotic fluid AFP is 20,000 U/L, and the maternal serum level is 20 U/L".   *Callen USG for Obs & Gynae 5/e, p 42.*

9. **Ans. is b, c, and e, i.e. Diabetic patients have ↑ AFP level; MSAFP is unrelated to period of gestation; and Increased in Down syndrome**

Ref. Williams 23/e, p 289-291; Dutta Obs. 7/e, p 106; Fernando Arias 3/e, p 454 for option 'b', p 40 for option c

As discussed earlier, levels of AFP are decreased in diabetics and Down syndrome (Trisomy 21) hence options b and e are incorrect.

"The maternal serum concentration of AFP increases during pregnancy and reaches a peak between 28 and 32 weeks"

Fernando Arias 3/e, p 40

This means option c is incorrect.

Option a and d are correct.

10. **Ans. is a, i.e. Major source in fetal life is yolk sac**   *Ref. Williams 23/e, p 288; Dutta Obs. 7/e, p 106*

As discussed earlier:

"AFP is synthesized early in gestation by the fetal yolk sac and later by the fetal GIT and liver."

—*Williams 23/e, p 288*

- No where it is given that major source is yolk sac, so this statement *(option "a")* is partially correct.
- AFP levels are not increased in Wilms tumour (i.e. **option "b"** is incorrect).
- Maximum level of AFP in:
  - Fetal serum is at 13 weeks
  - Amniotic fluid is at 13 weeks
  - Maternal serum is at 28-32 weeks.   —*Dutta Obs. 6/e, p 107; Fernando Arias 3/e, p 40*

So, option 'c' is incorrect.

- Half life of AFP is 3.5 days (internet) so, *option 'd'* is wrong.

Amongst all the options given - *Option 'a'* is the best bet.

11. **Ans. is b, i.e. Trisomy 21**   *Ref. Williams Obs. 25/e, p 287; Fernando Arias 2/e, p 38*

Low levels of MSAFP (< 0.25 MOM) are seen in:

Devils: Diabetes mellitus
G: Gestational trophoblastic disease
O: Overestimated gestational age
    Maternal Obesity
A: Abortion
T: Trisomy

Note: The list given in the *Williams Obs. 25/e, p 291* — *Includes fetal death both in causes of increased and decreased AFP. But Fernando Arias 2/e, p 38 specifically includes — IUD in the causes of increased AFP and Blighted ovum/Abortion in the causes of decreased AFP.*

12. **Ans. is d, i.e. Ectopic pregnancy**   *Ref. Williams Obs. 23/e, p 63, 64*

13. **Ans. is d and e, i.e. Rh-incompatibility; and Down syndrome**   *Ref. Williams Obs. 25/e, p 103; Dutta Obs. 9/e, p 54*

hCG levels:

Caught you, I know some of you must have instantly answered *"Down's syndrome"*. But my dear friends read the question very carefully. It says decreased hCG levels and not decreased AFP levels.

hCG levels:

Increased	Decreased	
Multiple fetuses[Q]		
Erythroblastosis fetalis associated with fetal hemolytic anemia	a.	Impending spontaneous abortion[Q]
Down syndrome[Q]	b.	Other trisomies viz. 18, 13
Choriocarcinoma[Q]	c.	Ectopic pregnancy
Hydatidiform mole[Q]		

14. Ans. is a, b and c, i.e. H. mole, Choriocarcinoma and Ectopic pregnancy

Ref. Shaw 14/e, p 231, 235, 380; Dutta Obs. 7/e, p 59

β-hCG levels are helpful in monitoring:

a. H. mole:

"A method of detecting the persistent mole and development of choriocarcinoma is by estimating hCG is the serum urine".

—Shaw 14/e, p 231

b. Choriocarcinoma:

β-hCG is a specific marker for choriocarcinoma.

The levels of β–hCG are monitored following chemotherapy and complete regression of tumor is indicated when three consecutive weekly radioimmunoassays of hCG in serum are negative. *—Shaw 14/e, p 235*

c. Ectopic pregrancy:

In case of unruptured ectopic pregnancy which is managed medically with methotrexate or by conservative surgery- monitoring is done by estimating β-hCG levels.

"Following conservative surgery or medical treatment, estimation of β-hCG should be done weekly till the value becomes < 5.0 mIU/ml" *—Dutta Obs 6/e, p 191*

d. Endodermal sinus tumor:

'These tumors are yolk sac tumors and their markers are Alpha fetoprotein and antitrypsin so their levels and not beta-hCG. So hCG levels are not used for monitoring. *—Shaw 14/e, p 380*

15. Ans. is a, i.e. Open spina bifida *Ref. Dutta Obs. 7/e, p 106; Fernando Arias 2/e, p 36*

Amniotic fluid Acetylcholinesterase level is elevated in open neural tube defect:

- It has a better diagnostic value than AFP.
- In case of suspected neural tube defect, on Amniocentesis, if amniotic fluid AFP levels are raised but Acetyl- cholinesterase levels are normal, patient should be reassured that elevated AFP levels are probably caused by fetal blood contamination but, if acetylcholinesterase is also elevated along with AFP it is indicative of NTD.
- It also helps to distinguish between neural tube defect and abdominal wall defects (both of which cause elevated MSAFP):
  – Acetylcholinesterase is raised in open NTD, but is low in abdominal wall defects.
  – In patients with NTD, the ratio of acetylcholinesterase to butyrylcholinesterase levels is 0.14 or more. In case of abdominal wall defects this ratio is less than 0.14.

16. Ans. is d, i.e. Pseudocholinesterase *Ref. Fernando Arias 2/e, p 35, 36; Sheila Balakrishnan, p 603*

In patients with elevated amniotic fluid AFP to differentiate between NTD and abdominal wall defect, acetylcholinesterase and pseudocholinesterase are measured:

Marker	Neural tube defect	Abdominal wall defect
• Acetylcholinesterase	• High	• Low
• Pseudocholinesterase (Butyl cholinesterase)	• Low	• High
• Ratio of ACh/pseudocholinesterase	• > 0.14	• < 0.14

 Also Know: Amniotic fluid levels of 17 hydroxyprogesterone are raised in congenital adrenal hyperplasia.

17. Ans. is d, i.e. Between 11–13 weeks

Ref. Harrison 17/e, p 409; Williams Obs. 22/e, p 329, 23/e, p 300, Dutta Obs. 9/e, p 104

"CVS is the second most common procedure for genetic prenatal diagnosis. Because this procedure is routinely performed at about 10 to 12 weeks of gestation, it allows for an earlier detection of abnormalities and a safer pregnancy termination, if desired." *—Harrison 17/e, p 409*

"Biopsy of chorionic villi is generally performed at 10 to 13 weeks." *—Williams 25/e, p 300*

"CVS is usually performed between 11 and 14 weeks." *—Fernando Arias 4/e, p 8*

18. Ans. is c, i.e. Oromandibular limb defects *Ref. Williams Obs. 21/e, p 990; 22/e, p 330, 23/e, p 300*

"Chorionic villous sampling is usually performed at 10-13 weeks and is associated with several complications but studies suggests that limb reduction and oromandibular limb hypogenesis is more common, if CVS is done before 9 weeks. So, CVS is done after 9 weeks because it is more safe." *—Williams Obs. 21/e, p 990*

"The frequency of oromandibular limb hypogenesis, however was increased after CVS, when the procedure was performed before 9 weeks." *—Williams Obs. 22/e, p 330*

"It was shown that limb reduction defects were associated with CVS performed earlier in gestation—typically around 7 weeks."

—*Williams 23/e, p 300*

19. Ans. is a, i.e. Tay-Sachs disease

Ref. JB Sharma TB of Obs pg 161; Williams Obs 25/e, p 296

Ref. Operative Obs and Gynae by Randhir Puri, Narendra Malhotra 1/e, p 261, 262; Obs. and Gynae Beckmann 5/e, p 45

In chorionic villous biopsy, trophoblastic tissue is obtained from the chorionic villi, followed by biochemical or molecular (DNA) analysis or chromosomal analysis of this tissue to diagnose various conditions.

Conditions which require molecular or DNA analysis	Conditions which require biochemical analysis
• Hemoglobinopathies	• Tay Sach's disease
• Sickle cell disease	• Niemann Pick disease
• Alpha thalassemia	• Gaucher's disease
• Beta thalassemia	• Urea cycle defects
• Hemophilia A or B	• Amino acid disorder
• Duchenne muscular dystrophy	• Congenital adrenal hyperplasia
• Cystic fibrosis	• Phenylketonuria
• Alpha-1 antitrypsin deficiency	
• Tay Sach's disease	

For diagnosis of Tay Sach's disease biochemical analysis and DNA analysis of chorionic villous sample is done (not DNA analysis). For rest all options only DNA analyses would do that is why I am picking that option.

20. Ans. is c, i.e. Neural tube defect

Chorionic villi sampling cannot detect structural abnormalities like neural tube defect.

"The indications of CVS and amniocentesis are usually the same, however disorders that specifically require analysis of amniotic fluid liquor such as neural tube defects are not amenable to prenatal diagnosis by CVS."

Ref. Obs. and Gynae Beckman 5/e, p 45

21. Ans. is a, b and d, i.e. Strongly associated with fasciomandibular defects; Done in 10-12 weeks; and Done to diagnose genetic disorders

Ref. Dutta Obs. 7/e, p 107

Remember after CVS:
• Anti-D immunoglobulin 50 m gm IM should be administered to a Rh-negative woman.

22. Ans. is b, i.e. Always done as a blind procedure

Ref. Williams Obs. 25/e, p 297–298

23. Ans. is b, i.e. 16-20 weeks

Best time to do amniocentesis is between 15–20 weeks.

24. Ans. is b, i.e. 1000 IU/mL

Ref. Dutta Obs. 7/e, p 642

Critical titre of hCG:

β-hCG level (mIU/ml)	Structure visible	TVS/TAS
• 1000-1200	Gestational sac	TVS
• 6000	Gestational Sac	TAS

25. Ans. is a, i.e. 6.0-6.5 weeks

Ref. USG in Obs. and Gynae. Callen 4/e, p 119, 120

When the question says—cardiac activity is earliest detected at—it means they are asking about TVS—Transvaginal sonography.

On TVS, cardiac activity is seen at 6 weeks.

 Remember: If the question says cardiac activity is detected at and does not specify TVS or TAS: Then it is TAS—so then answer is 7–8 weeks.

So earliest cardiac activity can be detected between 6 to 6.5 weeks.

26. Ans. is a, i.e. Yolk sac

Ref. Dutta Obs. 7/e, p 642

See the text for explanation.

27. Ans. is a, i.e. USG for cardiac activity *Ref. Dutta Obs. 7/e, p 147*

- With transvaginal scanning, cardiac activity is reliably seen in the uterus by 6 weeks, and by TAS cardiac activity by 7 weeks, cardiac activity confirms pregnancy.
- The level of hCG are not the best confirmatory test for pregnancy as hCG in plasma and urine are strikingly increased in women with hydatiform mole.
- Bimanual palpation can only detect uterine enlargement but the cause of uterine enlargement can only be detected by ultrasound.
- Confirmation of cardiac activity by Doppler can be done only at 10 weeks and not 6 weeks.

28. Ans. is b, i.e. Ectopic gestation *Ref. USG in Obs. and Gynae by Callen 4/e, p 127*

A pseudogestational sac is seen in a patient with an ectopic pregnancy.

Pseudogestational sac:

Character	True gestational sac	Pseudogestational sac
• Location within the uterus	Eccentric	Central
• Shape	Round and regular in outline	Irregular
• Double ring sign due to chorion	Present	Absent
• Identification of structures: yolk sac, fetal pole	Present	Absent
• Increase in sac size	1 mm/day	Absent

29. Ans. is a, i.e. Anencephaly

Ref. Williams Obs. 21/e, p 1120; USG in Obs. and Gynae by Callen 4/e, p 284, Fernando Arias 3/e, p 64, 66, 69

As discussed in the chapter, anencephaly can be diagnosed as early as 10 weeks/first trimester in experienced hards.

Microcephaly: *Ref. USG in Obs and Gynae Callen 4/e, p 298, 299*

- It is decreased head size.
- In these patients both brain mass and total cell number are reduced.
- There is disproportion in size between the skull and face.
- It is difficult to recognize this anomaly by ultrasound – A head circumference below 2 SD from the mean is used as a diagnostic criteria in midtrimester scan.

Holoprosencephaly is the presence of a single centrally placed cerebral ventricle and may be associated with midline abnormalities of the face.

With the use of vaginal probe it can be recognised in the beginning of midtrimester.

> ***Also Know:*** Encephalocele can also be recognised in first trimester and is seen as a bony defect with protrusion of the brain tissue and meninges. Occipital encephaloceles are commonest. A genetic association of encephalocele and polycystic kidney and is called Meckel-Gruber syndrome, which is an autosomal recessive disorder.

30. Ans. is a, i.e. Biparietal diameter *Ref. Williams Obs. 24/e, p 198; USG in Obs. and Gynae by Callen 4/e, p 208*

"In the second trimester the BPD most accurately reflects the gestational age, with a variation of 7 to 10 day."

Ref. Williams 24/e, p 198

Prediction of fetal gestational age using ultrasound biometric parameters

Ref. Bedside Obs/Gynae by Richa Saxena, p 191

Period of gestation	Ultrasound parameter to be used
8 weeks to 12 weeks	Crown-rump length measurement
Second trimester	BPD, HC
Third trimester	Femur length

Note: In brachycephaly or Dolichocephaly – HC is better parameter in 2nd trimester than BPD as HC is unaffected by the shape of fetal head.

31. Ans. is d, i.e. IUGR

As discussed in the text Doppler of middle cerebral artery is useful in IUGR.

32. Ans. is c, i.e. Fetal hypoxia

33. Ans. is c, i.e. Variable deceleration

34. Ans. is a, i.e. Head compression *Ref. Dutta Obs. 9/e, p 569*

"Deceleration is defined as a decrease in fetal heart rate below the base line by 15 beats per minute or more."

Three basic patterns of deceleration are observed, each of which has a diagnostic significance:

FHR pattern	Feature	Seen in
Early deceleration	Deceleration coincidences with a contraction Uniform onset, i.e. gradual takes > 30 sec and recovery Magnitude rarely >40 bpm	Head compression Not associated with fetal hypoxia
Late deceleration	Begins at or after the contraction peak and touches baseline only after contraction Uniform onset, i.e. gradual takes > 30 secs and recovery May be of low magnitude 10-20 bpm	Uteroplacental insufficiency, Fetal hypoxia. It is an ominous finding
Variable deceleration	Variable relationship to contraction Ragged waveform. Abrupt in onset < 30 sec Variable magnitude	Umbilical cord compression M/C type of deceleration

35. Ans. is a, i.e. Two fetal heart rate accelerations are noted in 20 minutes

Ref. Dutta Obs. 7/e, p 108, 109; Williams Obs. 23/e, p 338; Fernando Arias 3/e, p 17, 18

See the text for explanation.

36. Ans. is d, i.e. Proceed to biophysical profile *Ref. Management of High Risk Pregnancy, Manjupuri, SS Trivedi, p 62*

Non Stress Test is a screening test done when a female complains of decreased fetal movement.

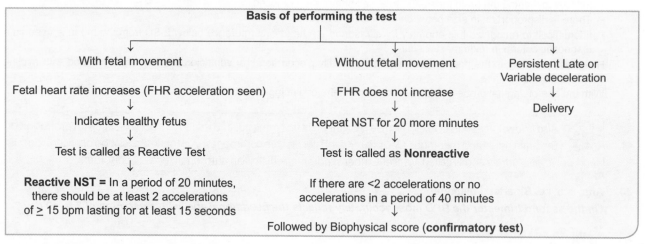

Basis of performing the test

With fetal movement	Without fetal movement	Persistent Late or Variable deceleration
Fetal heart rate increases (FHR acceleration seen) ↓	FHR does not increase ↓	↓ Delivery
Indicates healthy fetus ↓	Repeat NST for 20 more minutes ↓	
Test is called as Reactive Test ↓	Test is called as **Nonreactive** ↓	
Reactive NST = In a period of 20 minutes, there should be at least 2 accelerations of ≥ 15 bpm lasting for at least 15 seconds	If there are <2 accelerations or no accelerations in a period of 40 minutes ↓ Followed by Biophysical score (**confirmatory test**)	

37. Ans. is b, i.e. 72 hours *Ref. Williams Obs. 23/e, p 339*

Intervals between NST testing

"The interval between tests is arbitrarily set at 7 days. According to ACOG, more frequent testing is advocated for women with post-term pregnancy, type I diabetes mellitus, IUGR or gestational hypertension. In these circumstances some investigators recommend twice weekly (i.e. after 72 hours) with additional testing performed for maternal or fetal deterioration regardless of the time elapsed since the last test. Others recommend NST daily. Generally daily NST is recommended with severe preeclampsia remote from term."

This text I have given from *Williams*.

Reading the above text it is evident that, in severe preeclampsia - testing should be done daily.

For the rest of the high risk pregnancies twice weekly testing can be done (i.e. ≈ after 72 hours).

This is my way of looking at things because in clinical practice also we perform NST weekly or twice weekly.

38. Ans. is b, i.e. Oxytocin challenge test *Ref. Dutta Obs. 7/e, p 109*

39. Ans. is a, b and e, i.e. Fetal movements, Respiratory movements, Fetal heart rate accelerations

Ref. Williams 23/e, p 339, 340; Dutta Obs. 7/e, p 109

Manning: proposed a method using 5 fetal biophysical variables[Q] to assess the status of fetal well-being antenatally. These 5 variables together are called as Biophysical Profile (BPP)/Biophysical score

- Fetal **T**one
- Fetal **B**reathing Movements (seen in 30 minutes)
- Fetal gross body **M**ovements (seen in 30 minutes)
- **A**mniotic Fluid Volume
- **N**on stress test (i.e. option 'e' of Q. 39—fetal heart rate acceleration)

Mnemonic: Remember: TBM - (Tuberculosis meningitis) Always Notorious for these variables.

40. Ans. is c, i.e. Fetal Scalp blood pH > 7.3

Ref. Dutta Obs. 7/e, p 612, 613, William Obs. 23/e, p 426

- Normal fetal scalp pH ranges from 7.25 to 7.35.
- Fetal hypoxia is indicated by 'acidosis' or fall in fetal scalp pH to values below normal (Not by increase).
- It is used to corroborate the significance of fetal CTG (Cardiotocography).

Interpretation of Fetal Scalp blood sampling

	pH	Action
Normal	> 7.25	Reassuring
Pre-acidosis	7.20-7.25	Repeat in 30 min
Acidosis	< 7.20	Immediate delivery

Meconium staining: It has always been said meconium indicates fetal distress but it is seen that meconium may also be seen in fetuses which are not acidemic at birth.

"The high incidence of meconium observed in the amniotic fluid during labor often represents fetal passage of gastrointestinal contents in conjunction with normal physiological process. Although normal such meconium becomes an environmental hazard when fetal acidemia supervenes.'

Ref. Williams Obs. 23/e, p 432

Fetal movements: both decreased as well as excessive fetal movements are ominous features.

Fetal heart rate:

"Fetal distress on CTG is characterised by tachycardia or bradycardia, reduced FHR variability, deceleration and absence of acceleration."

Ref. Dutta Obs. 6/e, p 613

 Also Know: Cut off for oxygen saturation for diagnosing fetal distress is < 30%.
- Oxygen saturation > 30% even in presence of non reassuring FHR tracing indicates normal fetal oxygenation.

41. Ans. is a, i.e. NST with AFI

Ref. Williams Obs 24/e, p 342-344

Modified biophysical score consists of NST or vibroacoustic non stress test and estimation of amniotic fluid volume using AFI (<5 is considered abnormal). It takes 10 minutes to perform the score and is used as a screening test.

42. Ans. is a, i.e. Neural tube defect

Ref. Williams Obs. 23/e, p 354, 355

Signs of Spina bifida on Ultrasound

- Small biparietal diameter.
- Ventriculomegaly.
- Frontal bone scalloping or the so called *lemon sign*.
- Elongation and downward displacement of the cerebellum-the so called *banana sign*.
- Effacement or obliteration of the cisterna magna.

43. Ans. is a, i.e. Amniocentesis

This patient has H/O 2 kids with thalassemia major, hence definitive diagnosis is needed in this pregnancy. At 18 weeks, definitive diagnostic test is amniocentesis. Cordocentesis is difficult to perform before 20 weeks: "Before 20 weeks it is difficult to visualize the cord insertion and cord lumen is narrow."

Ref. JB Sharma, Obstetrics p 162

44. Ans. is d, i.e. 4000

Ref. Williams Obs 24/e, p 1104

- Folate Requirement in normal pregnancy: 4 micrograms
- Folate requirement in pregnancy with previous history of neural tube defects: 4 mg.

45. Ans. is c, i.e. hCG levels

hCG can be detected in maternal blood as early as 8 days following fertilisation/day 22 of menstrual cycle 15 days before missed period by immunoassay.

USG can detect cardiac activity as early as 6 weeks of pregnancy by TVS.

46. **Ans. is All**   *Ref. Dutta Obs 7/e, p 607; 8/e, p 690*

Stillbirth is birth of a newborn after 28 completed weeks (weighing 1000 g or more) when the baby does not breathe or show any sign of life after delivery.

Important causes of stillbirth:

Important causes of stillbirths and main interventions		
Causes	**Percent**	**Proven interventions**
Birth asphyxia and trauma	30	Skilled attendant at birth. Effective management of obstetric complications
Pregnancy complications (placental abruption, preeclampsia, diabetes mellitus)	30	Prepregnancy care, effective management of pregnancy complications
Fetal congenital malformations and chromosomal anomalies	15	Preconceptional genetic counseling, prenatal diagnosis
Infection	5	Effective care during pregnancy and labor. Clean delivery
Cause unknown	20	

Prematurity is a common cause of stillbirth.   *—Reddy 32/e, p 417.*

47. **Ans. is a, b and c, i.e. Twin, Down syndrome and Choriocarcinoma**   *Ref. Williams 25/e, p 103; Dutta Obs 9/e, p 54*

Increased	Decreased
Multiple fetuses[Q]	a. Ectopic pregnancy[Q]
Erythroblastosis fetalis due to fetal hemolytic anemia	b. Impending spontaneous abortion[Q]
Down syndrome[Q]	c. Other trisomies viz. 18, 13
Choriocarcinoma[Q]	
Hydatidiform mole[Q]	

48. **Ans. is a, i.e. 100%**   *Ref. Fernando Arias 3/e, p 34*

Recurrent Risk of Down's syndrome

Chromosome Constitution				
Affected child	**Father**	**Mother**	**Risk of the Offspring**	
Trisomy 21 (nondisjunction)	N	N	Mother < 30 years in present pregnancy	2 – 3%
			Mother > 30 years; had Down baby before 30 years of age	Risk at mothers age + 1%
			Mother >30 years; had Down baby after 30 years age	Risk at mother's age
Translocations 14/21, 15/21,	N	C		12%
13/21, 21/22	C	N		2–3%
Translocations	**N**	**C**		**100%**
21/21 called as balanced	**C**	**N**		**100%**
translocation				
Mosaic	N	N		2–3%

C = Carrier; N = normal.

 Remember: A funda – In balanced translocation (21/21), the risk of recurrence in subsequent pregnancy is 100% — regardless of the fact whether mother/father is a carrier.

49. Ans. is c, i.e. All in reproductive age groups. *Ref. Williams Obs. 23/e, p 296, Fernando arias 2/e, p 26*

Most important factor for Down syndrome is maternal age

As age of mother increases risk of down syndrome increases. Current recommendations for screening of Down syndrome are universal screening, i.e. it should be done in all pregnant females of all age.

In 30 years	: 1 in 1000
In 35 years	: 1 in 350
In 40 years	: 1 in 100
45 years	: 1 in 30

50. Ans. is a, c and e, i.e Nuchal translucency, PAPP-A and β-hCG *Ref. Williams Obs 24/e*

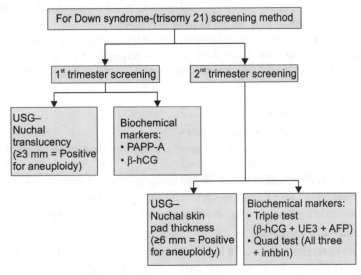

51. Ans. is c, i.e. Human placental lactogen (HPL) *Ref. Dutta Obs 9/e, p 103*

Discussed in preceding text

52. Ans. is a, i.e. Beta hCG and PAPPA

53. Ans. is a, i.e. Down's syndrome *Ref. Fernando arias 3/e, p 38, USG in obs & gynae by colleen 4/e, p 41*

In the options we have Down syndrome as well trisomy 18 as, discussed in preceding text, in both these conditions NT is raised still the better option is Down syndrome.

My answer is based on the following lines from USG in Obs. and Gynae by Callen.

"Johnson et al showed that simple nuchal translucency between 10 and 14 weeks were associated with a 60% incidence of abnormal karyotypes-mostly trisomy 21. Unlike the second trimester experience, in which large cystic hygromas were most often associated with Turner syndrome, the 45X karyotype represented a minority of the karyotype abnormalities in the group of fetuses with first trimester nuchal translucency thickening."

 Remember:

- Nuchal translucency (NT) is a sonographic marker of Down syndrome/aneuploidy in first trimester whereas nuchal fold thickness (NFT > 5 mm) is the most important sonographic marker of aneuploidy in the second trimester.
- Absent nasal bone is another marker of Down syndrome in 1st trimester. Nasal bone is absent in 68.8% of fetuses with Down syndrome.

54. Ans. is d, i.e. Amniocentesis

55. Ans. is c, i.e. Chorionic villous biopsy *Ref. Ghai 6/e, p 604, Fernando arias 3/e, p 44, 45*

As discussed earlier—the best way of diagnosing Down syndrome in present pregnancy is by karyotyping of the fetus. The sample for which can be obtained by chorionic villous biopsy in the first trimester and Amniocentesis in the second trimester.

In a Nut shell remember:

	1st trimester	2nd trimester
Screening test	Nuchal translucency + β-hCG + PAPP-A, i.e. combined test	Quad test/Triple test
Diagnostic test (karyotyping)	Chronic villi sampling	Amniocentesis

56.   Ans. is c, i.e. Karyotyping *Ref. Williams 23/e, p 267-269; Fernando Arias 3/e, p 34*

When a pregnant woman has a history of previous child with Down syndrome, it becomes important to know the type of chromosomal constitution, not only in that particular child but also in the parents because the risk of recurrence in future pregnancy depends on all these factors (as shown in Table in Ans. 48).

Karyotyping of Mrs. Annadural has already been done and a translocation variety of Down's detected. Risk of recurrence however does not depend on mother's karyotype alone, but it also depends on the father's karyotype. Father's karyotyping is therefore the test of choice prior to next pregnancy to determine the risk of recurrence.

57.   Ans. is b, i.e. Amniocentesis

58.   Ans. is d, i.e. Chorionic villous biopsy *Ref. Fernando Arias 3/e, p 27, Dutta Obs. 7/e, p 108, 494.*

In patients with previous history of Down syndrome –

"The risk of recurrence is greater than the risk of genetic diagnosis and these patients should be advised to seek genetic counseling and to have a genetic diagnosis." *Ref. Fernando Arias 3/e, p 27*

Therefore amniocentesis /Chorionic villous biopsy should be done.

In Q57 patient is 18 weeks pregnant therefore we will do Amniocentesis.

In Q58 since Amniocentesis is not given in options therefore chorionic villous biopsy is the answer of choice.

59.   Ans. is c, i.e. Chorionic villus sampling *Ref. Fernando Arias 3/e, p 38-40, Williams Obs. 23/e, p 300*

Friends – In Patients with previous H/O Down's syndrome the only confirmatory test, which tells us with 100% reliability of the chances of Down's syndrome in present pregnancy is **"Karyotyping".**

The sample for karyotyping can be obtained in first-trimester by – chorionic villi sampling and in 2nd trimester by amniocentesis.

So obviously we will think of marking option 'c' i.e. chorionic villi sampling as the correct answer but, the question specifically mentions that patient is 9 weeks pregnant and we all know that if CVS is done before 10 weeks– it can lead to limb reduction defects and oromandibular defects in the fetus. Therefore, some people argue CVS is not the correct thing to do at this stage.

Read for yourself what Williams has to say on this issue.

"Early reports of an association between CVS and limb. Reduction defects and oromandibular limb hypogenesis caused a great deal of concern (Burton, 1992; Firth, 1991, 1994; Hsieh, 1995, and all their colleagues). Subsequently, it was shown that limb-reduction defects were associated with CVS performed earlier in gestation—typically around 7 weeks" *Ref. Williams Obs 23/e, p 300*

60.   Ans. is b, i.e. Choroid plexus cyst *Ref. Ultrasound of Fetal Synd. by Benacerraf 1/e, p 404, 405, 413; USG in Obs. & Gyane by Callen 4/e, p 44; Williams Obs 23/e, p 295.*

Single umbilical artery and, diaphragmatic hernia are seen in USG of Down syndrome.

"Several investigators have suggested that choroids plexus cysts are also associated with an increased risk of trisomy 21. However, our group demonstrated that the frequency of choroids plexus cysts among fetuses with trisomy 21 was the same as that among fetuses without trisomy 21, suggesting that the presence of choroid plexus cysts should not increase a patient's calculated risk of having a fetus with Down syndrome.

This is in agreement with the work from Gupta and co-worker, who reported a 1 in 880 risk of Down syndrome among fetuses with isolated choroids plexus cysts detected antenatally." *Ref. Ultrasound of Fetal Synd. by Benacerraf 1/e, p 404, 505*

"The presence of a cyst in the choroids plexus in an axial view through the upper portion of fetal head has been correlated with the increased risk of Trisomy 18" —*Management of High Risk Pregnancy by SS Trivedi, Manju Puri, p 12*

- Choroid plexus cysts are found to be associated with trisomy 18 (occurring in nearly 30% of cases of trisomy 18).
- Choroid plexus cysts are also found in 0.7 to 3.6% of normal second trimester fetuses.

Structural malformation	Aneuploidy risk	Associated with
1. Cystic hygroma	50–70	Turners ,Trisomy 21, 18, 13; Triploidy
2. Holoprosencephaly	30–40	Trisomy 21, 18, 13; Turners.
3. Ventriculomegaly	5–25	Trisomy 21, 18, 13; Turners.
4. Dandy Walker malformation	40%	Trisomy 21, 18, 13; Turners.
5. Omphalocele	30–50	Trisomy 18, 13, 21, Triploidy
6. Duodenal atresia	30	Trisomy 21
7. Choroid plexus cyst	30%	Trisomy 18
8. Diaphragmatic hernia	5–15	Trisomy 18, 13, 21
9. Esophageal atresia	10–15	Trisomy 18, 21
10. Cleft up palate	5–15	Trisomy 18, 13

61. Ans. is d, i.e. Anencephaly *Ref. Williams 24/e, p 201*

The ultrasound appearance (absence of cranial vault and varying amount of brain) is classically seen in anencephaly of fetus.

62. Ans. is b, i.e. Amniotic sac and yolk sac *Ref: Williams 24/e p 170*

A double bleb sign is a sonographic feature where there is visualization of a gestational sac containing a yolk sac and amniotic sac giving an appearance of two small bubbles. The embryonic disc is located between the two bubbles. It is an important feature of an intrauterine pregnancy and thus distinguishes a pregnancy form a pseudogestational sac or decidual cast cyst.

Double bleb sign
• Visualization of a **gestational sac** containing a **yolk sac and amniotic sac** giving an **appearance of two small bubbles**[Q]
• Feature of an **intrauterine pregnancy**[Q]
• **Distinguishes a pregnancy from a pseudogestational sac** or **decidual cast cyst**[Q].

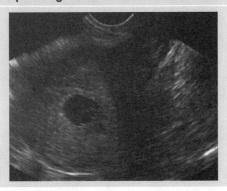

63. Ans. is a, i.e. Anencephaly *(Ref Williams Obs 24/e, pg 201)*

Anencephaly can be detected in the late first trimester.

Earliest it can be detected by 10 weeks and best by 14 weeks on USG

64. Ans. is d, i.e. Drop in fetal heart rate to less than 70 bpm for 60 seconds

Classification of variable deceleration

Deceleration	Definition
Mild variable deceleration	>80 bpm irrespective of duration, or <30 seconds irrespective of depth or between FHR-70 to 80 bpm lasting for 60 seconds
Moderate variable deceleration	>70 bpm lasting for 30 to 60 seconds or between FHR-70 to 80 bpm lasting for > 60 seconds
Severe variable deceleration	< 70 bpm lasting for 60 seconds

65. **Ans. is b, i.e. Estimation of PAAP-A and βhCG** *(Ref: J B Sharma textbook of Obs 1/e, pg 155, Williams 24/e pg 290)*
    First Trimester Screening
    - It uses PAPP-A (lower in Down syndrome) and free β-hCG (higher in Down's syndrome) b/w 11 and 14 weeks
    - It can detects 62% Down's syndrome pregnancies with a 5% false-positive rate.
    - In Downs syndrome hCG levels are higher approx. 2.0 MOM and PAPP-A levels are lower approx. 0.5 MOM . With Trisomy 18 and 13 levels of both analytes are lower.

66. **Ans. is a and b, i.e. Hypertension and Anaemia**
    (Ref: Dutta Obs 8th/255,303; J B Sharma 1st/541; William Obs 24th /1156)

    "Acne usually improves in pregnancy"—*J B Sharma 1st ed, pg 543*

    "There are no obvious adverse effects of rheumatoid arthritis on pregnancy outcome. The disease improves in majority (90%) of women during pregnancy"—*J B Sharma 1st ed pg 541*

    "Up to 90 percent of women with rheumatoid arthritis will experience improvement during pregnancy"—*William Obs 24th ed, pg 1178*

    "Hypertension is one of the common medical complications of pregnancy"—*Dutta Obs 8th ed pg 255*

    "Anemia is the commonest haematological disorder that may occur in pregnancy, the others being rhesus isoimmunisation and blood coagulation disorders"—*Dutta Obs 8th ed pg 303.*

    > *Note:* T helper cells 2 increase and its cytokines i.e Interleukin 4 and 6 also increase in pregnancy hence SLE flares during pregnancy whereas T Helper cells 1 and its cytokines i.e IL 2 and interferon gamma decrease during pregnancy so Rheumatoid arthritis improves in pregnancy.

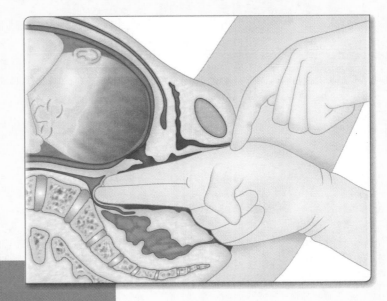

2

Section

Labor

Pelvis and Fetal Skull

PELVIS

ANATOMY

- The pelvis is composed of four bones—sacrum, coccyx, and two innominate bones.
- Each innominate bone is formed by the fusion of three bones—ilium, ischium and pubis.
- **Pelvic joint:** There are four joints in the pelvis namely the symphysis pubis, sacroiliac joint (left and right) and the sacrococcygeal joint (Table 7.1).

Table 7.1: Joints in the pelvis

Joints	Types
Symphysis pubis	Fibrocartilaginous joint
Sacroiliac joint	Synovial joint
Sacrococcygeal joint	Synovial hinge joint

- The pelvis is divided anatomically into false pelvis and true pelvis by the pelvis brim (Fig. 7.1).
- **The boundries of pelvic brim or inlet** (from posterior to anterior) are—sacral promontory, sacral alae, sacroiliac joint, iliopectineal lines, iliopectineal eminence, upper border of superior pubic rami, pubic tubercle, pubic crest and upper border of pubic symphysis (Fig. 7.2).
  - **False pelvis:** False pelvis lies above the pelvic brim and has no obstetrical significance
  - **True pelvis:** True pelvis lies below the pelvic brim and plays an important role in childbirth and delivery.

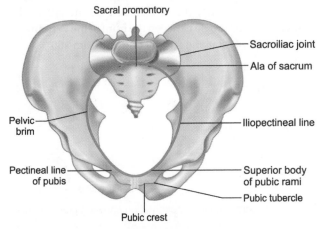

Fig. 7.1: Boundaries of the pelvic brim

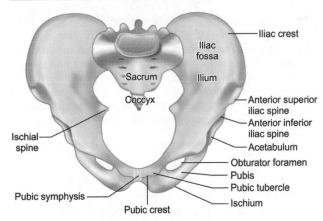

Fig. 7.2: Anterior view of maternal pelvis

The true pelvis forms a bony canal through which the fetus passes at the time of labor. It is formed by the symphysis pubis anteriorly and sacrum and coccyx posteriorly.

The true pelvis can be divided into three parts—Pelvic Inlet, Cavity and Outlet.

- Pelvic inlet lies @ level of pelvic brim
- Pelvic cavity lies @ level of ischial spine
- Pelvic outlet lies @ level of ischial tuberosity

Pelvic Inlet (Superior Strait)

- Pelvic inlet is transverse oval in shape in the most common variety of pelvis (gynecoid pelvis)
- It is narrowest in anteroposterior dimension and widest in transverse dimension
- The plane of the pelvic inlet (also known as superior straight) is not horizontal, but is tilted forwards due to oblique articulation of the pelvis with femur bone. It makes an angle of 55 degree with the horizontal. This angle is known as the **angle of inclination**. Radiographically, this angle can be measured by measuring the angle between the front of the vertebra L5 and plane of inlet and subtracting this from 180°.

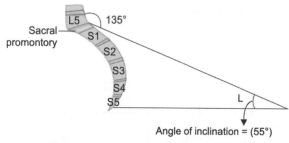

Fig. 7.3: Diagrammatic representation showing plane of inlet

Key Concept

Increase in the angle of inclination (also known as the high inclination) has obstetric significance because this may result in delayed engagement of the fetal head and delay in descent of fetal head. Increase in the angle of inclination also favors **occipitoposterior position**.
On the other hand, reduction in the angle of inclination (also known as **low inclination**) may not have any obstetric significance.

The axis of the pelvic inlet is an imaginary line drawn perpendicular to the plane of inlet in the midline. It is in downwards and backwards direction. Upon extension, this line passes through the umbilicus anteriorly and through the coccyx posteriorly.

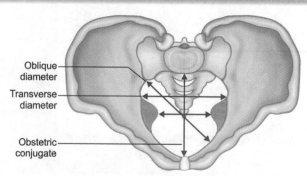

Fig. 7.4: Superior view of pelvic inlet

Key Concept

For the proper descent and engagement of fetal head, it is important that the uterine axis coincides with the axis of inlet.

Diameters of the Pelvic Inlet

Anteroposterior Diameter

- **True conjugate or anatomical conjugate** (11 cm) (Fig. 7.5): This is measured from the **midpoint of sacral promontory** to the **upper border of pubic symphysis**.

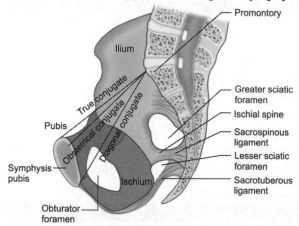

Fig. 7.5: The innominate bone is composed of the pubis (brown), ischium (red), and ilium (blue). Of the three anteroposterior diameters of the pelvic inlet, only the diagonal conjugate can be measured clinically. The important obstetrical conjugate is derived by subtracting 1.5 cm from the diagonal conjugate.

- **Obstetric conjugate** (10 to 10.5 cm): It is the most important anteroposterior diameter of the pelvic inlet[Q] as it is the one through which the fetus must pass:
  - It is the smallest anteroposterior diameter[Q].
  - It is measured from middle symphysis pubis to **the middle of the sacral promontory**[Q].
  - For normal vaginal delivery obstetric conjugate must measure 10 cm or more[Q].
  - The pelvic inlet is considered to be contracted, if obstetric conjugate is less than 10 cm.[Q]

- It cannot be measured clinically but can be estimated by subtracting 1.5 to 2 cm from the diagonal conjugate.
- **Diagonal conjugate** (12 cm): It is measured from the midpoint of sacral promontory to the lower border of pubic symphysis.
- Out of three AP diameters of pelvic inlet, only diagonal conjugate can be assessed clinically during the late pregnancy or at the time of the labor (Fig. 7.6).

 Note: Since diagonal conjugate can be measured clinically. If it is 'x' ions, then obstetric conjugate will be (x – 2 cm) and true conjugate (x – 1 cm).

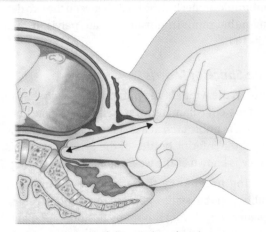

Fig. 7.6: Measurement of diagonal conjugate

Transverse Diameter of Pelvic Inlet (13 cm)

It is the distance between the farthest two points on the iliopectineal line (Fig. 7.4). It is perpendicular to obstetric conjugate. It is the largest diameter of the pelvic inlet and lies 4 cm anterior to the sacral promontory and 7 cm behind the symphysis.

Posterior sagittal diameter of the inlet (Fig. 7.7) is the distance between sacral promontory and the point where obstetric conjugate and transverse diameter intersect each other. *Ref. Williams Obs. 24/e, p 32*

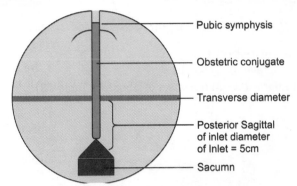

- Pubic symphysis
- Obstetric conjugate
- Transverse diameter
- Posterior Sagittal of inlet diameter of Inlet = 5cm
- Sacumn

Fig. 7.7: Posterior sagittal diameter of inlet

Oblique Diameters of Pelvic Inlet

There are two oblique diameters, right and left (12 cm). The right oblique diameter passes from right sacroiliac joint to the left iliopubic eminence, whereas the left diameter passes from left sacroiliac joint to the right iliopubic eminence.

Pelvic Cavity

The pelvic cavity is almost round in shape and is bounded above by the pelvic brim and below by the plane of least pelvic dimension, anteriorly by the symphysis pubis and posteriorly by sacrum.

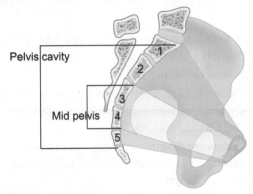

Fig. 7.8: Pelvic cavity and midpelvis at the junction of S_4 and S_5 or tip of sacrum

 Remember: The diameters of pelvic cavity both AP and transverse are 12 cm each.

Midpelvis (Fig. 7.8)

- The midpelvis is measured at the level of the ischial spine, also called the **midplane or plane of least pelvic dimension**.
- The plane of least pelvic dimension extends from the lower border of pubic symphysis to the tip of ischial spines laterally and to the junction of fourth and fifth sacral vertebra posteriorly.

Significance of ischial spine:
- Internal rotation occurs at this level.[Q]
- It marks the beginning of the forward curve of the pelvic axis.[Q]
- Most cases of deep transverse arrest occur here.[Q]
- Ischial spines represent zero station of the head.[Q]
- External os lies at this level.[Q]

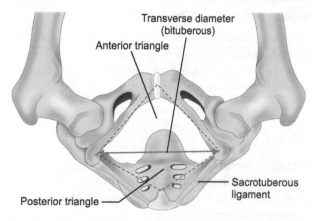

Fig. 7.9: Measurement of transverse diameter of the outlet

Besides these: It corresponds to origin of levator ani muscle[Q] and is a landmark used for pudendal block[Q].

- **Diameters of midpelvis:**
  - AP diameter of midpelvis: It extends from the junction of S_4 and S_5 vertebra to lower body of pubic symphysis. It is 11.5 to 12 cm (Fig. 7.8).
  - **Transverse diameter or bispinous or interspinous diameter.** It is the distance between the ischial spines. Normal = 10 cm.

 Key Concept

The interspinous diameter is usually the smallest pelvic diameter and in case of obstructed labor is particularly important.

  - Posterior sagittal diameter of midpelvis = 4 to 5 cm.

Pelvic Outlet

- It lies at the level of ischial tuberosity.
- **Anatomical pelvic outlet:** It is a lozenge or Rhombus shaped cavity bounded by anterior border of symphysis pubis, pubic arch, ischial tuberosities, sacrotuberous ligaments, sacrospinous ligaments and tip of coccyx.
- **Plane of anatomical outlet:** It passes along with the boundaries of the anatomical outlet and consists of two triangular planes with a common base which is the bituberous diameter (Fig. 7.9).

- Clinically three diameters of pelvic outlet are important:
  - **Anteroposterior:** It extends from the lower border of the symphysis pubis to the tip of the coccyx. It measures between 11.5 to 13.5 cm depending on the position of coccyx.
  - **Transverse — Syn: Intertuberous** diameter (11 cm or 4¼″): It is measured between inner borders of ischial tuberosities.
  - **Posterior sagittal diameter (7 cm or more):** It extends from the tip of the sacrum to the center of bituberous diameter.
- **Subpubic angle:** It is the angle between the two descending pubic rami. In normal female pelvis, it measures 90°–100°. *Ref. Williams Obs. 24/e, p 33*

Waste Space of Morris

Normally, the width of the pubic arch is such that a round disk of 9.4 cm (diameter of a well-flexed head) can pass through the pubic arch at a distance of 1 cm from the midpoint of the inferior border of the symphysis pubis. This distance is known as the **waste space of Morris** (Fig. 7.10).

During pregnancy there is increase in width and mobility of pubic symphysis due to hormone **relaxin and progesterone**. During lithotomy position, AP diameter of outlet is increased by 1.5 cm.

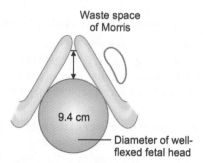

Fig. 7.10: Waste space of Morris

ASSESSMENT OF PELVIS

Time of assessment:
Primigravida = 37 weeks
Multigravida = At the onset of labor (*See* Table 7.2).

Table 7.2

Assessment of	Method	Comment
Pelvic inlet **Diagonal conjugate**	Measured by trying to reach the sacral promontory 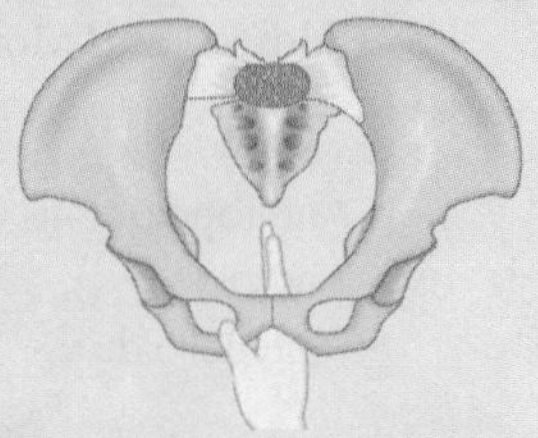 Fig. 7.11: Measurement of diagonal conjugate	In a contracted pelvis sacral promontory can be easily touched with fingers. Also substract 2 cm from diagonal conjugate to get obstetrical conjugate. If OC is < 10 cm–then pelvic inlet is said **to be contracted**
Pelvic cavity **Ischial spines**	They are felt on each side with two fingers 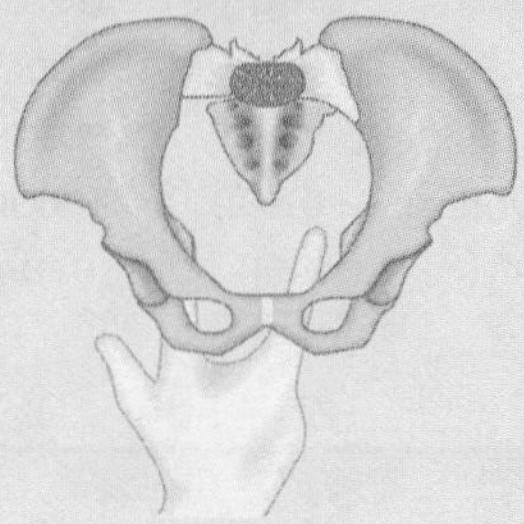 Fig. 7.12: Pelvic cavity	If ischial spines are prominent, they decrease transverse diameter of midpelvis. Interspinous diameter is said to be reduced if both the sides ischial spines can be touched simultaneously with two fingers of the hand
Sidewall	They are felt by fingers on both sides	They are parallel and divergent in normal pelvis. They are convergent in contracted pelvis at midpelvis
Pelvic outlet • Subpubic arch	It is felt on both sides of pubic symphysis (Fig. 7.12) 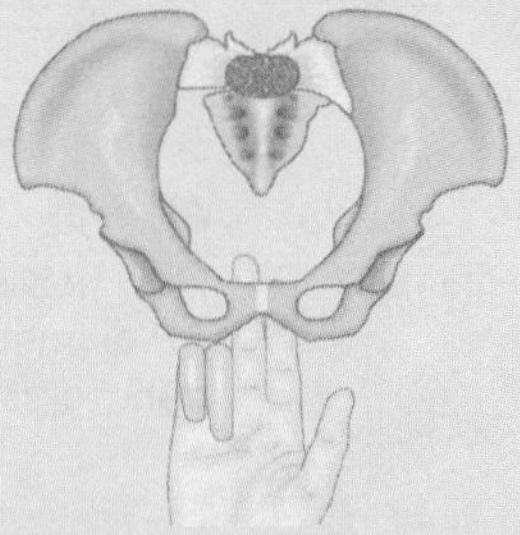 Fig. 7.13: Subpubic arch	It is rounded and spacious and easily allows two fingers
• Transverse diameter outlet (intertuberous diameter) or TDO	It can be assessed by placing four knuckles of wrist between the two ischial tuberosities (Fig. 7.13) 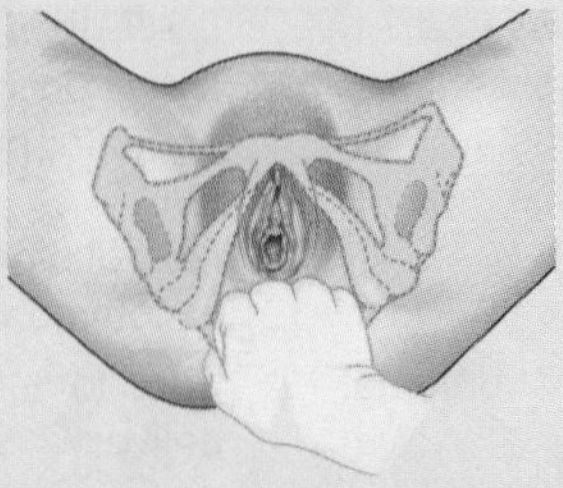 Fig. 7.14: Transverse diameter of outlet	Normally four knuckles can easily negotiate in a normal pelvis. If Transverse diameter of outlet is four knuckles tight or less than four knuckles means it is a contracted pelvis

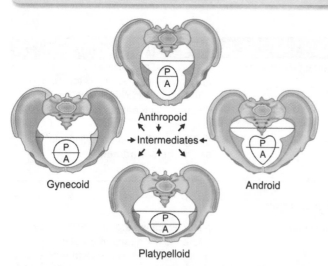

Fig. 7.15: The four parent pelvic types of the Caldwell-Moloy classification. A line passing through the widest transverse diameter divides the inlets into posterior (P) and anterior (A) segments

VARIETIES OF PELVIS

On the basis of shape of the inlet, the pelvis can be of four types:

Caldwell and Mohoy classification

Gynecoid	50%
Anthropoid	25%
Android	20%
Platypelloid	5%

Also Know: In the pelvis, the posterior segment determines the type of pelvis whereas the anterior segment determines the tendency. These are both determined because many pelvis are not pure but of mixed variety. For example a gynecoid pelvis with android tendency means posterior pelvis is gynecoid and the anterior pelvis is android shaped.

Table 7.3: Characteristic of each type of pelvis

Characteristic	Gynecoid pelvis	Android pelvis	Anthropoid pelvis	Platypelloid pelvis
Intro	Female type (M/C variety)	Male type pelvis	Ape like pelvis	Flat pelvis (least common variety)
Shape of inlet	Transverse oval	Heart shape	AP oval	Flat Bowl like
Relationship of transverse diam to AP diam of inlet	Transverse diameter of inlet is slightly bigger than AP diameter	Transverse diam is > AP diam	Only pelvis with - AP diameter > transverse diameter	Pelvis with - Transverse diameter>>> (much more than AP diameter)
Subpubic angle	90°	< 90°		
Pelvic side wall	Straight and parallel	Convergert	Narrow	Divergent
Ischial spine	Not prominent	Prominent	Not prominent	Not prominent
Obstetric outcome	Normal female pelvis No difficulty in engagement. M/C position of head LOT/LOA	Engagement is delayed Deep transverse arrest/persistent occipito posterior position common	Diam of engagement is AP diam Direct occipito posterior position is M/C. Nonrotation is common	Head engages in transverse diameter with marked asynclitism Engaging diameter is supersub parietal diam (18.5 cm) instead of usual biparietal diam (9.5).
Type of delivery	Normal delivery	Difficult instrumental delivery	Face to pubes delivery	If head is able to negotiate the inlet by means of asynclitism then normal labor otherwise cesarean section

Important One Liners

Remember the following points on pelvis (most of the questions are asked on them).

- Normal female pelvis – Gynecoid pelvis[Q].
- Male type pelvis – Android pelvis[Q].
- Most common type of pelvis – Gynecoid pelvis[Q].
- Least common type pelvis – Platypelloid pelvis[Q].
- The only pelvis with AP diameter more than transverse diameter – Anthropoid pelvis[Q].
- Face to pubes delivery is most common in Anthropoid pelvis[Q].
- Direct occipitoposterior position is most common in Anthropoid pelvis[Q].
- Persistent occipitoposterior position is most common in Android pelvis[Q].
- Deep transverse arrest/Nonrotation/Dystocia is most common in Android pelvis[Q].
- Broad flat pelvis – Platypelloid pelvis[Q].
- Transverse diameter is much more than AP diameter–Platypelloid pelvis[Q].
- Engagement by exaggerated posterior asynclitism occurs in Platypelloid pelvis[Q].
- Super subparietal instead of biparietal diameter engages in Platypelloid pelvis[Q].

IMPORTANT DIFFERENCES BETWEEN MALE AND FEMALE PELVIS

Android pelvis (Male)	Gynecoid pelvis (Female)
• Inlet: Heart shaped	• Transverse oval in shape
• Sidewalls convergent	• Sidewalls parallel
• Deep and narrow pelvis	• Shallow pelvis
• Ischial spines are prominent	• Ischial spines are not prominent
• Subpubic angle—acute	• Subpubic angle—obtuse 90–100°
• Preauricular sulcus absent	• Preauricular sulcus present
• Greater siatic notch narrow	• Greater siatic notch broad

CONTRACTED PELVIS

- A pelvis is said to be contracted if any of its major diameters are shortened by 0.5 cm or more.
- In contracted pelvis: Mode of delivery is always cesarean section.
- **It is a recurring indication for cesarean section.**

Types of Contracted Pelvis

- **Rachitic pelvis:** Seen in rickets. Here, in the inlet there is shortening of true and obstetric conjugate and widening of transverse diameter
- **Triradiate pelvis**
- **Osteomalacic pelvis**
- **Naegele's pelvis:** If one ala of sacral bone is absent.[Q]
- **Robert's pelvis:** If both ala of sacral bone are absent.[Q]

Contraction of Pelvis can Occur at 3 Levels

1. At the level of inlet:

i. Inlet is said to be contracted: if obstetric conjugate is < 10 cm
   Mild = obstetric conjugate < 10 cm (9.5–10 cm)
   transverse diameter < 12 cm
   Moderate = obstetric conjugate = 7.5–9.5 cm
   Severe = obstetric conjugate < 7.5 cm
   (Rare)
ii. Or inlet is also contracted if transverse diameter is < 12 cm *Ref. Williams Obs. 25/e, p 448*

2. At the level of midpelvis:

Midpelvis is said to be contracted when

- Interspinous diameter bispinous diameter < 8 cm
  Ref. Williams Obs. 25/e, p 449
- When sum of interspinous and posterior sagittal diameter of midpelvis is < 13.5 cm
  Ref. Williams Obs. 25/e, p 449

  (Normal = Interspinous diameter = 10.5
  Posterior sagittal diameter of midpelvis = 5 cm
  ∴ Sum = 15.5 cm)

Midpelvis should be suspected to be contracted when Interischial diameter or bispinous diamter is < 10 cm.
Ref. Williams Obs. 25/e, p 449

3. At the level of outlet:

- Outlet is said to be contracted when intertuberous diameter is < 8 cm *Ref. Williams Obs. 25/e, p 449*

Thomas dictum: If sum of bistuberous diameter and posterior sagittal diameter of outlet is < 15 cm then pelvis is said to be contracted and cesarean is needed.

Management of Contracted Pelvis

- Always cesarean section (elective at 38 weeks)
- Only in case of mild inlet contraction trial of labor can be done.

TRIAL OF LABOR

- This is not synonymous with trial of scar or VBAC (vaginal birth after cesarean)
- It means allowing labor in a mild degree of contracted pelvis, when contraction is only at the level of inlet. This is done in hospital setting with the expectation of vaginal delivery. But if it fails, cesarean section should be done immediately.
- Trial of labor is the best management of CPD at the level of inlet.

Contraindications of Trial of Labor

- Severe degree of contracted pelvis
- Pelvic contraction at midpelvis or outlet
- Previous cesarean section
- Elderly primigravida, bad obstetric history
- Malpresentation
- Previous failed trial of labor
- Severe PIH, diabetes and cardiac disease

CEPHALOPELVIC DISPROPORTION

- The term means that either the fetus is too big or pelvis small for this pregnancy only
- The term CPD and contracted pelvis are not synonymous
- If a female has CPD in this pregnancy—it does not mean next time also she will definitely have CPD here
- CPD is not a recurring cause of cesarean section (whereas contracted pelvis is a recurring cause)
- **Assessment of CPD can be done by abdominal method or by Muller-Kerr method.**

 Important One Liners

- Best method of pelvis assessment/CPD is Trial of labor > clinical assessment
- Best radiological method of pelvis assessment/CPD is MRI > CT > X-ray
- In females with height less than 140 cm, contracted pelvis should be suspected
- In a female with mildly contracted pelvic inlet: Management of choice is—**Trial of labor** but if this female had a previous cesarean then Trial of Labor is contradicted
- In a female with moderate on severe inlet contracted or pelvis with outlet or midpelvis contraction
- Management of choice is—Cesarean section.

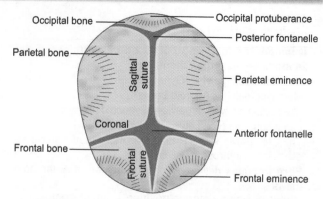

Fig. 7.16: Bones, sutures and fontanelles on fetal skull as viewed from above with head partially deflexed

FETAL SKULL AND DIAMETERS

SUTURES

- The **sagittal or longitudinal suture** lies between two parietal bones (Fig. 7.16).
- The **coronal sutures** run, between parietal and frontal bones on either side.
- The **frontal suture lies** between two frontal bones.
- The **lambdoid sutures** separate the occipital bone and the two parietal bones.
- **Importance:** (i) These sutures are of a great obstetric importance as they allow gliding movements of one bone over the other (moulding), causing a small variation in the shape of the foetal head necessary to negotiate the maternal pelvis. (ii) In addition, the digital palpation of the sagittal suture during labor while performing an internal examination gives important information regarding the internal rotation of the head and the manner of engagement of the head (synclitism or asynclitism).

FONTANELLE

- **Wide gap in the suture line is called as fontanelle**.
- At the time of birth, fetal skull has 6 fontanelle[Q], out of which two are of obstetric significance: (1) Anterior fontanelle or bregma and (2) Posterior fontanelle or lambda.

Anterior Fontanelle

- It is formed by joining of the four sutures in the midplane.
- The sutures are anteriorly frontal, posteriorly sagittal and on either side, coronal. It is diamond shaped.
- Its anteroposterior and transverse diameters measure approximately 3 cm each.

- The floor is formed by a membrane and it becomes ossified 18 months after birth.
- It becomes pathological, if it fails to ossify even after 24 months.

Posterior Fontanelle

- It is formed by junction of three suture lines—sagittal suture anteriorly and lambdoid suture on either side.
- It is triangular in shape
- It measures about 1.2 × 1.2 cm (1/2″ × 1/2″).
- The posterior fontanelle ossifies within 2–3 months of birth. The floor of posterior fontanelle is covered by a membrane. So ossification of posterior fontanelle is intramembranous ossification.

Sagittal Fontanelle

- It is inconsistent in its presence. When present, it is situated on the sagittal suture at the junction of anterior two-thirds and posterior one-third.
- It has got no clinical importance.

PRESENTING PARTS OF FETAL SKULL

These include the following:

- **Vertex:** This is a quadrangular area bounded anteriorly by bregma (anterior fontanel) and coronal sutures; and posteriorly by lambda (posterior fontanel) and lambdoid sutures; and laterally by arbitrary lines passing through the parietal eminences. When vertex is the presenting part, fetal head lies in complete flexion.
- **Brow:** This is an area bounded on one side by root of nose and supraorbital ridges and other side by the bregma and coronal sutures. The fetal head lies midway between full flexion and full extension in this presentation.
- **Face:** This is an area bounded on one side by the root of the nose along with the supraorbital ridges and other side by the junction of the chin or floor of mouth with the neck. Fetal head is fully extended during this presentation.
- Some other parts of fetal skull, which are of significance, include the following:
  - **Sinciput:** Area in front of the anterior fontanel corresponding to the forehead.
  - **Occiput:** Area limited to occipital bone.
  - **Mentum:** Chin of the fetus.
  - **Parietal eminences:** Prominent eminences on each of the parietal bones.
  - **Subocciput:** This is the junction of fetal neck and occiput, sometimes also known as the nape of the neck.
  - **Submentum:** This is the junction between the neck and chin.

IMPORTANT DIAMETERS OF FETAL SKULL

Anteroposterior Diameters

These diameters are described in Table 7.3 and shown in Figure 7.17.

The important AP diameters of fetal skull are:

Presenting part	Engaging AP diameter	Measurement in cm
Vertex (completely flexed head)	**Suboccipito-breg-matic (SOB)**	9.5 cm
Brow presentation (**partial extension**)	Mento vertical	14 cm
Face presentation Mento anterior position	Submento-bregmatic	9.5 cm
Mento posterior	Submento-vertical	11.5 cm

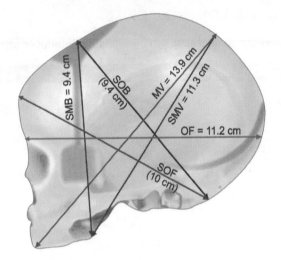

Fig. 7.17: Diameters of fetal skull

Transverse Diameters

The transverse diameters are:

- **Biparietal diameter (9.5 cm):** It extends between the two parietal eminences. This diameter nearly always engages.
- **Supersubparietal diameter (8.5 cm):** It extends from a point placed below one parietal eminence to a point placed above the other parietal eminence of the opposite side.
- **Bitemporal diameter (8 cm):** Distance between the anteroinferior ends of the coronal sutures.
- **Bimastoid diameter (7.5 cm):** Distance between the tips of the mastoid process. This diameter is nearly incompressible.

Mnemonic

- Remember the mnemonic "**Mi**ss **Ti**na **S**o **Pretty**" for transverse diameter when they are arranged in ascending order of their size

 Miss = **Bim**astoid diameter = 7.5 cm. (smallest)
 Tina = **Bit**emporal diameter = 8 cm.
 So = **S**uper subparietal diameter = 8.5 cm.
 Pretty = **Bip**arietal diameter = 9.5 cm. (Largest)

Remember:

- AP diameters of the skull are always bigger than transverse diameters.
- The longest AP diameter of fetal skull is Mentovertical diameter (14 cm).
- The second longest AP diameter is Submentovertical = Occipitofrontal = 11.5 cm.

Key Concept

- In Brow presentation—diameter of engagement is mentovertical diameter which is 14 cm. It is the largest diameter, hence in Brow presentation, always cesarean section has to be done.
- In anencephaly, skull of the fetus is absent but face is normal.
  ∴ M/c presentation in anencephaly is face presentation.

SWELLING ON FETAL SKULL

A swelling on fetal skull can be cephalhematoma or caput succedaneum or a meningocele.

Caput succedaneum	Cephalhematoma
Fig. 7.18: Formation of caput succedaneum	Fig. 7.19: Cephalhematoma
• It is a localised swelling of scalp due to effusion of serum above the periosteum.	• It is collection of blood due below the periosteum
• It is due to stagnation of fetal head in one position for a long time	• It is due traumatic instrumental delivery
• Diffuse swelling	• Sharply circumscribed swelling
• Soft and pits on pressure	• Soft but does not pit on pressure
• Present above the periosteum	• Present under the periosteum
• Can cross suture lines	• Cannot cross suture lines
• Present at birth and starts regressing immediately to disappear in a few hours	• Appears sometime after birth, grows larger and disappears after a week
• Never associated with fracture and jaundice	• Can be associated with fracture and jaundice

Note: A cephalhematoma should never be drained. Cephalhematoma can be differentiated from meningocele as transillumination test and impulse of coughing is absent in cephalhematoma (they are present in meningocele).

New Pattern Questions

N1. Conjugate of the diagonal is 'a' cm, obstetric conjugate will be:
a. a + 1 cm
b. a + 2 cm
c. a – 1 cm
d. a – 2 cm

N2. Dystocia dystrophia syndrome is seen in:
a. Android pelvis
b. Platypelloid pelvis
c. Anthropoid
d. Gynecoid pelvis

N3. The following are the features of "dystocia dystrophica syndrome" *except*:
a. The patient is stockily built with short thighs
b. They have normal fertility
c. Android pelvis is common
d. Often have difficult labour

N4. Information obtained by lateral plate X-ray pelvimetry are all *except*:
a. Sacral curve
b. True conjugate
c. Bispinous diameter
d. Inclination of the pelvis

N5. CPD is best assessed by:
a. CT scan
b. Ultrasound
c. Radio pelvimetry
d. Pelvic assessment

N6. If both the ala of the sacral bone are absent, pelvis is called as:
a. Naegele pelvis
b. Robert pelvis
c. Triradiate pelvis
d. Rachitic pelvis

N7. Adequacy of pelvis for labor is best judged by:
a. Clinical pelvimetry
b. X-ray pelvimetry
c. CT scan
d. Trial of labor

N8. Most important diameter of pelvis during labor is:
a. Interspinous diameter
b. Oblique diameter of inlet
c. AP diameter of outlet
d. Intertuberous diameter

N9. M/C cause of true CPD in developing countries is:
a. Occipito posterior position
b. Malpresentations
c. Rickets
d. Trauma

N10. CPD in absence of gross pelvic abnormality can be diagnosed by:
a. Ht of mother < 158 cm
b. Trial of labor
c. X-ray pelvimetry
d. Pelvic examination

N11. Which of the following is true for cephalhematoma?
a. Tension varies on crying
b. May cause jaundice
c. Edematous fluid
d. Cross suture lines

N12. Classification of types of pelvis is:
a. Page classification
b. Mohoy classification
c. Caldwell and Mohoy classification
d. O Sullivan classification

Previous Year Questions

1. **The smallest diameter of the true pelvis is:** [AI 05]
   a. Interspinous diameter
   b. Diagonal conjugate
   c. True conjugate
   d. Intertuberous diameter

2. **Most important diameter of pelvis during labour is:** [PGI June 02]
   a. Interspinous diameter of outlet
   b. Oblique diameter of inlet
   c. AP diameter of outlet
   d. Intertubercular diameter

3. **Female pelvis as compared to the male pelvis has all *except*:** [PGI Dec 01]
   a. Narrow sciatic notch
   b. Shallow and wide symphysis pubis
   c. Subpubic angle is acute
   d. Light and graceful structure
   e. Preauricular sulcus is larger

4. **The shortest diameter of fetal head is:** [AIIMS May 06]
   a. Biparietal diameter
   b. Suboccipitofrontal diameter
   c. Occipitofrontal diameter
   d. Bitemporal diameter

5. **Which type of pelvis is associated with increased incidence of 'face to pubis' delivery?** [AI 97]
   a. Gynecoid pelvis
   b. Anthropoid pelvis
   c. Android pelvis
   d. Platypelloid pelvis

6. **AP diameter is maximum in which type of pelvis?**
   a. Platypelloid   b. Android   [PGI June 97]
   c. Anthropoid   d. Gynecoid

7. **Triradiate pelvis is see in:** [PGI Dec 97]
   a. Rickets
   b. Chondrodystrophy
   c. Osteoporosis
   d. Hyperparathyroidism

8. **One of the following features can be used to define contracted pelvis:** [AI 97]
   a. Transverse diameter of inlet is 10 cm
   b. AP diameter of inlet is 12 cm
   c. Platypelloid pelvis
   d. Gynecoid pelvis

9. **Shortest diameter is:** [AI 02]
   a. Diagonal conjugate
   b. Obstetric conjugate
   c. True conjugate
   d. All are equal

10. **Longest diameter of fetal skull is:** [AI 04]
    a. Biparietal
    b. Bitemporal
    c. Occipito temporal
    d. Submentovertical

11. **Critical obstetric conjugate for trial of labour is:** [AIIMS Nov 05]
    a. 8.5 cm   b. 9.0 cm
    c. 9.5 cm   d. 10.0 cm

12. **The shortest AP diameter of pelvic inlet:**
    a. True conjugate   [AIIMS Nov 15]
    b. Obstetric conjugate
    c. Anatomical conjugate
    d. Bituberous conjugate

13. **The characteristics of caput succedaneum include all of the following *except*:** [AI 11]
    a. Crosses midline
    b. Crosses the suture line
    c. It does not disappear within 2–3 days
    d. It is a diffuse edematous swelling of the soft tissues of the scalp

14. **The number of fontanelles present in a newborn child is:** [AI 2000]
    a. 1   b. 2
    c. 4   d. 6

15. **Longest fetal diameter is:**
    a. Biparietal   b. Suboccipito bregmatic
    c. Occipito frontal   d. Mentovertical

Answers with Explanations to New Pattern Questions

N1. Ans. is d, i.e. (a –2) cm   *Ref. Williams Obs. 24/e, p 32*

Obstetric conjugate cannot be measured clinically but can be diagnosed by substracting 1.5–2 cm from diagonal conjugate. Hence if diagnonal cojugate is 'a' cm obstetric conjugate will be (a –2) cm

- Obstetric conjugate normally measures 10 cm or more[Q].
- *The pelvic inlet is considered to be contracted, if obstetric conjugate is less than 10 cm.[Q]*

N2. Ans. is a, i.e. Android pelvis   *Ref. Dutta Obs 9/e, p 327*

N3. Ans. is b, i.e. They have normal fertility

Dystocia dystrophia syndrome: It is charactersied by the following features:

- The patient is stockily built with bull neck, broad shoulder and short thigh.
- She is obese with a male distribution of hairs.
- *Pelvis is of the android type.*
- Occipitoposterior position is common.
- They are usually subfertile, having dysmenorrhoea, oligomenorrhoea or irregular period
- There is increased incidence of preeclampsia and a tendency for postmaturity during pregnancy.
- During labour, inertia is common and there is a tendency for deep transverse arrest or outlet dystocia leading to either increased incidence of difficult instrumental delivery or cesarean section.
- There are increase chances of lactation failure during purperium.

N4. Ans. is c, i.e. Bispinous diameter   *Ref. Dutta Obs. 9/e, p 329*

Bispinous diameter can be measured by anteroposterior view and not on lateral view of X-ray pelvimetry.

 Note: AP view can give the accurate measurement of transverse diameter of inlet and bispinous diameter.

 X-ray pelvimetry is of limited value in the diagnosis of pelvic contraction or cephalopelvic disproportion. Apart from pelvic capacity there are several other factors involved in successful vaginal delivery. These are the fetal size, presentation, position and the force of uterine contractions. X-ray pelvimetry cannot assess the other factors. It cannot reliably predict the likelihood of vaginal delivery neither in breech presentation nor in cases with previous cesarean section.

- **X-ray pelvimetry is useful** in cases with fractured pelvis and for the important diameters which are inaccessible to clinical examination.
- *Techniques:* For complete evaluation of the pelvis, three views are taken—anteroposterior, lateral and outlet. But commonly, X-ray pelvimetry is restricted to only the erect lateral view (the femoral head and acetabular margins must be superimposed) which gives most of the useful information. Anteroposterior view can give the accurate measurement of the transverse diameter of the inlet and bispinous diameter.
- **Hazards of X-ray pelvimetry** includes radiation exposure to the mother and the fetus. With conventional X-ray pelvimetry radiation exposure to the gonads is about 885 millirad. So it is restricted to selected cases only.

N5 Ans. is d, i.e. Pelvic assessment   *Ref. Dutta Obs. 9/e, p 329*

 IOC for detecting CPD or pelvic assessment or adequacy is – MRI.

Best method of detecting CPD–Trial of labor > MRI > manual pelvic assessment.

Pelvic assessment is done at 37 weeks in primigravida and at the onset of labor in multigravida.

N6. Ans. is b, i.e. Robert pelvis

Ref. Dutta Obs. 9/e, p 326

- If one ala is absent–pelvis is called Naegle's pelvis.
- If both ala of saccumb are absent-pelvis is called as Robert's pelvis.
- Both are varieties of contracted pelvis and in both cesarean section is done.

N7. Ans. is d, i.e. Trial of labor
Adequacy of pelvis is best assessed by Trial of labor (as discussed in Ans. 5).

N8. Ans. is a, i.e. Interspinous diameter
This is because it is the smallest diameter of the pelvis.

N9. Ans. is c, i.e. Rickets
CPD can be true or relative.
True CPD: Is relatively rare and occurs when the presenting part of the fetus is too big or pelvis is too small (pelvic dystocia). Pelvis dystocia is uncommon in developed countries but may occur after trauma. In developing countries, it is seen in vit D deficiency and rickets.
Relative CPD: is M/C and is associated with fetal malposition (occiptio posterior position or brow presentation).

N10. Ans. is b, i.e. Trial of labor
Discussed earlier.

N11. Ans. is b, i.e. May cause jaundice
Cephalhematoma is collection of blood below the periosterum (option c is incorrect, hence it cannot cross suture lines) (Option d is incorrect)
Tension varies with crying is a feature of meningocle, not cephalhematoma.
Since there is blood in cephalhematoma, hence it can cause jaundice, i.e. option b is correct.

N12. Ans. is c, i.e. Caldwell and Mohoy classification
See the text for explanation.

Answers with Explanations to Previous Year Questions

1. **Ans. is a, i.e. Interspinous diameter** *Ref. Williams Obs. 24/e, p 32-33*

   Friends, we have mugged up pelvis in detail for our undergraduate exams but for PGME exams you need not mug up each and everything about pelvis. All you need to know are some of the important diameters, which I am listing below.

   Diameters of Pelvis

Diameter	Inlet	Midpelvis	Outlet
Anteroposterior	Obstetric conjugate -10–10.5 cm	11–11.5 cm	11.5–13.5 cm
	True conjugate -11 cm Diagonal conjugate -12 cm		
Oblique	12 cm		
Transverse	13	Interspinous diameter 10 cm	Intertuberus diameter 11 cm

   Posterior sagittal diameter of outlet: It is an important diameter in case of obstructed labour caused by narrowing of the midpelvis or pelvic out let as the prognosis for vaginal delivery depends on the length of posterior sagittal diameter. Posterior sagittal diameter extends from tip of coccyx to a right angle intersection with a line between the ischial tuberosities. It usually exceed 7.5 cm.

   IOC for detecting CPD or pelvic assessment or adequacy is – MRI.

   Best method of detecting CPD–Trial of labor > MRI > manual pelvic assessment.

    Remember:

• Longest diameter of pelvis	– Transverse diameter of inlet and anteroposterior diameter of anatomic outlet[Q].
• Shortest major diameter of pelvis	– Interspinous diameter
• Longest AP diameter of inlet	– Diagonal conjugate[Q]
• Shortest AP diameter of inlet	– Obstetric conjugate[Q]
• Only AP diameter measured clinically	– Diagonal conjugate[Q]
• Crtical obstetric conjugate	– 10 cm (i.e. if obstetric conjugate is less than 10 cm vaginal delivery is not possible)

2. **Ans. is a, i.e. Interspinous diameter of the outlet** *Ref. Williams Obs. 24/e, p 33; Dutta Obs. 9/e, p 82*

   Interspinous diameter is the distance between the two ischial spines and is the smallest diameter of the pelvis = 10 cm or slightly greater. It corresponds to the transverse diameter of midpelvis (i.e. plane of least pelvis dimensions).

3. **Ans. is a and c, i.e. Narrow sciatic notch and Subpubic angle is acute**

   See the text for explanation.

4. **Ans. is d, i.e. Bitemporal diameter** *Ref. Dutta Obs. 9/e, p 77*

   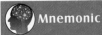 **Mnemonic**

   Remember friends: Always transverse diameters of the fetal skull are smaller than Anteroposterior diameters.

   Amongst the given options: Biparietal and bitemporal diameters are transverse diameters, whereas suboccipitofrontal and occipitofrontal are anteroposterior diameters.

Self Assessment & Review: Obstetrics

Now, the choice is between bitemporal and biparietal diameters.

For memorizing this: learn a mnemonic, where transverse diameter are arranged in ascending order of their size.

Miss	=	**Bima**stoid diameter	=	7.5 cm
Tina	=	**Bit**emporal diameter	=	8 cm
S	=	**S**uper subparietal diameter	=	8.5 cm
Pretty	=	**Bip**arietal diameter	=	9.5 cm

So, our answer is bitemporal diameter (8 cm)

 Remember:

In AP diameters:
- The longest AP diameter of fetal skull is mentovertical diameter = 14 cm
- The second longest AP diameter is submentovertical = Occipitofrontal = 11.5 cm.

5. **Ans. is b, i.e. Anthropoid pelvis** *Ref. Dutta Obs. 9/e, p 325, Table 24.1, 8/e, p 403, Table 24.2*

As discussed in the text in Table 7.2 face-to-pubis delivery is common in anthropoid pelvis.

6. **Ans. is c, i.e. Anthropoid** *Ref. Dutta Obs. 9/e, p 325, Table 24.1, 8/e, p 403, Table 24.2, 24.12*

 Remember:

The following points on pelvis (most of the questions are asked on them):
- Normal female pelvis – *Gynaecoid pelvis*[Q].
- Male type pelvis – *Android pelvis*[Q].
- Most common type of pelvis – *Gynaecoid pelvis*[Q].
- Least common type pelvis – *Platypelloid pelvis*[Q].
- The only pelvis with AP diameter more than transverse diameter – *Anthropoid pelvis*[Q].
- Face to pubes delivery is most common in *Anthropoid pelvis*[Q].
- Direct occipitoposterior position is most common in *Anthropoid pelvis*[Q].
- Persistent occipitoposterior position is most common in *Android pelvis*[Q].
- Deep transverse arrest/ Nonrotation/dystocia is most common in *Android pelvis*[Q].
- Broad flat pelvis – *Platypelloid pelvis*[Q].
- Transverse diameter is much more than AP diameter – *Platypelloid pelvis*[Q].
- Engagement by exaggerated posterior asynclitism occurs in *Platypelloid pelvis*[Q].
- Super subparietal instead of biparietal diameter engages in *Platypelloid pelvis*[Q].

7. **Ans. is c, i.e. Osteoporosis**

Osteomalacia or deficiency of Calcium and Vitamin D shows triradiate pelvis. Since osteomalacia is not given here we are going for osteoporosis.

8. **Ans. is a, i.e. Transverse diameter of inlet is 10 cm** *Ref. Dutta Obs. 7/e, p 345, 8/e, p 409; Williams 24/e, p 426*

Normal pelvic diameters

	Inlet	Midpelvis	Outlet
AP diameter	TC = 11 cm OC = 10 to 10.5 cm DC = 12 cm	11–12 cm (11.5 according to willams)	11.5 cm 13.5 cm
Oblique diameter	12 cm	✗	✗
Transverse diameter	13 cm	Interspinous diameter = 10 cm	Bituberous diameter 11 cm
Posterior sagittal diameter	5 cm	5 cm	7 cm

In contracted pelvis

Inlet: (i)   Obstetric conjugate < 10 cm

           (ii) Transverse diameter < 12 cm (in Question it is given Transverse diameter < 10 cm)

Midpelvis: (i)   Contraction suspected if interspinous diameter < 10 cm

                 100% confirmed contracted pelivs if interspinous diameter < 8 cm

           (ii) Sum of interspinous diameter and posterior sagittal diameter is < 13.5 cm

Outlet: (i)   If interspinous diameter < 8 cm

           (ii) Sum of bituberous and posterior sagittal diameter of outlet is < 15 cm.

9.   **Ans. is b, i.e. Obstetric conjugate**   *Ref. Dutta Obs. 9/e, p 80-81*

    Anteroposterior diameters of the pelvic inlet.

Diameters	Feature	Measurement
Obstetric conjugate	• It is the distance between the midpoint of the sacral promontory to prominent bony projection in the midline on the inner surface of the symphysis pubis. • It is the smallest AP diameter of pelvic inlet. • It is the diameter through which the fetus must pass. • It can not be measured clinically, but can be derived by substracting 1.5 cm from diagonal conjugate.	10–10.5 cm
True conjugate (Anatomical conjugate)	• It is the distance between the midpoint of the sacral promontory to the inner margin of the upper border of symphysis pubis. • It has no obstetrical significance.	11 cm
Diagonal conjugate	• It is the distance between the midpoint of the sacral promontory to the lower border of symphysis pubis. • Its importance as that it can be measured clinically.	12 cm

10.   **Ans. is d, i.e. Submentovertical**   *Ref. Dutta Obs 9/e p 77-78*

    Remember:

Smallest diameter	Longest diameter
I[st] = Bimastoid diameter	I[st] = Mento vertical
II[nd] = Bitemporal diameter	II[nd] = Submento vertical/occipitofrontal

11.   **Ans. is d, i.e. 10 cm**   *Ref. Williams Obs. 24/e, p 463*

    Critical obstetric conjugate is the minimum length of obstetric conjugate below which vaginal delivery is not possible and that is 10 cm.

12.   **Ans. is b, i.e. Obstetric conjugate**

    See the text for explanation.

13.   **Ans. is c, i.e. It does not disappear within 2–3 days**   *Ref. JB Sharma Textbook of Obs. p 88-89*

    Caput succedaneum disappears within 2–3 days.

14.   **Ans. is d, i.e. 6**

    At the time of birth, number of fontanelles present in a newborn are 6.   *Ref. Dutta Obs. 9/e, p 77*

15.   **Ans. is d, i.e. Mentovertical**

    As discussed, Anterioposterio diameters are longer than transverse diameters.

    The longest AP diameter is Mentovertical diameter (14 cm).

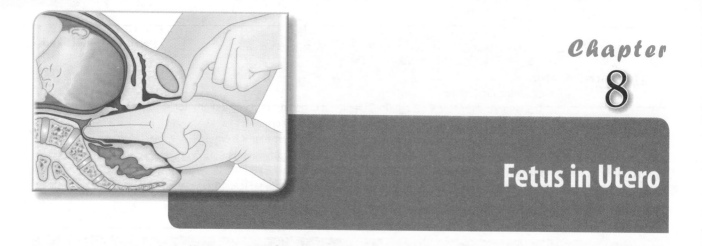

8

Fetus in Utero

 Chapter at a Glance

- Fetal Lie
- Reasons for Higher Frequency of Longitudinal Lie
- Presentation
- Reasons for Higher Frequency of Cephalic Presentation
- Presenting Part
- Denominator
- Position

- Fetal Attitude or Posture or Habitus
- Diagnosis of Fetal Presentation and Position
  - Abdominal Palpation
  - Engagement
  - Diagnosis
  - Auscultation
  - Clinical Importance

FETAL LIE (FIGS. 8.1A TO C)

Fetal lie is the relationship between the long axis of the fetus to the long axis of the uterine avoid. It can be longitudinal, transverse or oblique. When the long axis of the fetus and uterine ovoid correspond, the lie is said to be longitudinal which is seen in **99-99.5% cases**.

When the fetal axis and the maternal axis may cross at 45°, the lie is said to be oblique. It is unstable and almost always becomes longitudinal or transverse during the course of labor.

When fetal axis and maternal axis cross at 90° the lie is said to be transverse lie. The **transverse and oblique lies are present in about 0.5% cases.**

 Note: Management of transverse lie during labour is always cesarean section whether baby is alive or dead.

REASONS FOR HIGHER FREQUENCY OF LONGITUDINAL LIE

The fetus being in the attitude of universal flexion has the shape of an ovoid with 25 cm length. Uterus also has ovoid shape. Hence, the longitudinal axis of the fetal ovoid accommodates well in the longitudinal axis of the uterine ovoid causing higher frequency of longitudinal lie.

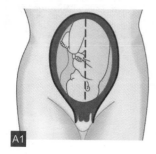 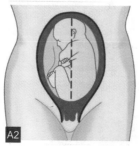 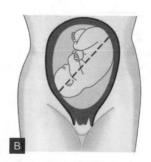 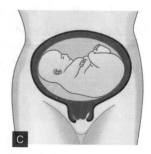

Figs. 8.1A to C: Diagrammatic representation of various fetal lies (A1) longitudinal lie with cephalic presentation; (A2) longitudinal lie with breech presentation; (B) oblique lie; (C) transverse lie

PRESENTATION

Presentation is the part of the fetus which lies over the pelvic inlet and occupies the lower pole of the uterus. In longitudinal lie: presentation can be cephalic (when head is lower pole) or breech (when buttocks are in lower pole). Cephalic presentation is seen in 96.8% cases while breech presentation is seen in 2.7-3.0% cases. Shoulder presentation is seen in transverse lie in 0.3-0.5% cases. When more than one part of the fetus is present, it is called **compound presentation** (e.g. head with hand) and is seen in 0.1% cases.

 Note: Management of shoulder presentation is caesarean section.

REASONS FOR HIGHER FREQUENCY OF CEPHALIC PRESENTATION

The larger and bulkier podalic pole (breech with flexed thighs) is accommodated in broad and roomier fundus. The smaller and compact fetal head is accommodated in narrow lower pole. The effect of gravity also causes heavier head to lie in the lower pole of uterus.

PRESENTING PART

The presenting part is the most dependent part of the fetal body which is foremost within the birth canal or in closest proximity to it. It is felt first through the cervix on vaginal examination. Hence, in cephalic presentation, the presenting part is either vertex seen in 96% cases (most common), face (0.5%) or brow (0.01%) as per the degree of flexion of the head.

DENOMINATOR

Denominator is an arbitrary chosen fixed bony point on the presenting part of fetus which lies in various quadrants of the maternal pelvis and determines the position.

POSITION

Position is the relationship of the denominator to the different quadrants of the pelvis of mother. The pelvis is divided into 8 equal segments of 45° each (total 360°). Thus, 8 positions are possible with each presenting part (Fig. 8.2)

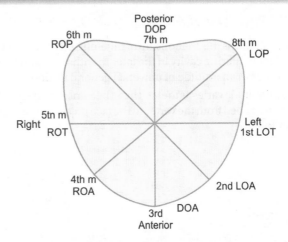

Fig. 8.2: Different positions of fetus during labor

- Vaginal delivery is said 'Normal vaginal delivery if position of fetus is from (1) to (5)
- From position (6) to (8) it is called occipito posterior position
- M/c position of fetus—LOT > LOA

In most cases, the vertex enters the pelvis with the sagittal suture lying in the transverse pelvic diameter. The fetus enters the pelvis in the *left occiput transverse (LOT)* position more commonly than *right occiput transverse (ROT)* position (Caldwell, 1934). In *occiput anterior positions—LOA or ROA*—either the head enters the pelvis with the occiput rotated 45 degrees anteriorly from the transverse position, or this rotation occurs subsequently. The mechanism of labor in all these presentations is usually similar.

- M/c position during labor—LOT > LOA
- M/c occipito anterior position—LOA
- M/c occipito posterior position—ROP
- M/c position in breech = LSA (left sacro anterior)
- M/c position in face – LMA (left mento anterior)

Table 8.1: Presentations and denominators in different positions

Presentation/Position	Denominator
1. Vertex presentation	Occiput
i. Occipito-anterior position	Occiput
ii. Occipito-posterior position	Occiput
2. Face presentation	Mentum (chin)
3. Brow presentation	Sinciput
4. Breech presentation	Sacrum
5. Shoulder presentation (transverse lie)	Acromian process of scapula

FETAL ATTITUDE OR POSTURE OR HABITUS

Fetal attitude is the relationship of different fetal parts to one another in uterine cavity in the later months of pregnancy. Fetus lies in an attitude of universal general flexion.

The attitude varies as the fetal head becomes progressively more extended from the vertex to the face presentation (Figs. 8.3A to D).

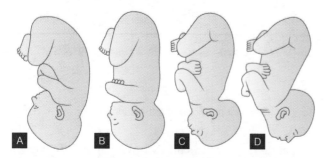

Figs. 8.3A to D: Changes in fetal attitudes in relation to fetal vertex with the degrees of flexion. (A) Vertex presentation with flexed head; (B) Vertex presentation with deflexed head; (C) Brow presentation; (D) Face presentation

DIAGNOSIS OF FETAL PRESENTATION AND POSITION

Abdominal Palpation

Leopold's Maneuvers: Abdominal examination can be conducted systematically employing the four maneuvers described by Leopold.

Leopold's first maneuver or fundal grip (Fig. 8.4A): The fundus is palpated with both hands to identify the fetal pole (breech or head) occupying the uterine fundus. In majority of cases of cephalic presentation (97%), the breech is felt at fundus as a large, soft, irregular nodular mass, which is not ballotable. In a minority (3%) with breech presentation, head is felt at the fundus as hard, smooth, round, compact, mobile and ballotable part. In transverse lie the grip is usually empty.

Leopold's second maneuver or lateral grip (Fig. 8.4B): After the determination of fetal lie, the hands are placed on either side of maternal abdomen to locate fetal back and limbs. On one side, a hard resistant structure is felt—the back—and on the other, numerous small, irregular, mobile parts are felt—the fetal extremities (limbs). By noting whether the back is directed anteriorly, transversely or posteriorly, the orientation and position of the fetus can be made out. Thus, if back is felt on the left side which is more common, the position is usually left occipito-anterior (LOA) or left occipito-transverse (LOT). If the back is felt on the right side, the position is usually right occipito-anterior (ROA) or right occipito-transverse (ROT).

Leopold's third maneuver (Fig. 8.4C): It is also called second pelvic grip or Pawlik's grip or maneuver and is performed facing mother's face. Using thumb and fingers of the right hand, the lower portion of the maternal abdomen is grasped just above the symphysis pubis. If the presenting part is not engaged, a mobile mass will be felt, usually the head. However, the findings from this maneuver are simply indicative that the lower fetal pole is in the pelvis and details are then defined by the last (fourth) maneuver. In transverse lie, this grip is empty. *This grip being uncomfortable for the woman should be performed gently.*

Leopold's fourth maneuver (Fig. 8.4D): It is also called first pelvic grip. The examiner faces the mother's feet and with the tips of the first three fingers of each hand exert deep pressure in the direction of the axis of the pelvic inlet parallel to inguinal ligament. *This pelvic grip is favored by obstetricians as this is the most comfortable for the woman and gives maximum information.*

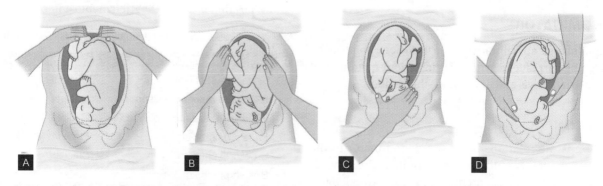

Figs. 8.4A to D: Abdominal palpation using Leopold's maneuvers: (A) Leopold's first maneuver; (B) Leopold's second maneuver; (C) Leopold's third maneuver; (D) Leopold's fourth maneuver

Engagement

When the largest transverse diameter of the head (the biparietal) has crossed the pelvic brim, the head is stated to be engaged.

Diagnosis

First pelvic grip:

- Both the sincipital and occipital poles are not felt abdominally as they have entered the pelvis.
- Inability to reach below the head and divergence of the fingers of both the hands on the lower abdomen indicate engaged head (Fig. 8.5A). Ability to reach below the head and convergence of the fingers below the fetal head is indicative of non-engaged head (Fig. 8.5B).

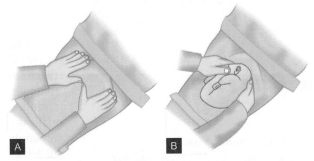

Figs. 8.5A and B: (A) Abdominal palpation in engaged head; Fingers diverging; (B) Abdominal palpation in non-engaged head; Fingers converging

Crichton's Method of Assessing Fetal Head Descent in Fifths by Abdominal Palpation

Progressive descent of the fetal head can be assessed abdominally by estimating the number of 'fifths' of the head above the pelvic brim (Crichton method): When one/fifth above only the sinciput can be felt abdominally and head is said to be engaged and nought fifths represents a head entirely in the pelvis with no poles felt abdominally.

Auscultation

The fetal heart sound is best heard through the back (left scapular region) in vertex and breech presentation where the convex portion of the back is in contact with the uterine wall. However, in face presentation, the heart sounds are heard through the fetal chest. *The fetal heart sound is best heard below the umbilicus in cephalic presentation and around the umbilicus in breech presentation.* The usual position of fetal heart best heard in different presentations is shown (Fig. 8.7).

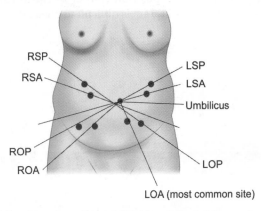

Fig. 8.7: Usual position of fetal heart in various vertex and breech presentation
Glossary clockwise: ROA: Right occipito-posterior position
ROP: Right occipito-posterior position
RSA: Right sacro-anterior position
RSP: Right sacro-posterior position
LSP: Left sacro-posterior position
LSA: Left sacro-anterior position
LOP: Left occipito-posterior position
LOA: Left occipito-anterior position

Clinical Importance

Engagement of the head usually excludes cephalopelvic disproportion, as the head is considered the best pelvimeter.

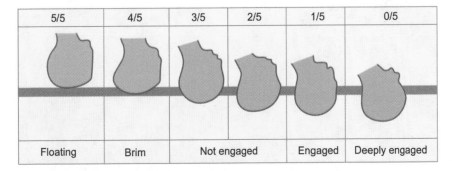

Fig. 8.6: Crichton method of assessing fetal head descent

It has been taught traditionally that engagement of fetal head occurs by 38 weeks in primigravidas. In clinical practice, it may not happen and the engagement often occurs between 38-41 weeks or even during labor. In multiparas, the engagement usually occurs late, in first stage of labor after the rupture of the membranes.

Causes of non-engagement of fetal heard at term in primigravidas.

- Cephalopelvic disproportion due to android, anthropoid or contracted pelvis, large head or both.
- Occipito-posterior position (larger occipito frontal diameter which is 11.5 cm is difficult to engage).

- Hydramnios
- Hydrocephalus with too large diameter of head is unable to engage.
- Placenta previa preventing descent of head
- Pelvis masses like ovarian cyst, subserous or cervical fibroid impacted in the pouch of Douglas preventing engagement of head.
- High assimilation (inclination) pelvis causes delayed engagement of fetal head.
- Unknown cause

New Pattern Questions

N1. Denominator refers to:
- a. Part of presentation which lies over the Int. os
- b. Relation of different parts of fetus to one another
- c. Bony fixed point of reference on presenting part
- d. Part of fetus lying in the lower segment of uterus

N2. When fetus is in attitude of flexion, presentation is:
- a. Vertex
- b. Brow
- c. Cephalic
- d. Face

N3. Head of fetus is engaged if:
- a. 4/5 is palpable
- b. 3/5 is palpable
- c. 2/5 is palpable
- d. 1/5 is palpable

N4. M/c presenting part is:
- a. Cephalic
- b. Vertex
- c. Face
- d. Brow

N5. Cesarean section is mandatory in following presentation:
- a. Cephalic
- b. Vertex
- c. Face
- d. Brow

N6. When fetus is in attitude of flexion, the presenting part is:
- a. Vertex
- b. Face
- c. Brow
- d. Breech

Previous Year Questions

1. Commonest cause of nonengagement at term, in primi is: [PGI June 98]
   a. CPD
   b. Hydramnios
   c. Brow presentation
   d. Breech

2. Which of the following Leopold's grip is shown in the image?
   a. Pawlick's grip
   b. Pelvic
   c. Fundal
   d. Abdominal

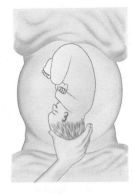

Answers with Explanations to New Pattern Questions

N1. Ans. is c, i.e. Bony fixed point of reference on presenting part
See the text for explanation.

N2. Ans. is c, i.e. Cephalic
Read the question carefully—they are asking presentation, hence answer will be cephalic. If they would have asked presenting part then answer would be vertex.

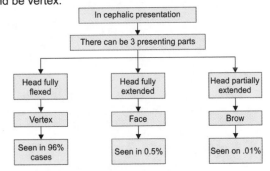

N3. Ans. is d, i.e. 1/5 is palpable
As per Crichton method head of fetus is said to be engaged if 1/5 or less is palpable per abdominally.

N4. Ans. is b, i.e. Vertex

> *Remember*:
> M/c lie: longitudinal
> M/c presentation: cephalic
> M/c presenting part: vertex

N5. Ans. is d, i.e. Brow

In brow presentation, the engaging diameter is mentovertical diameter which is 14 cms. 14 cms cannot pass through cervix and hence caesarean section is mandatory in brow presentation.

N6. Ans. is a, i.e. Vertex

When head is fully flexed, the presenting part is vertex.

Answers with Explanations to Previous Year Questions

1. **Ans. is a, i.e. CPD** *Ref. Dutta Obs. 7/e, p 81, 82, 352*
   - *Engagement is said to occur when the greatest transverse diameter of the presenting part, has passed through the pelvic inlet. In all cephalic presentations, the greatest transverse diameter is always the biparietal.*
   - Engagement occurs in multipara with commencement of labour[Q] in the late Ist stage after rupture of membranes and in Nullipara during the last few weeks of pregnancy, i.e. ≈ 38 weeks
   - In primi's the *most common* cause of non engagement at term is deflexed head or occipitoposterior position followed by cephalopelvic disproportion (CPD).[Q]
   - Since deflexed head or occipitoposterior is not given in option, we will go for CPD as the answer.

2. **Ans. is a, i.e. Pawlick's grip.**
   Leopold third maneuver is done facing the patients face and with one hand. It is called second pelvic grip or Pawlik grip. Leopold fourth maneuver is done facing the patients feet and with both hands. It is called first pelvic grip. In the figure one hand is used and examiner is facing patients face… Hence it is pawlik grip or leopold third maneuver.

Normal and Abnormal Labor

PHASES OF PARTURITION

Now friends, don't confuse phases of parturition with stages of Labor.

• These are 4 phases of parturition (like 4 stages of labor)

Phases	Event included	Main role
Phase 1	Uterine quiescence, i.e. entire pregnancy cervical softening begins in phase 1	Progesterone hCG Nitric oxide Prostacyclin
Phase 2	Uterine activation/ uterus gets prepared for labour Includes cervical Ripening and lightening and formation of lower uterine segment from isthmus	• Withdraw of progesterone • Myometrial changes i.e. increase in oxytocin receptors, gap junction proteins and comexin 43 • Fetal endocrine changes (below) • Estrogen • Hyaluronan
Phase 3	Begins with onset of Labor and includes all 3 stages of labor	• Prostaglandin • Oxytocin • Estrogen • Inflammatory cell activation • Endothelin
Phase 4	**Period after delivery Includes**: Stage 4 of labor and Involution of uterus Puerperium	Oxytocin Endothelin

 Note: The number of oxytocin receptors increase in myometrium in phase 2 i.e. towards end of pregnancy but role of oxytocin in phase 2 is uncertain

• Oxytocin plays a major role in stage 2 of labor (phase 3 of parturition) and puerperium (phase 4 of parturition)
• Fetal endocrine changes which occur in phase 2 of parturition are:
  1. Human fetal hypothalamic pituitary adrenal placental axis is a critical component for normal labor.
  2. Placenta near term releases CRH which acts like ACTH and stimulates fetal adrenal gland to produce DHEAS and cortisol. (Fig. 9.1)

This DHEAS is used by placenta to synthesize estrogen

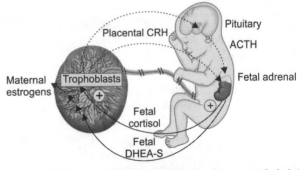

Fig. 9.1: The placental-fetal adrenal endocrine cascade in late gestation, placental corticotropin-releasing hormone (CRH) stimulates fetal adrenal production of ehydroepiandrosterone sulfate (DHEA-S) and cortisol. The latter stimulates production of placental CRH, which leads to a feed-forward cascade that enhances adrenal steroid hormone production. ACTH = adrenocorticotropic hormone.

PHYSIOLOGY OF LABOR

Labor

Series of events that take place in the genital organs in an effort to expel the viable products of conception (fetus, placenta and the membranes) out of the womb through the vagina into the outer world is called as labor, **a parturient** is a patient in labor and parturition is the process of giving birth.

Normal Labor (EUTOCIA): Labor is called normal if it fulfills the following criteria. (1) Spontaneous in onset and at term. (2) With vertex presentation. (3) Without undue prolongation. (4) Natural termination with minimal aids. (5) Without having any complications affecting the health of the mother and/or the baby.

Abnormal Labor (DYSTOCIA): Any deviation from the definition of normal labor is called Abnormal labor.

Prelabor

- It is the premonitory stage of labor and begins 2–3 weeks before the onset of true labor in primigravida and a few days before in multipara.
- It is associated with an increase in oxytocin receptors in myometrium.
- The changes seen during pre labor are:
  - *Lightening*: i.e. the decrease in fundal height seen at term. This is due to the formation of the lower segment of the uterus which allows the presenting part to descend into the pelvis. It brings a sense of relief to the mother.
  - *Cervical ripening,* i.e. softening of the cervix.
  - *False labor pains (see Table 9.1).*

Table 9.1: Differences between true labor pains and false labor pains

Features	True labor pains	False labor pains
Cervical changes (dilatation and effacement)	Present	Absent
Frequency and duration of contractions	Regular and gradually increase	Irregular
Pain	Lower abdomen and back, radiating to thighs	Lower abdomen only Not formed
Bag of water	Formed	Absent
Show	Present	No
Relief with enema/sedation	No	Yes

MECHANISMS RESPONSIBLE FOR ONSET OF LABOR (SEE FIGURE 9.2)

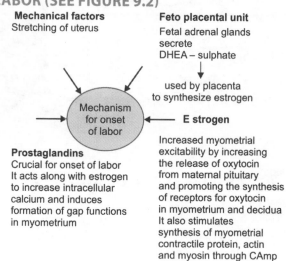

Fig. 9.2: Mechanism of onset of Labor

TRUE LABOR

- Oneset of True labor is characterized by:
- Appearance of true labor pain (Table 9.1)
- Appearance of show

True labor (i.e. phase 3 of parturition.) is divided into four functional stages:

Stages of True Labor

First stage: It starts with onset of true labor pain and ends with full dilatation of cervix (10 cm).[Q]

Second stage: It starts with full dilatation of cervix and ends with expulsion of fetus from birth canal. Duration is 0 minutes to 1 hour in primi and 30 minutes in multipara.

Third stage: It begins after expulsion of fetus and ends with expulsion of placenta and membranes (after births). Duration is about 15–25 minutes in both primi & multipara if it is managed passively. The duration is, however, reduced to 5 minutes in active management.

Fourth stage: 1 hour observation period after the delivery of placenta. Physiological chills are experienced by the mother in this stage.[Q]

Uterine Contractions

- Throughout pregnancy, a pregnant female experiences irregular involuntary spasmodic contractions which are painless and do not lead to dilation of cervix. These are called as **Braxton Hicks contractions**.

- During labor: The contractions are painful and lead to dilatation of cervix.
- The **pacemaker of uterine** contractions is situated **at the cornu (the right pacemaker** predominates over the left).
- **Contractions spread from** pacemaker area throughout uterus **at 2 cm/sec**, depolarizing the whole organ **within 15 secs.**
- Contractions are **predominant over the fundus.**

Table 9.2: Intrauterine pressure

Event	Intrauterine pressure
• Contractions are palpable	10 mm of Hg
• Contractions are painful	15 mm of Hg
• Cervix dilates	15 mm of Hg
• Fundus cannot be indented	40 mm of Hg
• 1st stage of Labor	40–50 mm of Hg
• 2nd and 3rd	100–120 mm of Hg

- **Adequate uterine contractions** refer to 3 contractions in 10 mins each lasting for 45 secs and causing Intrauterine pressure of 65–75 mm of Hg or 220 montevideo unit.
- **Tachysystole** is defined as more than 5 contractions in 10 mins (averaged over 30 minutes).
- **Term Tachysystole can be applied to spontaneous or induced labor.** When tachysystole causes fetal distress it is called as **Hyperstimulation.**
- The term **hyperstimulation** has been abandoned now.

Also Know:
Units for measuring uterine contractions:
1. mm of Hg
2. Montevideo unit (MV unit)

- 1 montevideo unit = Intensity of uterine contraction × number of contractions in 10 minutes.

For example, if a female experiences 3 contraction in 10 minutes with pressure of 60 mm of Hg.

Montevideo unit (MV unit) will be = 3 × 60 = 180 MV units

Note: Clinical labor commences with 80–120 MV units.
Uterine activity is 200–225 MV units in established labor.

Abnormal Uterine Action

1. **M/C: Hypotonic contractions:** (also k/a uterine inertia). Number of contractions are < 3 in 10 minutes lasting for < 45 secs and < 180 montevideo units. Management is to Augment labor by amniotony (ARM) or oxytocin.
2. **Excessive contractions:** It can result in **precipitate labor, i.e. entire process of delivery completed in less than 3 hours.**

Requirement for Normal Labor

For normal labor to occur, the 3 most important things are:
1. Push, i.e. uterine contractions
2. Passage, i.e. normal pelvis
3. Passenger, i.e. fetus

IMPORTANT CONCEPTS IN STAGES OF LABOR

FIRST STAGE OF LABOR

It begins with the onset of True Labor pains and ends with full dilatation of cervix.

First stage of labor, i.e. the stage of cervical effacement and dilatation is further divided into 2 phases (Table 9.3).

Table 9.3: Differences between latent and active phase

Latent phase preparatory division	Active phase dilatational division
• It starts at the point at which the mother perceives true labor pains and ends when cervix is 5 cm dilated.	• It begins with cervical dilatation of ≥ 6 with regular uterine contractions. (Williams **25/e pg 433**) • Gynaecologists and Society for Maternal-Fetal Medicine (2016c) has redefine active labor to begin at 6 cm.
• Its duration in nulliparous is 12 hours (avg 8.6 hours)[Q] and 8 hours (avg 5.6 hours) in multiparous females.[Q]	• Normal minimum cervical dilatation rate of 1.2 cm/hr for nulliparous[Q] and 1.5 cm/hr for parous women[Q]. **According to WHO Minimum dilatation should be 1 cm/hr**[Q]
• Mainly concerned with cervical effacement and dilatation	• Mainly concerned with cervical dilatation and descent of fetal head • Descent of fetal head: • Nulliparous = 1 cm/hr • Multiparous = 2 ch/hr

Abnormality of Latent Phase

Prolonged Latent Phase

Latent phase is said to be prolonged if it is :
- Greater than 20 hours in nullipara.[Q]
- Greater than 14 hours in multipara.[Q]

Causes of Prolonged Latent Phase

- Excessive sedation or epidural analgesia.
- Poor cervical conditions (e.g., Thick, uneffaced or undilated).
- False labor (*most common* cause in multipara).

Management

> **Therapeutic Rest**
>
> 15 mg of morphine is given intramuscularly. Most of the patients are asleep within 1 hour and awake 4 to 5 hours later, in active labor or in no labor.

Abnormalities of Active Phase

- Active phase as we have discussed earlier, begins when cervix is ≥ 6 cms dilated.
- The 2 main events in active phase are
  - Dilatation of cervix
  - Descent of fetal head

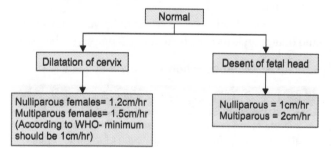

Protracted Active Phase

If dilatation or descent is less than above said values.

Management of Protracted Active Phase

1. Rule out cephalopelvic disproportion
2. Rule out occipitoposterior posterior position
3. After ruling them out, augment labor by doing artificial rupture of membranes and starting oxytocin IV infusion. If Contraction are not sufficient

> **Artificial rupture of membrane**
> - It is a method of augmenting labor (i.e. accelerating labor)
> - Done using Kocher's artery forceps
>
> **Immediate beneficial effects of ARM**
> - Lowering of the blood pressure in pre-eclampsia-eclampsia.
> - Relief of maternal distress in hydramnios.
> - Control of bleeding in APH.
> - Relief of tension in abruptioplacentae and initiation of labour.

Contd...

Contd...

> These benefits are to be weighed against the risks involved in the indications for which the method is adopted.
>
> **Hazards of ARM**
> - Chance of umbilical cord prolapse — The risk is low with engaged head or rupture of membranes with head fixed to the brim.
> - Amnionitis
> - Accidental injury to the placenta, cervix or uterus, fetal parts or vasa-previa
> - Liquor amnio embolism (rare)
>
> **Conditions where ARM (artificial rupture of membranes) is contraindicated:**
> 1. Intrauterine fetal death
> 2. Maternal HIV
> 3. Active genital herpes infection.
>   **Note:** In chronic hydramnios, controlled ARM is done and not just simple ARM as sudden decompression can lead to abruptio placenta.

Active Phase Arrest

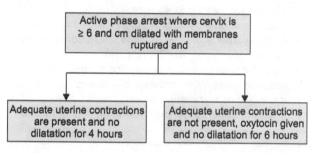

 Remember: Diagnosis of arrest, should only be made after membranes are ruptured.

Recent Updates

> **Obstetric Care Consensus Committee** *Williams 25/e*
> There are **four recommendations by the** Consensus Committee (2016) applicable to management of the first stage labor.
>
> - **The first admonishes** against cesarean delivery in the latent phase of labor. Specifically, a prolonged latent phase is not an indication for cesarean delivery. This guideline is not new and is traceable to the work of Friedman (1954), on which traditional tenets are based.
> - **The second** directive, too, is conventional practice. It recommends against cesarean delivery if labor is progressive but slow---A *protraction disorder*. This instance is typically managed with observation, assessment of uterine activity, and stimulation of contractions as needed.

Recent Updates

- **A third instruction** addresses the cervical dilation threshold that serves to herald active labor. Namely, a cervical dilation of 6 cm—not 4 cm—is now the recommended threshold. Thus, before this threshold, standards for active phase progress should not be applied.
- **A fourth stipulation** notes that cesarean delivery for active phase arrest should be reserved for women at or beyond 6 cm of dilation with ruptured membranes who fail to progress despite 4 hours of adequate uterine activity, or at least 6 hours of oxytocin administration with inadequate contractions and no cervical change.

Management

Cesarean section

Concept Box

Friends so that you understand the different problems which can occur during 1st stage of labor and their management, lets look at a few clinical situations:

1st situation

A G$_2$P$_1$ is admitted in labor at 8 am on Monday.
P/V findings = Cervix 2 cm dilated, 20% effaced
At 10 pm findings are: Cervix = 3 cm dilated, 60% effaced
FHR = Regular, 140–146 bpm
Membranes = intact
What is the next step in management

Solution

- This female is multiparous
- Stage of labor = Latent phase (as cervix is < 6 cm dilated)
- Total duration = 8 am to 10 pm = 14 hours

Latent phase is said to be prolonged if it is 14 hours in multiparous female.
Hence diagnosis is: Prolonged latent phase
Management: Sedation/Therapeutic rest.

2nd situation

A G$_2$P$_1$ is admitted in labor at 8 am on Monday.
P/V findings = Cervix 2 cm dilated, 20% effaced
At 12 pm (midnoon): Cervix 6 cm dilated 80% effaced
At 3 pm = Cervix 8 cm dilated, membranes intact
FHR is 140, Regular uterine contractions are present.
What is the next step in management

Solution

Here again,
Female is multiparous.
When she was admitted, she was in latest phase (cervix 2 cm dilated) but it ended in 4 hours (at 12 pm = cervix is 6 cm dilated). Hence latent phase was normal. Now she came in active phase at 12 pm. Since she is a multigravida, dilatation of cervix should be 1.5 cm/hr (In 3 hours = 4.5 cm, already at 12 pm she is 6 cm dilated therefore by 3 pm she should be 6 + 4.5 = 10 cm, i.e. fully dilated). But here she is only 8 cm dilated, i.e. it is a case of protracted active phase. Management should be ARM followed by oxytocin.

3rd situation

3. A G$_2$P$_1$ female is admitted in labor at 8 am on Monday.
P/V findings = Cervix 6 cm dilated, 100% effaced
Membranes ruptured, No meconium
FHR = 140–148 bpm, Regular uterine contractions = Adequate
At 12 pm (midnoon): Same findings.
        Next step in management.

Solution

Now here patient is:
- Multiparous
- She is admitted in active phase (cervix 6 cm dilated) at 8 am At 12 pm inspite of good uterine contractions and membranes ruptured, there is no dilatation for 4 hours, hence diagnosis is arrest of active phase.

Management is cesarean section.

SECOND STAGE OF LABOR

It begins from full dilatation of cervix and ends with expulsion of fetus.

In the second stage, the expulsive efforts by a woman play more important role than uterine contractions.

Prolonged Second Stage

Second stage			
	Normal	Prolonged without epidural	Prolonged with epidural
Nulli-parous	1 hr (50 mins as per Williams 25/e pg 434)	2 hrs (+1 for arrest)	3 hrs (+1 for arrest)
Multi-parous	30 mins (20 mins Williams 25/e pg 434)	1 hr (+1 for arrest)	2 hrs (+1 for arrest)

Causes of Prolonged Second Stage Include

1. Small pelvis
2. Large fetus
3. Impaired expulsive efforts from conduction analgesia or sedative.

Management of Prolonged Second Stage of Labour

It depends on station of fetal head.

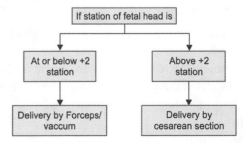

Second Stage Arrest

	Without Epidural	With Epidural
Nulliparous	3 hours	4 hours
Multiparous	2 hours	3 hours

Management

Second stage arrest is synonymous to obstructed labor and should be managed by doing cesarean section.

Moulding of fetal head and caput formation begins in second stage arrest.

Moulding

> **Definition: Moulding is the change in the shape of the fetal head while passing through the resistant birth canal during labor.**
> The cranial bones are connected by membrane and this allows considerable shifting or sliding of each bone to accommodate to the maternal pelvis. Usually the frontal and occipital bones pass under the parietal bone. Thee is compression of the presenting diameter with compensatory bulging of the diameter at right angle.

For example, in occipito-anterior presentation, the head is compressed in the presenting suboccipito-bregmatic diameter and elongated in the mento-vertical diameter. In normal labor, 0.5–1 cm of moulding is normal.

Grading

According to the severity of compression and thereby extent of overlapping, moulding is divided into:

- **Grade 1 (+).** The bones touch each other but do not overlap.
- **Grade 2 (++).** The bones overlap but are easily separable (reducible overlapping)
- **Grade 3 (+++).** Fixed, irreducible overlapping. It is usually pathological.

Clinical Significance

1. Some amount of moulding is physiological and is beneficial.
2. Severe moulding (Grade 3) seen in obstructed labor is pathological. It can lead to intracranial hemorrhage.
3. The site of moulding gives information about the position of the head.

New Concept: *Williams 25/e*

Emergency Medical Treatment and Labor Act—EMTALA

- The definition of an emergency conditions makes specific reference to a pregnant woman who is having contractions.
- Labor is defined as the process of childbirth beginning with the latent phase of labor continuing through delivery of the placenta.
- A woman experiencing contractions is in true labor unless a physician certifies that after a reasonable time of observation the woman is in false labor.
- A woman in true labor is considered unstable for interhospital transfer purposes until the newborn and placenta are delivered. A stable woman may, however, be transferred at the direction of the patient or by a physician who certifies that the benefits of treatment at another facility outweigh the transfer risks.
- Physicians and hospitals violating these federal requirements are subject to civil penalties and termination from participation in the Medicare program.

THIRD STAGE OF LABOR

Third stage of labor extends from the birth of child to complete expulsion of placenta and membranes and contraction and retraction of uterus.

All details of this stage are discussed in next chapter.

MECHANISM OF LABOR

Mechanism of normal labor is defined as the manner in which the fetus adjusts itself to pass through the parturient canal with minimal difficulty.

There are 8 cardinal movements of the head in normal labor.

- Every – Engagement (Synclitic or Asynclitic)
- Decent – Descent
- Female – Flexion
- I – Internal rotation
- Choose to – Crowning
- Employ – Extension
- Rises – Restitution
- Extremely – External rotation

> **Mnemonic**
>
> Every Decent Female I Choose to and Employ Rises Extremely.

Engagement

- *Engagement is said to occur when the greatest transverse diameter of the presenting part, has passed through the pelvic inlet. In all cephalic presentations, the greatest transverse diameter is generally the biparietal (Fig. 9.3).*

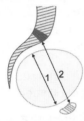

Fig. 9.3: Engagement in vertex showing that the BPD (1) has passed through the pelvic inlet, (2) and the lowermost part of the head is at the level of the ischial spines.

- Engagement occurs in Multipara with commencement of labor[Q] in the late Ist stage after rupture of membranes and in Nullipara during the last few weeks of pregnancy 38 weeks.
- In primi's the *most common* cause of non engagement at term is deflexed head, occipitoposterior position followed by cephalopelvic disproportion (CPD).[Q]

Causes of nonengagement of head in a nullipara at term:

- Malpresentations[Q]/Occipitoposterior position/deflexed head
- Cephalopelvic disproportion[Q]
- Placenta previa[Q]/Tumours in the lower segment[Q]

- Tumours of the fetal neck[Q]/Cord around the neck[Q]/ Hydrocephalus[Q]
- Polyhydramnios[Q]
- Distended bladder and rectum.[Q]

- Engagement of head rules out CPD at the level of pelvic inlet.
- If head is engaged, it means head is at 'O' station.
- Per abdominally 1/5th or less of head is palpable.

Engagement can be:

Synclitic	Asynclitic	
When sagittal suture of the head of fetus lies in the transverse diameter of pelvic inlet (midway between the pubic symphysis and the sacral promontory) It occurs in 25% cases	*Anterior:* Sagittal suture is defected towards sacral promontory. Also k/a anterior parietal presentaion/ **Naegeles obliquity.** It occurs commonly in **Multipara** Mnemonic: ANM	*Posterior:* Sagittal suture is defected towards pubic symphysis, the posterior parietal bone thus becomes the leading part. Also k/a **Litzman obliquity/ parietal presentation** It occurs commonly in **nulliparous** women.

 Important One Liners

- Engagement occurs with marked asynclitism in platypelloid pileus.

Engaging Diameter

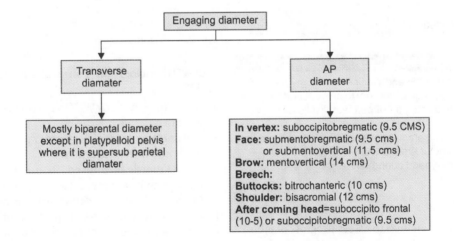

In vertex: suboccipitobregmatic (9.5 CMS)
Face: submentobregmatic (9.5 cms)
         or submentovertical (11.5 cms)
Brow: mentovertical (14 cms)
Breech:
Buttocks: bitrochanteric (10 cms)
Shoulder: bisacromial (12 cms)
After coming head=suboccipito frontal (10-5) or suboccipitobregmatic (9.5 cms)

Other Important points to Remember:

M/C position at the beginning of labor = LOT > LOA during rotation

- Internal rotation occurs at the level of ischial spine
- Occiput moves by 2/8th of a circle in LOT position and shoulders by 1/8th of a circle. Their is torsion of neck.
- Head of fetus is delivered by movement of extension.
- Restitution is untwisting of neck back by 45°. The occiput turns towards the mothers left thigh in LOA position and towards right thigh in ROA position.
- External rotation
  - External rotation is a continuation of movement of restitution by another 45°. Actually it is the outward manifestation of internal rotation of shoulder from oblique diameter to AP diameter.
  - After external rotation the occiput of the baby will occupy the original position @ which labor began. Hence in LOT position Occiput = is at LOT Position Face of the baby is towards mothers right thigh
  - Anterior shoulder of baby is delivered first and then posterior shoulder
  - Delivery of rest of the body is by lateral flexion.

- The most important step in delivery is delivery of fetal head.
- For delivery of fetal head---**Modified Ritgen Maneuver is done (Fig. 9.4)**
- In this maneuver gloved fingers beneath a draped towel exert form and pressure on fetal chin through the perineum just in front of coccyx. Concurrently other hand presses against occiput. It allows controlled delivery of head.

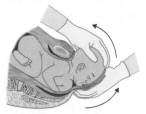

Fig. 9.4: Ritgen maneuver

Methods to Prevent Perineal Tear

- WHO does not recommend routine episotomy for all females undergoing vaginal delivery to prevent perineal tear
- WHO recommends support of perineum while delivery **head of fetus**
- Use of modified Ritgen maneuver for delivery of head so that smaller diameter emerges out
- Maintain flexion of head during delivery.

PARTOGRAM

Partogram is the best method to assess progress of labor.

- *Partogram is the graphical recording of stages of labor including cervical dilatation, descent and rotation of the head.*

Various partographs have been made and it is essential to have their detailed knowledge:

1st: Friedman Curve (1954) (Fig. 9.5)
- Friedman divided the first stage of labor into 2 phases: Latest phase and Active phase
- Active phase as per Friedman began at ≥ 3 cm

The pattern of cervical dilatation during the latent and active phase of normal labor is a sigmoid curve.

Friedman subdivided the active phase into:
- Acceleration phase – 3-4 cm of cervical dilatation
- Phase of maximum slope – 4-9 cm
- Deceleration phase – 9-10 cm

2nd: The second partograph was introduced by **Philpott and Castle in 1972.**

They introduced the concept of alert line and action line. Labor is said to be progressing normally till it remains to the left of alert line.

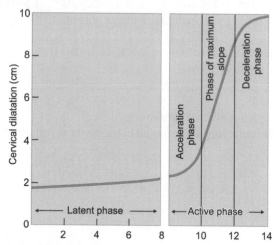

Fig. 9.5: Friedman curve.

3rd: WHO partograph-Composite Partograph (Fig. 9.6A and B)

- It was introduced by WHO a part of the Safe Motherhood initiative.
- The *main purpose* of the partogram is to *avoid prolonged labor* and *intervene timely.*
- Once labor is diagnosed, its progress is charted on a partogram by abdominal and vaginal examination.

  Cervical dilatation and descent of the head (which are the best parameters to assess the progress of labor) are plotted on Y axis and time in hours is plotted on X axis.

- The latent phase of labor is up to **3 cm** dilatation, and should not be more than **8 hours**. In the active phase which extends from 3 cm to complete cervical dilatation, labor is expected to progress at the rate of at least 1 cm cervical dilatation per hour which corresponds to the *alert line*.
- The *action line* is drawn 4 hours to the right and parallel to the alert line in the *WHO partogram*.
- Labour is considered normal as long as the progress of cervical dilatation is to the left of the alert line.

- Prolonged labor is diagnosed, once the alert line is crossed, i.e., there is a shift to the right.
- **If the patient is in a peripheral hospital, once the alert line is crossed, it is an indication for referral to a higher centre for extra vigilance.**
- If action line is crossed, it is an indication for some action.

  Thus, the partogram can be used to identify an abnormal labor pattern and to indicate the correct time for intervention by means of the alert and action lines.

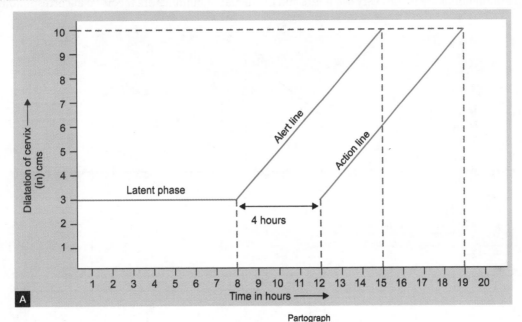

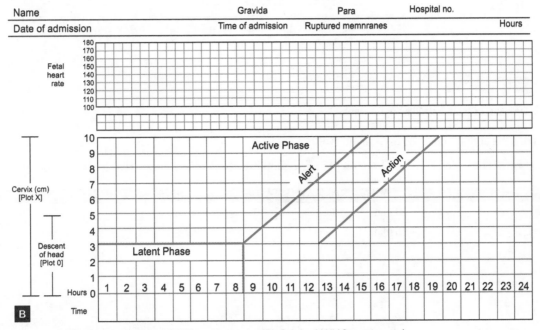

Figs. 9.6A and B: (A) Drawing of original WHO partograph; (B) Original WHO pantograph

Modified WHO Partograph (Figs. 9.7A and B)

In this partograph two changes occurred:

1. Latent phase was removed
2. Active phase begins at 4 cms

How to use a Partograph

Graphical record of cervical dilatation Marked with X begin at 4 cms: The first vaginal examination is done on admission. Subsequent examinations are made every 0–4 hours and the dilatation findings are recorded at corresponding hours.

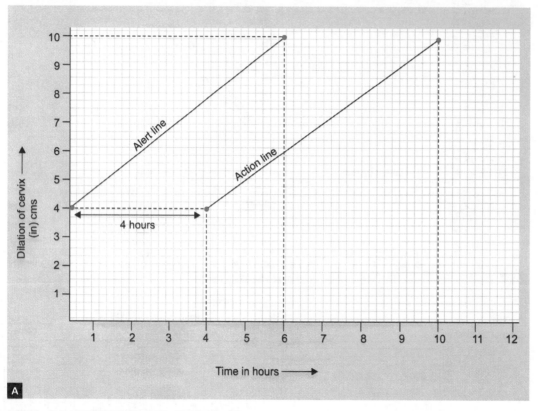

Fig. 9.7A: Drawing of modified WHO partograph.

Time: Record the actual time at 30 minute interval.

Fetal heart rate is recorded at half an hour on the partogram but checked as follows: (williams 25/e pg 436)

	Low-risk	High-risk
1st state	30 mins	15 mins
2nd state	15 mins	5 mins

Liquor amnii. If the membranes are intact, it is recorded as 'I'. If there is rupture of membranes (ROM), is time is also recorded. In this case if the liquor amnii is clear it is recorded as 'C', if it is meconium stained, it is recorded as 'M' and if it is blood stained, it is recorded as 'B'.

Moulding. Degree of moulding is recorded as + or ++ or +++.

Descent of head is recorded as the number of fifths of head above the pelvic brim being plotted on the graph.

Uterine contractions can be assessed with electronic monitoring or manually noted every 30 minutes. This graph consists of a vertical column of five squares. The squares are shaded according to the number of contractions per 10 minutes. The density of shading (faint: < 20 seconds, slightly dark: 20–40 seconds, dark: > 40 seconds) also denotes the intensity of contractions.

Oxytocin. If oxytocin infusion has been started then the time at which the infusion has started, charted every 30 minutes.

Maternal Monitoring

- Temperature, pulse, and blood pressure are evaluated at least every 4 hours.
- If membranes have been ruptured for many hours before labor onset or if there is a borderline temperature elevation, the temperature is checked hourly.

Note: Although uterine contractions are usually assessed with electronic monitoring, they can be quantitatively and qualitatively evaluated manually. With the palm of the hand resting lightly on the uterus, the time of contraction onset is determined. Its intensity is gauged from the degree of firmness the uterus achieves. At the acme of effective contractions, the finger or thumb cannot readily indent the uterus during a firm contraction. The time at which the contraction disappears is noted next. This sequence is repeated to evaluate the frequency, duration, and intensity of contractions.

- During the first stage of labor, the need for subsequent vaginal examinations to monitor cervical change and presenting part position will vary considerably.
- When the membranes rupture, an examination to exclude cord prolapse is performed expeditiously if the fetal head was not definitely engaged at the previous examination.
- The fetal heart rate is also checked immediately and during the next uterine contraction to help detect occult umbilical cord compression.
- At Parkland Hospital, periodic pelvic examinations are typically performed at 2- to 3-hour intervals to evaluate labor progress. Evidence implicating the number of vaginal examinations in infection-related morbidity is conflicting.

Indications for Partogram

- All primigravidas
- High-risk pregnancies
- Malpositions (occipito-posterior) and malpresentations are given trial of vaginal delivery
- Trial of labor in mildly contracted pelvic inlet.

Paperless Partogram

Dr. Aloke Debdas from Jamshedpur has developed a simple to use paperless partogram in which alert estimated time of delivery (ETD) is calculated in active labor considering 1 cm/hour dilatation while action is taken 4 hours after estimated time of delivery.

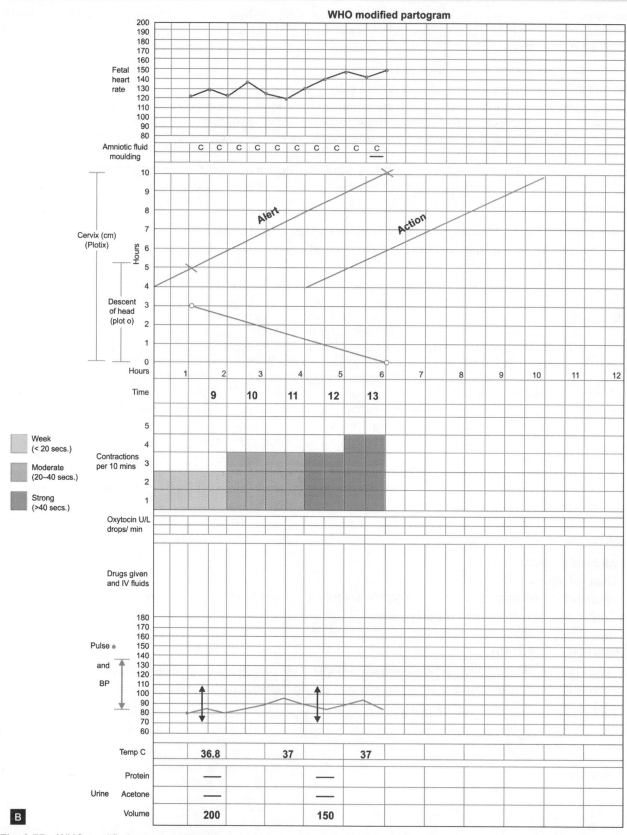

Fig. 9.7B: WHO modified actual partograph.

PAIN PATHWAY IN LABOR (FIG. 9.8)

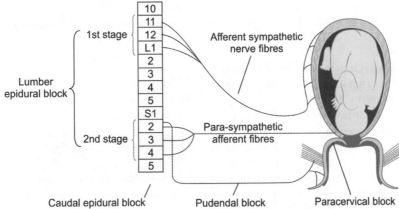

Fig. 9.8: Pain pathway in labor.

 Remember:

- Pain during early stage of labor is due to uterine contraction, hence felt along T10–L1 (Nerve supply of uterus).
- Pain during later stages of labor is due to cervical dilatation therefore felt along S2–S4 (Nerve supply of cervix).
- Therefore for painless Labor-Epidural block should be given from segment T10 onwards.
- Perineum is supplied by pudendal nerve.
- Therefore for applying instruments like forceps, pudendal nerve block should be used.

Management of Pain During Labor

Pudendal nerve block:

- *Pudendal nerve arises from:* S2, S3, S4 and therefore pudendal nerve block -will block S2, S3, S4, nerve roots.
- It is used for perineal analgesia and relaxation.
- **Anaesthesia** used is 20 ml of 1% lignocaine/lidocaine
- **Route** Transvaginal and perineal route
- **Site :** Pudendal nerve is blocked just above the tip of ischial spine

 Note: The ligament pierced for Pudendal Nerve block is sacrospinous ligament.

- **Indications:**
  - Prior to application of forceps or vacuum
  - To suture vaginal lacerations
  - In Assisted breech delivery

Paracervical block:

Paracervical block
- ***Basis of use:*** Sensory nerve fibres from the uterus fuse bilaterally at the 4-6 O' clock and 6-8 O' clock position around the cervix in the region of cervico vaginal junction.
- In para cervical block, 5-10 mL of 1% lidocaine is injected into these areas to interrupt the sensory input from the cervix and uterus.
- **It relieves the pain of uterine contractions**Q
- Since the block is given in lateral fornix so it anesthetizes upper 1/3rd of vagina also.Q
- It is not useful at the time of episiotomy as lower part of vagina is not anesthetized.
- It is no longer considered safe as it causes fetal bradycardia.Q

Epidural block:

When complete relief of pain is needed throughout labor, epidural analgesia is the safest and simplest method for procuring it.

Advantages of regional anesthesia
- The patient is awake and can enjoy the birth time
- Newborn apgar score generally good
- Lowered risk of maternal aspiration
- Postoperative pain control is better.

For complete analgesia during labor a block from T10 to the S5 dermatomes is needed. For cesarean delivery a block from T4 is needed.

- Repeated doses (top ups) of 4 to 5 mL of 0.5 percent bupivacaine or 1 percent lignocaine are used to maintain analgesia.

- Epidural analgesia, as a general rule should be given when labor is well established.
- Maternal hydration should be adequate.
- The women is kept in semilateral position to avoid aortocaval compression.
- **Epidural analgesia is specially beneficial** in cases like pregnancy induced hypertension, breech presentation, twin pregnancy and preterm labor.
- Previous cesarean section is not a contraindication.
- Epidural analgesia when used there is no change in duration of first stage of labor. But second stage of labor appears to be prolonged. This might lead to frequent need of instrumental delivery like forceps or ventouse

Contraindications of Epidural Analgesia	Complications of Epidural Analgesia
• Maternal coagulopathy or anticoagulant therapy • Supine hypotension • Hypovolemia • Neurological diseases • Spinal deformity or chronic low back pain • Skin infection at the injection site • Refractory maternal Hypotension • Maternal coagulopathy • Thrombocytopenia • LMW hepain with 12 hours of labor • Untreated maternal bacteremia or skin infection. • Increased ICT due to mass lesion	• Hypotension due to sympathetic blockade. Parturient should be well hydrated with (IL) crystalloid solution beforehand • Pain at the insertion site. Back pain • Postspinal headache due to leakage of cerebrospinal fluid through the needle hole in the dura • Total spinal due to inadvertent administration of the drug in the subarachnoid space • Injury to nerves, convulsions, pyrexia • Ineffective analgesia

INDUCTION OF LABOR

Induction: Implies stimulation of contractions before the spontaneous onset of labor.

Indications for Induction of Labour

- Membrane rupture without labor
- Gestational hypertension
- Oligohydramnios
- Non reassuring fetal heart rate
- Post term pregnancy
- Medical conditions of mother like chronic hypertension and diabetes.

Often the cervix is closed and uneffaced ∴ labor induction is commenced by first making cervix soft, the process is called as **cervical ripening.**

 Note: This is anterior term:
- **Augmentation of labor** which means increasing the strength of uterine contractions such that labor progresses fast.

 Before labor is induced, **Bishop scoring is** done to assess whether induction will be successful or not.

Bishop Score

Bishop score is a quantitative method for prediction of successful induction of labor.

 Mnemonic

Delhi Police Employed Special Commandos
It includes the following parameters:
Delhi = Cervical **D**ilatation (**most important parameter**)
—*Dutta 9/e p 485*
Police = Cervical **P**osition
Employed = Cervical **E**ffacement
Special = Head **S**tation
Commandos = Cervical **C**onsistency
(For detail, see Table 9.4)

- Induction of labor is successful with a score of 9 or more which clinically would mean cervix 2 cm dilated, 80% effaced, soft, mid position and with fetal occiput at station.
- A score of < 4 means ripening of cervix is indicated before inducing labor.

Modified Bishop Score

In an effort to increased predictability of successful induction and to reduce associated morbidity, several modification have been proposed to Bishop's original pelvic scoring system. Burrnett (1966) proposed what has become known as the modified Bishop score (Table 9.5). In this scoring cervical effacement has been replaced by dilatation of cervix and each category given a maximum score of 2, for a total maximum score of 10.

Nearly 90% of patients with scores of 6 to 8 were delivered within 6 hours. The outcome of patients with scores of less than 6 was unpredictable.

 Mnemonic

Delhi Police Left Special Commandos
It includes the following parameters:
Delhi = Cervical **D**ilatation (**most important parameter**)
Police = Cervical **P**osition
Left = Cervical **L**ength
Special = Head **S**tation
Commandos = Cervical **C**onsistency
(For detail, see Table 9.5)

Table 9.4: Bishop scoring in detail

Score	Dilatation (cm)	Effacement (%)	Station*	Cervical Consistency	Cervical Position
0	Closed	0 – 30	– 3	Firm	Posterior
1	1 – 2	40 – 50	– 2	Medium	Midposition
2	3 – 4	60 – 70	– 1, 0	Soft	Anterior
3	≥ 5	> 80	+1, +2	—	—

* Station reflects a –3 to +3 scale.

Table 9.5: Modified Bishop scoring in detail

Score	Dilatation (cm)	Length of cervix	Station*	Cervical Consistency	Cervical Position
0	0	2 cm	– 2	Firm	Posterior
1	1 cm	1 cm	– 1	Soft	Midposition
2	> 2 cm	< 0.5 cm	0	Soft and stretchable	Anterior

Risks of Induction of Labor (See Table 9.6)

Table 9.6: Risk of IOL

Risk	Comment
Increased chance of caesarean delivery	This risk is more in Nulliparous females
Chorioamionitis	Risk is more if ARM (Amniotomy) is done to augment labor
Rupture of prior uterine incision	Risk is more with prostaglandins "**ACOG-2017** recommends against the use of prostaglandin for pre induction cervical ripening or labor induction in women with prior uterine incision.
Uterine atony and associated PPH	

Factors Affecting Induction Success

Favourable factors

Young age
Multiparity
BMI < 30
Favourable cervix
Birthweight < 3.5 Kg

Cervical Ripening

- It occurs in phase 2 of parturition normally i.e. weeks/days before labor
- During the transformation the cervical matrix changes its total amount of glycosamino glycans (which are large polysaccharides) and proteoglycans (which are proteins bound to these glycosaminoglycans.

Commonly Used Agents for Preinduction Cervical Ripening

Method of ripening	Dosage	Comment
PGE2 dinoprostone	Local application of gel (2.5 mL syringe with 0.5 mg dinoprostone)	Gel is deposited just below internal OS
		Gel can be repeated after 6 hours
		Maximum 3 doses in 24 hours
		Side effect: Tachysystole
		1-5% cases
PGE1 (Misoprostol)	Vaginally-Dose 25 μg (1/4 of 100 mcg tablet) Orally 50-100 mcg Repeat after 3 -6 hrs	ACOG recommends its use for cervical ripening Higher dose of vaginal misoprost is associated with decreased need of oxytocin but has higher chances of tachysystole

Method of ripening	Dosage	Comment
Nitric oxide Donor, like Isosorbide, mononitrate and glyceral nitrate		These are less effective than PGE2/PGE1
Mechanical techniques: Transcervical catheter or Hygroscopic cervical dilators	30 mL balloon Laminaria test	Improve Bischop score rapidly 80 mL balloon more effective

Method of Induction and Augmentation

PGE1	Oral = 100 mcg Vaginal = 25 mcg Repeated 6 hrs interval	Oxytocin should be given 6 hrs after misoprost Studies have shown 75 mcg oral misoprost repeated @ 4 hours for a maximum of 2 doses to be safe and effective for labor augmentation
Oxytocin	10-20 mIu/L given by infusion or 1/m never in bolus)	It is used for augmentation of labor
ARM (early used for induction of labor)	Done using kocher's forceps	Also called Amniotomy
		Used for augmentation of labor

 Also Know:

Ferguson reflex: mechanical stretching of the cervix enhances uterine activity. In many species including humans manipulation of the cervix and stripping of fetal membranes leads to an increase in blood levels of prostaglandins.
Prostaglandins are very useful both for ripening of cervix and for induction of labor.

 Important points on prostaglandins:

- The gold standard agent for cervical ripening is PGE_2, i.e. dinoprost gel
- The gold standard agent for inducing labour is PGE_2
- The analogue of prostaglandin recently approved by ACOG for cervical ripening-PGE_1 (misoprost)
- The analogue of prostaglandin which is contraindicated in scarred uterus and should not be used in previous LSCS patients-PGE_1
- The analogue of prostaglandin which is not used for inducing labour-*PGF-2 alpha*
- The analogue of prostaglandin which is used in PPH-*PGF-2 alpha*

Contraindications of Induction of Labor

They include all those conditions that preclude spontaneous labor and vaginal delivery.

 Mnemonic

Absolute contraindication of induction of labor
- Severe degree of contracted pelvis
- Cancer cervix
- Cord prolapse in early labor
- Major malpresentations like transverse lie, brow, mentoposterior face
- Previous uterine scar of hysterotomy, classical cesarean section, repair of uterine rupture
- Active genital herpes
- Grade II posterior, grade III and Grade IV placenta previa

Relative contraindication
- Fetal distress
- Cervical fibroid
- Impacted ovarian cyst in pouch of Douglas .

New Pattern Questions

N1. Which of the following trigger onset of labour?
   a. ACTH in mother   b. ACTH in fetus
   c. Prostaglandin   d. Oxytocin

N2. Engagement of fetal head is with reference to:
   a. Biparietal diameter b. Bitemporal diameter
   c. Occipitofrontal diameter
   d. Suboccipitofrontal diameter

N3. All of the following are included in first stage of labor except:
   a. Effacement of Cx b. Dilatation of Cx
   c. Crowning of fetal head
   d. Descent of head

N4. All of the following are indications for induction of labor except:
   a. PROM   b. Oligohydramnios
   c. Gestational Hypertension
   d. Placenta previa

N5. During active labour cervical dilatation per hour in primi is:
   a. 1.2 cm   b. 1.5 cm
   c. 1.7 cm   d. 2 cm

N6. Bag of membrane ruptures:
   a. Before full dilatation of cervix
   b. After full dilatation of cervix
   c. After head is engaged
   d. With excessive show

N7. Percentage of women who deliver on the expected date of delivery:
   a. 4%   b. 15%
   c. 35%   d. 70%

N8. Pressure of normal uterine contractions is between 190–300 units. Which unit is being referred to here?
   a. Montevideo units b. mm of Hg
   c. cm of water   d. Joules/kg

N9. Intrauterine pressure is raised during labour to:
   a. First stage — 40–50 mm Hg
   b. Second stage — 100–120 mm Hg
   c. Third stage — 100–120 mm Hg
   d. All of the above

N10. All are true about origin and propagation of contractions except:
   a. The right pacemaker predominates over left
   b. Intensity of propagation is greatest at cervix
   c. The contraction spreads from pacemaker towards cervix
   d. Speed of contraction is 2 cm/sec

N11. During the active phase of labour, the minimum effective dilatation of the cervix in primigravida should be at the rate of:
   a. 0.5 cm/hour   b. 1 cm/hour
   c. 1.5 cm/hour   d. 2 cm/hour

N12. Factors which help in descent of the presenting part during labour are all except:
   a. Uterine contraction and retraction
   b. Straightening of the fetal axis
   c. Bearing down efforts
   d. Resistance from the pelvic floor

N13. The prerequisites for internal rotation of the head are all except:
   a. Well-flexed head
   b. Efficient uterine contraction
   c. Favourable shape of the pelvis
   d. Tone of the abdominal muscles

N14. The following statement is true for internal rotation of the head:
   a. Rotation occurs mostly in the cervix
   b. In majority rotation occurs in the pelvic floor
   c. Rotation occurs commonly after crowning of the head
   d. Rotation is earlier in primipara than multipara

N15. The perineal injury can be prevented in normal labour by all except:
   a. Maintaining flexion of the head
   b. Timely episiotomy as a routine
   c. Slow delivery of the head in between contractions
   d. Effective perineal guard

N16. Ritgen maneuver is done in:
   a. Shoulder dystocia
   b. For delivery of head in breech presentation
   c. For delivery of legs in breech
   d. For delivery of head in normal labour

N17. Uterine contractions are clinically palpable when there intensity is more than?
   a. 10 mm of Hg   b. 15 mm of Hg
   c. 20 mm of Hg   d. 40 mm of Hg

N18. Which does not influence the factor in progress of labor is:
   a. Parity of female   b. BMI of female
   c. Fetal sex   d. Number of fetuses
   e. None of the above

N19. The nerve roots blocked in pudendal nerve block is:
   a. L1,2,3   b. L2,3
   c. S2,3,4   d. S4

N20. Paracervical block relieves pain from all but one of the following:
   a. Pain from dilatation of the cervix
   b. Uterine pain
   c. Relives pain from the lower third of vagina and episiotomy can be performed
   d. Relieve pain from the upper third of vagina

N21. A 35-year-old pregnant female at 40 weeks gestational age presents with pain and regular uterine contractions every 4–5 min. ON arrival, the patient is in a lot of pain and requesting relief immediately. Her cervix is 5 cm dilated. What is the most appropriate method of pain control for this patient?
a. Intramuscular morphine
b. Pudendal block
c. Local block   d. Epidural block

N22. True regarding hypertonic dysfunction of labor is:
a. M/C associated with occipitoposterior position
b. Oxytocin administration is beneficial with occipito pestonion position
c. Occurs in of 1st stage of labor
d. Leads to rapid dilatation of cervix

N23. CPD in absence of gross pelvic abnormality can be diagnosed by:
a. Ht of mother < 158 cms
b. Trial of labor
c. X-ray pelvimetry   d. Pelvic examination

N24. When fetus is in attitude of flexion, presentation is:
a. Vertex   b. Brow
c. Cephalic   d. Face

N25. Most important component of Bishop score:
a. Position   b. Dilatation
c. Station   d. Effacement

N26. A 25-year-old women whose antenatal period was uncomplicated is in labour. She has a single foetus in cephalic presentation. The head is not engaged. The foetal heart rate is 150 beats per minute. The cervical dilatation is 5 cm, the membranes are absent and the pelvis is adequate. It is decided to perform a caesarean section immediately.

Which one of the following findings is the most likely cause for this decision?
a. Approximation of the suture lines
b. Palpation of the anterior fontanelle and the sagittal suture
c. Palpation of the eyes, nose and mouth
d. Palpation of the frontal bones and the supraorbital ridges

N27. A woman undergoes induction of labour with amniotomy followed by an oxytocin infusion at a period of amenorrhoea of 41 weeks. Six hours later she is getting 4 contractions per 10 minutes and the foetal heart rate drops to 100 beats per minute.

What is the first step in the management?
a. Administer oxygen to the mother
b. Change the position of the mother
c. Perform a cardiotocograph
d. Stop the oxytocin infusion

N28. As per recent guidelines active phase of labor begins at
a. 3 cms   b. 4 cms
c. 5 cms   d. 6 cms

N29. Prolonged latent phase in a primigravida is
a. > 12 hrs   b. > 14 hrs
c. > 18 hrs   d. > 20 hrs

N30. Protractive active phase in nullipara is:
a. Dilatation < 1 cm/hr
b. Dilatation < 1.2 cm/hr
c. Dilatation < 1.5 cm/hr
d. Dilatation < 1.8 cm/hr

N31. Protracted active phase with respect to descent is:
a. Descent < 1 cm/hr in nullipara
b. Descent < 1 cm/hr in multipara
c. Descent < 2 cm/hr in nullipara
d. Descent < 3 cm/hr in multipara

N32. Not a contraindication for induction of labor:
a. Herpes infection   b. Heart disease
c. Cancer cervix   d. Hysterotomy scan

N33. Bishop score for inducing labor:
a. ≥ 3   b. ≥ 5
c. ≥ 6   d. ≥ 8

N34. Uterine tachysystole is:
a. More than 5 contraction in 5 minute period
b. More than 5 contraction in 10 minute period
c. More than 10 contraction in 5 minute period
d. More than 10 contraction in 10 minute period

N35. Dose of vaginal misoprost recommended by ACOG for induction of labor:
a. 25 mcg   b. 50 mcg
c. 75 mcg   d. 100 mcg

N36. Controlled ARM is done:
a. IUD   b. Maternal HIV infection
c. Polyhydramnios   d. Genital herpes

N37. False statement regarding Ferguson reflex:
a. Mechanical stretching of cervix enhances uterine activity
b. Not seen in humans
c. Release of oxytocin may be the cause
d. Associated with increased to levels of PGF-2α

N38. Moderate uterine contraction should last for:
a. 20-40 secs   b. < 10 secs
c. 10-20 secs   d. > 40 secs

N39. Phase 4 of parturition refers to:
a. 1 hour observation period after delivery of placenta
b. Puerperium
c. 3 stages of labor   d. Both a and b

N40. Uterotonic in parturition phase 3 include:
a. Oxytocin   b. CRH
c. Nitric oxide   d. hCG

N41. All are true regarding oxytocin except:
a. The number of oxytocin receptors increase in myometrium and decidual tissue near end of gestation
b. It plays a major role in phase 2 of parturition
c. It plays a major role in stage 2 of labor
d. Levels are elevated in phase 3 of parturition and in early puerperium

N42. Ripening of cervix occurs in:
a. Phase 1 of parturition
b. Phase 2 of parturition
c. Phase 3 of parturition
d. Phase 4 of parturition

N43. Phase 2 of parturition includes all except:
a. Cervical softening
b. Cervical ripening
c. Lightening
d. Formation of lower uterine segment from isthmus

Previous Year Questions

1. Cardinal movements of labour are:
[PGI 00, Dec. 00]
a. Engagement → descent → flexion → internal rotation → extension → restitution → external rotation → expulsion
b. Engagement → flexion → descent → internal rotation → extension → expulsion
c. Engagement → flexion → descent → external rotation → expulsion
d. Engagement → extension → internal rotation → external rotation → expulsion

2. Which cardinal movements occur during labour?
a. Flexion   b. Extension   [PGI June 08]
c. Internal rotation   d. Descent
e. Asynclitisms

3. Duration of latent phase of labour is affected by:
a. Early use of conduction anaesthesia and sedation
b. Unripe cervix   [PGI Dec 00]
c. Hypertonic uterine contraction
d. Pre-eclampsia

4. Prolong latent phase is/are seen in: [PGI May 2010]
a. Placenta praevia
b. Unripe cervix
c. Abruptio placentae
d. Excessive sedation
e. Early epidural analgesia

5. A female at 37 weeks of gestation has mild labour pains for 10 hours and cervix is persistently 1 cm dilated but non effaced. What will be the next appropriate management?   [AIIMS Nov 08]
a. Sedation and wait   b. Augmentation with oxytocin
c. Cesarean section   d. Amniotomy

6. 37 weeks primi with uterine contraction for 10 hours, cervix is 1 cm dilated and poorly effaced management is: [AI 2011]
a. Cesarean section   b. Amniotomy
c. Oxytocin drip   d. Sedation and wait

7. Commonest cause of nonengagement at term, in primi is: [PGI June 98]
a. CPD
b. Hydramnios
c. Brow presentation
d. Breech

8. True labour pain includes all except:
a. Painful uterine contraction   [PGI June 09]
b. Short vagina
c. Formation of the bag of waters
d. Progressive descent of presenting part
e. Cervical dilatation

9. Pain in early labor is limited to dermatomes:
a. $T_{10} - L_1$ b. $S_1 - S_3$ [AIIMS Nov 09]
c. $L_4 - L_5$ d. $L_2 - L_3$

10. Assessment of progress of labour is best done by:
a. Station of head   b. Rupture of membrane
c. Contraction of uterus   [PGI Dec 97]
d. Partogram

11. Mrs AR G3 P1LIA a full term pregnant female is admitted in labor. On examination, she has uterine contractions 2 in 10 minutes, lasting for 30-35 seconds.

On P/A examination 3/5th of the head is palpable per abdomen.

On P/V examination-cervix is 4 cm dilated, membranes intact.

On repeat examination 4 hours later, cervix is 5 cm dilated, station is unchanged, and cervicograph remains to the right of the alert line. Which of the following statements is true?   [AIIMS]
a. The head was engaged at the time of presentation
b. Her cervicographical progress is satisfactory
c. Her cervicographical status suggests intervention
d. On repeat examination, her cervicograph would have touched the action line

12. Induction at term is not done in: [AI 08]
a. Hypertension   b. DM
c. Heart disease   d. Renal disease

13. In bishop score all are included except: [AI 07]
a. Effacement of cervix
b. Dilatation of cervix
c. Station of head
d. Interspinal diameter

14. Bishop's score includes: [PGI Nov 07/PGI June 98]
a. Dilatation of cervix b. Effacement
c. Cervical softening d. Condition of os
e. Position of head

15. **All of the following are used for induction of labour, except:** [AIIMS May 04]
    a. PG F$_2$ α tablet
    b. PG E$_1$ tablet
    c. PG E$_2$ gel
    d. Misoprostol

16. **All of the following drugs are effective for cervical ripening during pregnancy except:** [AI 04]
    a. Prostaglandin E2
    b. Oxytocin
    c. Progesterone
    d. Misoprostol

17. **ARM is contraindicated in:** [PGI Dec 98]
    a. Placenta previa
    b. Hydramnios
    c. Accidental hemorrhage
    d. Twins

18. **Benefits of surgical induction (ARM) are all except:** [AI 06]
    a. Lowers the blood pressure in preeclampsia
    b. Relieves the maternal distress in hydramnios
    c. Decreases incidence of amnionitis
    d. Reduces the need of caesarean section

19. **All of the following are true about augmentation of labor except:** [AIIMS Nov 14]
    a. Twin pregnancy precludes the use of oxytocin
    b. Ammiotomy decreases the need for oxytocin use
    c. Methods of augmentation does not increase the risk of operational management
    d. Associated with a risk of uterine hyperstimulation

20. **Indication for induction of labour is:** [AIIMS Nov 05]
    a. Placenta previa
    b. PIH at term
    c. Heart disease at term
    d. Breech

21. **Best method of induction of labour in hydramnios:**
    a. High rupture of the membranes [AI 08]
    b. Low rupture of the membranes
    c. Abdominal amniocentesis followed by stabilising oxytocin drip
    d. Prostaglandins

22. **Which one of the following methods for induction of labour should not be used in patient with previous lower segment caesarean section?** [AIIMS May 07]
    a. Prostaglandin gel
    b. Prostaglandin tablet
    c. Stripping of the membrane
    d. Oxytocin drip

23. **Feature of false labor:** [PGI May 2015]
    a. Steady intensity of pain
    b. Cervical dilation
    c. Discomfort is in the back and abdomen
    d. Intervals remain long
    e. Discomfort usually is relieved by sedation

24. **The following graph represents the stages of labor. Which of the following statements is true about the graph C?** [AIIMS Nov 2016]

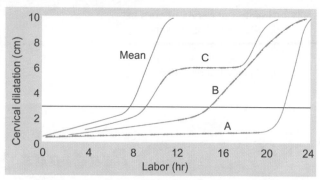

    a. Secondary arrest after progression of labor
    b. Prolonged active phase of labor
    c. Prolonged latent phase/primary arrest of labor
    d. Normal labor in a primigravida

25. **A 38 weeks primigravida presented to the labor room with minimal labor pains and contraction. On examination, the cervix is 2 cm dilated and 50% effaced. The heart rate of the patient is 86/min and blood pressure is 126/76 mm Hg. What should be done next?** [AIIMS Nov 2016]
    a. Induce labor by artificial rupture of membranes
    b. Give oxytocin to augment labor
    c. Sedate the patient by and give phenergan to decrease labor pains
    d. Observe the patient and wait for increase in uterine contractions

26. **All of the following are true regarding partogram except:** [AIIMS MAY 2016]
    a. Right side of alert line indicates referral to FRU
    b. There is 4 hours difference between action line and alert line
    c. Each small square in partograph equals to an hour
    d. Partograph is to be plotted once the cervical dilation reaches 4 cms

27. **A primigravida came to the labor room at 40 weeks + 5 days gestation for induction of labor. On per vaginal examination, the cervix is 1 cm dilated and 30% effaced. The vertex is at –1 station and the cervix is soft and posterior. What will be the modified bishop score for this lady?** [AIIMS May 2016]
    a. 0
    b. 3
    c. 5
    d. 8

28. **Mrs. S (G2 L1) presented to the hospital in labor pains. On examination she had 3 uterine contractions of 20 seconds in 10 minutes, cervical dilation 6 cm and HR 145 bpm. What is the stage of labor?**
    [AIIMS Nov 2017]
    a. Stage I
    b. Stage II
    c. Stage III
    d. Stage IV

29. **When a patient in labor presents to us for the first time, where on the partograph will we plot the cervical dilation.** [AIIMS Nov 2017]
    a. Left of alert line
    b. Between alert and action line

c. Right of action line
d. Right of alert line

30. **In the gynae labor room, the scissor shown in the diagram was used: Identify** [AIIMS Nov 2017]
   a. Episiotomy scissor b. Dissection scissor
   c. Stitch scissor   d. Mayo scissor

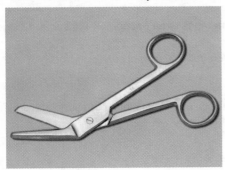

31. **According to WHO guidelines, which of the following is true about management of second stage of labor?**
   [AIIMS May 2017]
   a. Manual support of perineum to maintain continuous deflexion of head
   b. Episiotomy should be performed as a routine
   c. A warm cloth should be applied to the perineum to prevent trauma
   d. Delivery should be ideally performed in a lithotomy position

32. **A midwife at a PHC is monitoring pregnancy and maintaining the partograph of pregnancy progression. At how much cervical dilation should the partograph plotting be started?**
   [AIIMS May 2017]
   a. 2 cm   b. 8 cm
   c. 4 cm   d. 6 cm

Answers with Explanations to New Pattern Questions

N1.   Ans. is b, i.e. ACTH in fetus.   *Ref. Williams 24/e, p 108–109*

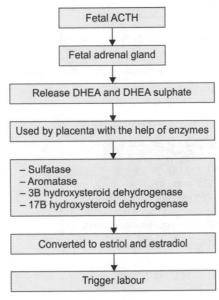

N2.   Ans. is a, i.e. Biparietal diameter
Engagement is said to occur when the largest transverse diameter of fetal head crosses the pelvic inlet.
Largest transverse diameter of fetal head is: Biparietal diameter.

N3.   Ans. is c, i.e. Crowning of fetal head
Crowning is a cardinal movement of labor, which occurs during second stage.

N4.   Ans. is d, i.e. Placenta previa
In placenta previa, in all cases IOL is not done in all cases, some are managed expectantly as discussed is chapter on APH

N5. **Ans. is a, i.e. 1.2 cm**

Labour is said to active when:

- Cervix is dilated to at least ≥ 6 cm.[Q]
- Regular uterine contractions are present.[Q]
- Rate of dilatation is at least 1.2 cm/hr[Q] for nulliparous and 1.5 cm/hr[Q] for parous women.

N6. **Ans. is b, i.e. After full dilatation of cervix**   *Ref. Dutta Obs. 7/e, p 130*

Membranes usually rupture after full dilatation of cervix or sometimes even beyond, in the second stage.

Early Rupture of Membranes:

- *Rupture of membranes any time after the onset of labour but before full dilatation of cervix.*

Premature Rupture of Membrane:

- *Rupture of membranes before the onset of labour.*
- Sometimes the membranes remain intact until completion of delivery, the fetus is then born surrounded by them and the portion covering the head of the newborn infant is known as the *Caul.*

N7. **Ans. is a, i.e. 4%**   *Ref. Dutta Obs. 7/e, p 113*

Expected date of delivery is calculated using Naegele's rule, i.e.

- EDD is 9 months + 7 days calculated from the 1st day of last menstrual period.
- This rulme is based on a normal 28 days cycle.
- In case of women with longer cycle additional number of days that the cycle extends beyond 28 days is added.

Based on the formula, labour starts approximately:

- On the expected date in 4% cases.
- One week on either side in 50% cases.
- 2 weeks earlier and 1 week later in 80% cases.

N8. **Ans. is a, i.e. Montevideo units**   *Ref. Williams Obs, 23/e, p 437*

1 montevideo unit = Intensity of constraction x number of contractions in 10 mins.

Montevideo unit is to define uterine activity.

As per this:

Clinical labour usually commences when uterine activity reaches values between 80–120 Montevideo units (This translates into approximate 3 contractions of 40 mm of Hg every 10 minutes).

During labour—Normal uterine contractions are between 190–300 Montevideo units

(At the time of delivery it is 300 Montevideo units)

N9. **Ans. is d, i.e. All of the above**

Intrauterine pressure during labor:

Stage	Pressure
• 1st	• 40–50 mm Hg
• 2nd	• 100–120 mm Hg
• 3rd	• 100–120 mm Hg

N10. **Ans. is b, i.e. Intensity of propogation is greatest at cervix**

Intensity is greatest at fundus of uterus.

See the text explanation.

N11. **Ans. is b, i.e. 1 cm/hour**   *Ref. Dutta Obs. 7/e, p 130*

See the text explanation.

N12. **Ans. is d, i.e. Resistance from the pelvic floor**   *Ref. Dutta Obs. 7/e, p 124*

Descent: Descent is a continuous process provided there is no undue bony or soft tissue obstruction. It is slow or insignificant in first stage but pronounced in second stage. It is completed with the expulsion of the fetus. In primigravidae, with prior engagement of the head, there is practically no descent in first stage; while in multiparae, descent starts with engagement. Head is expected to reach the pelvic floor by the time the cervix is fully dilated.

Factors facilitating descent are—(1) uterine contraction and retraction, (2) bearing down efforts and (3) straightening of the fetal ovoid specially after rupture of the membranes.

Note: Resistance offered by the pelvic floor promotes flexion of head and not descent.

N13. Ans. is d, i.e. Tone of the abdominal muscles *Ref. Dutta Obs. 7/e, p 125*

N14. Ans. is b, i.e. In majority rotation occurs in the pelvic floor

The prerequisites of anterior internal rotation of the head are well-flexed head, efficient uterine contraction, favourable shape at the midpelvic plane and tone of the levator ani muscles.

The level at which internal rotation occurs is variable. Rotation in the cervix although favorable occurs less frequently. In majority of cases, rotation occurs at the pelvic floor. Internal rotation occurs earlier in multipara than primipara Rarely, it occurs as late as crowning of the head.

N15. Ans. is b, i.e. Timely episiotomy as a routine *Ref. Williams Obs. 23/e, p 395 and Dutta Obs. 7/e, p 137*

Now if you have ever been to labor ward and assisted or even seen a normal delivery, you know all the options given in the question are done to prevent perineal laceration.

The controversy lies in option, b i.e. whether routine episiotomy should be performed: Well read for yourself what williams has to say on this issue.

"There once was considerable controversy concerning whether an episiotomy should be cut routinely. It is now clear that an episiotomy will increase the risk of a tear into the external anal sphincter or the rectum or both. Conversely, anterior tears involving the urethra and labia are more common in women in whom an episiotomy is not cut. Most, advocate individualization and do not routinely perform episiotomy." —Williams Obs 23/e, p 395

Hence option b is incorrect.

> **Steps done for prevention of perineal laceration (Ref. Dutta Obs 7/e p 125):** More attention should be paid not to the perineum but to the controlled delivery of the head.
> - Delivery by early extension is to be avoided. Flexion of the sub-occiput comes under the symphysis pubis so that lesser suboccipitofrontal 10 cm (4") diameter emerges out of the introitus.
> - Spontaneous forcible delivery of the head is to be avoided by assuring the patient not to bear down during contractions.
> - To deliver the head in between contractions.
> - To perform timely episiotomy (when indicated not routine).
> - To take care during delivery of the shoulders as the wider bisacromial diameter (12 cm) emerges out of the introitus.

N16. Ans. is d, i.e. For delivery of head in normal labour *Ref. Dutta Obs. 4/e, p 137; Williams 23/e, p 395*

Ritgen (Ritzen) maneuver is done for delivery of head in normal labour to allow controlled delivery of the head.

When the head distends the vulva and perineum enough to open the vaginal introitus to a diameter of 5 cm of more, a towel-draped, gloved hand may be used to exert forward pressure on the chin of the fetus through the perineum just in front of the coccyx. Concurrently, the other hand exerts pressure superiorly against the occiput.

This maneuver allows controlled delivery of the head. It also favors neck extension so that the head is delivered with its smallest diameters passing through the introitus and over the perineum.

N17. Ans. is a, i.e. 10 mm of Hg *Ref Williams 24/e, p 498*

- Uterine contractions are palpable when intensity exceeds 10 mm of Hg.
- Uterine contractions become painful when intensity exceeds 15 mm of Hg.
- Minimum intrauterine pressure required for cervical dilatation = 15 mm of Hg.
- Intrauterine pressure at which uterus becomes so hard that it cannot be indented by figure – 40 mm of Hg.
- Uterine contractions are called adequate when they generate an IUP of 200–220 Montevideo units.

N18. Ans. is e, i.e. None of the above *Ref. High Risk Pregnancy Fernando Arias 4/e, p 338*

Factors affecting progress of labor:
- **Parity of female:** In multiparous females progress of labor is fast.
- **CPD:** If CPD is present, progress of labor is slow.
- **BMI:** In obese females, progress of labor is slow.
- **Gestation at age:** Increasing gestational age also shows progress of labor.
- **Fetal sex:** Male gender is associated with statistically longer active first stage.
- **Twin pregnancy:** Is also associated with slower progress of labor.

N19. Ans. is c, i.e. S2,3,4

Ref. Dutta Obs 7/e, p 518

- Pudendal nerve arises from: $S_{2,3,4}$ roots
- Pudendal block will block these roots

N20. Ans. is c, i.e. Relieves pain from the lower third of Vagina and episiotomy can be performed

Ref Dutta Obs 7/e, p 517-518 and William 23/e, p 450

- Paracervical block relieves pain from upper third of Vagina, not lower third.

N21. Ans. is d, i.e. Epidural block

Ref. Williams 24/e, p 513

When complete relief of pain is needed throughout labor, epidural analgesia is safest and simplest.

N22. Ans. is a, i.e. M/C associated with occipitoposterior position

Ref. Fernando Arias 4/e, p 33

Hypertonic uterine dysfunction:

Labor Dysfunction:

Can be described as Hypotonic or Hypertonic

Hypertonic uterine dysfunction:

- It is rare spontaneous event (occuring in I in 3000 labors)
- M/C associated with **late active phase dysfunction (not latent phase).** In active phase also- it occurs during late phase, i.e when cervix is almost 7 cm dilated.
- The labor curve shows a decelerative or arrest pattern from 7 cm to 10 cm.
- M/C cause (in 30 % cases) is occipitoposterior position.
- M/C in Nulliparous females.
- Hypertonic uterine dysfunction means- the uterine contractions are incoordinated and increased in frequency (4–5 per 10 minutes) without a rest period in between. The baseline tone is also increased.
- Since the M/C cause is OP position, hence wait and watch policy should be adopted.
- Attention should be paid towards maternal hydration status.
- Oxytoin infusion can be considered but it can lead to hyperstimulation/tachysystole.

Hypotonic dysfunction:

- Refers to the presence of inadequate uterine contractions.
- It is also seen in active phase- but early active phase, i.e poor progress is seen between 4 to 7 cm dilatation
- M/C in Nulliparous females.

N23. Ans. is b, i.e. Trial of labor

Best method to rule out CPD is Trial of labor.
Best investigation is MRI.

N24. Ans. is c, i.e. Cephalic

Read the question carefully—they are asking presentation, hence answer will be cephalic. If they would have asked presenting part then answer would be vertex.

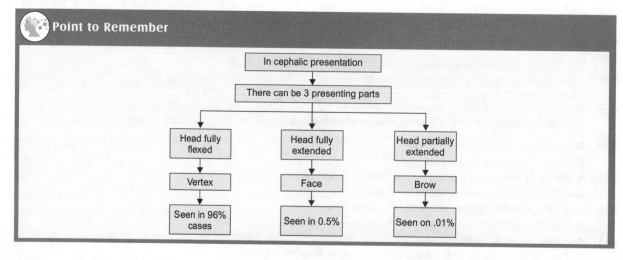

N25. Ans. is b, i.e. Dilatation

The most important component of Bishop score is dilatation of **cervix**.

N26. Ans. is d, i.e. Palpation of the frontal bones and the supraorbital ridges

Part palpated	Presenting part
• Anterior fontanelle, sagittal suture and posterior fontanelle	• Vertex
• Anterior fontanelle, frontal bone, sagittal suture, supraorbital ridges or root of nose	• Brow
• Supraorbital ridges, Eyes, nose, mouth and chin	• Face

Amongst these presenting parts:

It is absolutely essential to do cesarean section in Brow because in brow, engaging diameter is Mentovertical diameter (14 cms), which cannot pass through cervix.

Hence in Brow always cesarean is done. Thus during labor if obstetrician palpates, supraorbital ridges and frontal bone she should understand, it is brow presentation and take patient for cesarean immediately.

N27. Ans. is d, i.e. Stop the oxytocin infusion

The first step in the management is to stop the oxytocin drip, as this may reverse the foetal bradycardia, which may be due to excessive uterine contractions caused by oxytocin. (Note this patient is having 4 uterine contractions in 10 minutes) Next oxygen is administered to the mother and a cardiotocograph is performed. The position of the mother should be changed to relieve cord compression if present. Vaginal examination is done to determine the stage of labour in order to decide the mode of delivery, if foetal distress persists after the initial treatment.

N28. Ans. is d, i.e. 6 cm

See text for explanation

N29. Ans. is d, i.e. > 20 hours

See text for explanation

N30. Ans. is b, i.e. Dilatation < 1.2 cm/hr

See text for explanation

N31. Ans. is a, i.e. Descent < 1 cm/hour in nullipara

See text for explanation

N32. Ans. is b, i.e. Heart disease

See text for explanation

N33. Ans. is d, i.e. ≥ 8

See text for explanation

N34. Ans. is b, i.e. More than 5 contraction in 10 minute period

See text for explanation

N35. Ans. is a, i.e. 25 mcg

See text for explanation

N36. Ans. is c, i.e. Polyhydramnios:

In case of polyhydramnios to prevent abruptio from sudden rupturing of membranes, controlled ARM is done.

N37. Ans. is b, i.e. Not seen in humans

See text for explanation

N38. Ans. is a, i.e. 20–40 seconds

See text for explanation

N39. Ans. is d, i.e. Both a and b

See text for explanation

N40. Ans. is a, i.e. Oxytocin

See text for explanation

N41. Ans. is b, i.e. It plays a major role in phase 2 of parturition

See text for explanation

N42. Ans. is b, i.e. Phase 2 of parturition

See text for explanation

N43. Ans. is a, i.e. Cervical softening

Answers with Explanations to Previous Year Questions

1. **Ans. is a, i.e. Engagement → descent → flexion → internal rotation → extension → restitution → external rotation → expulsion**

2. **Ans. is a, b, c, d and e, i.e. Flexion, Extension, Internal rotation, Descent and Asynclitism** *Ref. Dutta Obs. 7/e, p 128*

   Series of events that take place in the genital organs in an effort to expel the viable products of conception out of the womb through the vagina into the outer world is called as *Labour.*

   Mechanism of normal labour is defined as the manner in which the fetus adjusts itself to pass through the parturient canal with minimal difficulty.

   There are 8 cardinal movements of the head in normal labour.

   - **Every** – Engagement (Synclitic or Asynclitic)
   - **Decent** – Descent
   - **Female** – Flexion
   - **I** – Internal rotation
   - **Choose to** – Crowning
   - **Employ** – Extension
   - **Rises** – Restitution
   - **Extremely** – External rotation

    Mnemonic

   Every Decent Female I Choose to and Employ Rises Extremely.

    Also Know: **Other questions asked on cardinal movements:**
   - Most common presentation – cephalic (95%).
   - Most common presenting part – vertex.
   - In normal labour, the head enters the pelvis more commonly through the transverse diameter[Q] (75% cases) or oblique diameters (20% cases) (IInd most common) and AP diameter (5% cases) at the onset of labour[Q].
   - The most common position *(i.e. relation of occiput to quadrant of pelvis)* is left occipito-transverse[Q] followed by Left occipito anterior position (Ref Williams Obs. 23/e p 378).
   - The engaging diameter of head is Suboccipito bregmatic diameter (9.5 cm) or[Q]
     In slight deflexion is Sub occipito frontal (10 cm).[Q]
   - Internal rotation of fetal head occurs the level of ischial spine.
   - In a vertex delivery the babys head is delivered by extension, whereas in breech it is born by flexion.
   - Best time for giving episiotomy is after crowning has occured.

3. **Ans. is a and b, i.e. Early use of conduction anaesthesia and sedation; and Unripe cervix**

4. **Ans. is b, d and e, i.e. Unripe cervix, Excessive sedation and Early epidural analgesia**
   Ref. Fernando Arias 3/e, p 376; Williams Obs. 24/e, p 446, 23/e, p 386-388

   Read the text for explanation.

5. **Ans. is a, i.e. Sedation and wait** *Ref. Fernando Arias 3/e, p 376*

6. **Ans. is d, i.e. Sedation and wait** *Ref. Fernando Arias 3/e, p 376*
   - The patient is presenting at 37 weeks with mild labor pains for 10 hours. Cervix is 1 cms dilated and is not effaced. Now this can either be a case of false labor pains or it can be prolonged latent phase of labor.

   False labor can be differentiated from latent phase of labor by therapetuic rest, i.e. patient is sedated with morphine.

Patient in false labor	Patient in latent phase
↓	↓
Sleeps for a few hours and wakes-up without contractions	Continues contracting and show cervical changes following the rest

So the correct option is Sedate and Wait.

7. **Ans. is a, i.e. CPD**　　　　　　　　　　　　　　　　　　　*Ref. Dutta Obs. 7/e, p 81, 82, 352*

- ***Engagement is said to occur when the greatest transverse diameter of the presenting part, has passed through the pelvic inlet. In all cephalic presentations, the greatest transverse diameter is always the biparietal.***
- Engagement occurs in multipara with commencement of labour[Q] in the late Ist stage after rupture of membranes and in Nullipara during the last few weeks of pregnancy, i.e. ≈ 38 weeks
- In primi's the *most common* cause of non engagement at term is deflexed head or occipitoposterior position followed by cephalopelvic disproportion (CPD).[Q]
- Since deflexed head or occipitoposterior is not given in option, we will go for CPD as the answer.

8. **Ans. is b, i.e. Short vagina**　　　　　　　　　　　　　　　　*Ref. Dutta Obs. 7/e, p 117*

Differences between true and false labour pains.

Features	True labour pains	False labour pains
Cervical changes (dilatation & effacement)	Present	Absent
Frequency and duration of contractions	Regular and gradually increase	Irregular
Pain	Lower abdomen and back, radiating to thighs	Lower abdomen only
Bag of water	Formed	Not formed
Show	Present	Absent
Relief with enema/sedation	No	No

9. **Ans. is a, i.e. $T_{10} - L_1$**　　　　　　　　　　　　　　　　*Ref: Dutta Obs 7/e, p 117*

In the early stages of labour pain is mainly uterine in origin because of painful uterine contraction

"The pain of uterine contractions is distributed along the cutaneous nerve distribution of T_{10} to L_1

Ref. Dutta Obs, 6/e, p 118

In later stages pain is due to dilatation of the cervix.

"The pain of cervical dilatation and stretching is referred to the back through sacral plexus."

Ref. Dutta Obs, 6/e, p 118

10. **Ans. is d, i.e. Partogram**　　　　*Ref. Dutta Obs. 7/e, p 530, Williams Obs. 23/e, p 406*

Partogram is the best method to assess progress of labour.

11. **Ans. is d, i.e. On repeat examination, her cervicograph would have touched the action line**　　*Ref: Read below*

In this patient at the beginning of the labor, three fifths of the head was palpable , which indicates head is not engaged as head is said to be engaged only if 1/5th is palpable per abdomen.

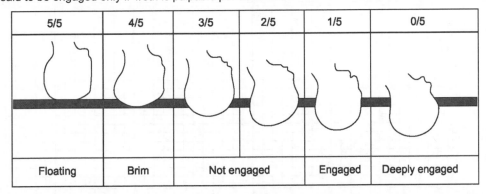

5/5	4/5	3/5	2/5	1/5	0/5
Floating	Brim	Not engaged	Engaged	Deeply engaged	

Crichton's method of assessing fetal head descent in fifths by abdominal palpation

Progressive descent of the fetal head can be assessed abdominally by estimating the number of "fifths " of the head above the pelvic brim(Crichton method): When one/fifth above, only the sinciput can be felt abdominally and head is said to be engaged and noughtfifths represents a head entirely in the pelvis with no poles felt abdominally.

- Now in this female lets draw the partograph-remember in partograph on Y-axis, dilatation of cervix and descent of fetal head are noted and on X-axis time is noted in hours. If we measure only cervical dilatation, the term cervicograph can be used instead, thus both the terms mean approximately the same (for example if you see the partogram drawn in Dutta 7/e, p 403..they have used the term cervicograph instead of partograph...so don't get confused.)

- Another important thing to remember is –we use modified partogram proposed by WHO for all purposes and not any other partogram.

- **Now lets draw the partograph related to this patient**

- Mrs AR is coming to us with dilatation of cervix 4 cm i.e. she comes in active phase-so directly I am plotting her dilatation on the alert line now 4 hours later her dilatation is 5 cm, so next I have plotted that.

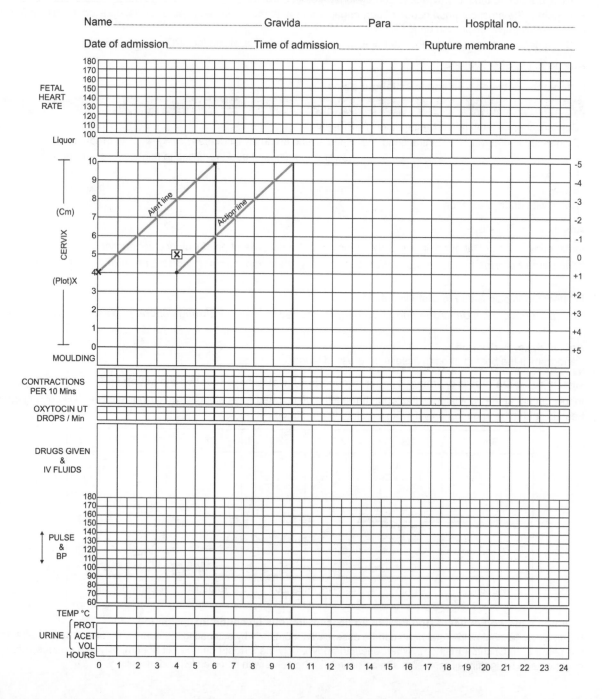

- As you can see from the graph Mrs AR progress is unsatisfactory as it lies towards the right of alert line, so the obstetrician should get alerted that some intervention may be needed. (Not immediately needed) & on repeat examination her cervicograph would touch action line.

12. Ans. is None
Ref. John Hopkins Manual of Obs and Gynae 4/e, p 77; COGDT 10/e, p 209, 210; Dutta Obs. 7/e, p 522; Williams 24/e, p 523

I have already discussed in text, contradictions of induction of labour.

As far as Heart disease is concerned:

It is no more taken as a contraindication for induction of labour:

Heart disease-"induction is generally safe" *—Williams Obs. 23/e, p 962*

This is an older question where heart disease was taken a contraindication for IOL but nowadays it is not, so our answer is none.

13. Ans. is d, i.e. Interspinal diameter

14. Ans. is a, b, c and e, i.e. Dilatation of cervix; Effacement; Cervical softening; and Position of head
Ref. Williams Obs. 22/e, p 537; 23/e, p 502; COGDT 10/e, p 209; Dutta Obs. 7/e, p 523

Bishop score is a quantitative method for prediction of successful induction of labour.

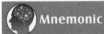 **Mnemonic**

It includes the following parameters:
D = Cervical **D**ilatation (**most important parameter**)
P = Cervical **P**osition
E = Cervical **E**ffacement
S = Head **S**tation
C = Cervical **C**onsistency
Mnemonic: **D**elhi **P**olice **E**mployed **S**pecial **C**ommandos.

 Note: In modified Bishop score cervical effacement has been replaced by dilatation of cervix.

15. Ans. is a, i.e. PGF$_2\alpha$ tablet

16. Ans. is c, i.e. Progesterone *Ref. Dutta Obs. 7/e, p 524; Fernando Arias 3/e, p 284-286; Williams Obs. 24/e, p 525*

Ripening of cervix is changing the cervical matrix from sol to gel state by dissolving the collagen bundles. Ultimately the cervix becomes soft.

Techniques for cervical ripening: *Ref. Williams Obs. 24/e, p 525*

Pharmacological method	Nonpharmacological method

• Prostaglandin
  – *Dinoprostone gel (PGE$_2$)* - it is the gold standard for cervical ripening
  – Misoprostol (PGE1) tablet - vaginal or oral
• Steroid receptor antagonist
  – Mifepristone
  – Onapristone
• Relaxin
• Glyceryl trinitrate, isosorbide mononitrate
• Oxytocin
	• Stripping the membrane
	• Mechanical dilators:
	  – Osmotic dilators
	  – Balloon catheter/Transcervical catheter placed through internal os
	• Extra-amniotic saline infusion
	Ref. Dutta Obs. 7/e, p 524

Prostaglandins are very useful both for ripening of cervix and for induction of labour.

 Important points on prostaglandins:
- The gold standard agent for cervical ripening is *PGE$_2$* i.e dinoprost gel
- The gold standard agent for inducing labour is *PGE$_2$*

Contd...

Contd...

> - The analogue of prostaglandin recently approved by ACOG for cervical ripening-*PGE$_1$* (misoprost)
> - The analogue of prostaglandin which is contraindicated in scarred uterus and should not be used in previous LSCS patients-*PGE$_1$*
> - The analogue of prostaglandin which is not used for inducing labour-*PGF-2 alpha*
> - The analogue of prostaglandin which is used in PPH-*PGF-2 alpha*

17. Ans. is b, i.e. Hydramnios *Ref. Dutta Obs 7/e, p 525*

18. Ans. is c, i.e. Decreases incidence of amnionitis *Ref. Dutta Obs. 9/e, p 487-488*

- ARM is a method for inducing and augmenting labour.
- It involves rupturing the membranes overlying the cervix using a Kocher's forcep[Q].
- It is applicable when cervix is partially dilated and bischop score is high.

Advantages:
- Promotes labour by stimulating release of endogenous prostaglandins.
- Encourages application of the fetal head to the cervix.
- Colour of the liquor can be observed and meconium staining ruled out.
- Permits the use of fetal scalp electrode for intrapartum fetal surveillance.

Disadvantages:
- If performed before the presenting part is well fixed, so it can lead to cord prolapse.
- ARM can lead to-infection if frequent vaginal examinations are performed.
- It can cause abruption in case of polyhydramnios.
- Rarely it can lead to liquor amni embolism

Contraindications:

• Intrauterine fetal death[Q]	• Maternal AIDS
• Genital active herpes infection	• Chronic hydramnios[Q] (In chronic hydrominos controlled ARM is done and not just simple ARM — as sudden decompression can lead to abruptioplacentae)

> *Also Know:*
> - ARM and stripping of membranes are different. Stripping of Membranes is the digital separation of membranes from the wall of the cervix and lower uterine segment.
> - Immediately after ARM fetal heart sounds should be auscultated.
> - Transient changes in the fetal heart rate, can occur due to resettlement of the cord after the liquor flows out.
> - Early and variable deceleration[Q] of fetal heart rate is relatively common with amniotomy.

19. Ans. is a, i.e. Twin pregnancy precludes the use of oxytocin *Ref. Williams 24/e, p 530-532*

Lets analyse each option:

Option b: Amniotomy decreases the need for oxytocin use

"Route and associates found that amniotomy with oxytocin augmentation for arrested active-phase labor shortened the time to delivery by 44 minutes compared with that of oxytocin alone". —*Williams 24/e, p 532*

Thus option b is correct.

Option c: Methods of augmentation does not increase the risk of operational management.

"Amniotomy does not alter the route of delivery" —*Williams 24/e, p 532*

Thus option c is correct.

Option d: Assiciated with risk of uterine hyperstimulation.

Dutta 7/e, p499: Clearly mentions-uterine hyperstimulation is an observed side effect of oxytocin, i.e. option d is correct

Thus by exclusion our answer is 'a', i.e.

Twin pregnancy precludes the use of oxytocin

This is incorrect as proved by the following lines of williams

In twin pregnancy

"Provided women with twins meet all criteria for oxytocin administration, it may be used" —*Williams 24/e, p 916*

20. Ans. is b, i.e. PIH at term

Ref. Dutta Obs. 7/e, p 522; COGDT 10/e, p 209, John Hopkins Manual of Obs and Gynae 4/e, p 77.

Indications of Induction of Labour

Williams 24/e, p 523

Maternal	Fetal
• Preeclampsia/eclampsia	• Intrauterine fetal death
• Maternal medical complications like	• IUGR
– Diabetes mellitus	• Prolonged pregnancy
– Chronic renal disease	• Rh incompatibility
• Abruptio placenta	• Lethal malformation
• Premature rupture of membrane	• Unstable lie after correction into longitudinal lie (versions)
• Chorioamnionitis	• Fetus with major congenital anomaly
• Chronic hydramnios/Oligohydromnios	• Nonreassuring fetal status

Note:

- Major degree of placenta previa is a contraindication for IOL.
- We are not taking heart disease as our answer because although induction of labour is not contraindicated in it but then it is not an indication also. No where it is given that heart disease is an indication for induction of labour, everywhere it is mentioned that IOL is safe or can be done.

21. Ans. is c, i.e. Abdominal amniocentesis followed by stabilising oxytocin drip   *Ref. Dutta Obs 7/e, p 215*

Artificial rupture of membranes is C/I in polyhydramnios as it leads to sudden decompression of uterus which can cause abruptio placenta.

Method of induction in these patients is:

Amniocentesis → drainage of good amount of liquor → to check the favorable lie and presentation of the fetus → a stabilising oxytocin infusion is started → low rupture of the membranes is done when the lie becomes stable and the presenting part gets fixed to the pelvis. This will minimize sudden decompression with separation of the placenta, change in lie of the fetus and cord prolapse.

22. Ans. is b, i.e. Prostaglandin tablet   *Ref. Dutta Obs. 7/e, p 524; Fernando Arias 3/e, p 286*

Prostglandin tablet is misoprostol (PGE$_1$) which is contraindicated in women with previous cesarean births.

Misoprostol

It is an analogue of Prostaglandin E$_1$.

Indications:

- Medical abortion in the first trimester of pregnancy.
- Evacuation of uterus in case of anembryonic pregnancies or early fetal demise.
- Ripening of cervix prior to second trimester abortions.
- Ripening of cervix and induction of labour in term pregnancies.
- For treatment and prevention of postpartum bleeding.

Pharmakokinetics:

- It is available in tablet form.
- Metabolized in liver.

Complication:

Nausea, vomiting, diarrhea.

- Uterine hyperstimulation.
- Tachysystole
- Meconium passage
- Possibly uterine rupture

Contraindication:

- Women with previous uterine surgery particularly cesarean section.

23. **Ans. is a, d and e, i.e Steady intensity of pain, Intervals remain long and Discomfort usually is relieved by sedation**

Ref. Dutta 7/e, p 117

False labor pains are either constant or irregular. They do not have regular, rhythmic character seen in True labor pains, (i.e. option a is correct).

The interval between contractions or pain progressively decreases in true labor pains whereas it remains long and constant in false labor, (i.e. option d is correct).

False labor pain do not lead to cervical dilatation and does not radiate to back, (i.e. options b and c are incorrect)

False labor pains are relieved by sedation or enema, (i.e. option e is correct).

24. **Ans. is a, i.e. Secondary arrest after progression of labor**

Now friends—first you should know how to read this graph.

If you see their is a horizontal line shown which corresponds to 3 cms, i.e. in this graph-active phase is beginning at 3 cms. In the graph line marked as '**mean**'—means normal graph.

In the graph marked as mean, the patient is reaching 3 cms at 8 hrs, i.e. latent phase ends at 8 hrs and active phase begins. Now in active phase minimum dilatation should be 1 cm/hr i.e. from 3 cms to 10 cms it should take maximum 7 hrs, i.e. 8 + 7 = 15 hrs. Now if you see the patient reached 10 cms (full dilatation) well within the time i.e. at 12 hrs. Now keeping this mind let's analyze:

Graph A

In graph A—patient is reaching 3 cms i.e. active phase at 20 hrs or more, which means latent phase is prolonged. As prolonged latent phase in:

- Nulliparous = 20 hrs
- Multiparous = 14 hrs

So graph A shows prolonged latent phase

Graph B

Latent phase (i.e. uptil 3 cms dilatation) occurred at 14 hrs. Then from 3 cms to 10 cms the patient is taking around 10 hours (14 to 24 hrs) whereas this 7 cms of dilation should have been completed in maximum 7 hours @ 1 cm/hr. This means here active phase is getting prolonged.

Graph C

The latent phase ended at 8 hours. Then the patient dilated till 6 cms @ 10–11 hours.

Now from 11 to 16 hours she is 6 cms dilated, i.e. 4 hours have passed and still there is no dilatation. Now since nothing has been mentioned about membranes, I am assuming they are ruptured.

So it is a case of active phase arrest i.e. secondary arrest after progression of labor.

25. **Ans. is d, i.e. Observe the patient and want for increase in uterine contractions**

This patient is a primi@38 weeks with dilatation of cervix 2 cms and 50% effaced. So the patient may be in latent phase (D/D is false labor pains). Now to differentiate between latent phase and false labor pains sedation could be given but the option says give phenergan. Use of phenergan is not recommended these days during labor as it leads to neonatal respiratory depression.

Phenergan can be detected in cord blood within 1.5 minutes of administration and equilibrates with maternal blood within 15 minutes hence the best answer is observe the patient.

26. **Ans. is c, i.e. Each small square in partograph represents an hour.**

As discussed and shown in Fig. 9.4A each small square represents 30 mins and not an hour. Rest all options are correct.

27. **Ans. is c, i.e. 5**

Ref: Williams 24/e p 525-526; Dutta 7/e p 722

Cervical Station: –1 means score of 2; Cervical Dilatation: 1 cm means score of 1; Effacement: 30% means score of 0; Cervix Position: Posterior means 0 as score; Consistency: Soft means score is 2. Hence, Bishop Score becomes 5.

Bishop Scoring System Used for Assessment of Inducibility					
			Cervical Factor		
Score	Dilatation (cm)	Effacement (%)	Station (–3 to +2)	Consistency	Position
0	Closed	0–30	–3	Firm	Posterior
1	1–2	40–50	–2	Medium	Midposition
2	3–4	60–70	–1	Soft	Anterior
3	≥ 5	≥ 80	+1, +2	–	–

28. Ans. is a, i.e. Stage I

As discussed in chapter 7 of the book, first stage of labor is from the time when a female starts perceiving true labor pains and uptil 10 cm of dilatation.

29. Ans. is a, i.e. Left of alert line

In a partograph the patients labor should be represented to the left of alert line as discussed in Chapter 9

30. Ans. is a, i.e. Episiotomy scissor

Mayo scissor:

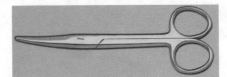

Mayo scissors have semi-blunt ends, a feature that distinguishes them from most other surgical scissors.

Straight-bladed Mayo scissors are designed for cutting body tissues near the surface of a wound. As straight-bladed Mayo scissors are also used for cutting sutures, they are also referred to as "suture scissors".

Curved-bladed Mayo scissors allow deeper penetration into the wound than the type with straight blades. The curved style of

Mayo scissor is used to cut thick tissues such as those found in the uterus, muscles, breast, and foot. Mayo scissors used for dissection are placed in tissue with the tips closed.

Episiotomy scissors

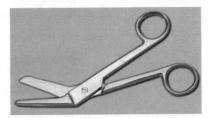

It is bent on the edge. The blade with the blunt tip goes inside the vagina

31. Ans. is a, i.e. Manual support of perineum to maintain continuous deflexion of head

Friends WHO does not recommend universal episiotomy for second stage of labor but it recommends giving support to the perineum (Ritgen maneuver) while delivering the head of the fetus.

"*Conduct the delivery with support for the perineum to avoid tears, and use of episiotomy only where a tear is very likely*." WHO guideline.

Also know- Ritgen maneuver

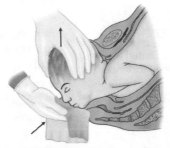

Ritgen maneuver is an obstetric procedure used to control delivery of the fetal head. It involves applying upward pressure from the coccygeal region to extend the head during actual delivery, thereby protecting the musculature of the perineum. In Ritgen maneuver the fetal chin is reached for between the anus and coccyx and pulled interiorly, while using the fingers of the other hand on the fetal occiput to control speed of delivery. The Ritgen maneuver is called modified (Jönsson 2008) when performed during a contraction, rather than between contractions as originally recommended.

32. Ans. is c, i.e. 4 cm

In Modified WHO partograph –latent phase is absent and plotting begins at 4 cm of dilatation of cervix.

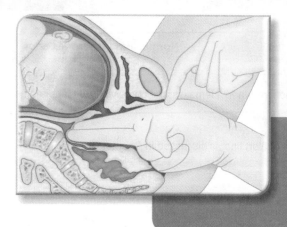

Chapter 10

Third Stage of Labor and its Complications

Chapter at a Glance

- ➢ Third Stage of Labor
- ➢ Active Management of Third Stage of Labor
- ➢ Complications of Third Stage of Labor
- ➢ Postpartum Hemorrhage
- ➢ Atonic PPH Management
- ➢ Management of Traumatic PPH

- • Vaginal and Vulval Hematoma
- • Perineal Tears
- • Retained Placenta
- • Morbidly Adherent Placenta
- ➢ Uterine Inversion
- ➢ Amniotic Fluid Embolism

THIRD STAGE OF LABOR

- • As discussed in the previous chapter, it is concerned with the expulsion of placenta, after the expulsion of baby.
- • Average time taken = (15–20 minutes).
- • With active management of third stage of labor (AMTSL) Time taken = 5 mins.
- • If time taken is more than 30 minutes—it is called as **Prolonged 3rd stage of labor on Retained placenta.**

Key Concept

- • In AMTSL, placental separation is actively facilitated and uterine contraction are initiated to reduce the incidence of third stage complications (like PPH)
- • In AMTSL—Duration of third stage reduced (to 5 minutes)
⇓
Less bleeding
⇓
Less chances of PPH
⇓
Less maternal mortality
Hence active management of Third Stage of labor is preferred these days.

Signs of Placental Separation (Table 10.1)

Table 10.1:

Per abdomen	Per vaginal
• Uterus becomes globular, firm and ballottable **(earliest sign to appear)**	• Sudden gush of blood
	• Permanent lengthening of cord
• Fundal height is slightly raised as the separated placenta comes down in lower segment and uterus rests over it **(Schroeder's sign)**	
• Slight suprapubic bulging may be seen due to separated placenta distending the lower segment	
• On pushing the uterus cephalad with a hand on the abdomen, the cord no longer recedes **(Kustner's sign)**	

Methods of Placental Separation (Figs. 10.1A and B)

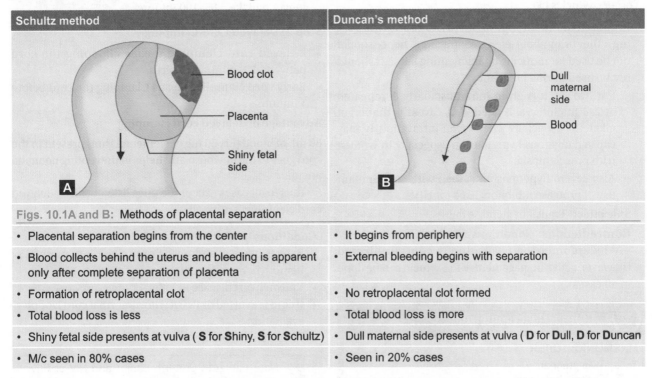

Figs. 10.1A and B: Methods of placental separation

Schultz method	Duncan's method
• Placental separation begins from the center	• It begins from periphery
• Blood collects behind the uterus and bleeding is apparent only after complete separation of placenta	• External bleeding begins with separation
• Formation of retroplacental clot	• No retroplacental clot formed
• Total blood loss is less	• Total blood loss is more
• Shiny fetal side presents at vulva (**S** for **S**hiny, **S** for **S**chultz)	• Dull maternal side presents at vulva (**D** for **D**ull, **D** for **D**uncan
• M/c seen in 80% cases	• Seen in 20% cases

Note: Separation of placenta is along decidua spongiosum (intermediate spongy layer of the decidua basalis).

Average Blood Loss during Deliveries

- After vaginal delivery: 500 mL
- After cesarean section: 1000 mL
- After twin vaginal delivery: 1000 mL
- After cesarean hysterectomy: 1500 mL

ACTIVE MANAGEMENT OF THIRD STAGE OF LABOR

Components of Active Management of Third Stage of Labor (AMTSL)

1. Use of oxytocic after the birth of baby
2. Delayed cord clamping (≥ 1–3 minutes)
3. Delivery of placenta by controlled cord traction
4. Intermittent uterine tone assessment (Note: Uterine massage is no longer a part of AMTSL as per the latest guidelines of WHO).

Details of Each Component of AMTSL

Step 1: Use of Oxytocics

- *Oxytocin:* It is **the preferred drug and the drug recommended by WHO** for preventing PPH.

  Dose = 10 units IM or IV infusion

Route	Onset of action	Duration of action
I/M Bolus	Within 3 mins	3 hours
I/V infusion	Immediate	1 hour

Note: Oxytocin should not be given as IV bolus due to risk of marked transient fall in BP, abrupt increase in cardiac output, myocardial ischemia and chest pain.

- Oxytocin is synthesized in the paraventricular nucleus of hypothalamus
- It is nonapeptide
- Synthetic oxytocin is octapeptide
- Half life = 3–5 minutes
- Oxytocin loses its effectiveness unless it is stored at 2°–8° C
- At room temperature its shelf life is 3 months
- It is the **hormone responsible for milk ejection**
- It increases uterine contractions physiologically and law of polarity is maintained hence it is used for inducing labor and augmenting labor also.

If oxytocin is not available then WHO recommends use of other oxytocics like:

i. **Ergometrine (0.25 mg) or methylergometrine (0.2 mg):** They bring about tetanic contractions, hence should not be used for inducing or augmenting labor. It should not be used during pregnancy.
   – For AMTSL it is given intramuscularly & repeated at 2–4 hrs interval if needed. A caveat is that ergot alkaloids especially when given intravenously may cause dangerous hypertension especially in women with preeclampsia.
   – Also severe hypertension is seen with concomitant use of protease inhibitors used for HIV.

   Side effect: Transient increase in BP.

   Contradictions: Conditions in which ergometrine/ methylergometrine is absolutely contraindicated (however, active management with oxytocin can be done in all cases).

 C/I for methylergometrine

MNEMONIC: TOPER

T	:	Twin pregnancy
O	:	Organic heart disease
P	:	Preeclampsia
E	:	Eclampsia
R	:	Rh negative female

ii. **Inj PGF-2α (Carboprost, Hembate): Dose 250 mcg I/M.** It is contraindicated **in bronchial asthma patients.** It acts mainly on myometrium of uterus hence used in AMTSL and in PPH but not in inducing labor.

iii. **PGE1-misoprostol:** Available as tablet. WHO recommends use of 600 mcg orally for preventing PPH, i.e. during active management of third stage of labor. PGE1 can act on both cervix and uterus and hence is used for:

   a. Ripening of cervix (25 cg every 3–6 hours orally or vaginally)
   b. Inducing labor
   c. AMTSL
   d. For treating PPH

   Side effects: Nausea, vomiting, abdominal pain, shivering or hyperpyrexia, hypotension. It is contraindicated in previous cesarean patients.

iv. **Syntometrine:** It is 5 units of oxytocin and 0.5 mg methergine. It is expensive.

v. **Carbetocin:** Dose 100 mcg I/V over 1 minute for AMTSL, i.e. for preventing PPH. It is an analogue of oxytocin and

has action similar to oxytocin. Its advantage is, it has longer half life = 85–100 minute

Step 2: Delayed Cord Clamping

- Delayed cord clamping means clamping the cord between 1–3 minutes of birth
- **Early cord clamping** means Clamping the cord before 1 minute

Advantage of delayed cord clamping

80 mL of blood (i.e. 50 mg of elemental iron) present in the cord goes to the newborn and helps in preventing neonatal anemia.

Thus in all cases except the ones listed below—delayed cord clamping is advised.

Conditions in which early cord clamping is done:
- Baby is hypoxic and needs resuscitation or mother is hemodynamically unstable
- Known heart disease in baby
- If cord is avulsed or IUGR with abnormal cord Doppler evaluation
- Rh negative female

 Note: Earlier in preterm babies and HIV-positive mothers, early cord clamping was advised, but now delayed cord clamping is done in them also.

Step 3: Delivery of Placenta by Controlled Cord Traction (Modified Brandt-Andrews Technique) (Fig. 10.2)

Here with one hand uterus is pushed upwards and backwards and with other hand traction is given to cord in downward and forward direction in a steady and slow manner, until complete expulsion of the placenta occurs.

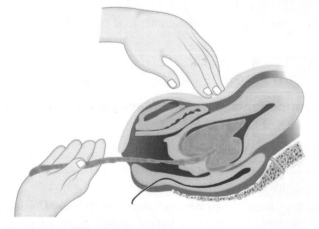

Fig. 10.2 Modified Brandt-Andrews technique

Note:
- If the placenta is undelivered after 30 minutes, it is called "Retained placenta".
- Controlled cord traction is only recommended by WHO if skilled birth attendant is available, otherwise not.

Step 4: Intermittent Uterine Tone Assessment
- After delivery for early identification of uterine atony, tone assessment is recommended for all births (uterine massage is now not a component of AMTSL).

Remember: Most important component of AMTSL is the use of oxytocic

COMPLICATIONS OF THIRD STAGE OF LABOR

POSTPARTUM HEMORRHAGE

Postpartum Hemorrhage (PPH) is blood loss of more than 500 ml from the genital tract following vaginal delivery and more than 1000 mL following cesarean.

Note: PPH is said to be minor if blood loss is between 500–1000 mL and major if it is >1000 mL and severe if it is > 2L.

According to ACOG - *PPH is defined as a drop in hematocrit of 10%.*

Types of PPH

Table 10.2: Types of PPH

Primary PPH	Secondary PPH
• Hemorrhage occurring within 24 hours following child birth • Most common cause: Atonic PPH	• Hemorrhage occurring after 24 hours and up to 12 weeks postpartum • Most common cause: Retained placenta

Causes of PPH

Table 10.3: Causes of PPH = 4T's

Atonic PPH (Tone)	**It is the most common cause of primary PPH accounting for 90% of cases.** The bleeding occurs as the blood vessels are not obliterated by contraction and retraction of uterine muscle fibres

Contd...

Contd...

Traumatic PPH (Trauma)	Genital tract injuries like: Lacerations of the cervix, vagina and perineum; hematomas Colporrhexis and Rupture uterus
Coagulopathy (Thrombin)	Disseminated intravascular coagulation (DIC) and hypofibrinogenemia are rare causes of PPH
Other causes (Tissue)	Retained products of conception. Retained placenta like lead to mainly secondary PPH

Remember: 4T's

Risk Factors for PPH (Table 10.4)

Table 10.4: Predisposing factors of PPH

Atonic PPH	Traumatic PPH	Blood coagulopathy
• Grand multipara^Q • Malnutrition/Anemia • Previous H/o atonic PPH • Antepartum hemorrhage (Placenta previa, placenta abruptio) • Overdistended uterus due to multiple pregnancy^Q, hydramnios^Q and macrosomia^Q • *Obesity* • Precipitate labor (labor < 3 hours) and prolonged labor^Q (>12 hours) • Mismanaged third stage of labor • Inadvertent use of oxytocin • Use of general/epidural anesthesia especially halothane • Retained placental fragments • Morbidly adherent placenta • Fibroid uterus	• Instrumental delivery • Vaginal birth after cesarean • Face to pubis delivery • Precipitate labor	• Abruption • Sepsis • Intrauterine death • Severe preeclampsia • HELLP syndrome

 Important One Liners

- M/C cause of PPH = Atonic uterus
- M/C cause of primary PPH = Atonic uterus
- M/C cause of secondary PPH = Retained placenta
- Structural placental abnormalities which can lead to PPH = succenturiate placenta/placenta bilobata.

Diagnosis of PPH

$$\text{Shock Index} = \frac{HR}{\text{systolic BP}}$$

- Normal value = 0.5–0.7
- This has been used in intensive treatment units and trauma centre as a guide to estimate the amount of blood loss.
- If it increases above 0.9–1.1 then intensive resuscitation may be required.

Obstetric shock index (OSI):

- During pregnancy its normal value = 0.7–0.8
- OSI >1–indicates massive haemorrhage and need for blood transfusion.

Urgency Grid: Based on OSI and shock index an urgency grid has been proposed (See Table 10.5).

Management of PPH

Step 1: General Measures: Including Resuscitative Measures + Investigations + Confirmation of Diagnosis

- The first and basic step in the management of PPH is resuscitation of the patient which includes:
  - Securing I/V lines
  - Volume restoration by crystalloids (normal saline/ Ringer lactate)
  - Oxygen inhalation
  - Crossmatching and arranging for blood.

- At the same time investigations like Blood group, Hemoglobin, Clotting time, Coagulation profile, Electrolytes should be sent.

The Cause of PPH, i.e., whether it is atonic (abdominal palpation) or traumatic should be looked and managed accordingly. This can be known by palpating the uterus perabdominally. If uterus can be palpated, it means tone of uterus is normal, i.e. it is a case of traumatic PPH. If uterus cannot be palpated per abdominally, it means atonic PPH.

Management of Atonic PPH

1. Medical Management

Once the diagnosis of atonic PPH has been made uterotonic agents are given to increase the tone of uterus (Table 10.6).

2. Mechanical Methods

If medical methods fail then mechanical methods are adopted.

a. **Uterine massage and bimanual compression (Fig. 10.3):** Uterine massage has been removed from active management of Third stage of Labor, (i.e. it is no longer a measure to prevent PPH). **It is now recommended by WHO as a measure to treat PPH**.

Table 10.5: Degree of blood loss and clinical findings in obstetric hemorrhage–the urgency grid

Loss of blood volume/ % of blood volume	Systelic BP	Symptoms and signs	OSI	Degree of shock urgency
500–100 mL 10–15%	Normal BP	Palpitation, mild tachycardia, dizziness	< 1	Compensated
1000–1500 mL 15–30%	Slight fall in SBP (SBP = 80–100 mm of Hg). A, rise in diastolic BP leading to increased pulse pressure	Weakness, marked tachycardia, sweating	> 1	Mild grade 3
1500–200 30–40%	Moderate fall in SBP (70–80 mm of Hg)	Restlessness, marked tachycardia, pallor, oliguria	> 1.5	Moderate grade 2
> 2000 mL > 40%	Marked fall in SBP (50–70 mm of Hg)	Collapse, air hunger, anuria	> 2	Severe grade 1

Table 10.6: Uterotonic drugs

Uterotonic drug	Dosage	Comment
• Oxytocin	10–20 units In 500 mL of normal saline @ 40–60 drops/minute	Never give oxytocin, I/V bolus
• Carbetocin (synthetic oxytocin analogue)	100 mcg I/V	More effective than oxytocin
• Ergometrine/ methylergometrine	0.25 mg I/M or I/V 0.2 mg I/M or I/V It can be repeated every 15 minutes	

• 15 methyl PGF-2α **(Carboprost)**	250 mcg
	I/M or intra myometrially and repeated after 15 minutes for maximum 8 doses
		• May cause diarrhea, hypertension vomiting, fever tachycardia pyrexia
		• It is C/I in asthmatics, as it leads to bronchospasm
		• It is also C/I in patients with risk of amniotic fluid embolism
		• **Relative C/I**
		  – Renal disease
		  – Liver disease
		  – Cardiac disease

• Misoprostol (PGE1)	**800 mcg sublingual**^{Q}	• Can cause hyperpyrexia • Can be given safely in asthmatics
• Dinoprostone (PGE2)	20 mg per rectum or per vagina every 2 hrs	Can cause diarrhea
• Tranexamic acid	500 mg I/V or I/M	It is recommended if above drugs fail to control bleeding

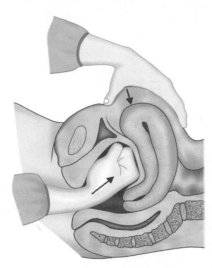

Fig. 10.3: Bimanual compression of the uterus

b. **Intrauterine packing (tamponade):** Done under GA using-5-metre-long gauze soaked in antiseptic solution.

However current WHO recommendations do not recommend uterine packing for treating PPH.

c. **Balloon tamponade (Fig. 10.4):** Using condom catheter or Sengstaken-Blakemore esophageal catheter or **Bakri balloon catheter.**

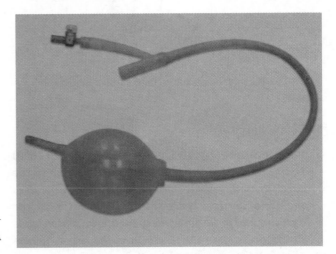

Fig. 10.4: Intrauterine Bakri balloon for postpartum hemorrhage

 Note: The Bakri Balloon catheter is filled **with 300–500 mL of warm saline and kept till 12–24 hrs.**

d. **Military anti-shock garment or treatment (MAST):**
It is a giant BP cuff that applies external counter pressure to
legs and abdomen such that blood returns to vital organs
and stabilizes the BP.

MAST: Use is recommended by WHO—as a temporary
method till appropriate care is available.

When mechanical methods fail—then surgical methods are adopted.

3. Surgical Methods

Surgical methods

If family is not completed
- Application of B lynch sutures (Fig. 10.5)
- Radiographic embolization of pelvic vessels (COGDT 10/ed p 481)
- Uterine and ovarian artery ligation
- Internal iliac artery ligation (anterior division)
  ↓
  If these methods fail then hysterectomy is done as final resort.

Family is completed
↓
Subtotal hysterectomy/supracervical
hysterectomy

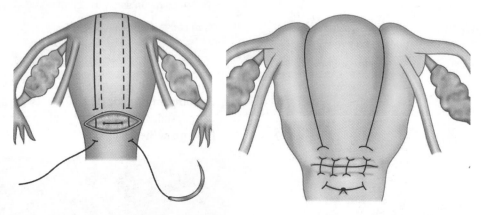

Fig. 10.5: B Lynch brace suture for control of atonic PPH

Details of Surgical method.

- *B Lynch Suture (Fig. 10.5) (Christopher B Lynch 1997)
  is an alternative to vessel ligation technique in the
  surgical management of PPH. B Lynch suture involves
  the use of vertical brace sutures, which appose the
  anterior and posterior walls of the uterus, which leads
  to compression of the fundus and the lower uterine
  segment, thereby controlling the hemorrhage.*

  – The main advantage is that it is very easy to perform
    and may obviate the need for a hysterectomy.
  – It is commonly performed at cesarean section but can
    also be done after vaginal delivery.

- *Application of block sutures (multiple square
  sutures):* The anterior and posterior uterine walls are
  approximated until no space is left in uterine cavity using
  block sutures/multiple squares.

Other sutures which can be used: in PPH
Hayman suture
Cho square
Gunshella suture.

- *Uterine and ovarian artery ligation:* It is easier than
  internal iliac artery ligation and can be tried as the first
  resort.

- **Uterine artery ligation is done at the level of internal OS (Fig. 10.6).**

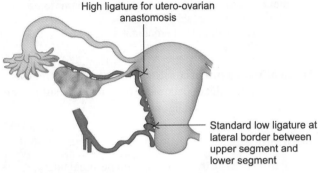

Fig. 10.6: Uterine and ovarian artery ligation

- **Internal iliac artery ligation (anterior division Fig. 10.7):** It should be considered before hysterectomy, especially in nullipara, as the uterus can be preserved. The artery is ligated about *5 cm from common iliac artery.* It will ensure that posterior division is not included in the ligature, as it may lead to loss of lower limb sensation (femoral artery and dorsalis pedis artery are branches of posterior division).

 Note: **When B/L internal iliac artery ligation is done:**
  a. Pulse pressure reduces by 85%.
  b. Blood flow reduces by 50%
  c. Mean arterial pressure reduces by 25%

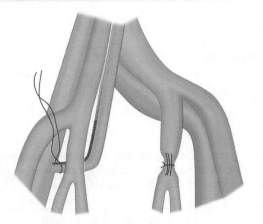

Fig. 10.7: Internal iliac artery ligation

- *Arterial embolisation:* Done when patient is hemodynamically stable and good radiological facilities are available. Under fluoroscopic guidance femoral artery is catheterised, the bleeding vessel identified and embolisation is carried out using gel foam.
- *Subtotal hysterectomy:* It is the most definitive method of controlling PPH and should be the last resort.

In subtotal hysterectomy, only uterus is removed. Cervix is not removed. This is done to give a better quality of sexual life to the female.

WHO RECOMMENDATIONS FOR TREATMENT OF PPH (2012)

1. I/V oxytocin is the recommended drug to treat PPH. If it is unavailable or if bleeding continues even after giving oxytocin, then I/V ergometrine, syntometrine (oxytocin + ergometrine), sublingual misoprost (800 mcg) or carboprost can be used.
2. Use of Tranexamic acid is recommended if other uterotonics fail.
3. For initial resuscitation isotonic crystalloids is recommended as compared to colloids.
4. Uterine massage is recommended for treatment of PPH (not AMTSL).
5. If woman does not respond to treatment using oxytocics or if oxytocics are unavailable, use of intrauterine balloon tamponade is recommended for the treatment of PPH due to uterine atony.
6. If bleeding still does not stop—**following temporary measures are recommended till appropriate care is available in the form of surgical intervention.**

  - Bimanual compression
  - External aortic compression
  - Anti-shock garment (MAST)

   Note: Uterine packing is not recommended by WHO.

7. Surgical interventions and uterine artery embolization are all recommended by WHO for treating atonic PPH.

Table 10.7: Management algorithm for PPH (HEMOSTASIS) Proposed by Chandraharan and Arulkumaran (based on WHO)

H	Ask for help and hands on uterus
E	Establish aetiology, ensure ABC, ensure availability of blood and ecobolics (drugs that contract the uterus)
M	Massage of uterus
O	Oxytocin infusion/Prostaglandins
S	Shift to theatre—aortic pressure or antishock garment. or bimanual compression (as temporary method)
T	Tamponade balloon (consider tranexemic acid 1 gm)

Contd...

Contd...

A	Apply compression suture—B lynch suture
S	Systemic pelvic devascularization—uterine/internal iliac artery/ovarian artery ligation
I	Interventional radiology—embolization
S	Subtotal/total hysterectomy

MANAGEMENT OF TRAUMATIC PPH

- **2nd M/C cause of PPH** is Genital tract trauma
- Traumatic PPH can be due to perineal tear, hematoma, cervical tear or uterine rupture.

Pelvic Hematoma (Fig. 10.8)

- M/C site for pelvic hematoma—vulva
- M/C artery to form vulval hematoma—Pudendal A
- M/C artery to form vagina hematoma—Uterine A and its branches
- M/C symptom—pain, inability to pass urine.

Local examination:

Bluish tender swelling

Management:

- A small hematoma (< 3 cm) is managed conservatively using cold compress and analgesics.

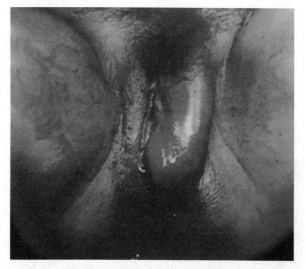

Fig. 10.8: Left sided anterior perineal triangle hematoma associated with a vaginal laceration following spontaneous delivery in a woman with consumptive coagulopathy form acute fatty liver of pregnancy.

Indications for surgical management of hematoma:
- Hemodynamic instability
- Increasing size of the hematoma
- Extensive pain.

Surgical Management consists of drainage of clot followed by obliteration of dead space using deep mattress suture and if bleeder is present, put figure of 8 suture.

Perineal Tear

The tears involving the perineum are perineal tears.

Classification of perineal tears and obstetric anal sphincter injury (RCOG 2007).

Grade	Description
1st degree	Tear involving vaginal epithelium or skin only
2nd degree	Tear involving both vaginal skin and muscles (mediolateral episiotomy corresponds to 2nd degree perineal tear)
3rd degree Grade 3a Grade 3b Grade 3c	Involvement of anal sphincter Tear of < 50% of external anal sphincter Tear of ≥ 50% of external anal sphincter Tear of external and internal anal sphincter
4th degree	Third degree tear along with involvement of anal epithelium

Ways to Prevent Perineal Tear

- **Ritgen maneuver** (promoting flexion of fetal head with left hand and supporting perineum with right hand)
- Episiotomy—Not routinely commended

Amongst these methods—the only method approved by WHO to be used routinely is support of perineum while delivering head (Modified Ritgen maneuver)

Note: Instrumental delivery can lead to perineal tear but ventouse delivery is associated with less perineal trauma as compared to forceps delivery.

Management of Perineal Tear

First and Second Degree Tear

- Repaired in labor room.
- Using analgesia (preferably epidural analgesia)
- Technique:

Vaginal mucosa repaired [using vicryl (polygalactin suture), interrupted or continuous suture] site - begin from 1 cm above the apex

⇩

Muscles bulbospongiosus superual tawlvenre peasli muscles repaired
(Same vicryl - continuous sutures)

⇩

Vaginal skin
(Same vicryl - interrupted Mattress suture)

Third and Fourth Degree Tear (OASIS)

- It is medical emergency
- Repair should be done immediately
- Repair is done in OT under general anesthesia
- Technique:

1st repair—Anal epithelium (using vicryl) or PDS suture

⇩

Internal anal sphincter repaired
Using polydioxanone suture
PDS suture (prolene suture) or vicryl, by end-to-end anastomosis

⇩

External anal sphincter repaired
Using polydiaxanone suture (prolene suture) by either end-to-end anastomis (M/C used) or overlapping technique (Best suited for 3C type of perineal tear)

⇩

Then repair same like 1st degree and 2nd degree tear
Vaginal mucosa

⇩

Vaginal muscles

⇩

Skin

 Note: Pregnancy should be avoided preferably for an year but atleast for 6 months after 3rd or 4th degree perineal tear repair.

- In future these females can have vaginal delivery with or without episiotomy.
- ACOG 2016 recommends a single shot of antiseptic at the time of repair

Cervical Tears

M/c site = 3 o'clock position followed by 9 o'clock position.
Mgt: Repair using vicryl.

RETAINED PLACENTA

Types

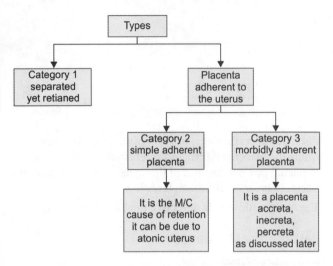

Management of Retained Placenta (Category 1 and 2) as Recommended by WHO

1. **Initial step:** If placenta does not expel spontaneously, WHO recommends use of oxytocin (10 IU I/M or I/V) and controlled cord traction for 30 minutes if vitals are stable as the first measure.

   That means a total wait for 60 minutes before manual removable of placenta is attempted (Williams Obs 25/e pg 52). **If brisk bleeding over in between then immediate MRP is done.**

 Note: WHO does not recommend the use of following drugs for retained placenta management.
- Ergometrine
- Dinoprost

Manual removal of placenta (MRP)
- Done in OT
- Under general anesthesia
- A single dose of antibiotic (ampicillin/1st generation antibiotic) is given
- After the procedure – I/V oxytocin infusion is given.

PLACENTA ACCRETA/MORBIDLY ADHERENT PLACENTA

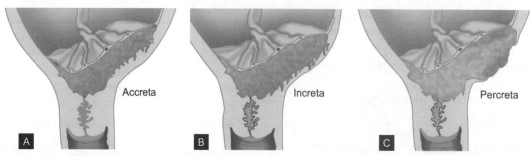

Figs. 10.9A to C: Morbidly adherent placentas: (A) Placenta accreta, (B) Placenta increta, (C) Placenta percreta

Placenta accreta is a type of morbidly adherent placenta where the placenta is firmly adherent to the uterine wall due to partial or total absence of the decidua basalis[Q] and the fibrinoid layer i.e. Nitabuch layer[Q].

The main aetiology is defective decidua formation.

Pathological Findings

- Absence of decidua basalis
- Absence of Nitabuch's fibrinoid layer

Classification/Variants

- **Placenta accreta:** Chorionic villi are attached to the superficial myometrium (Fig. 10.9A).
- **Placenta increta:** villi invade deep in the myometrium (Fig. 10.9B).
- **Placenta percreta**: villi penetrate the full thickness myometrium and reach up to the serosal layer (Fig. 10.9C).

Risk Factors

- M/C risk factor is placenta previa in present pregnancy (Note: previous H/o placenta previa is not a risk factor[Q])
- History of operative interference like:
  - Previous cesarean section (2nd M/c risk factor)
  - Previous curettage
  - Previous manual removal
  - Previously treated Asherman syndrome
  - Synaechiolysis
  - Myomectomy
- Multiparity
- Advanced maternal age > 35 years

 Note: Highest rise of adherent placenta is in a case of placenta previa in present pregnancy with previous H/o cesarean section (11% risk).
- It is also seen that in females with βhcg and AFP raised levels the chances of morbidly adherent placenta are high

Diagnosis

At the Time of Delivery

It is made mostly during attempted manual removal of placenta when the plane of cleavage between the placenta and uterine wall cannot be made out.[Q]

Prior to Delivery

Presumptive diagnosis may be made by:

- **Transvaginal sonography:**
  Features suggestive of placenta accreta are:

  - Visualization of **irregular vascular sinuses with turbulent flow,** i.e. large placental lakes are seen (Fig. 10.10)
  - Myometrial thickness less than 1 mm
  - **Absence of the subplacental sonolucent zone**[Q] (which represents the normal decidua basalis).

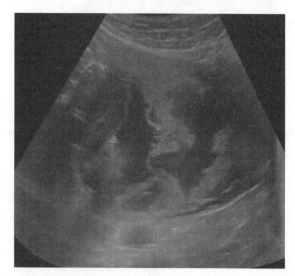

Fig. 10.10: Transabdominal sonogram of placental percreta shows multiple and massive placental 'lakes' or 'lactunae'.

- **Doppler imaging-shows:**
  - A distance less than 1 mm between the uterine serosal bladder interface and retroplacental vessels (Fig. 10.11)

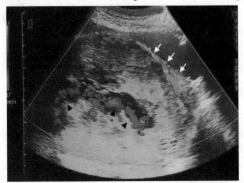

Fig. 10.11: Transvaginal sonogram and Doppler of placental invasion with a morbidly adherent placenta. Retroplacental vessels (white arrows) invade the myometrium and obscure the bladder-serosal interface. Abnormal intraplacental venous lakes (black arrowheads) are commonly seen in this setting.

  - Presence of large intraplacental lakes (Fig. 10.11)
  - It is useful in making diagnosis
- **C: MRI** Findings: Uterine bulging
  - Heterogeneous signal intensity within basic intraplacental bands.

ACOG recommends use of MRI if sonography results are inconclusive or if there is posterior previa

Complications

- Excessive bleeding
- Shock
- Sepsis
- Uterine inversion

Management

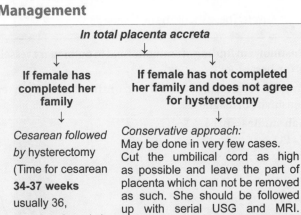

In total placenta accreta	
If female has completed her family	**If female has not completed her family and does not agree for hysterectomy**
Cesarean followed by hysterectomy (Time for cesarean **34-37 weeks** usually 36, completed weeks)	*Conservative approach:* May be done in very few cases. Cut the umbilical cord as high as possible and leave the part of placenta which can not be removed as such. She should be followed up with serial USG and MRI. Follow-up with only BhCG levels is not recommended. The patient should be given antibiotics and methotrexate in hope of autolysis.

UTERINE INVERSION

- Uterine inversion is a condition in which there is inside out turning of the uterus.
- *It is a rare cause of postpartum collapse but collapse occurs suddenly after labor.*

Aetiology

- **Mismanagement of the third stage (M/C cause):** Attempting to deliver a placenta by cord traction that has not yet separated (Crede's method).
- Spontaneous inversion can occur with an atonic uterus (in 40% cases).
- Placenta accreta is a rare cause.

Clinical Features

- **Patient present with shock immediately after delivery,** degree of shock being out of proportion to the amount of bleeding.
- Shock is both neurogenic (initially) and later haemorrhagic because uterus becomes atonic.
- Bleeding is due to attempts to detach the placenta before correcting the inversion.
- Vaginal examination reveals a soft, globular swelling in the vagina or cervical canal.
- On abdominal palpation, the fundus of the uterus is felt to be absent[Q].

M/c cause of death: In patient of uterine inversion is hemorrhagic shock.

 Important One Liners

- A patient after delivery goes into shock—Most probable cause is–Answer: PPH.
- A patient after delivery goes immediately, into shock—Most probable cause is–Answer: Uterine inversion
- A patient after delivery goes into unexplained shock—Most probable cause-Answer: Amniotic fluid embolism.

Management

- Resuscitation and replacement of inverted uterus should be done simultaneously.
- **Manual replacement:** First step, if diagnosis is made immediately. The part which comes out first, i.e fundus, the uterus should be last to reposit. After replacing oxytocics should be given to promote contraction. This is called as **'Johnsons maneuver'** (ACOG 2006).

Varieties (See Fig. 10.12)

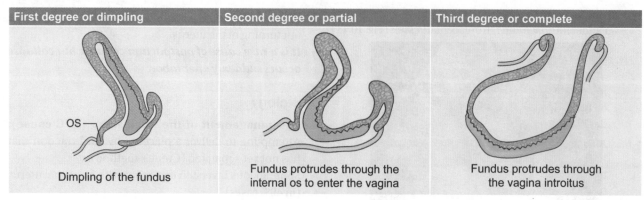

First degree or dimpling	Second degree or partial	Third degree or complete
OS Dimpling of the fundus	Fundus protrudes through the internal os to enter the vagina	Fundus protrudes through the vagina introitus

Fig. 10.12: Grading of uterine inversion

- **Hydrostatic O sullivan method:** It is done if Johnson maneuver fails. Warm saline is run into vagina with labia apposed to prevent leakage. The vagina balloons with the fluid and the inversion corrects on its own.
- Surgery-is done if above measures fail.

    A. Vaginal approach:
      i. Spinelli method
      ii. Kustner method

    B. Abdominal approach
      i. Huntington method
      ii. Robinson method
      iii. Haultain method

AMNIOTIC FLUID EMBOLISM

- It is an inevitable cause of maternal mortality
- It is a rare condition
- It is a complex condition characterized by abrupt onset of pulmonary embolism, shock and DIC due to entering of amniotic fluid into maternal circulation.
- **Most consistent risk factors are:**
    - Increased maternal age
    - Induction of labor
- **Time of event:**
    - During labor
    - During caesarean section
    - After vaginal delivery
    - During 2nd trimester MTP
- **Diagnosis is clinical** and one of exclusion classically it presents during labor or immediately after labor with sudden onset maternal collapse associated with tachypnea, cyanosis, hypotension, altered mental status and DIC.

US and UK have recommended the following 4 criteria for diagnosis of AFE all of which should be met

1. Acute hypotension or cardiac arrest
2. Acute hypoxia
3. Coagulopathy or severe haemorrhage in absence of other explanation
4. All these occurring during labor, caesarean section, dilatation and evacuation or within 30 minutes post partum. With no other explanation to these findings.

 Note: These should be no fever > 38°C

Postmortem finding of amniotic fluid in pulmonary vessels is the best proof.

Immunostaining with TKH-2 antibodies increases sensitivity of diagnosis.

Lab studies = pH $\downarrow$
$PO_2 \downarrow$
$PCO_2 \uparrow$

New Pattern Questions

N1. Living ligature of the uterus is:
   a. Endometrium
   b. Middle layer of myometrium
   c. Inner layer of myometrium
   d. Perimetrium

N2. All are signs of placental separation *except*:
   a. Lengthening of cord
   b. Gushing of blood
   c. Suprapubic bulge
   d. Increase of BP

N3. M/c cause of maternal death immediately after delivery:
   a. Amniotic fluid embolism
   b. PPH
   c. Uterine inversion
   d. Pulmonary embolism

N4. All of the following steps are recommended by WHO for preventing PPH *except*:
   a. Inj oxytocin 10 IU I/V infusion
   b. Uterine massage
   c. Delivery of placenta by controlled cord traction
   d. Intermittent assessment of uterine tone

N5. All of the following methods are recommended by WHO for treatment of PPH *except*:
   a. Uterine packing
   b. Bimanual compression
   c. Use of military anti-shock garment
   d. Balloon tamponade

N6. Identify the suture shown plate–used for management of PPH:

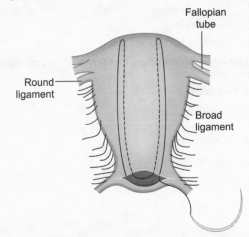

   a. B Lynch suture   b. Hayman suture
   c. Chi square suture   d. Gunshella suture

N7. All of the following are used in management of PPH *except*:
   a. Blood
   b. FFP
   c. Cryoprecipitate
   d. NOVO-T

N8. Which of the following test can be used to detect severity of PPH?
   a. Shock index
   b. Clot amplitude
   c. Maximum clot firmness
   d. All of the above

N9. M/c cause of death in a patient with uterine inversion:
   a. Neurogenic shock
   b. Haemorrhagic shock
   c. Pulmonary embolism
   d. Amniotic fluid embolism

N10. The following statements are related to obstetric inversion:
   a. It is usually insidious in onset
   b. It is usually acute
   c. It is usually incomplete
   d. In majority, it is spontaneous in nature

N11. Which one of the following is not an operation for uterine inversion?
   a. O sullivan
   b. Haultain
   c. Spincelli
   d. Fentoni

N12. Common cause of retained placenta:
   a. Atonic uterus
   b. Constriction ring
   c. Placenta accreta
   d. Poor voluntary expulsive effort

N13. A 30-year-old G3P2 woman delivered a term baby and started bleeding after delivery. She was given in fluids but bleeding did not stop. The EMO advised blood transfusion. After how many blood transfusions should be given FFP:
   a. 1   b. 2
   c. 3   d. 4

N14. The triple P procedure for placenta percreta involves all except:
   a. Pelvic devascularization
   b. Placental localization using USG
   c. Peripartum hysterectomy
   d. Myometrial excision for placental nonseparation

N15. A P$_3$ female has had a normal vaginal delivery in a peripheral hospital with the delivery of anterior shoulder of baby, 5U of oxytocin was given I/V and controlled cord traction applied soon after it. The placenta is not delivered after 30 minutes - Vitals of patient are stable. What is the most appropriate management?
   a. Adminster 0.5 mg ergometrine and wait for 30 more minutes
   b. Commence oxytocin infusion and observe further for a period of 30 minutes
   c. Commence oxytocin infusion and proceed to manual removal of placenta
   d. Give intraumbilical vein injection of oxytocin

N16. A P$_3$ female who had normal vaginal delivery develops PPH. The third stage was managed actively and placenta and membranes were expelled completely. What is the first step in management?
   a. Carry out uterine massage
   b. Insert two 14G cannula and start I/V fluids
   c. Give oxytocin infusion
   d. Palpate the uterus to determine its consistency

N17. A female bleeds profusely soon after delivery. Placenta and membranes were expelled I/V fluid initiated. Uterus is relaxed and fails to contract adequately after treatment with oxytocin drugs.

Her P/R = 120 beats/minute

B/P = 90/60 mm of Hg

What is the next appropriate step in management?
   a. Apply B lynch suture
   b. Carry out balloon tamponade
   c. Ligate internal iliac arteries
   d. Do hysterectomy

N18. A 35-year-old grand multipara starts bleeding profusely soon after delivery. Following steps were done:
   • IV lines secured
   • Resuscitation commenced
   • Oxytocins given
   • Balloon tamponade done

While these steps were being done 4 units of blood were transfused. But still her vitals are:

BP = 80/50 mm of Hg

P/R = 130 beats/minute

What is the next step in management?
   a. Insert B lynch suture
   b. Ligate internal iliac artery
   c. Perform hysterectomy
   d. Transfuse factor VIIa

N19. A woman complains of severe pain in vagina after vaginal delivery. O/E – she is pale, her P/R = 110 beats/minute, B/P = 100/60 mm of Hg. Vaginal examination reveals a large soft boggy mass on right lateral vaginal wall. What is the most appropriate treatment?
   a. Analgesics and observation
   b. Tight vaginal packing
   c. Drain and insert a figure of 8 suture
   d. Drain and explore for bleeding vessels

N20. All of the following methods are recommended by WHO in the treatment of PPH as temporary methods till appropriate care arrives *except*:
   a. Military antishock treatment
   b. Bimanual compression of the uterus
   c. Uterus packing
   d. External aorta compression

N21. All of the following can lead to secondary PPH except:
   a. Retained bits of placental tissue
   b. Parametritis
   c. Placental polyp
   d Coagulation disorder

N22. Risk factors for PPH are all except:
   a. Macrosomia
   b. Twin pregnancy
   c. Nuliparity
   d. Previous H/O PPH

N23. The most potent drug to control PPH amongst the options:
   a. Oxytocin
   b. Misoprost
   c. Carboprost
   d. Dinoprostone

Previous Year Questions

1. **Which is not included in active management of Third stage of Labor?** [AI 08]
   a. Uterotonic within 1 minute of delivery
   b. Immediate clamping, cutting and ligation of cord
   c. General massage of uterus
   d. Controlled cord traction

2. **Which is not included in active management of 3rd stage in labor to prevent PPH?** [AIIMS May 2013]
   a. Direct oxytocin injection after delivery of shoulder
   b. Immediate cutting and cord clamping
   c. Prophylactic misoprostol
   d. Controlled and sustained cord traction

3. **Early cord clamping is indicated in all except:**
   a. HIV positive females
   b. Birth asphyxia
   c. IUGR
   d. Cord avulsion

4. **The dose of misoprostol in emergent management of PPH:** [AIIMS Nov 2015]
   a. 200 mcg   b. 400 mcg
   c. 600 mcg   d. 800 mcg

5. **Carbetocin dose for PPH is:** [AIIMS May 2015]
   a. 100 microgram IV   b. 50 microgram IV
   c. 150 microgram IV   d. 250 microgram

6. **Most common cause of postpartum hemorrhage is:** [AIIMS Feb 97]
   a. Uterine atony   b. Retained products
   c. Trauma   d. Bleeding disorders

7. **The following complications during pregnancy increase the risk of postpartum hemorrhage (PPH) except:** [AI 06]
   a. Hypertension   b. Macrosomia
   c. Twin pregnancy   d. Hydramnios

8. **Atonic uterus is more common in:** [PGI Dec 97]
   a. Cesarean section   b. Multigravida
   c. Primigravida   d. Breech delivery

9. **All of the following are used in the treatment of postpartum hemorrhage except:** [AI 03; AIIMS May 02]
   a. Misoprostol   b. Mifepristone
   c. Carboprost   d. Methylergometrine

10. **Treatment of postpartum hemorrhage is all except:** [AIIMS Dec 97]
    a. Oxytocin   b. Syntometrine
    c. Oestrogen   d. Prostaglandins

11. **Which of the drug is not commonly used in PPH?**
    a. Mifepristone   b. Misoprostol [AI 08]
    c. Oxytocin   d. Ergotamine

12. **Massive PPH may warrant following interventions:**
    a. Hysterectomy [PGI Dec 09]
    b. Thermal endometrial ablation
    c. Internal iliac A. ligation
    d. Balloon tamponade
    e. Uterine artery embolisation

13. **B Lynch suture is applied on:** [AI 03]
    a. Cervix   b. Uterus
    c. Fallopian tube   d. Ovaries

14. **True regarding PPH:** [PGI Nov 07]
    a. Type B Lynch suture used
    b. With new advances both atonic and traumatic PPH can be reduced
    c. More common in multipara
    d. Associated with polyhydramnios
    e. Mifepristone used

15. **A 30-year-old G3P2 woman with a history of hypertension presents to the birthing floor in labor. Following a prolonged labor and delivery with no fetal complications, she continues to bleed vaginally but remains afebrile. On bimanual examination, her uterus is soft, boggy, and enlarged. There are no visible lacerations. Uterine massage only slightly decreases the hemorrhage, and oxytocin is only mildly effective.**

    Which of the following is the next best step in mgt?
    a. Dilatation and curettage
    b. PGF2α   c. Methylergometrine
    d. Misoprost   e. Platelet transfusion

16. **True about placenta accreta is:** [AIIMS Nov 99]
    a. Seen in cesarean scar
    b. Removal should be done under GA in piecemeal
    c. Chorionic villi invade serosa
    d. It is an etiological factor for amniotic fluid embolism

17. **Which is not a common cause of Placenta Accreta?**
    a. Previous LSCS [AI 08/MP 09]
    b. Previous curettage
    c. Previous myomectomy
    d. Previous placenta previa/abrupto placenta

18. **Placenta accreta is associated with:** [PGI June 08]
    a. Placenta previa   b. Uterine scar
    c. Multiple pregnancy   d. Multipara
    e. Uterine malformation

19. **Minimum duration between onset of symptoms and death is seen in:** [AI 09]
    a. APH   b. PPH
    c. Septicemia   d. Obstructed labor

20. **A patient went into shock immediately after normal delivery, likely cause is:** [AIIMS Nov 2010]
    a. Amniotic fluid embolism [AIIMS May 2013]
    b. PPH   c. Uterine inversion
    d. Eclampsia

21. All of the following drugs are used for prevention and treatment of PPH *except*: [PGI May 2013]
    a. Misoprostol   b. Oxytocin
    c. Ergometrine   d. Carboprost
    e. Mifepristone

22. A female presents with significant blood loss due to postpartum haemorrhage (PPH). What would be the shock index (HR/systolic BP)? [AIIMS Nov 12]
    a. 0.7–0.9   b. 0.5-0.7
    c. 0.9-1.1   d. 0.1–0.5

23. Perineal tear should be repaired: [AIIMS May 95]
    a. 24 hrs later   b. 48 hrs later
    c. 36 hrs later   d. Immediately

24. All are true regarding Duncan's placental separation *except*:
    a. Peripheral separation
    b. Maternal surface presents at vulva
    c. More blood loss
    d. Most common method of separation

25. A 22 years old gravida 3 para 2 lady delivers a normal child followed by delivery of an intact placenta. Following delivery, the lady develops severe per vaginal bleeding after 30 minutes. On table sonogram revealed retained placental tissue. What is the suspected type of placenta? [AIIMS May 2016]
    a. Membranous placenta
    b. Placenta fenestrae
    c. Placenta accreta
    d. Placenta succenturiata

26. What dose of misoprostol is used orally to control bleeding in post partum hemorrhage? [AIIMS November 2016]
    a. 400 micrograms
    b. 600 micrograms
    c. 800 micrograms
    d. 1000 micrograms

27. What is the maximum capacity of Bakri balloon which is used in post partum hemorrhage?
    a. 200 mL   b. 300 mL [AIIMS Nov 2016]
    c. 500 mL   d. 1000 mL

28. Which of the drugs must be available in labor room while giving narcotics for pain? [AIIMS Nov 2017]
    a. Fentanyl   b. Naloxone
    c. Pheniramine   d. Morphine

Answers with Explanations to New Pattern Questions

N1. Ans. is b, i.e. Middle layer of myometrium

The middle layer of myometrium is called as **Living Ligature as** it has fibers running in criss cross manner. Thus when uterus contracts after delivery, these fibers contract and the blood vessels constrict.

N2. Ans. is d, i.e. Increase of BP

See the text for explanation.

N3. Ans. is b, i.e. PPH

M/c cause of death after delivery is PPH.

N4. Ans. is b, i.e. Uterine massage   *Ref. JB Sharma Obs, Pg 218*

Prevention of PPH in other words means active management of third stage of labor (AMTSL).

Earlier uterine massage was included in AMTSL, but now WHO does not recommend uterine massage as a component of AMTSL.

Uterine massage is now recommended by WHO in the treatment of PPH.

N5. Ans. is a, i.e. Uterine packing   *Ref. JB Sharma Obs, Pg 341*

WHO does not recommend uterine packing in the management of PPH.

For more details, see the text.

N6. Ans. is a, i.e. B Lynch suture

The sutures shown in the figure, are B Lynch sutures–applied on uterus for managing PPH.

N7. Ans. is d, i.e. NOVO-T   *Ref. Fernando Arias 4/e, p 393*

For fluid resuscitation after PPH following are used:

> - Colloids and crystalloids
> - Blood
> - Fresh frozen plasma–to correct clotting factor deficiency given, if 4U of blood has been given or, if PT>1.5
> - Cryoprecipitate
> - Platelets (if platelet count < 50,000 or, if 4 units of blood have been transfused).

NOVO-T is activated factor 7. Its role is well, established in hemophilia. Activated factor VII (NOVOT) acts by binding with tissue factor to augment intrinsic clotting pathway by activating factor IX and X. However its role is obstetrical haemorrhage is uncertain and moreover it is not used in these cases due to risk of thromboembolic events like MI.

N8. Ans. is a, i.e. Shock index

Clot amplitude and clot firmness are done in DIC.

N9. Ans. is b, i.e. Hemorrhagic shock

Shock in uterine inversion is initially neurogenic (vasovagal), with inversion uterus becomes atonic and bleeding occurs which leads to hemorrhagic shock.

M/c cause of death in uterine inversion - haemorrhagic shock.

N10. Ans. is b, i.e. It is usually acute *Ref. Williams Obs. 23/e, p 780, 781; Dutta Obs. 9/e, p 395*

- Uterine inversion is a condition in which there is inside out turning of the uterus.
- *It is a rare cause of postpartum collapse but collapse occurs suddenly after labor.*
- **It is acute in onset.**[Q] *Ref. Dutta Obs. 9/e, p 395*
- **Mostly uterine inversion is complete, i.e. of third degree**
- **Most common cause of uterine inversion is mismanagement of the third stage of labor**
- Spontaneous inversion can occur with an atonic uterus (in 40% cases).
- Placenta accreta is a rare cause of uterine inversion.

N11. Ans. is d, i.e. Fentoni *Ref. Dutta Obs. 7/e, p 422; IAN Donald Obstetrics 7/e, p 592*

Surgical Procedures to Correct Uterine Inversion

Vaginal operations	Abdominal operations	Hydrostatic method
• Spincelli	• Huntingtons procedures	• O sullivan method
• Kustner	• Haultain	• Oguch method
• Oejo	• Robinson	

N12. Ans. is a, i.e. Atonic uterus *Ref. JB Sharma Obs, Pg 343*

M/C cause of retained placenta is a simply adherent placenta. This is due to mainly atonic uterus.

N13. Ans. is d, i.e. 4 *Ref. Practical Guide to High Risk Pregnancy – Fernando Arias 4/e, p 395*

- The most important initial resuscitating step of PPH is fluid management. Till blood is not available this is done using colloids and crystalloids which although replaces fluid but worsens existing coagulopathy.
- Therefore blood transfusion should be followed by transfusion of fresh frozen plasma and platelets. This is done after 4 units of blood transfusion i.e. ratio of FFP : Platelets: RBC = 1:1:4. These days latest recommendations for massive PPH are 1:1:1, i.e. after every unit of blood transfusion, 1 unit of FFP and 1 unit of platelets should be given to correct the ongoing coagulopathy. But this is still to be implemented.

N14. Ans. is c, i.e. Peripartum hysterectomy *Ref. Fernando Arias 4/e, p 396*

> Triple P procedure has been developed for placenta percreta as a conservative surgical alternative to peripartum hysterectomy. It consists of following 3 steps:
> 1. Perioperative placental localization and delivery of fetus via transverse uterine incision above the upper border of placenta.
> 2. Pelvic devascularization
> 3. Placental nonseparation is dealt with myometrial excision and reconstruction of uterine wall.

N15. Ans. is b, i.e. Commence oxytocin infusion and observe further for a period of 30 minutes

For this question - Read what JB Sharma Pg 342 says—

"WHO states that in the absence of haemorrhage, the women should be observed for a further 30 minutes following initial 30 minutes before manual removal of placenta (MRP) is attempted."   *TB of obstetric, JB Sharma Pg 342*

Since in this question - vitals of patient are stable we can wait for 30 minutes more after starting I/V oxytocin infusion.

"There is insufficient evidence to recommend the use of intraumbilical vein injection of oxytocin as a treatment for retained placenta (WHO-2012)".

N16. Ans. is b, i.e. Insert two 14G cannula and start IV fluids

This patient has developed PPH but always the first step in management - when any patient comes with bleeding is - general resuscitation which includes inserting two 14G cannulae and starting I/V fluids.

N17. Ans. is b, i.e. Carry out balloon tamponade

In this case, initial resuscitation has been done, oxytocin has been given next logical step is balloon tamponade before attempting any surgical procedure.

N18. Ans. is c, i.e. Perform hysterectomy

Friends, management of PPH has to individualised in each case. In this question, oxytocin and balloon tamponade have failed incontrolling PPH. Inspite of giving 4 units of blood, her vitals are unstable.

She is a grand multipara ∴ instead of trying any conservative surgery like B lynch suture or ligation of internal iliac artery. I will straight away perform hysterectomy.

N19. Ans. is c, i.e. Drain and insert a figure of 8 suture

This patient is having soft, boggy mass on right lateral wall of vagina, i.e. she has vaginal hematoma. The hematoma has led to unstable Vitals. This is an indication for the surgical management of hematoma, i.e. put a drain and insert figure of 8 suture. Indications for the surgical management of hematoma are as follows:

1. Hemodynamic instability
2. Increasing size of hematoma
3. Extensive pain

N20. Ans. is c, i.e. Uterus packing

WHO recommends following methods as temporary method till appropriate care arrives
1. Military anti-shock garments
2. Binamal compression of uterus
3. External aorta compression

It does not recommend uterine packing rather as a temporary measure nor as permanent method.

N21. Ans. is d, i.e. Coagulation disorder   *Ref. JB Sharma Textbook of Obs Pg 342)*
Causes of Secondary PPH

1. **Placental causes**
   i. Retained bits of placenta
   ii. Subinvolution of placental site
   iii. Placenta accreta

2. **Infections**
   i. Endometritis
   ii. Myometritis
   iii. Parametritis
   iv. Infection at vulvo vaginal laceration

3. **Miscellaneous causes**
   i. Chorio carcinoma
   ii. Infected fibroid
   iii. Placental polyp
   iv. Cervical cancer
   v. Uterine inversion

N22. Ans. is c, i.e. Nulliparity   *Ref. JB Sharma Obs Pg 335*
Risk factors for PPH

Table 10.6: Risk factors for postpartum hemorrhage

Factors in history	Antepartum factors	Intrapartum factors	Miscellaneous causes

• Advanced maternal age	• Overdistended uterus
	  – Multiple pregnancy
	  – Large-sized fetus
	  – Polyhydramnios
		• Induction of labor	• Sepsis

• Multiparity, anemia, malnutrition	• Antepartum haemorrhage	• Prolonged labor	
• Previous PPH	• Chorioamnionitis	• Precipitate labor	

• Previous placenta previa or accrete		• Instrumental delivery, operative manipulations	
• Bleeding and coagulation disorders		• Rupture uterus	
• Fibroid uterus		• Genital tract trauma	
		• Non judicious use of oxytocics, sedatives, etc.	

N23. Ans. is c, i.e. Carboprost

Amongst all drugs, the most potent drug to control PPH is carboprost

Answers with Explanations to Previous Year Questions

1. Ans. is b, i.e. Immediate clamping, cutting and ligation of cord

2. Ans. is b, i.e. Immediate cutting and cord clamping *Ref. JB Sharma Obs, Pg 218)*

Friends, Q1 is old question when uterine massage was included in active management of third stage of labor.

3. Ans. is a, i.e. HIV positive females

Indications of early cord clamping

- Maternal or fetal instability – if either needs resuscitation
- IUGR baby with abnormal Doppler evaluation
- Known heart disease in baby
- If cord is avulsed

4. Ans. is d, i.e 800 mcg *Ref. JB Sharma Obs, Pg 338, 341*

Dose of misoprost for preventing PPH (i.e. AMTSL) = 600 mcg orally.
Dose of misoprost for treating PPH = 800 mcg sublingually

5. Ans. is a, i.e. 100 micrograms I/V

Dose of carbetocin = 100 mcg I/V in PPH
Dose of carboplast = 250 mcg I/M in PPH

6. Ans. is a, i.e. Uterine atony *Ref. Dutta Obs. 7/e, p 410*

- Most common cause of PPH or primary PPH is Atonic uterus
- Most common cause of secondary PPH is retained placenta

7. Ans. is a, i.e. Hypertension *Ref. Dutta Obs. 7/e, p 411*

8. Ans. is b, i.e. Multigravida *Ref. Dutta Obs. 7/e, p 411*

Friends, in the text question I have listed the predisposing factors for Atonic PPH. The list is long, but I remember I did not use any mnemonic for memorising it during my undergraduate and postgraduate exams. I memorized it by:

Obstetric history which points towards PPH:

- Grand multipara[Q] due to laxed abdomen
- H/o atonic PPH[Q] or adherant placenta

Examination findings which point towards PPH:

Obesity:

- Malnutrition and/or anemia
- Overdistended uterus due to:
  – Hydramnios[Q]
  – Multiple pregnancy[Q]
  – Macrosomia[Q]
- Gynaecological disorders:
  – Fibroid uterus
  – Uterine malformations

Factors increasing the risk of PPH at the time of delivery:

- Precipitate labor
- Prolonged labor
- Inadvertent use of oxytocics
- Use of general anaesthesia
- Mismanagement of third stage of labor
- Retained placental bits.

As far as hypertension *(Option 'a')* is concerned.

 Remember: Hypertension can lead to Antepartum hemorrhage (abruptio placenta), but not PPH.

9. **Ans. is b, i.e. Mifepristone**

10. **Ans. is c, i.e. Oestrogen**

11. **Ans. is a, i.e. Mifepristone**   *Ref. Dutta Obs. 7/e, p 415, 416; Williams Obs. 23/e, p 775; COGDT 10/e, p 481; Munro Kerr's 10/e, p 426, 427*

Atonicity is the most common cause of PPH. Any drug which increases the tone of uterus or the force of contraction is used to control PPH and is called oxytocic or uterotonic.

Commonly used oxytocics in the management of PPH are:

- Oxytocin/Carbetocin
- Methergin
- Syntometrine – oxytocin + methylorgonovine
- 15 methyl $PGF_{2\alpha}$ (carboprost)
- Misoprostol (PGE_1)

12. **Ans. is a, c, d, and e, i.e. Hysterectomy; Internal iliac A. ligation; Balloon tamponade and Uterine artery embolisation.**
    Discussed in detail in the text

13. **Ans. is b, i.e. Uterus**   *Ref. COGDT 10/e, p 482, 483*
    Already explained

14. **Ans. is a, b, c and d, i.e. Type B Lynch suture used; With new advances both atonic and traumatic PPH can be reduced; More common in multipara; and Associated with polyhydramnios**   *Ref. Dutta Obs. 7/e, p 411, 412, 417*

    - PPH is more common in multipara due to laxed abdomen and associated factors like adherent placenta and anemia (i.e., *option "c"* is correct).
    - Overdistension of uterus as in multiple pregnancy, hydraminos and large baby also lead to PPH (i.e., *option "d"* is correct).
    - Incidence of atonic and traumatic PPH can be reduced with new advances or rather by intelligent anticipation, skilled supervision, prompt detection and effective institution of therapy.   *—Dutta Obs. 6/e, p 413*
    - B Lynch suture are used for management of PPH (Dutta Obs. 7/e, p 418). **(For more details about B lynch suture, see answer)**
    - Mifepristone is not used in the management of PPH.

15. **Ans. is b, i.e PGF2α**

    This is a case of Atonic PPH as the patient has presented with vaginal bleeding immediately after delivery and uterus is not palpable per abdominally, i.e it has lost its tone.

In Atonic PPH the first step in management should be uterotonic agents like oxytocin or methylergometrine and if bleeding is not controlled by using either of it, straightaway PGF2α i.e carboprost should be used.

>
> *Note:*
> • If patient would have been an asthamatic then our answer would have been misoprostol since PGF2α is contraindicated in asthamatics.
> • If patient would have presented 24 hours after delivery then the answer would have been Dilatation and curettage as the most common cause of secondary PPH, is retained placental bits.

16. **Ans. is a, i.e. Seen in cesarean scar** *Ref. Dutta Obs. 7/e, p 419*

17. **Ans. is d, i.e. Previous placenta previa/abruptio placenta** *Ref. Dutta Obs. 7/e, p 419*

18. **Ans. is a, b and d, i.e. Placenta previa; Uterine scar; and Multipara** *Ref. Dutta Obs. 7/e, p 419;*
    Risk factors for placenta accreta: *Williams Obs. 23/e, p 776, 777; Munro Kerr's 10/e, p 432, 434*

    • Present placenta previa
    • Previous H/o cesarean section
    • Previous curettage
    • Previous manual removal of placenta
    • Previously treated Asherman syndrome
    • Myomectomy
    • Multiparity
    • Advanced materal age > 35 years

19. **Ans. is b, i.e. PPH** *Ref: Textbook of Prenatal Medicine by Kurjak and Chervenak 2/e, p 1945*

    Friends – the most common of rapid death in obstetrics is PPH. In PPH, we can lose a patient within minute
    "In sharp contrast to APH, which usually claims life after 10 hrs if left untreated. PPH kills swiftly often in less than 2 hrs if not properly treated" *—Textbook of Perinatal Medicine 2/e, p 1945.*

20. **Ans. is c, i.e. Uterine inversion** *Ref. Sheila Balakrishna, Textbook of Obs 1/e, p 489, 490, 491*

    Friends this is one of those questions where we can derive the answer by excluding other options as very little information has been provided to us.

    Sudden post partum collapse – may be seen in all the four cases viz – amniotic fluid embolism, PPH, uterine inversion and eclampsia.

    But in case of PPH antecedent H/O excessive blood loss, in eclampsia – H/O antecedent convulsions and in amniotic fluid embolism – H/O abrupt onset of respiratory distress before collapse should be present, which is not given in the question so these options are being excluded.

    The clinical picture of acute inversion occurring in the third stage of labor is characterised by shock and haemorrhage, the shock being out of proportion to the bleeding.

    Since this a problem which occurs due to mismanaged third stage of labor, patient doesnot have any complain in the antenatal period or during labor.

    Uterine inversion – ***"It should be suspected whenever a woman has unexplained postpartum collapse".***
    Textbook of Obs, Sheila Balakrishnan, p 489

>
> **Note:** Although PPH is a more common cause of postpartum collapse than uterine inversion, but still the word 'shock immediately after normal delivery' prompts me to choose uterine inversion as the answer.

>
> *Remember:*
> • If Q says-A female presents with shock after delivery: Most probable cause – Answer is PPH
> • If Q says – A female presents with shock immediately after delivery. Most probable cause–Answer is uterine inversion.

21. **Ans. is e, i.e. Mifepristone**

    Repeat

22. **Ans. is c, i.e. 0.9 to 1.1**   *Ref. Fernando Arias 4/e, p 391*

    - **Shock index = heartrate/systolic BP**
    - Normal = 0.5–0.7
    - If it becomes 0.9–1.1 it indicates massive blood loss and need for intensive resuscitation.

23. **Ans. is d, i.e. Immediately**   *Ref. Dutta Obs. 7/e, p 422, 423*

    Management of Perineal tears:

    Recent tear should be repaired immediately following the delivery of the placenta.[Q]

    In cases of delay beyond 24 hours, the complete tear should be repaired after 3 months.[Q]

24. **Ans. is d, i.e. Most common method of separation**   *Ref: Williams obs 23/e, p 147*

    See the text for explanation   *Ref: JB Sharma obs p 205*

25. **Ans. is d, i.e. Placenta succenturiata**   *Ref: Williams 24/e p117*

    If whole placenta come out and still USG shows retained placental tissue it is succenturiate placenta

26. **Ans. is c, i.e. 800 micrograms**

    WHO Recommends use of 800 mcg of misoprost sublingually or orally to treat PPH.

27. **Ans. is c, i.e. 500 mL**

    Maximum capacity of Bakri balloon catheter is 500 mL
    Initially it should be filled to 200 mL.

28. **Ans. is b, i.e. Naloxone**   *(Ref Dutta Obs 9/e, pg 479)*

    In a labor room when opioid narcotics are being given, to reverse the respiratory depression induced by them, naloxone should be available. It is given to the mother 0.4 mg IV in labor .

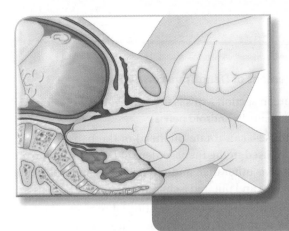

11

Malpresentations

Chapter at a Glance

- ➤ Malpositions
- ➤ Occipito-posterior Position
- ➤ Malpresentations
- ➤ Face Presentation
- ➤ Brow Presentation

- ➤ Breech Presentation
- ➤ Transverse Lie
- ➤ Unstable Lie
- ➤ Cord Prolapse

MALPOSITIONS

- **Malposition** refers to any position of the vertex other than flexed occipito-anterior or occipito transverse.
- **M/C malposition is occipito-posterior position**.

OCCIPITO-POSTERIOR POSITION

- In a vertex presentation where the occiput is placed posteriorly over the sacroiliac joint or directly over the sacrum, it is called an occipito-posterior position.
- When the occiput is placed over the right sacroiliac joint, the position is called **right occipito-posterior (ROP)** and when placed over the left sacroiliac joint, is called **left occipito-posterior** (LOP) and when it points towards the sacrum, is called **direct occipito-posterior**.
- **M/C being Right occipito-posterior position as Dextro-rotation of the uterus and the presence of the sigmoid colon on the left, disfavor LOP position.**
- All the three positions may be primary (present before the onset of labor) or secondary (developing after labor starts.

Incidence

- At the onset of labor—10%
- During late stages of labor—only 2% as occipito-posterior positions rotate in 80–90% cases and become occipito anterior.

Etiology

- Mostly idiopathic.

- M/C cause of OP position—Anthropoid and android pelvis.
- It is M/C in nulliparous females (where as all the rest malpresentations are more common in multiparous females).
- Marked deflection of the fetal head, also favors posterior position of the vertex. The causes of deflexion are: (1) High pelvic inclination. (2) Attachment of the placenta on the anterior wall of the uterus (3) Primary brachycephaly.

Diagnosis

- There is delay in engagement of head-infact Occipito-posterior position is the M/c cause of non engagement of head at term in primigravida patients.
- Since the occipito-posterior position is due to deflexed head—the sinciput and occiput are at the same level.
- On P/V examination:
  - Elongated bag of membranes which is likely to rupture during examination.
  - The sagittal suture occupies any of the oblique diameters of the pelvis.
  - Posterior fontanelle is felt near the sacroiliac joint.
  - In right OP— the anterior fontanelle will be present on left anterior side and in left OP, the anterior fontanelle will be present on right anterior side.
  - In late labor, the diagnosis is often difficult because of caput formation which obliterates the sutures and fontanelles. In such cases, the ear is to be located and the unfolded pinna points towards the occiput.

Mechanism of Labor: In Favorable Circumstances

Engaging Diameter: In Deflexed Head-Occipitofrontal Diameter-11.5 cm

- In 90% cases normal delivery occurs as head moves through 3/8th of circle (Fig. 11.1).

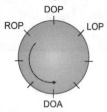

Fig. 11.1: Favorable rotation

So, when diagnosis of occipito-posterior presentation is made—labor is allowed to proceed in a manner similar to normal labor, in anticipation of normal vaginal delivery.

Hence the best management of occipito-posterior position when it is diagnosed during labor is—Wait and watch.

In Unfavorable Circumstances

Incomplete Forward Rotation (Fig. 11.2)

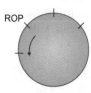

Fig. 11.2: Incomplete forward rotation

In this condition, the occiput rotates through 1/8th of a circle anteriorly and the sagittal suture comes to lie in the bispinous diameter. Thereafter, further anterior rotation is unlikely and arrest in this position is called **deep transverse arrest**.

Deep transverse arrest is defined as the head is deep into the cavity; the sagittal suture is placed in the transverse bispinous diameter and there is no progress in descent of the head even after 1/2–1 hour following full dilatation of the cervix.

 Important One Liners

- Deep transverse arrest occurs at the level of ischial spine.
- Deep transverse arrest is more common in pelvis in which ischial spines are prominent, i.e. in Android pelvis.

Management of Deep Transverse Arrest

1. Cesarean section—this is the management of choice, if DTA occurs in android pelvis.
2. Ventouse—can rotate the head of the baby, hence it can be used in the management of DTA, if it occurs in any pelvis other than android pelvis (as android pelvis has sharp and pointed ischial spine).
3. Manual rotation and application of forceps—forceps per se cannot rotate fetal head, but if manual rotation of the fetal head is done, then delivery can be done by forceps.
4. Forceps rotation and delivery with Kielland—**the only forceps which can rotate the fetal head is Kielland forceps but it is outdated these days**.

Note: Operative vaginal delivery for DTA should only be performed by a skilled obstetrician. Otherwise cesarean delivery is always preferred for all kinds of arrest.

Oblique Posterior Arrest

- It is due to Non-rotation of fetal head and is also called as **persistent occipito-posterior position**
- **M/C in anthropoid pelvis** (as in this pelvis, transverse diameter of the pelvis is narrow, so fetal head does not rotate at all)

Malrotation

- In extreme cases there will be malrotation—instead of turning forward fetus turns backward and comes to lie in **direct occipito-posterior position** (Fig. 11.3).
- **It is M/C in anthropoid pelvis** (as AP diameter of this pelvis is the biggest diameter)

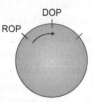

Fig. 11.3: Malrotation

- In case of anthropoid pelvis, **Face to pubis delivery occurs (as AP diameter is the largest diameter)**
- Final delivery in this case is still by extension
- Perineal tears and moulding more common
- In unfavorable circumstances, i.e. in all other types of pelvis, if malrotation occurs, arrest occurs called as **deep sacral arrest**
- **Management of deep sacral arrest** is cesarean section.

MALPRESENTATIONS

All presentations of the fetus other than the vertex are called as malpresentations.

- **M/C malpresentation is Breech.**

FACE PRESENTATION

- The presenting part is the face
- **There is abnormal attitude in face presentation,** i.e. normally there is flexion of fetal head but in face presentation, there is extension
- The denominator is mentum
- **The commonest position is left mento-anterior (LMA)**
- M/C seen in multiparous females
- M/C pelvis—in which it is seen—platypelloid pelvis
- M/C cause—anencephaly
- Incidence—1 in 500 to 1 in 2,000 deliveries.
- **In mento-anterior (seen in 60–80% cases)**—vaginal delivery is possible. It can be detected during labor by chin facing anteriorly.
  - The engaging diameter of the head is **submento-bregmatic (9.5 cm)** in fully extended head or **submentovertical** (11.5 cm) in partially extended head
  - Engagement is delayed
  - The head is born by flexion instead of extension.

- **In mentoposterior (seen in 20–25% cases)**—if it is detected in early labor, best management is to wait and watch because in 20-30% cases mentoposterior become mentoanterior and delivery occurs but if it is detected in late labor then cesarean section has to be done.

BROW PRESENTATION

- It is the rarest presentation, it is seen in partial extension of head
- Causes of brow presentation are same as for face presentation, i.e. multiparity, platypelloid pelvis and anencephaly or fetal macrosomia
- Engaging diameter—Mentovertical (14 cm)
- There is no mechanism of labor
- Diagnosed on P/V by palpating supraorbital ridges and anterior fontanelle
- Delivery is by cesarean section.

BREECH PRESENTATION

- In breech presentation, the lie is longitudinal and the podalic pole presents at the pelvic brim
- It is the commonest malpresentation
- Incidence: The incidence is about 20% at 28th week and drops to 5% at 34th week and to 3–4% at term. Thus in 3 out of 4, spontaneous correction into vertex presentation occurs by 34th week.

Causes of Breech

Causes of Breech Presentation
Most common cause-prematurity.
Other Causes: *Factors preventing spontaneous version:*
- Breech with extended legs
- Twins
- Oligohydramnios
- Congenital malformation of uterus like septate on bicornuate uterus
- Short cord
- IUD of fetus

Favorable adaptation:
  - Hydrocephalus
  - Placenta previa
  - Cornual-fundal attachment of the placenta[Q]
  - Contracted pelvis

Undue mobility of the fetus:
  - Hydramnios[Q]
  - Multipara[Q] with lax abdominal wall

 Also Know:

Recurrent breech: When breech recurs in 3 or more consecutive pregnancies, it is called haibitual or recurrent breech
Causes:
- Congenital malformation of uterus (septate or bicornuate)
- Repeated cornual-fundal attachment of the placenta.

Varieties of Breech

1. **Complete breech/flexed breech:** The normal attitude of full flexion is maintained. The thighs are flexed at the hips and the legs at the knees. The presenting part consists of two buttocks, external genitalia and two feet. It is commonly present in multipara. Overall incidence is 10%. Chances of cord prolapse-6%.

2. **Breech with extended legs (Frank breech):** In this condition, the thighs are flexed on the trunk and the legs are extended at the knee joints. The presenting part consists of the two buttocks and external genitalia only. It is commonly present in primigravida. Overall incidence is about 70%. Chances of cord prolapse are least (0.5%). The increased prevalence in primigravida is due to tight abdominal wall.

3. **Knee presentation (rare):** Thighs are extended but the knees are flexed, bringing the knees down to present at the brim. Chances of cord prolapse are more in this case, hence in knee presentation cesarean section is preferred.

4. **Footling presentation:** Both the thighs and the legs are partially extended so the feet become the presenting part. Chances of cord prolapse are maximum 12%. In this condition cesarean section has to be done.

Chances of cord prolapse are Maximum in Transverse lie > Footling > Knee prentation breech > Frank > Flexed > Frank breech.

 Note: In case of breech normally the fetal head is flexed, but if head of the fetus is extended, it is called as **Stargazer breech**. Stargazer breech is an indication for doing cesarean section.

Management of Breech

It depends on whether the patient is presenting in antenatal period at ≥ 37 weeks of pregnancy or she is presenting in labor:

If patient presents with breech at >37 weeks external cephalic version can be tried.

External Cephalic Version

- OPD procedure
- No anesthesia needed but recent evidences support use of tocolytics (Terbutaline/Pethidine)—ACOG
- Should be done under continuous fetal monitoring
- Here the breech/transverse lie is tried to rotate per abdominally so that it converts to cephalic

 Prerequisite:
- Period of gestation ≥ 37 weeks (Williams Obs 25th/ ed pg 549)
- Liquor should be adequate
- Membranes should be intact
- There should be no contraindication for vaginal delivery.
- Facility of emergency cesarean section (ACOG 2016a)

Contraindication of ECV

Absolute contraindication

- Placenta previa
- Multifetal pregnancy
- Whenever vaginal delivery is C/I like contracted pelvis

Relative contraindication

- Early labor
- Oligohydramnios
- Rupture of membranes
- Known case of nuchal cord
- Structural uterine abnormalities
- Fetal growth restriction
- Prior assumption on its risks Previous cesarean section

Complications of ECV

- Fetal compromise
- Placental abruption

Chances of emergency cesarean section with ECV = 0.5%

If patient comes in late labor or if external cephalic version is unsuccessful/contraindicated:

In this case there are 3 options:
1. Assisted breech delivery
2. Breech extraction
3. Cesarean section

1. Assisted Breech Delivery

- Vaginal delivery can be done in breech only if Zatuchni-Andros score is > 4.
- If it is < 4, then cesarean delivery is indicated.
- In assisted breech delivery, vaginal delivery of breech is allowed to progress and at whichever stage, breech gets stuck, the obstetrician performs some maneuver to deliver that part.

Mechanism of Labor in Breech

- Lie-longitudinal
- Presentation-podalic
- Denominator-sacrum
- M/C position-left sacroanterior.

General Principles in Breech Delivery

- Labor should be carried out in specialized units
- Induction of labor is best avoided
- In prolonged second stage, it is not advisable to rupture membranes due to the risk of cord prolapse and not by oxytocin also because strong contractions produced by oxytocin can cause descent of soft breech even if there is fetopelvic disproportion, with resultant difficulties in delivery of head
- Delay in first or second stage is regarded as a sign of feto-pelvic disproportion and requires cesarean section.

Delivery of Breech Occurs at 3 Levels

1. **Delivery of Buttocks:** The diameter of engagement of the **buttock is one of the oblique diameters of the inlet**. The engaging diameter is bitrochanteric (10 cm).

- Always give episiotomy in breech.
- The best time for episiotomy is when the perineum is distendedand thinned by the breech as it is 'climbing' the perineum.
- If buttocks do not deliver spontaneously-the maneuver used by obstetricians are:
  - **Groin traction (Fig. 11.4)**
  - **Pinard maneuver (Figs. 11.5A to C)**—used for delivery of extended legs. In Pinard maneuver, the middle and the index fingers are carried up to the popliteal fossa (Remember P for pinard, P for popliteal fossa). It is then pressed and abducted so that the fetal leg is flexed. The fetal foot is then grasped at the ankle and leg delivered.

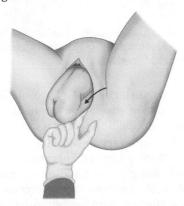

Fig. 11.4: Delivery of the extended leg by abduction at the knee

- Soon after the trunk up to the umbilicus is born
- The umbilical cord is now to be pulled down and mobilized to one side of the sacral bay to minimize compression

---

- To prevent cord from shrivelling—Wrap the baby in warm towel after delivery of body and before delivery of head-this is called as **Savage technique**.

---

2. **Delivery of Shoulders:**

- The engaging diameter is bisacromial diameter (12 cm).
- **Shoulder engages in the same oblique diameter as that occupied by the buttocks** at the brim soon after the delivery of the breech
- If the shoulders do not deliver spontaneously because of the extended arms or nuchal displacement of arms **Lovset maneuver** is done where using femoro-pelvic grip, the trunk of the baby is rotated so that shoulders occupy anteroposterior diameter of the pelvis **(Figs. 11.6A to C)**.

3. **Delivery of after-coming head of breech:**

- **Engagement occurs through the opposite oblique diameter as that occupied by the buttocks**

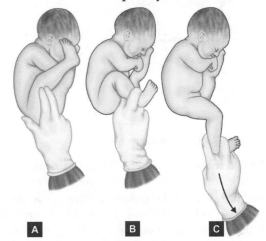

Figs. 11.5A to C: Pinard's maneuver—(A) Flexion and abduction of popliteal fossa; (B) To catch, hold the ankle; (C) To pull down by movement of abduction

- The engaging diameter of the head is suboccipitofrontal (10 cm)
- This is the most important stage of delivery. Not more than 10 minutes (preferably) should elapse between delivery of umbilicus and head to reduce the chances of fetal sphyxia
- **Maneuvers used for delivery of after-coming head are**
  - **Burns-Marshall technique**—Let baby hang by its weight. The assistant gives suprapubic pressure with every contaction in downward and backward direction

(kristeller maneuver) and then the obstetrician takes the feet towards mother's abdomen. It is the most commonly used method (Figs. 11.7A and B).

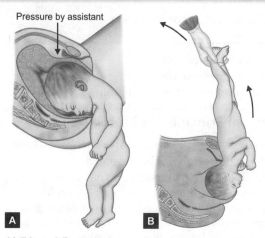

Figs. 11.7A and B: (A) Delivery of after-coming head by Burns-Marshall method; (B) Continuation of the Burns-Marshall method

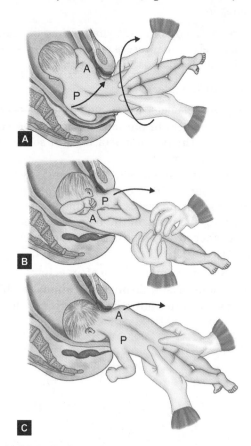

Figs. 11.6A to C: Lovset's maneuver

– **Bracht maneuver**—Do not let the baby hang by its weight, rest same as Burn-Marshall method
– **Malar flexion and shoulder traction—Mauriceau-Smellie-veit technique (Figs. 11.8A and B)**—The baby is placed on the supinated left forearm (preferred) with the limbs hanging on either sides. The middle and index fingers of the left hand are placed over the malar bones on either sides (modification of the original method where the index finger was introduced inside the mouth). This maintains flexion of the head. The ring and little fingers of the pronated right hand are placed on the child's right shoulder, the index finger is placed on the left shoulder and the middle finger is placed on the suboccipital region. Traction is now given in downward and backward direction till the nape of the neck is visible under the pubic arch. The assistant gives suprapubic pressure during the period to maintain flexion.

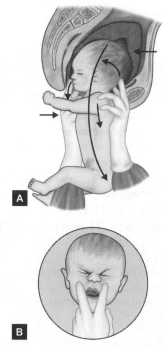

Figs. 11.8A and B: Delivery of the after-coming head by malar flexion and shoulder traction—(A) Original Mauriceau-Smellie-Veit; (B) Modification (preferred)

– **Wigand-Martin technique**—Here one finger in baby mouth and 2 on cheeks and no shoulder traction is given just suprapubic pressure is used.
• **Forceps**: Any ordinary mid cavity forceps like **Das forceps** or **Neville Barney Forceps** can be used for delivery of after-coming head of breech. There are specially designed forceps—**Pipers forceps** (with absent pelvic curve) for this purpose, but usually they are not available in India.

Complications of Breech

Maternal	Fetal
• Genital tract laceration	• Prematurity
• Extension of episiotomy	• Increased risk of congenital anomalies
• Perineal tear	• Umbilical cord prolapse
	• Birth tranova including fracture of clavicle, humerus and femur
	• Brachial plexus injury
	• Hematoma of sternocleidomastoid
	• Genital injury
	• Some complications are inherent to breech position rather than breech delivery—e.g. dysplasia of hip is most common in breech than cephalic presentation

Also Know:

Sometimes in breech presentation, the after-coming head rotates posteriorly. So that the face is behind the pubis, this condition is difficult to deliver and is called Chin to pubis rotation. **Prague maneuver** is used for delivery of occipito-posterior of head in breech.

2. Breech Extraction

- When part or the entire body of the fetus is extracted by the obstetrician under general anesthesia without any effort by the patient it is called breech extraction.
- It is rarely done these days as it produces trauma to the fetus and the mother.
- Its only indication is delivery of the second twin if it is transverse lie and internal podalic version is successful.

3. Cesarean Section

The rates of term breech vaginal delivery are decreasing as more and more studies are showing that planned cesarean delivery is associated with lower risk of perinatal mortality compared to planed vaginal delivery. As it is in preterm breech we prefer cesaran. So overall cesarean is being done for Breech

Factors Favouring Elective Cesarean in Breech

- Footling/knee presentation
- Stargazer breech
- Preterm breech (here external cephalic version is avoided. Cesarean delivery is usually performed when fetal weight is <2500 gm)
- The SOGC committee states that vaginal breech delivery is reasonable if weight of fetus > 2500g
- Breech with baby weight more than 3.8 to 4 kg
- Twin with first breech
- Breech with previous cesarean
- Breech with any other complication of pregnancy—Placenta previa, PIH
- Breech score 3 or less

- Breech with postmaturity >40 weeks as induction of labor is best avoided.
- Primi with breech-**relative indication**.

Indications for emergency cesarean section

- Prolonged first or second stage of labor
- Cord prolapse
- Fetal distress
- If footling or knee presentation are detected during labor

TRANSVERSE LIE

- Lie-transverse
- Presentation—shoulder
- When the long axis of the fetus lies perpendicularly to the maternal spine or centralized uterine axis, it is called transverse lie. But more commonly, the fetal axis is placed oblique to the maternal spine and is then called oblique lie.
- The position is determined by the direction of the back which is the denominator. The position may be:
  - **Dorsoanterior** which is the commonest (60%)
  - **Dorsoposterior**.
- The incidence is about 1 in 200 births

- M/c cause—prematurity > platypelloid pelvis > multiparity

- Other causes are—twins—(it is more common for the second baby than the first one to be in transverse position), hydramnios, contracted pelvis, placenta previa, pelvic tumor, congenital malformation of the uterus—arcuate or subseptate
- No mechanism of labor
- **Diagnosis:**
  - The fundal height is less than the period of amenorrhea
  - Fundal grip—Fetal pole (breech or head) is not palpable
  - Pelvic grip—The lower pole of the uterus is found empty. This, however, is evident only during pregnancy but during labor, it may be occupied by the shoulder
  - During labor on P/V examination—The characteristic landmarks are the feeling of the ribs and intercostal

spaces **(grid iron feel)**. On occasion, the arm is found prolapsed.

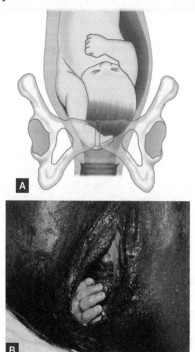

Figs. 11.9A and B: Compound presentation. (A) The left hand is lying in front of the vertex. With further labor, the hand and arm may retract from the birth canal, and the head may then descend normally; (B) Photograph of a small 34-week fetus with a compound presentation that delivered uneventfully with the hand presenting first.

> *Note:* It should be remembered that the findings of a prolapsed arm is confined not only to transverse lie but it may also be associated with compound presentation.

- Determination of position: The thumb of the prolapsed hand, when supinated, points toward the head, the palm corresponds to the ventral aspect.

Management

- Management of transverse lie or shoulder presentation is always cesarean, whether baby alive or dead

> *Note:* With cesarean delivery, because neither feet nor head of fetus occupies lower uterine segment a low transverse increase may lead to difficult extraction hence vertical hysterectomy incision is preferred

- If it recognized in pregnancy—External Cephalic Version can be tried.

> *Note:* In modern day obstetrics, destructive procedures are not done for managing transverse lie. Earlier the destructive procedure done for transverse lie were— decapitation and evisceration.

Twin with Transverse Lie

- If first twin is transverse lie—management is cesarean section
- If second twin is transverse lie—First twin is delivered by vaginal delivery and then general anesthesia given to mother in OT followed by internal podalic version to make the fetus breech. Then breech is delivered by breech extraction.

Corpora conduplicata: If fetus is less than 800 gm, preterm and IUD—spontaneous expulsion can occur as thoracic wall below the shoulder appears at the vulva. Then head and thorax pass through the cavity and fetus is expelled by doubling up.

> *Remember: With transverse lie > Footling > knee presentation*

Guidelines for the Management of Transverse Lie

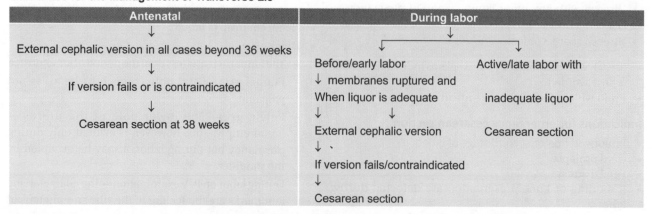

Antenatal	During labor
↓	↓ ↓
External cephalic version in all cases beyond 36 weeks	Before/early labor Active/late labor with
↓	↓ membranes ruptured and
If version fails or is contraindicated	When liquor is adequate inadequate liquor
↓	↓ ↓
Cesarean section at 38 weeks	External cephalic version Cesarean section
	↓
	If version fails/contraindicated
	↓
	Cesarean section

UNSTABLE LIE

This is a condition where the presentation of the fetus is constantly changed even beyond 36th week of pregnancy when it should have been stabilized.

Causes

The causes are those which prevent the presenting part to remain fixed in the lower pole of the uterus:

- Grand multipara (commonest cause)
- Polyhydramnios
- Contracted pelvis
- Placenta previa
- Pelvic tumor.

 Note: Oligohydramnios and uterine malformations can lead to malpresentations but not unstable lie.

Management

The patient is to be admitted at 37th completed week. Premature or early rupture of the membranes with cord prolapse is the real danger.

Treatment: Elective cesarean section is done in majority of the cases.

 Note: M/C cause of fetal death in unstable lie is cord prolapse.

Stabilizing induction of labor: External cephalic version is done (if not contraindicated) after 37 weeks → oxytocin infusion is started to initiate effective uterine contractions. This is followed by low rupture of the membranes (amniotomy). Labor is monitored for successful vaginal delivery. This procedure may be done even after the spontaneous onset of labor.

CORD PROLAPSE

Cord Prolapse: Cord prolapse is the condition where the umbilical cord lies below the presenting part after rupture of membranes.

- **In cord presentation**, the membranes are intact
- **In occult cord prolapse,** the cord is by the side of the presenting part, but not felt by the examining fingers

Maximum chances of cord prolapse are with—Transverse lie> footling> knee> complete breech>frank breech

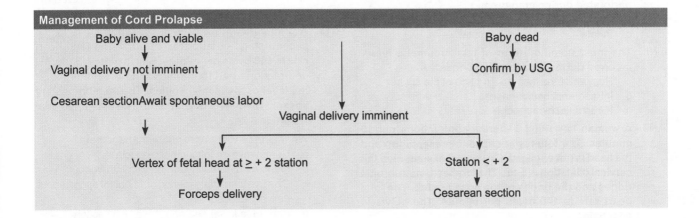

Management of Cord Prolapse

Baby alive and viable → Vaginal delivery not imminent → Cesarean sectionAwait spontaneous labor

Baby dead → Confirm by USG

Vaginal delivery imminent → Vertex of fetal head at ≥ + 2 station → Forceps delivery

Station < + 2 → Cesarean section

New Pattern Questions

N1. In deep transverse arrest, all of the following can be done *except:*
  a. Cesarean section   b. Vacuum extraction
  c. Kielland forceps   d. Wrigley's forceps

N2. In case of IVD with transverse are, following can be done *except*:
  a. Decapitation   b. Evisceration
  c. Craniotomy   d. Cesarean section

N3. Face to pubis delivery occurs in which position?
  a. Occipito sacral position
  b. Mentoanterior
  c. Mentoposterior   d. Blow presentation

N4. Least chances of cord prolapse are seen with:
  a. Frank breech   b. Complete breech
  c. Footling   d. Knee

N5. In left oblique breech presentation, head engages in:
  a. Right oblique diameter
  b. Left oblique
  c. Right transverse   d. Left transverse

N6. In transverse lie, the presentation is:
  a. Vertex   b. Breech
  c. Brow   d. Shoulder

N7. In an after-coming head the following bone is perforated during craniotomy:
  a. Occiput   b. Parietal
  c. Palate   d. Frontal

N8. The most common form of fetal traumatic injury incurred during breach extraction is:
  a. Rupture of the liver b. Rupture of the spleen
  c. Intraadrenal hemorrhage
  d. Intracranial hemorrhage

N9. A woman is getting 3 uterine contractions per 10 minutes. The fetus is in cephalic presentation and the head is not engaged. On vaginal examination the cervical dilatation is 5 cm. The forehead, supraorbital ridges and the bridge of the nose are felt. The fetal heart rate is 140 beats per minute. The pelvis is adequate.

What is the most appropriate treatment?
  a. Allow labor to continue without interference for 4 hours
  b. Carryout manual rotation of the head after full dilatation of the cervix
  c. Perform a cesarean section as soon as possible
  d. Perform an amniotomy and commence an oxytocin infusion

N10. ECV is absolutely contraindicated in all *except:*
  a. Previous LSCS scar
  b. Severe preeclampsia
  c. Placenta previa   d. Septate uterus

N11. A multipara is admitted to the ward at a period of amenorrhea of 40 weeks. The uterus is relaxed and there are no uterine contractions. The fetus is in the transverse lie. The cervical os is closed. She has no other pregnancy complications. The ultrasound scan does not reveal any other abnormalities and the cardiotocography is normal.

What is the most appropriate management?
  a. Perform a lower segment cesarean section
  b. Perform an external cephalic version soon after onset of labor
  c. Perform an external cephalic version immediately
  d. Perform an internal version during the second stage of labor

N12. A second para is admitted in advanced labor at a period of amenorrhea of 40 weeks. She has a single fetus in the transverse lie. The fetal heart beat is absent. On vaginal examination the cervix is fully dilated. The presenting part is the shoulder.

What is the most appropriate management?
  a. Await spontaneous delivery of the dead fetus
  b. Perform a cesarean section immediately
  c. Perform a decapitation operation
  d. Perform an external cephalic version

N13. A primipara with a breech presentation is in the second stage of labor for 2 hours. The fetal heart rate is 140 beats per minute. She is getting 3 uterine contractions per 10 minutes. The breech is felt at the level of the ischial spines. The membranes are absent. The pelvis is adequate. The estimated fetal weight is 3 kg.

What is the most appropriate management?
  a. Commence an infusion of oxytocin
  b. Improve maternal hydration with intravenous fluids
  c. Observe for a further period of 1 hour for spontaneous delivery to occur
  d. Perform a lower segment cesarean section

N14. A 40-year-old primipara who has been infertile for 12 years attends the antenatal clinic of 37 weeks. The fetus is in breech presentation. The estimated fetal weight is 3 kg. The pregnancy is otherwise uncomplicated. The pelvis is adequate.

What is the best management option?
  a. Await spontaneous onset of labor and normal vaginal delivery
  b. Perform a cesarean section at 39 weeks
  c. Perform a cesarean section, if labor becomes prolonged
  d. Perform an external cephalic version

N15. A 28-year-old primipara attends the antenatal clinic at a period of amenorrhea of 35 weeks. She has a single fetus in breech presentation. Ultrasound scan confirms breech presentation. No other abnormalities are detected. She is 5' 3" in height. Her pregnancy is otherwise uncomplicated.

What is the next step in the management?
a. Allow a normal vaginal delivery
b. Induce labor, if not delivered by 41 weeks
c. Perform an elective cesarean section at 39 weeks
d. Perform an external cephalic version at 36 weeks

N16. A 30-year-old G1P1001 patient comes to see you in office of 37 weeks gestational age for her routine OB visit. Her 1st pregnancy resulted in a vaginal delivery of a 9-lb, 8-oz baby boy after 30 minutes of pushing. On doing Leopold maneuvers during this office visit, you determine that the fetus is breech. Vaginal examination demonstrate that the cervix is 50% effaced and 1–2 cm dilated. The presenting breech is high out of pelvis. The estimated fetal weight is about 7 lb. you send the patient for a USG which confirms a fetus with a frank breech prestation. There is a normal amount of amniotic fluid present, and the head is well-flexed. As the patient's obstetrician, you offer all the following possible management plans *except*:
a. Allow the patient to undergo a vaginal breech delivery whenever she goes into labor
b. Send the patient to labor and delivery immediately for an emergent LSCS
c. Schedule a LSCS at or after 39 weeks gestation age
d. Schedule an external cephalic version in next few days

N17. In a case of direct occipito-posterior position (face to pubis delivery) most commonly encountered problem is:
a. Intracranial injury   b. Cephalhematoma
c. Paraurethral tears   d. Complete perineal tears

N18. Deep transverse arrest is seen in all *except*:
a. Android pelvis   b. Epidural analgesia
c. Transverse lie   d. Uterine inertia

N19. A 30-years-old primipara in labor with transverse lie. Treatment of choice is:
a. Internal cephalic version
b. Emergency cesarean section
c. Wait and watch
d. External cephalic version

N20. The complications of shoulder presentations are all of the following *except*:
a. Fetal death   b. Uterine rupture
c. Obstructed labor   d. Shoulder dystocia

N21. In case of unstable lie of fetus, the placenta is usually:
a. Cornual   b. Lateral wall
c. Fundus   d. Placenta in lower segment

N22. The following statements are related to occipito-posterior *except*:
a. Malrotation of occiput may cause occipito acral arrest
b. 10% cases are associated with anthropoid-or android pelvis
c. Incomplete forward rotation of occiput may cause deep transverse arrest
d. Nonrotation of occiput may cause are associated

N23. The following are related to face presentation *except*:
a. The commonest position is LMA
b. Engaging diameter is submentobregmatic
c. The diameter distending the vulval outlet is mentovertical
d. During moulding, there is elongation of occipitofrontal diameter

N24. In which fetal presentation vaginal delivery can be expected?
a. Face presentation when the chin lies direct to the sacrum
b. Brow presentation
c. Shoulder presentation
d. Face presentation when the chin lies under the symphysis pubis

N25. For the deep transverse arrest all are correct *except*:
a. Head is deep into the pelvic cavity
b. Sagittal suture lies in the bispinous diameter
c. There is no progress at least for 1 hour following full dilatation of the cervix
d. Delivery should be done by immediate cesarean section

N26. Which of the following is correctly matched in breech delivery?

A.	Lovset's maneuver	1.	After-coming head of breech
B.	Burn-Marshall method	2.	Shoulder delivery
C.	Prague maneuver	3.	OP position head
D.	Groin traction	4.	Delivery of breech

a. A = 3   B = 1   C = 4   D = 2
b. A = 2   B = 1   C = 3   D = 4
c. A = 2   B = 1   C = 4   D = 3
d. A = 3   B = 1   C = 2   D = 4

N27. Procedure to be performed in the case of arrest of after-coming head due to contracted pelvis in breech:
a. Craniotomy   b. Decapitation
c. Zavanelli maneuver   d. Cleidotomy

Previous Year Questions

1. **The commonest cause of breech presentation is:** [AIIMS May 03, AI 97]
   a. Prematurity b. Hydrocephalus
   c. Placenta previa d. Polyhydramnios

2. **All of the following are associated with breech presentation at normal full-term pregnancy, *except*:**
   a. Placenta accreta [AI 02]
   b. Fetal malformation
   c. Uterine anomaly
   d. Cornual implantation of placenta

3. **Causes of breech presentation are:** [PGI June 03]
   a. Hydrocephalus b. Oligohydramnios
   c. Pelvic contracture d. Placenta previa

4. **Best method to deliver arms in breech:** [PGI June 98]
   a. Lovset's method b. Smellie-Veit
   c. Pinard's maneuver d. Any of the above

5. **The after-coming head of breech, chin to pubis is delivered by:** [PGI Dec 98]
   a. Maricelli technique
   b. Burns-Marshall method
   c. Lovest's method
   d. Manual rotation and extraction by Piper's forceps

6. **Techniques of delivery of after-coming head in breech presentation:** [PGI June 07]
   a. Burns-Marshall method
   b. Forceps delivery
   c. Modified Mauriceau-Smellie-Veit technique
   d. Lovset's maneuver

7. **After-coming head of breech will have difficulty in delivery in all of the following conditions *except*:** [AIIMS Nov 06, Nov 03, Nov 11]
   a. Hydrocephalus b. Placenta previa
   c. Incomplete dilation of cervix
   d. Extension of head

8. **Cause of death in breech delivery:** [PGI 97]
   a. Intracranial hemorrhage
   b. Aspiration
   c. Atlantoaxial dislocation
   d. Asphyxia

9. **True about Frank breech:** [PGI Dec 02]
   a. Thigh extended, leg extended
   b. Thigh flexed, knee extended
   c. Both are flexed
   d. Buddha's attitude e. Common in primi

10. **Breech presentation with hydrocephalus is managed by:** [PGI June 02]
    a. Cesarean section
    b. Transabdominal decompression
    c. PV decompression
    d. Craniotomy of after-coming head

11. **In deep transverse arrest the delivery of baby is conducted by:** [PGI Dec 99]
    a. Cesarean section b. Vacuum extraction
    c. Keilland forcep
    d. Manual rotation and forcep delivery

12. **38 weeks primi in early labor with transverse presentation, TOC is:** [PGI Dec 98]
    a. Allow for cervical dilatation
    b. Internal podalic version
    c. LSCS d. Forceps

13. **A 30 years old multigravida presented with transverse lie with hand prolapse in IInd stage of labor with dead fetus. The treatment is:** [PGI June 03]
    a. Chemical cesarean section
    b. LSCS c. Craniotomy
    d. Decapitation e. Cleidotomy

14. **M/C type of breech presentation:**
    a. Frank breech b. Complete breech
    c. Footling d. Knee

15. **The commonest cause of occipito-posterior position of fetal head during labor is:** [AIIMS May 03]
    a. Maternal obesity b. Deflexion of fetal head
    c. Multiparity d. Android pelvis

16. **When in labor, a diagnosis of occipito-posterior presentation is made. The most appropriate management would be:** [AIIMS May 08/Nov 09]
    a. Emergency CS
    b. Wait and watch for progress of labor
    c. Early rupture of membranes
    d. Start oxytocin drip

17. **Causes of face presentation:** [PGI Dec 03]
    a. Anencephaly b. Prematurity
    c. Hydramnios d. Contracted pelvis
    e. Placenta previa

18. **Which favor face presentation?** [PGI Dec 09]
    a. Anencephaly b. Contracted pelvis
    c. Placenta praevia d. Thyroid swelling
    e. Bicornuate uterus

19. **On per vaginal examination, anterior fontanelle and supraorbital ridge is felt in the second stage of labor. The presentation is:** [AIIMS May 02]
    a. Brow presentation b. Deflexed head
    c. Flexed head d. Face presentation

20. Diameter of engagement in face presentation/ diameter in face presentation:
    a. Mentovertical   [PGI June 02, Dec 00, MP 08]
    b. Submentovertical
    c. Suboccipitobregmatic
    d. Submentobregmatic
    e. Suboccipitovertical

21. In brow presentation, presenting diameter (s) is/are:
                                    [PGI June 03]
    a. Submentovertical
    b. Occipitofrontal
    c. Mentovertical
    d. Suboccipitobregmatic
    e. Suboccipitofrontal

22. A multigravida with previous 2 normal deliveries presents with unstable lie of the fetus at 34 weeks gestation. What could be the most probable cause?
                                    [AIIMS Nov 12]
    a. Placenta previa   b. Oligohydramnios
    c. Uterine anomaly   d. Pelvic tumor

23. ECV is contraindicated in: [AI 07, RJ 08]
    a. Primi   b. Flexed breech
    c. Anemia   d. PIH

24. On external cephalic version, fetal bradycardia occurred. The next course of action is: [AP 97]
    a. Reversion to the original position immediately by external version
    b. Internal podalic version
    c. Cesarean section
    d. Rupture of the membranes

25. The complication that can occur with internal podalic version for transverse lie: [AI 08, AIIMS Nov 07]
    a. Uterine rupture   b. Uterine atony
    c. Cervical laceration d. Vaginal alceration

26. True about breech delivery:
    a. Vasa previa is a complication
    b. Fetal congenital malformation increases breech risk
    c. Increases fetal and maternal morbidity
    d. Oligohydramnios increases breech risk
    e. Increase risk of hip joint dislocation of baby

Answers with Explanations to New Pattern Questions

N1. **Ans. is d, i.e. Wrigleys forceps**

As discussed in the chapter, Deep Transverse Arrest occurs at the level of ischial spine and hence it cannot be managed by Wrigleys forceps which is an outlet forceps basically and forceps cannot rotate the head of body except Kielland forceps Rest all options can be done in DTA, i.e.

- Cesarean section
- Manual rotation
- Vacuum delivery
- Kielland forceps

N2. **Ans. is c, i.e. Craniotomy**

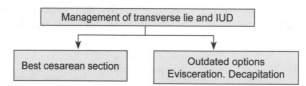

Decapitation:
- Decapitation earlier was done in case of dead fetus in obstructed labor with cephalic presentation (vertex, face or blow)
- After-coming head of breech
- Hydrocephalus even in living fetus

N3. **Ans. is a, i.e. Occipito sacral position**

Face to pubes delivery is done, if in occipito-posterior position, head rotates posteriorly and becomes direct occipito-posterior position.

N4. **Ans. is a, i.e. Frank breech**

Maximum chances of cord prolapse in breech are in footling presentation
Minimum chances of cord prolapse are in frank breech

N5. **Ans. is a, i.e. Right oblique diameter**

Head in breech, engages in opposite oblique diameter as that occupied by the buttocks. Since breech is in Left oblique hence head will engage in Right Oblique diameter

N6. **Ans. is d, i.e. Shoulder**

Presentation in transverse lie is shoulder presentation.

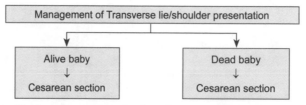

Dead baby in transverse lie with shoulder presentation is called as neglected shoulder presentation.

N7. **Ans. is a, i.e. Occiput**

Ref. Dutta Obs. 9/e, p 544

Craniotomy: It consists of perforating the fetal skull, evacuating the contents and then delivering rest of the fetal parts.

Indication:
- Delivery of a dead fetus in obstructed labor with a cephalic presentation (vertex, brow or face).
- Delivery of the arrested after-coming head in vaginal breech delivery.
- Hydrocephalus

Presenting part	Perforation site
Vertex	One or other parietal bone
Brow	Frontal bone
Face	Orbit or roof of the mouth
After-coming head in breech	Occipital bone

N8. **Ans. is d, i.e. Intracranial hemorrhage**   *Ref. Manual of Holand and Brews 16/e, p 190*

The most frequent single cause of death in breech presentation is intracranial haemorrhage due to tentorial tears, these tears are the result of sudden excessive pressure on the after-coming head and may be aptly described as the snapping of the internal "*grey-ropes*" of the cranium.

N9. **Ans. is c, i.e. Perform a cesarean section as soon as possible**

In the question, on per vaginal examination forehead, supra orbital ridges and bridge of nose are feet, i.e. it is brow presentation.

In Brow presentation, management is always cesarean section.

N10. **Ans is a, i.e. Previous LSCS scar**   *Ref. Fernando Arias 4/e, p 374; William 24/e, p 570*

Absolute Contraindications for ECV:
i.   Placenta previa or recent bleeding
ii. Multiple pregnancies
iii. H/O antepartum hemorrhage
iv. IUGR
v.   Severe preeclampsia and hypertension
vi. Rupture of membranes
vii. Known uterine malformation

> *"Prior uterine incision is a relative contraindication"*   *Ref. William 24/e, p 570*

N11. **Ans. is c, i.e. Perform an external cephalic version immediately**

The patient is presenting at 40 weeks with relaxed uterus with transverse lie.

There is no contraindication to external cephalic version and remember ECV can be done from 36 weeks onward uptil the end of latent phase of 1st stage of labor. So in this case ECV will be done immediately.

N12. **Ans. is b, i.e. Perform a cesarean section immediately**

In this case, patient is presenting in advanced labor with IUD and transverse lie
Management is immediate cesarean section

N13. **Ans. is d, i.e. Perform a lower segment cesarean section**

In the question patient is a primigravida,

She is in 2nd stage of labor for 2 hours with breech, i.e. it is a case of prolonged second stage of labor.

In case of breech, as discussed in the text,

In prolonged second stage, it is not advisable to rupture membranes due to the risk of cord prolapse and not by oxytocin because strong contractions produced by oxytocin can cause descent of soft breech even, if there is fetopelvic disproportion with resultant difficulty in delivery of fetal head.

In case of breech, delay in 1st or 2nd stage is regarded as a sign of fetopelvic disproportion and requires cesarean section.

N14. **Ans. is b, i.e. Perform cesarean section at 39 weeks.**

In this case, pregnancy is very precious as this female has been infertile for 12 years and then conceived, hence ECV should not be done and elective cesarean section should be done at 39 weeks.

N15. **Ans. is d, i.e. Perform an external cephalic version at 36 weeks**

In this female everything is normal, hence we can do ECV at 36 weeks.

N16. **Ans. is b, i.e. Send the patient to labor and delivery immediately for an emergent LSCS**

Now here patient has come for routine antenatal visit during which it was discovered that the fetus is breech.

Points worth noting are:
* Gestational age is 37 weeks.
* On vaginal examination the cervix is 50% effaced and 1-2 cm dilated.
* The presenting breech is high out of pelvis, i.e. it is not engaged and version can be attempted.

- The estimated fetal weight is about 7 lb (i.e. it is not much that vaginal breech delivery cannot be attempted).
- USG confirms fetus is in frank breech position, there is a normal amount of amniotic fluid present, and the head is well-flexed (all factors favoring version and vaginal breech delivery).
- Since patient is 37 weeks pregnant and presenting part is high out of the pelvis, amount of amniotic fluid is adequate so we can attempt external cephalic version and yes since version carries a risk of fetal distress and cesarean section. I will give the patient a chance to discuss with her family members and come back to me in a few days, if she wishes for external cephalic version (i.e. option d is correct).

Another option in this case would be to allow the patient to undergo a vaginal breech delivery whenever she goes into labor, i.e, option a is correct.

Now both version and vaginal breech delivery carry a risk to the fetus, so if patient refuses to take any risk I will advise her to go for an elective cesarean section at or after 39 weeks, but there is no need/indication for an emergency cesarean section immediately and hence option b is the answer.

N17. **Ans. is d, i.e. Complete perineal tears** *Ref. Dutta Obs. 7/e, p 370*

In face to pubis delivery → the most common complication is perineal tear as the occiput is posterior and thus the longer biparietal diameter (9.4 cm) distends the perineum rather than the smaller bitemporal diameter (8 cm). Hence in all such cases liberal episiotomy should be given.

N18. **Ans. is c, i.e. Transverse lie** *Ref. Dutta Obs. 9/e, p 349*

Deep transverse arrest is a complication of occipito-posterior position, how can it occur in transverse lie.

Causes of deep transverse arrest:
- Faulty pelvic architecture – Android pelvis
- Depression of the head
- Weak uterine contractions
- Laxity of pelvic floor muscles:
    - Epidural analgesia causes prolonged 2nd stage of labor.

> *In transverse lie; presenting part is shoulder; so no question of DTA of head.*

N19. **Ans. is b, i.e. Emergency cesarean section** *Ref. Dutta Obs. 9/e, p 372; Williams Obs. 22/e, p 510, 23/e, p 478*
- Patients in labor with transverse lie can be managed by external cephalic version followed by surgical rupture of the membrane.
- But it is important to note that the patient is a primigravida with age 30 years, i.e. elderly primi, so ECV is contraindicated.
- This patient requires an emergency cesarean section.

N20. **Ans. is d, i.e. Shoulder dystocia** *Ref. Dutta Obs. 9/e, p 370*

In neglected shoulder presentation there is a increased fetal loss due to:
- Cord prolapse
- Tonic contraction of uterus/obstructed labor
- Rupture of uterus

Maternal risk is increased due to:
- Dehydration ⎫
                ⎬ due to obstructed labor
- Ketoacidosis ⎭
- Septicemia; rupture uterus; hemorrhage; shock and peritonitis
- Shoulder dystocia is not a complication of neglected shoulder presentation.

N21. **Ans. is d, i.e. Placenta in lower segment** *Ref. Dutta Obs. 9/e, p 372*

Unstable Lie is seen in the placenta previa

N22. **Ans. is b, i.e. 10% cases are associated with anthropoid- or android pelvis** *Ref. Dutta Obs. 9/e, p 343*

All the options given in the question are correct, except – option b

"In more than 50%, the occipito-posterior position is associated with either anthropoid- or android pelvis"

—Dutta Obs 9/e, p 343

N23. **Ans. is c, i.e. The diameter distending the vulval outlet is mentovertical (14 cm)** *Ref. Dutta Obs. 7/e, p 388*

Face presentation:
- **The attitude** of the fetus shows complete flexion of the limbs with extension of the spine. **There is a complete extension of the head** so that the occiput is in contact with the back.

- **The denominator** is mentum.
- **The commonest position is left mento-anterior (LMA).**
- Face presentation present during pregnancy (primary) is rare, while that developing after the onset of labor (secondary) is common. It occurs more frequently seen in multipara (70%), like other malpresentations.
- Most common maternal cause is platypelloid pelvis and most common fetal cause is anencephaly.
- **The diameter of engagement** is the oblique diameter—right in LMA, left in RMA.
- **The engaging diameter of the head** is submentobregmatic 9.5 cm (3 3/4") in fully extended head or submento-vertical 11.5 cm (4 1/2") in partially extended head.
- **Engagement is delayed** because of long distance between the mentum and biparietal plane (7 cm).
- **The head is born by flexion:** (11.5 cm).
- Vaginal delivery is possible in mentoanterior positions but not in persistent mentoposterior.
- In mentoposterior during early stages of labor the policy of wait and watch should be adopted in hope of mentoposterior getting converted to mentoanterior spontaneously. Persistent mentoposterior position is an indication for doing cesarean section.

N24. Ans. is d, i.e. Face presentation when the chin lies under the symphysis pubis   *Ref. Dutta Obs. 9/e, p 365*

Vaginal delivery is not possible in:
- Brow presentation
- Shoulder presentation (transverse lie)
- Mentoposterior presentation of face (i.e. when chin lies directed to sacrum)

In mentoanterior, i.e. when chin lies under the symphysis pubis – vaginal delivery is possible.

N25. Ans. is d, i.e. Delivery should be done by immediate cesarean section   *Ref. Dutta Obs. 7/e, p 372*
In Deep Transverse arrest
- The head is engaged (option a)
- The sagittal suture lies in the transverse bispinous diameter (option b)
- Anterior fontanelle is palpable
- Faulty pelvic architecture
- Now in case DTA, cesarean is not the only option, although it is the best option if obstetrician is not well versed with other techniques.

> *Note:* Operative vaginal delivery for DTA should only be performed by a skilled obstetrician. Otherwise cesarean delivery is always preferred these days.

N26. Ans. is b, i.e. A = 2, B = 1, C = 3, D = 4   *Ref. Dutta Obs. 7/e, p 383, 384*

 Maneuver used in assisted breech delivery:

i. Delivery of head	– Burns-Marshall method[Q]
	– Wigand-Martin maneuver
	– Mauriceau-Smellie-Veit technique[Q]
	– Piper's forceps[Q]
ii. Extended legs	– Pinard's maneuver[Q]
	(Remember: P for popliteal fossa and P for Pinard's maneuver)
iii. Extended arm	– Lovset's method[Q]

Sometimes the head rotates posteriorly so that the face is behind the pubis. Delivery in this position is difficult and *'Prague maneuver'* may be tried.

N27. Ans is c, i.e. Zavanelli maneuver   *Ref. Williams, 24/e, p 567*
The last rescue for entrapped fetal head in term fetus is replacement of the fetus higher into the vagina and uterus followed by cesarean delivery. This is called as Zavanelli maneuver.
In preterm babies, last resort for entrapment of after-coming head of breech is-to give Duhrssen Incisions.

Answers with Explanations to Previous Year Questions

1. **Ans. is a, i.e. Prematurity** *Ref. Dutta Obs. 9/e, p 352*

2. **Ans. is a, i.e. Placenta accreta** *Ref. Dutta Obs. 9/e, p 352*

3. **Ans. is a, c and d, i.e. Hydrocephalus; Pelvic contracture; and Placenta previa** *Ref. Dutta Obs. 9/e, p 352*

   *At 28 weeks of pregnancy, approximately 20% of women have breech presentation. The fetus undergoes spontaneous version usually between 30th and 34th week. This corrects the breech position such that, at term **only 3% of pregnant women** have breech presentation.*

   Any maternal or fetal condition, which prevents this spontaneous version will result in a persistent breech presentation.

   Causes of Breech presentation
   Most common cause-prematurity.
   Incidence of breech at term 3%.
   Other Causes: ***Factors preventing spontaneous version—***
   - Breech with extended legs
   - Twins
   - Oligohydramnios
   - Congenital malformation of uterus like septate or bicornuate
   - Short cord
   - IUD of fetus

Favourable adaptation:	–	Hydrocephalus
	–	Placenta pralevia
	–	Cornual-fundal attachment of the placenta[Q]
	–	Contracted pelvis
Undue mobility of the fetus:	–	Hydramnios[Q]
	–	Multipara[Q] with lax abdominal wall

4. **Ans. is a, i.e. Lovset's method** *Ref. Dutta Obs. 9/e, p 359*

   Assisted Breech Delivery:
   - In breech delivery assistance may be required for:

i. Delivery of head	–	Burns-Marshall method[Q]
	–	Mauriceau-Smellie-Veit method[Q]
	–	**Piper's forceps[Q] or Neville-Barnes forceps**
ii. Extended legs	–	Pinard's maneuver[Q]
		(**Remember:** P for popliteal fossa and P for Pinard maneuver)
iii. Extended arm	–	Lovset's maneuver[Q]

   Sometimes the head rotates posteriorly so, that the face is behind the pubis. Delivery in this position is difficult and *'Prague maneuver'* may be tried.
   Also Know:
   - Best time for episiotomy in breech — Climbing of perineum.
   - Best time for episiotomy in vertex — Crowning of head.

5. **Ans. is d, i.e. Manual rotation and extraction by Piper's forceps**

   Ref. Dutta Obs. 9/e, p 363; Shiela Balakrishnan, p 455; Williams Obs. 22/e, p 578, 579, 23/e, p 537, 538

   - Sometimes in breech presentation, the after-coming head rotates posteriorly so that the face is behind the pubis, this condition is difficult to deliver and is called ***Chin to pubis rotation.***

- In this situation, manual rotation of fetal head and trunk is done as in malar flexion and shoulder traction and then head is delivered with forceps. In case of premature baby, the delivery of head may be completed as face to pubis by reversed malar flexion and shoulder traction (**Prague maneuver**) or by forceps.

6. **Ans. is a, b and c, i.e. Burn-Marshall method; Forceps delivery; and Modified Mauriceau-Smellie-Veit technique**
    Ref. Dutta Obs. 9/e, p 360-361

    Methods of delivery of after-coming head of breech:
    - Burns-Marshall technique
    - Mauriceau-Smellie-Veit technique
    - Piper's forcep or Neville Barnes forceps

     Note: Lovset's method is used for delivery of extended arms in breech.

7. **Ans. is b, i.e. Placenta previa**
    Ref. Williams Obs. 22/e, p 579, 24/e, p 567; Dutta Obs.

    Entrapment of the after-coming head occurs in the case of:
    - *Incompletely dilated cervix*
    - Hydrocephalus
    - *Extended head*/deflexed head
    - Contracted pelvis

    Management:
    - If head of preterm breech entraps—*'Duhrssen's incisions'* are placed over the cervix as descending cervical artery is present here (avoiding the 3 and 9'o clock position).
    - *Increase of full term head of breech*
    - Replacement of the fetus higher into the vagina and uterus followed by cesarean delivery *(Zavanelli maneuver).*

     Also Know:

    Impacted Breech:
    - Inspite of good uterine contractions and complete dilatation of the cervix, the breech fails to descend.
    - This occurs only in extended breech and is usually due to disproportion.
    - Impaction can occur at the inlet, cavity or outlet.
    - If within 30 min of full cervical dilation the breech does not descend and distend the perineum, cesarean section is done regardless of the level of impaction.

8. **Ans. is a, c and d, i.e. Intracranial hemorrhage; Atlantoaxial dislocation; and Asphyxia**
    Ref. Dutta Obs. 9/e, p 379
    - The risk of fetal mortality and morbidity are greatly increased in the vaginal breech delivery.
    - Fetal mortality is least in frank breech and maximum in footling presentation *(as the chances of cord prolapse are more).*
    - Gynecoid-and anthropoid pelvis are favorable for the after-coming head.
    - The fetal risk in multipara is no less than that of primigravida because of increased chances of cord prolapse associated with flexed breech which occurs in multipara.

    The main causes of increased perinatal mortality and morbidity in breech are:
    - Prematurity
    - Increased incidence of congenital anomalies.
    - **Birth asphyxia:**
      - Due to cord prolapse or cord compression.
      - Due to prolonged delivery and delay in the after-coming head.
    - **Birth trauma due to rough handling during delivery and failure to use the femoropelvic grip:**
      - *Intracranial hemorrhage* is due to uncontrolled delivery of the head and rupture of the veins of Galen or tentorial or falx tears. Skull fractures can also occur.
      - Fracture dislocation of cervical vertebra, *atlantoaxial dislocation* and occipital diastasis.
      - Cervical and brachial plexuses injuries including Erb's palsy.
      - Complete transection of the spinal cord.

– Sternocleidomastoid hematoma and later torticollis.
– Rupture of liver and spleen.
– Fracture of femur, clavicle or humerus.
– Damage to the fetal adrenals.
– Traumatised pharynx is due to the obstetrician's finger.

9. **Ans. is b and e, i.e. Thigh flexed, knee extended and Common in primi** *Ref. Dutta Obs. 7/e, p 374, 375*

Breech presentation			
Incomplete breech			*Complete/flexed breech*
Breech with extended legs (Frank breech)	**Footling presentation**	**Knee presentation**	• Full flexion attitude is maintained, the legs are flexed, knees and thighs flexed at hips
• Thighs are flexed on trunk and legs are extended at the knee joint^Q	• Both thighs and legs are partially extended	• Thighs are extended but knees are flexed	• Presenting part consists of two buttocks, external genitalia and feet
• Presenting part consists of two buttocks and external genitalia			• Commonly seen in multipara
• Common in primi^Q			

10. **Ans. is a, b, c and d, i.e. Cesarean section, Transabdominal decompression, PV decompression and Craniotomy of after-coming head** *Ref. Dutta Obs. 7/e, p 586; Williams Obs. 22/e, p 518, 23/e, p 480; Sheila Balakrishnan, p 470*

Management options in case of breech presentation with hydrocephalus.

Cephalocentesis: In this, excessive fluid is removed thereby reducing the fetal head size, allowing vaginal delivery.
—Williams Obs. 22/e, p 518, 23/e, p 480

It can be done:
• **Perabdomen:** A wide bore needle is inserted via the maternal abdomen into the fetal head after emptying the bladder. The transabdominal approach is used successfully in both cephalic and breech presentation.
• **Pervaginal:** With cephalic presentation, as soon as the cervix is dilated upto 3–4 cm, ventricles are tapped trans-vaginally with a wide bore needle. With breech presentation labor is allowed to progress upto delivery of trunk and shoulders. The needle is inserted transvaginally just below the anterior vaginal wall and into the after-coming head through the widened suture line.

Cesarean Section: Recommends all hydrocephalic fetuses should be delivered abdominally, whereas the use of cephalocentesis should be limited to fetuses with severe associated abnormalities. *Williams Obs. 23/e, p 481*

Craniotomy: is recommended, if the obstetrician is well versed with the technique and is applicable for the forecoming (vertex) and the after-coming head (breech) in case of hydrocephalus if fetus is dead.

 Note: In a hydrocephalic fetus if BPD is < 10 cm or, if head circumference is < 36 cm, vaginal delivery may be permitted. *—Williams 23/e, p 480*

11. **Ans. is a, b, c and d, i.e. Cesarean section; Vacuum extraction; Keilland forcep; and Manual rotation and forcep delivery** *Ref. Dutta Obs. 9/e, p 349; Williams 23/e, p 480*

See the text for explanation.

12. Ans. is c, i.e. LSCS *Ref. Dutta Obs. 9/e, p 372*

See the text for explanation

13. Ans. is b and d, i.e. LSCS; and Decapitation *Ref. Dutta Obs. 7/e, p 397, 585-587, Munrokerr 100/e, p 134, 135*

Patient is presenting with transverse lie with hand prolapse, i.e. baby is dead so it should be managed as dead baby with transverse lie.

Management in case of dead baby with transverse lie – Cesarean section even in such cases is much safer in the hands of those who are not conversant with destructive operations. *If the obstetrician is conversant with destructive operation,* decapitation or evisceration is to be done. —*Dutta Obs. 7/e, p 397*

During labor with fetus dead — in transverse lie *"In these circumstances, decapitation with the Blond-Heidler saw is the most appropriate treatment, if the skill exists to carry this out. In regions where there is less experience with such procedures, or where the mother may not accept this management, cesarean section may be preferable."*
—*Murnokerr 100/e, p 134, 135*

> *Note*: If this question is asked in AI/AIIMS where a single option is to be marked — go for option b, i.e. LSCS, because in present day obstetrics there is no role of destructive procedures.

14. Ans is a, i.e. Frank breech *Ref. Fernando Arias 4/e, p 375*

Varieties of breech:

* Complete
* Incomplete:
    - Frank breech (70%)
    - Footling breech
    - Knee breech

15. Ans. is d, i.e. Android pelvis *Ref. Dutta Obs 9/e, p 343*

In more than 50% cases, occipito-posterior position is associated with Anthropoid- or Android pelvis.

> *Remember:*
>
> * M/C cause of OP position — Android pelvis/Deflexed head.
> * All malpresentations are common in multiparous females except occipito-posterior which is common in nulliparous (Primigravida) females.
> * At the onset of labor — 15–20% cases are occipito-posterior
> * At the end of labor — 5% cases are occipitoposterior
> * M/C position in OP = Right is occipito-posterior position.

16. Ans. is b, i.e. Wait and watch for progress of labor
Ref. JB Sharma TB of Obs. p 284, Operative Obs and Gynae by Randhir Puri and Narendra Malhotra 1/e, p 173; Williams Obs 23/e, p 479

Occipito-posterior positions

'Expectant observation is practised initially as given time, most of the malposition will rotate anteriorly and the baby will be born spontaneously' *Ref. JB Sharma Obs. p 284*

"In practice about 5-10% of women admitted in labor with cephalic presentations present with occipito-posterior presentations. Given time and patience, many of these will rotate and get corrected to occipitoanterior position and deliver normally". —*Operative Obs and Gynae 1/e, p 173, Randhir Puri and Narendra Malhotra*

This explains that a careful wait and watch policy should be adopted for occipito-posterior position.

17. Ans. is a, b and d, i.e. Anencephaly, Prematurity; and Contracted pelvis *Ref. Dutta Obs. 9/e, p 364*

18. Ans is a, b and d, i.e. Anencephaly, Contracted pelvis and Thyroid Swelling *Ref. Dutta Obs. 9/e, p 364*

I know it is difficult to mug up the causes of different malpresentations. To help you out I am telling you an easy way to remember the causes of face presentation.

Causes of Face presentation:
 A. **Causes similar in face and breech presentation:**

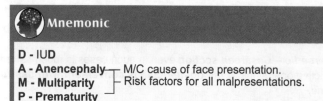

> **Mnemonic**
>
> **D - IUD**
> **A - Anencephaly** — M/C cause of face presentation.
> **M - Multiparity** — Risk factors for all malpresentations.
> **P - Prematurity**

 B. **Causes related to neck:**
 – **T**umor of neck (congenital branchocele, congenital goiter).
 – **T**wist of the cord round the neck.
 – Increased **t**one of extensor group of neck muscles.
 C. **Other causes:**
 – Lateral obliquity of uterus.
 – Platypelloid pelvis.

> *Remember*:
>
> • Most common congenital anomaly associated with face presentation is Anencephaly.[Q]
> • M/C cause of face presentation— Anencephaly.
> • M/C pelvis associated with face presentation — Platypelloid pelvis.

19. **Ans. is a, i.e. Brow presentation**   *Ref. Dutta Obs. 9/e, p 367*

Palpation on per vaginal examination	Presentation
• Occiput and posterior fontanelle (Anterior fontanelle not felt easily)	Vertex (Occipitoanterior position)
• Both fontanelle felt easily	Vertex (Occipito-posterior position)
• Anterior fontanelle (bregma) is felt at one end and root of nose (nasion) and orbital ridges at the other end of an oblique or transverse diameter	Brow
• Mouth with hard alveolar margins with nose, malar eminence, superior orbital ridges and mentum	Face

> *Also Know:*
> Face and Breech are often confused on palpation

On palpation, difference between face and breech presentations:

Face	Breech
• Mouth and malar eminences form a triangle	• Ischial tuberosities and anus are in a line
• Alveolar margins hard	• Anal margins soft
• Sucking effect of mouth	• Grip of anal sphincter
• No meconium staining	• Meconium staining on finger

20. **Ans. is b and d, i.e. Submentovertical; and Submentobregmatic**   *Ref. Dutta Obs. 7/e, p 389*

Presentation	Engaging Diameter
• Vertex (occipito anterior) • Occipito-posterior	• Suboccipitobregmatic • Suboccipito frontal (deflexed head) • Occipito frontal (further deflexed head)
• Face	• Submentovertical (partially extended head) • Submentobregmatic (in fully extended head)
• Brow	• Mentovertical

• Breech
  – Of breech
  – Of shoulder
  – Of head
	•
	• Bitrochanteric
	• Bisacromial
	• Suboccipito frontal

21. Ans. is c, i.e. Mentovertical   *Ref. Dutta Obs. 7/e, p 392*

Brow Presentation:
- Causes of brow presentation are same as for face presentation.
- Most common cause – Flat pelvis/Platypelloid pelvis.
- Engaging diameter – Mentovertical (14 cm).
- There is no mechanism of labor.
- Diagnosed on P/V by palpating supraorbital ridges and anterior fontanelle.
- Delivery is by cesarean section.

22. Ans. is a, i.e. Placenta previa   *Ref. Dutta Obs. 7/e, p 397*
- The presenting female is multipara with previous 2 normal deliveries and unstable lie.
- Lie refers to the relationship between the longitudinal axis of the fetus to that of the mother which may be longitudinal transverse or oblique.
- Unstable lie refers to the frequent changing of fetal lie and presentation even beyond 36th week of pregnancy.

Contributing factors:
- Grand multipara (M/C cause)
- **Placenta previa**
- Polyhydramnios   — Prevent engagements
- Pelvic inlet contracture and/or fetal macrosomia
- Pelvic tumors
- Uterine abnormalities (e.g. bicornuate uterus or uterine fibroids)
- Fetal anomaly (e.g. tumors of the neck or sacrum, hydrocephaly, abdominal distension).

Coming to the question- patient is a multigravida with previous 2 normal deliveries:
- As history of normal delivery is present, it rules out uterine anomaly.
- There are no signs and symptoms suggestive of pelvic tumor.
- Oligohydramnios does not cause unstable lie, it is caused by polyhydramnios.
- Thus in this patent most probable cause of unstable lie is placenta previa.

 Note: M/C cause of fetal death in unstable lie is cord prolapse.

23. Ans. is d. i.e. PIH   *Ref. Williams Obs 24/e, p 185*
See explanations of Q N10

24. Ans. is a, i.e. Reversion to the original position immediately by external version   *Ref. Dutta Obs. 9/e, p 542*
External cephalic version:
Is done to bring favorable cephalic pole in the lower pole of uterus.

Indications:
- Breech presentation
- Transverse lie

Procedure:
- The maneuver is carried out on or after 37 weeks under the effect of Terbutaline 0.25 mg SC or Isoxsuprine 50–100 µg IV. **Ultrasound** examination is done to confirm the diagnosis and adequacy of amniotic fluid volume. A reactive NST should precede the maneuver[Q]. Then ECV is attempted followed by a repeat NST after the procedure.
- A reactive NST should be obtained after completing the procedure[Q]. There may be undue bradycardia due to head compression which is expected to settle down by 10 minutes. If however, fetal bradycardia persists, the possibility of cord entanglement should be kept in mind and in such cases reversion is done.
- If version is successful the patient is observed for 30 minutes -
  - To allow for the fetal heart rate to settle down to normal.

If even after reversion, fetal distress persists—cesarean should be done.

25. Ans. is a, i.e. Uterine rupture   *Ref. Dutta Obs. 9/e, p 543, Munrokerr 100/e, p 292*

Internal podalic version (IPV):
- In modern obstetrics, there is no place for this procedure in a singleton pregnancy.
- Internal podalic version **is only used for the second twin when it is lying transversely and external version fails**[Q].

Prerequisites for IPV:
- The membranes should be intact or very recently ruptured in other words liquor should be adequate.
- The cervix should be fully dilated.
- Fetus must be living.

Anesthesia: General anesthesia[Q] (halothane).

Contraindications:
- Obstructed labor[Q]
- Membranes ruptured with all the liquor drained
- Previous cesarean section even if it is LSCS.
- Contracted pelvis.

Complications:

Maternal	Fetal
Placental abruption	Asphyxia
Rupture uterus	Cord prolapse
Increase morbidity	Intracranial hemorrhage

26. Ans. is b,c,d and e, i.e. Fetal congenital malformation increases breech risk, Increases fetal and maternal morbidity, Oligohydramnios increases breech risk, Increase risk of hip joint dislocation of baby

Ref. Williams Obs. 25/e, pg 542

See the text for explanation.

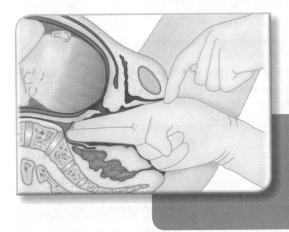

Chapter 12

Obstructed Labor and Intrauterine Death (IUD)

Chapter at a Glance

➤ Obstructed Labor
➤ Rupture Uterus

➤ Intrauterine Fetal Death (IUD)

OBSTRUCTED LABOR

Obstructed labor is one where in spite of good uterine contractions, the progressive descent of the presenting part is arrested due to mechanical obstruction. This may result either due to factors in the fetus or in the birth canal or both, so that further progress is almost impossible without assistance.

Incidence

In the developing countries, the prevalence is about 1–2% in the referral hospitals.

Causes

- **Fault in the passage:** Cephalopelvic disproportion and contracted pelvis are the common causes, cervical or broad ligament fibroid, impacted ovarian tumor.
- **Fault in the passenger:** Transverse lie, brow presentation, congenital malformations of the fetus—hydrocephalus (most common), fetal ascites, big baby, occipito-posterior position.

Clinical Feature

The mother is exhausted, dehydrated, tachypneic and acidotic breathing is present.

Per Abdominally

- Lower uterine segment is stretched
- The upper uterine segment is contracted tonically
- A Ring will be felt per abdominally called as **Bandl's ring (Retraction ring)**

- **Fetal heart sounds:** Fetal-distress or fetal heart sounds are absent as fetus might be dead.

Per Vaginally

- Dry, hot vagina
- Offensive purulent vaginal discharge may be present
- Fresh per vaginal bleeding present
- Caput/moulding may be seen
- The urethra is pressed between symphysis pubis and fetal head with inability to pass urine causing bladder distension. There may be hematuria due to hyperemia and trauma to bladder.

Obstructed labor is the most common cause of vesico-vaginal fistula in developing countries.

Prevention

Partographic management of labor and timely intervention can prevent it.

Management

- Resuscitation of the patient
  - Correction of dehydration and ketoacidosis
  - Antibiotics given

The two most important principles in management of obstructed labor are:

1. Never wait and watch in obstructed labor as it can lead to uterine rupture.
2. Never give oxytocin in obstructed labor

Obstetric management is always cesarean section whether fetus is dead or alive.

 Note: At cesarean section, it is essential to exclude rupture uterus.
Continuous bladder drainage must be done for atleast 10 days to prevent formation of a vesicovaginal fistula due to pressure necrosis.

 Remember: In obstructed labor, ring seen is Bandl's ring. There is another ring called as Schroeders ring seen in incoordinated uterine action.

	Constriction ring	Retraction ring/Bandl ring
Nature	It is a manifestation of localized incoordinate uterine contraction	It is an end result of tonic uterine contractions and retractions
Cause	Undue irritability of the uterus	Following obstructed labor
Situation	Usually at the junction of upper and lower segment but may occur in other places. Once formed the position does not alter	Always situated at the junction of upper and lower segment The position progressively moves upward
Uterus	Upper segment contracts and retracts with relaxation in between; lower segment remains thick and loose	Upper segment is tonically contracted with no relaxation. The wall becomes thicker; lower segment becomes distended and thinned out
Maternal condition	Almost unaffected unless the labor is prolonged	Features of maternal exhaustion, and sepsis appear
Abdominal examination	a. Uterus feels normal and nontender b. Fetal parts are easily felt c. **Ring is not felt** d. Round ligament is not felt e. FHS is usually present	a. Uterus is tense and tender b. Fetal parts not easily felt c. **Ring is felt** as a groove place obliquely d. Taut and tender round ligaments are felt e. FHS is usually absent
Vaginal examination	a. The lower segment is not pressed by the presenting part b. **Ring is felt** usually above the head c. Features of obstructed labor are absent	a. Lower segment is very much pressed by the presenting part b. **Ring cannot be felt vaginally** c. Features of obstructed labor are present
End result	a. Maternal exhaustion is a late feature	a. Maternal exhaustion and sepsis appear

RUPTURE UTERUS

Disruption in the continuity of all layers of is uterine (endometrium, myometrium and serosa) any time beyond 28 weeks of pregnancy is **called rupture of the uterus**. Small rupture to the wall of the uterus in early months is called perforation either due to instrumental or perforating hydatidiform mole.

There are 2 terms which need to be differentiated: uterine rupture and uterine dehiscence.

- **Uterine rupture/complete rupture:** All layers of the uterine wall give way. The fetus lies in the abdominal cavity and there is hemoperitoneum.
- **Uterine dehiscence/incomplete rupture:** Its an intraoperative finding. Here the serosa of the uterine wall remains intact. The fetus is still alive.

Rupture of the Uterus can be seen in:

1. As a result of obstructed labor
2. **Scar rupture:** Previous cesarean section scar rupture.

 Note: Classical cesarean or hysterotomy scar is more likely to rupture than lower segment section.

3. Injudicious administration of oxytocin
4. Use of prostaglandins for induction of abortion
5. Fall or blow on the abdomen
6. Internal podalic version

 The greatest risk factor for either complete or incomplete uterine rupture is prior cesarean delivery.

Time of Rupture

During labor: Spontaneous rupture during pregnancy **is usually complete, involves the upper segment** and usually occurs in later months of pregnancy.
During pregnancy: Classical cesarean or hysterotomy scar is likely to give way during later months of pregnancy. Lower segment scar rarely ruptures during pregnancy.

Signs of Uterine Rupture

- **First sign: Fetal bradycardia** followed by absent fetal heart sounds
- Maternal tachycardia and hypotension as there is maternal shock
- Uterine contractions stop suddenly.

Per Abdominally

- Tenderness present
- Distension
- Fetal parts are palpable superficially
- Fetal heart sounds are usually absent
- Uterus and fetus may be felt separate.

Vaginal Examination

- Hot dry vagina
- Recession of the presenting part, loss of station
- Vaginal bleeding
- Hematuria

 Also Know:

In a case of previous LSCS if pelvis is adequate and all conditions fostered vaginal delivery can be tried called as vaginal birth after cesarean while attempting VBAC. One should be aware of signs of impending rupture.

Signs of Impending Scar Rupture
- Fetal tachycardia
- Scar tenderness
- **Management of impending rupture:** Immediate cesarean section

Management of Rupture

Rupture is an emergency with immediate emergency with high maternal mortality and morbidity necessitating immediate resuscitation (fluids and blood) and laparotomy. For scar dehiscence, repair may be tried. Most of the ruptures need subtotal or total hysterectomy.

INTRAUTERINE FETAL DEATH (IUD)

Intrauterine fetal death is death of the fetus in utero after the period of viability (*after 22 weeks 2 > 500 gm by WHO) or when fetus weighs more than 500 gm.*

Diagnosis

IUD can be diagnosed clinically by:
- The size of the uterus less than the period of gestation.
- Liquor decreased.
- FHS absent.
- Fetal movements absent.
- Egg-shell crackling feel of the fetal head (*late feature*).

Ultrasound: Earliest diagnosis is possible by USG.

Diagnostic features:

- Absence of fetal cardiac activity on ultrasound scan (diagnostic).
- Decreased liquor amnii.
- *Spalding's sign i.e.,* overlapping of fetal skull bones due to shrinkage of cerebrum after fetal death.

Radiology:

- *Roberts sign:* Presence of gas in the fetal large vessels (earliest sign—seen 12 hours after fetal death).
- *Ball sign:* Crumpled up spine of the fetus or hyperflexion of the spine.
- *Spalding's sign:* Overlapping of fetal skull bones seen due to shrinkage of cerebrum after death of fetus. Seen around 7 days after death.

  Note: Spalding sign is seen both on USG and radiology (Fig. 12.1).

- Crowding of ribs (concertina effect)
- **Halo sign:** There is abnormal increase of the causal soft tissue as a result of maceration.

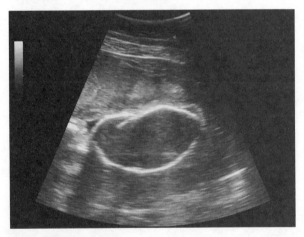

Fig. 12.1: Spalding sign

Sign	Interval after death
Roberts sign (gas in great vessels of fetus)	12 hours
Spalding sign, i.e. overlapping of skull bones of fetus	1 week
Ball sign (hyperflexion/ hyperextension of spine)	3-4 weeks

Management

In 80% cases of IUD, spontaneous expulsion occurs in 2 weeks. If spontaneous expulsion fails to occur within 2 weeks, intervention should be done.

But this type of expectant management, i.e. awaiting for spontaneous expulsion is now no longer done.

- Nowadays, the usual practice is to induce labor as soon as fetal death is diagnosed, because most women have a natural disinclination to carry a dead fetus within them.
- Labor can be induced by PGE_2 gel where to can ripen the cervix if Bishop score is < 6 and by oxytocin can be used if score is > 6. An alternative of PGE_2 is misoprostol phost.
- ARM is not done; due to the risk of infection.
- Cesarean section is avoided as far as possible in a dead fetus.
- Cesarean section with a dead fetus may sometimes be necessary in case of previous cesarean section, placenta previa and transverse lie.

Recent Updates

ACOG earlier recommended karyotyping of all still born fetuses, but procedures like CAM—Chromosomal microarray analysis (CAM) are now replacing standard karyotyping for chromosomal analysis of still born fetuses

- CMA does not require dividing cells and is reported to be more useful for evaluation of fetal death
- Any type of fetal or placental tissue or amniotic fluid can be submitted for genetic testing by CMA
- In females with H/O previous still births delivery/ induction is done at 39 weeks.[Q]

New Pattern Questions

N1. The following statements are related to the management of obstructed labor *except*:
a. There is no place of wait and watch policy
b. Dehydration and ketoacidosis should be promptly corrected
c. Oxytocin has got a definite place in the management
d. Uterus should be explored as a routine following delivery

N2. All of the following are features of obstructed labor *except*:
a. Hot dry vagina   b. Tonic contracted uterus
c. Bandl's ring
d. Unruptured membranes

N3. M/C fistula as a complication of obstructed labor:
a. Uretero vaginal fistula
b. Urethro vaginal fistula
c. VVF
d. Vesico uterine fistula

N4. A primigravida with full-term pregnancy in labor for 1 day is brought to casualty after dia handing. On examination she is dehydrated, slightly pale, pulse 100/min, BP120/80 mm Hg. Abdominal examination reveals a fundal height of 36 weeks, cephalic presentation, fetal heart absent, mild uterine contractions present. On P/V examination, cervix is fully dilated, head is at +1 station, caput with moulding present, pelvis adequate. Dirty, infected discharge is present. What would be the best management option after initial work-up?
a. Cesarean section
b. Oxytocin drip
c. Ventouse delivery
d. Craniotomy and vaginal delivery

N5. All are true about constriction ring *except*:
a. Also called Schroeder's ring
b. Can be caused by injudicious oxytocin use
c. Ring can be palpated per abdomen
d. Inhalation of amylnitrate relaxes the ring

N6. About constriction ring all are correct *except*:
a. The ring is always felt on abdominal examination
b. Usually situated around the neck of the fetus in cephalic presentation
c. There is no progress of labor
d. The ring is felt during cesarean section or forceps delivery or during manual removal of placenta

N7. Uterine rupture is least common with:
a. LSCS
b. Classical section
c. Inverted T-shaped incision
d. T-shaped incision

N8. In classical cesarean section more chances of rupture of uterus is in:
a. Upper uterine segment
b. Lower uterine segment
c. Uterocervical junction
d. Posterior uterine segment

N9. The following statements are related to rupture uterus *except*:
a. Lower segment scar rarely ruptures during pregnancy
b. In incomplete rupture the peritoneal coat remains intact
c. Classical cesarean scar often rupture during late pregnancy
d. Risk of lower segment scar rupture is high compared to classical scar rupture

N10. Robert sign is a sign of:
a. Down's syndrome of fetus
b. Gonadal agenesis in fetus
c. IUGR   d. IUD

N11. A patient at 22 weeks gestation is diagnosed as having IUD which occurred at 17 weeks but did not have a miscarriage. This patient is at increased risk for:
a. Septic abortion
b. Recurrent abortion
c. Consumptive coagulopathy with hypofibrinogenemia
d. Future infertility
e. Ectopic pregnancy

N12. Which is most likely complication of IUD?
a. Hypofibrinogenemia
b. Sterility
c. Cervical tear
d. None of the above

N13. A G_2P_{1+0} at 36 weeks of gestation has a H/O prior still birth at 37 weeks. The best time of delivery for the patient this time is:
a. Immediately   b. 37 weeks
c. 38 weeks   d. 39 weeks

N14. Intrauterine death at 36 weeks. Treatment is:
a. Continue up to term
b. Wait for spontaneous expulsion
c. Syntocinon + ARM
d. Hysterectomy
e. LSCS

N15. Early fetal death is death of fetus at:
a. 10 weeks   b. < 20 weeks
c. < 28 weeks   d. > 20 weeks

N16. In a patient with history of previous still birth, Optimum time of delivery is:
a. 37 weeks   b. 38 weeks
c. 39 weeks   d. 40 weeks

Previous Year Questions

1. **Indicators of impending uterine rupture during labor include all of the following** *except*:
   a. Fetal distress   [AI 06]
   b. Hematuria
   c. Fresh bleeding per vaginum
   d. Passage of meconium

2. **All are seen with scar dehiscence,** *except*:
   a. Maternal bradycardia   [AIIMS Nov 01]
   b. Fetal bradycardia
   c. Vaginal bleeding
   d. Hematuria

3. **Blood in urine in a patient in labor is diagnostic of:**
                                        [AIIMS May 08]
   a. Impending scar rupture
   b. Urethral injury
   c. Obstructed labor
   d. Cystitis

4. **Hematuria during labor in previous LSCS is sign of:**
                                        [AIIMS Nov 09]
   a. Impending rupture of scar
   b. Urethral trauma
   c. Prolong labor
   d. Sepsis

5. **A woman comes with obstructed labor and is grossly dehydrated. Investigations reveal fetal demise. What will be the management?** [AIIMS Nov 08]
   a. Craniotomy   b. Decapitation
   c. Cesarean section d. Forceps extraction

6. **30-year-old female comes with obstructed labor and is febrile and dehydrated with IUFD and cephalic presentation. Which is the best way to manage?**
                                        [AIIMS May 11]
   a. Craniotomy   b. Decapitation
   c. Cesarean section d. Forceps extraction

7. **Bandl's ring is also called as:**   [PGI June 98]
   a. Constriction ring b. Schroeder's ring
   c. Retraction ring   d. Cervical dystocia

8. **A multipara with previous LSCS comes at 38 weeks pregnancy in shock. Differential diagnosis includes:**
                                        [PGI June 06]
   a. Placenta previa
   b. Abruptio placenta
   c. Rupture uterus

9. **True about intrauterine fetal death (IUD):**
                                        [PGI Dec 03]
   a. Gas bubbles in great vessels
   b. Halo's sign +ve
   c. Overlapping of skull bone
   d. Decreased amniotic fluid volume

10. **USG sign of fetal death:**   [PGI June 01]
    a. 'Halo' sign of head
    b. Heart beat absent
    c. Spalding sign
    d. Hegar's sign

11. **Spalding's sign is seen in:**   [PGI June 99; Dec 98]
    a. Still born   b. Live born
    c. Premature   d. Dead born

12. **In a pregnant woman of 28 weeks gestation IUD is earliest demonstrated on X-ray by:** [PGI Dec 98]
    a. Increased flexion
    b. Overlapping of cranial bone
    c. Spalding's sign
    d. Gas in vessels

13. **Cause of death in breech delivery:** [PGI Dec 97]
    a. Intracranial hemorrhage
    b. Aspiration
    c. Atlanto axial dislocation
    d. Asphyxia

14. **In intrauterine death with transverse lie, the following are treatment options** *except*: [PGI June 99]
    a. Decapitation
    b. Evisceration
    c. Craniotomy
    d. Cesarean section

Answers with Explanations to New Pattern Questions

N1. **Ans. is c, i.e. Oxytocin has got a definite place in the management**   *Ref. Dutta Obs 9/e, p 380*

Principles for management of obstructed labor:

- **To relieve** the obstruction at the earliest by a safe delivery procedure (there is no place for wait and watch)
- **To combat** dehydration and ketoacidosis
- **To control sepsis.**

Remember:

- Before proceeding for definitive operative treatment, rupture of the uterus must be excluded.
- Oxytocin should never be used in management of obstructed labor.

'There is no place of wait and watch, neither is any scope of using oxytocin to stimulate uterine contraction'.

Ref. Dutta Obs 9/e, p 380

N2. **Ans. is d, i.e. Unruptured membranes**

All the options given in the question are features of obstructed labor except unruptured membranes. In case of obstructed labor, membranes are ruptured, vagina is hot and dry and there is foul smelling discharge.

N3. **Ans. is c, i.e. VVF**

M/C cause of VVF in developing countries is obstructed labor.

M/C fistula seen in obstructed labor is VVF.

N4. **Ans. is a, i.e. Cesarean section**   *Ref. Read below*

Well friends lets first analyse the condition of patient and then think about its management:

- Patient is primigravida
- On examination:
    - Dehydration is present
    - P/R is 100/min, i.e. tachycardia present.

P/A

- Fundal height-36 weeks
- Presentation-cephalic
- FHS-Absent
- Mild uterine contractions are present.

P/V

- Cervix-fully dilated
- Station = + 1
- Caput present
- Moulding present
- Dirty infected discharge is present.

Most importantly–Pelvis is adequate.

This patient is undoubtedly a case of obstructed labor. As we all know in nulliparous females in case of obstructed labor—a state of uterine exhaustion is reached manifested as weakened uterine conditions.

- In such cases, if oxytocin drip is given it may lead to rupture of uterus as lower segment is thinned out (i.e. **option 'b'** ruled out).
- Craniotomy and other destructive procedures are not carried out in modern obstetrics (i.e., **option 'd'** ruled out).

Management of obstructed labor is always cesarean section.

N5. **Ans. is c, i.e. Ring can be palpated per abdomen**   *Ref. Dutta Obs 9/e, p 338*

Constriction ring/Schroeder's can be palpated per vaginally and not per abdominally.

N6. **Ans. is a, i.e. The ring is always felt on abdominal examination**

See the text for explanation.

N7. Ans. is a, i.e. LSCS *Ref. Williams Obs. 22/e, p 611, 24/e, p 613 Table 31.3*

Estimated incidences of rupture of uterus with different types of incisions in case of cesarean section are:

Prior incision	Estimated rupture rate (%)
Classical	**4–9**
T-shaped	**4–9**
Low-vertical[a]	**1–7**
One low-transverse	**0.2–1.8**
Prior pre-term cesarean	"increased"
Prior uterine rupture	
• Lower segment	2–6
• Upper uterus	9–32

[a]See text for definition.

Data from the American College of Obstetricians and Gynecologists, 2013a; Cahill, 2010b; Chauhan, 2002; Landon, 2006; Macones, 2005; Martin, 1997; Miller, 1994; Sciscione, 2008; Society for Maternal-Fetal Medicine, 2012; Tahseen, 2010.

 Also Know:

In 1/3rd cases rupture of classical cesarean section scar occurs before labor (Spontaneous rupture during pregnancy).

N8. Ans. is a, i.e. Upper uterine segment *Ref. Dutta Obs. 9/e, p 401-402*

Types of rupture	Most common site involved
1. Spontaneous rupture during pregnancy	Upper segment
2. Rupture during labour due to non obstructive cause (as seen in grand multipara)	Fundal area (complete rupture)
3. Rupture during labour due to obstruction	Anterior lower segment transversely is the MC site
	It can extend upwards along the lateral uterine wall
4. Rupture of the scar:	
In classical cesarean section	Upper segment
In LSCS	Lower segment

N9. Ans. is d, i.e. Risk of lower segment scar rupture is high compared to classical scar rupture

Ref. Dutta Obs. 9/e, p 401

N10. Ans. is d, i.e. IUD

Robert sign is presence of gas in the great vessels. It is the first sign seen of IUD on USG.

N11. Ans. is c, i.e Consumptive coagulopathy with hypofibrinogenemia *Ref. Dutta Obs. 9/e, p 304, p 304*

Dead fetus, if retained for more than 4 to 5 weeks, release thromboplastin which leads to DIC (consumptive coagulopathy). In the question, the fetus has been dead and has been retained for five weeks so there are increased chances of DIC.

Obstetrical conditions leading to DIC

a. Septic abortion
b. IUD
c. Abruptio placentae
d. Amniotic fluid embolism
e. Severe preeclampsia, eclampsia. HELLP syndrome.

N12. Ans. is a, i.e. Hypofibrinogenemia *Ref. Dutta Obs. 9/e, p 304*

Complications of IUD

- Psychological upset.
- Uterine Infections. Once the membranes rapture
- *Blood coagulation disorder: If the fetus is retained for more than 4 weeks (as occurs in 10–20%) there is a possibility that thromboplastin from the dead fetus enters maternal circulation and leads to disseminated intravascular coagulopathy (DIC).*
- *During labor:* Uterine inertia, retained placenta and PPH.

Hypofibrinogenimia occurs due to gradual absorption of thromboplastin, liberated from the dead placenta and decidua, into the maternal circulation.

Remember:

- Critical level of fibrinogen is = 100 mg/ml.
- Hypofibrinogemia/defibrination is observed predominantly in:
  - Retained dead fetus
  - Rh-incompatibility.

N13. Ans. is d, i.e. 39 weeks *Ref. Williams 24/e, p 666*

In patients with history of previous still birth—delivery at 39 weeks is recommended by induction or by cesarean delivery (for those with contraindication to induction), irrespective of the gestational age at which previous still birth occured.

 Note: In all these patients antepartum fetal surveillance should begin at 32 weeks.

N14. Ans. is b, i.e. Wait for spontaneous expulsion *Ref. Dutta Obs. 9/e, p 304*

In 80% cases of IUD, spontaneous expulsion occurs in 2 weeks. If spontaneous expulsion fails to occur within 2 weeks, intervention should be done.
But this type of expectant management, i.e. awaiting for spontaneous expulsion is now no longer done.

- Nowadays, the usual practice is to induce labor as soon as fetal death is diagnosed, because most women have a natural disinclination to carry a dead fetus within them.
- Labor can be induced by oxytocin drip or PGE$_2$ gel can be used to ripen the cervix (but this is not given in option).
- ARM is not done; due to the risk of infection (i.e., *option 'b' ruled out*).
- Cesarean section is avoided as far as possible in a dead fetus.
- Cesarean section with a dead fetus may sometimes be necessary in case of previous cesarean section, placenta previa and transverse lie (i.e., *option 'e' ruled out*).

So still amongst the given options best is, Wait for spontaneous expulsion.

N15. Ans. is b, i.e. < 20 weeks *Ref. Williams 24/e, p 661*

The definition given in Williams for IUD says:

Williams 24/e p 661 says. ***"According to CDC and WHO—Fetal death means death prior to complete expulsion or extraction from the mother of a product of human conception irrespective of the duration of pregnancy and which is not an induced termination of pregnancy. The death is indicated by the fact that after such expulsion or extraction, the fetus does not breathe or show any other evidence of life such as beating of the heart, pulsation of the umbilical cord, or definite movement of voluntary muscles".***

Fetal mortality is divided into three periods: **Early**, < 20 completed weeks; **intermediate**, 20–27 weeks; and **late**, 28 weeks or more. The fetal death rate after 28 weeks has declined since 1990, whereas deaths from 20 to 27 weeks are largely unchanged.

N16. Ans. is c, i.e. 39 weeks *Ref. Williams 25/e, p 649*

All these females who have previous H/O still birth, the optimal time of delivery is 39 weeks and mode of delivery is vaginal delivery.

Answers with Explanations to Previous Year Questions

1. **Ans. is d, i.e. Passage of meconium**
   Ref. Munrokerr's 10/e, p 444,447; Dutta Obs. 9/e, p 328,
   Operative Obs and Gynae by Randhir Puri, Narendra Malhotra 1/e, p 203, COGDT 10/e, p 340

2. **Ans. is a, i.e. Maternal bradycardia**
   Ref. Dutta Obs. 7/e, p 328; Operative Obs and Gynae, Randhir Puri and Narendra Malhotra 1/e, p 202, 203

   In Q1 – Indicators of impending uterine rupture:
   Option a – Fetal distress (correct)
   Option b – Hematuria (correct)
   Option c – Fresh bleeding per vaginum (correct)
   Option d – Passage of meconium (+/-)

   In case of impending rupture when fetal distress occurs, it may be followed by passage of meconium but meconium passage occurs/is a sign of fetal distress and not impending rupture. Moreover these days, meconium passage is not even taken as a sign of fetal distress since fetus can pass meconium without fetal distress, e.g. postdatism.
   Hence the **correct option is d, i.e. passage of meconium.**

   In Q2 – All are seen with scar dehiscence, except:
   Option a – Maternal bradycardia
   Option b – Fetal bradycardia
   Option c – Vaginal bleeding
   Option d – Hematuria

   Remember – the following line of COGDT

   "There are no reliable signs of impending uterine rupture that occur before labor, although the sudden appearance of gross Hematuria is suggestive."
   —COGDT 10/e, p 340
   So we are left with 2 options – maternal bradycardia and fetal bradycardia.

   "Prolonged late and variable decelerations and bradycardia seen on FHR monitoring are the M/C and often the only manifestation of uterine rupture.
   —Williams Obs. 23/e, p 573

   "The most common sign of uterine rupture is a non reassuring fetal heart rate pattern with variable deceleration evolving into late decelerations, bradycardia and undetectable fetal heart rate pattern".
   —John Hopkins Manual of Obs. and Gynae 4/e, p 86

   Thus when impending rupture proceeds to complete rupture, fetal bradycardia occurs, so I am ruling out maternal bradycardia which never occurs, rather in case of scar dehiscence or uterine rupture, mother goes into shock so then is maternal tachycardia.

    Remember:

   - M/C sign of impending rupture: Fetal bradycardia
   - Most consistent sign of impending rupture: Fetal bradycardia

3. **Ans. is c, i.e. Obstructed labor**
   Ref. Dutta Obs. 9/e, p 379

   "In obstructed labor the bladder becomes an abdominal organ due to compression of urethra between the presenting part and symphysis pubis, the patient fails to empty the bladder. The transverse depression at the junction of the superior border of the bladder and the distended lower segment is often confused with the Bandl's ring. The bladder wall gets traumatized which may lead to blood stained urine, a common finding in obstructed labor.

    Also Know:

   Though hematuria can also indicate impending uterine rupture but for that obviously the patient should have a previous scar, atleast the question should say that patient has had a previous LSCS or something.

4. **Ans. is a, i.e. Impending rupture of scar**   *Ref. COGDT 10/e, p 340*

Now friends - here in the question it is asked specifically that hematuria is seen in a patient with previous LSCS during labor - which indicates **impending rupture of scar**.

"There are no reliable signs of impending uterine rupture that occurs before labor, although the sudden appearance of gross hematuria is suggestive."   *COGDT 10/e, p 340*

Here in this question obstructed labor is not given in the options, but even if it was given, I would have still opted for impending scar rupture as the question is specifically asking, in a case of previous LSCS.

5. **Ans. is c, i.e. Cesarean section**   *Ref. Textbook of Obstetrics Sheila Balakrishnan 1/e, p 474*

6. **Ans. is c, i.e. Cesarean section**   *Ref. Dutta 7/e, p 404, Textbook of Obs. Sheila Balakrishnan, p 479*

Always remember—two main principles in the management of obstructed labor are:

1. Never wait and watch
2. Never use oxytocin.

In case of obstructed labor there is a problem with either the passage or the passenger bur the uterus contracts adequately, so if we increase uterine contractions by giving oxytocin it will lead to uterine rupture.

Management of obstructed labor:

- Management of dehydration—by giving IV fluids
- Antibiotics are given to prevent infection
- Most important step is to relieve obstruction by either instrumental delivery or by doing LSCS. LSCS may even have to be done, if the baby is dead to relieve the obstruction otherwise uterine rupture can occur.

7. **Ans. is c, i.e. Retraction ring**   *Ref. Dutta Obs. 7/e, p 362*

Bandl's ring is retraction ring
Schroeder's ring is constriction ring

8. **Ans. is a, b and c, i.e. Placenta previa; Abruptio placenta; and Rupture uterus**   *Ref. Dutta Obs. 7/e, p 618*

Shock in Obstetrics:
Causes of shock during pregnancy

Hypovolemic shock	Septic shock	Cardiogenic shock	Neurogenic shock
Hemorrhagic shock - Ectopic pregnancy - Post abortal hemorrhage - Placenta previa - Abruptio placenta - PPH - Rupture of uterus - Obstetric surgery **Fluid loss shock** - Excessive vomiting - Excessive diarrhea - Diuresis - Too rapid removal of fluid - Supine hypotension syndrome due to IVC compression by gravid uterus - Shock associated with DIC	- Septic abortion - Chorioamnionitis - Pyelonephritis - Endometritis (Rare)	- Cardiac arrest - Myocardial infarction - Cardiac tamponade - Pulmonary embolism	- Spinal anesthesia - Aspiration of gastro-intestinal contents during general anes-thesia especially in cesarean section (Mendelson's syndrome)

9. **Ans. is a, b, c and d, i.e. Gas bubbles in great vessels; Halo's sign +ve; Overlapping of skull bone; and Decreased amniotic fluid volume**   *Ref. JB Sharma TB of Obs. p 476*

10. **Ans. is a, b and c, i.e. Halo sign, Heart beat absent and Spalding sign**

See the text for explanations

11. **Ans. is d, i.e. Dead born**   *Ref. Dutta Obs. 9/e, p 303; Sheila Balakrishnan, p 249; Reddy 26/e, p 378, 379*

Spalding sign: It is the irregular overlapping of the cranial bones on one another, due to liquefaction of the brain matter and softening of the ligamentous structures supporting the vault.

- *Appears 7 days after death.*
- Is evident on both ultrasound and radiology?
- Similar features may be found in extrauterine pregnancy with live fetus.

12. **Ans. is d, i.e. Gas in vessels** *Ref. Dutta Obs. 9/e, p 303; JB Sharma TB of Obs. p 475-476; Sheila Balakrishnan, p 249; Reddy 26/e, p 378, 379*

Sign	Interval after death
Roberts sign (gas in great vessels of fetus)	12 hours
Spalding sign, i.e. overlapping of skull bones of fetus	1 week
Ball sign (hyperflexion/hyperextension of spine)	3-4 weeks

13. **Ans. is a, i.e. Intracranial hemorrhage**   *Ref. Manual of Obs. by Holland and Brews 16/e, p 190*
    - Intracranial hemorrhage is the most common cause of fetal loss in breech and occurs due to tear of tentorium cerebelli and falx cerebri.
    - It is caused by traumatic delivery of the after coming head of breech or too rapid delivery of the soft head of a premature baby.

14. **Ans. is c, i.e. Craniotomy**   *Ref. Dutta Obs. 7/e, p 397*

> ***Management in case of dead baby with transverse lie – Cesarean section,*** is much safer in the hands of those who are not conversant with destructive operations. ***If the obstetrician is conversant with destructive operation,*** decapitation or evisceration is to be done.   —*Dutta Obs. 6/e, p 397*

- Destructive operations were done in the past in case of obstructed labor, when the fetus was dead or dying or grossly malformed.
- Today they are undertaken extremely rarely.
- Generally speaking, there is no place for destructive operations in modern day obstetrics.

Type	Indication	Procedure
Craniotomy	• Delivery of a dead fetus with cephalic presentation (vertex, brow or face) • Delivery of the arrested after coming head in breech • Interlocking head of twins	• Fetal skull is perforated, contents are evacuated and fetus delivered • *Perforation site:* – Vertex-parietal bone – Brow-frontal bone – Face-orbit or roof of the mouth – After coming head in breech-occipital bone.
Craniocentesis	• Hydrocephalus	• Per abdomen reduction of hydrocephalic head using a large bore needle
Decapitation	• ***Neglected shoulder presentation*** (If the neck is easily accessible) • Interlocking head of twins	• Fetal head is separated from the body, then the decapitated head and trunk are extracted through the vagina
Cleidotomy	• In case of shoulder dystocia when all measures have failed	• One or both clavicles are divided
Spondylotomy	• ***Neglected shoulder presentation***	• Vertebral column is divided
Embryotomy or Evisceration	• ***Neglected shoulder presentation*** • (If the neck is not easily accessible)	• Fetal abdomen is perforated and its contents are debulked

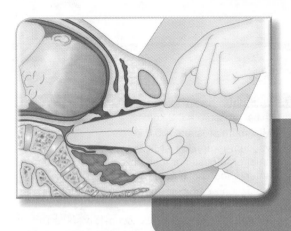

Operative Obstetrics

Chapter at a Glance

➢ Instrumental Delivery
➢ Forceps and Vacuum
➢ Episiotomy

➢ Cesarean Section
➢ VBAC/Trial of Scar

GENERAL CONSIDERATIONS ABOUT INSTRUMENTAL DELIVERY

Types of Forceps Application   *p402, My Obs 9/e*

Types of Procedure	Criteria
A High forceps	• Vertex not engaged • No longer used
B Mid forceps	• Head is engaged but presenting part/station is above +2
C Low forceps	• Station is below or at +2 station but has not yet reached the pelvic floor • Rotation can be more or less than 45°
D Outlet forceps	• Station is more than +2 below and fetal skull has reached the level of pelvic floor • Scalp is visible at the introitus without separating the labia

Contd...

Contd...

Types of Procedure	Criteria
	• Fetal skull has reached pelvic floor • Fetal head is at or on the perineum • Sagittal suture is in direct AP diameter or rotation is < 45°

 ### Important One Liners

• These days both forceps and vacuum are applied at or beyond +2 station.

• Wrigleys forceps is a type of outlet forceps available in India.

• Kielland forceps is a long forceps, used for high forceps application in the past, but these days it is outdated.

• Rest most of the varieties of forceps are low forceps.

	Forceps	Vacuum
Prerequisites	**F**-favorable position and station **O**-Os should be fully dilated **R**-membranes should be ruptured Head should be rotated **C**-uterus should be contracting **E**-episiotomy should be given, Bladder should be empty Head should be engaged **P**-no CPD, Pelvis should be adequate	Same as forceps, but it has 2 advantages 1. It can be applied even if head is not rotated 2. It can be applied when cervix is >/= 6 cm dilated (full dilatation is not required)

Contd...

Contd...

	Forceps	Vacuum
Pressure/Traction	Primi = 20 kgs Multi = 13 kgs	Initial pressure = 0.2 kg/cm² Maximum pressure = 0.8 kg/cm²
Application	Forceps is applied along occipitomental direction.	Vacuum is applied at flexion point which is 3 cm anterior to posterior fontanelle or 6 cm posterior to anterior fontanelle (see Fig. 13.4).
Indications	1. Maternal distress-mother is exhausted 2. Fetal distress-when station of fetal head is ≥ +2 3. Prolonged second stage of labor 4. Used prophylactically to cut short second stage of labor in heart disease patients/PIH/ postmaturity/small for date fetus/patients under epidural analgesia	Indications same as forceps but in fetal distress vacuum is not used. In heart disease patients, vacuum is preferred as for vacuum-lithotomy position is not necessary.
Presentations in which it can be used	Forceps can be used in all those presentations, where it is not necessary to do cesarean.	Vacuum cannot be used in presentation other than vertex (occipito anterior/posterior)

Advantage	**Remember:** Cesarean section is necessary in
	• Mentoposterior face presentation
	• Brow presentation
	• Transverse lie
	
	Hence presentations in which forceps can be applied-
	• Mentoanterior face presentation
	• After coming head of breech
	• Vertex occiptoanterior position
	• Occipitoposterior position
	Advantage of forceps over vacuum
	  i. It can be used for presentation other than vertex
	  ii. It can be used in preterm babies
	  iii. Can be used in fetal distress	

Absolute contraindications	• CPD/Contacted pelvis • HIV positive female • Osteogenesis imperfecta • Known coagulopathy in fetus	Same as forceps Also in preterm babies and fetal distress vacuum is a relative contraindication.
Complications	Leads to more of maternal injury Complete perineal tears are M/C **Complications more common with forceps:** • Facial nerve palsy • Brachial plexus injury • Depressed skull fracture • Corneal abrasion	Leads to more of fetal injury **Complications more common with vacuum:** • Cephalohematoma • Subgaleal hematoma • Retinal nerve injury • Sixth nerve palsy
Williams obs 25/e pg 555	*Note:* Intracranial hemorrhage of fetus rates are same with forceps, vaccum and cesarean section.	
Some rules	Maximum three attempts should be given with forceps. If in 3 pulls fetal head is undelivered, it is called as **failed forceps** which should be managed by cesarean section.	Maximum three attempts should be given with vacuum. If in 3 pulls fetal head is undelivered, it is called as **failed vacuum** which should be managed by cesarean section

Forceps

The forceps has following parts (Figs. 13.1A and B):

1. **Blade:** Each forcep has 2 blades, left and right. Mostly the blades are fenestrated for a better grip on fetal head except in Tucker-Mclane forcep which is solid. The blade has 2 curves:
   i. **Pelvic curve:** Present on edges of the blade conforms to the axis of birth canal. It forms a part of larger circle whose radius is 17.5 cm. The front of forceps is concave side of pelvic curve.
   ii. **Cephalic curve:** It is the curve on the flat surface of the blade which conforms to the shape of fetal head. The radius of curve is 11.5 cm.
2. **Shank:** It connects the blade with the handle and gives length to the forceps.
3. **Lock:** The blades articulate at the lock. Most of them are english locks.
4. **Handles:** The handles are opposed an articulation of the blade, length of handle is 12.5 cm.

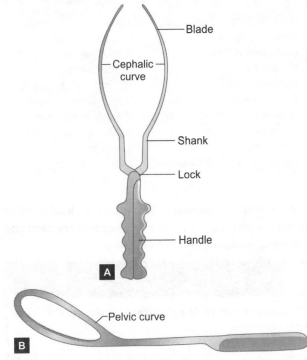

Figs. 13.1A and B: Curves of blade

Note:

- In India: Outlet forceps used is Wrigley's forceps (Fig. 13.2B).
- In India: mid cavity forceps used is Das forceps or Neville Barry forceps.

- The forceps which can rotate head of fetus - Kielland forceps (Fig. 13.3) and Barton forceps
- Forceps used to deliver after coming head of breech = Piper's forceps
- Left hand blade is introduced first
- Special features of Kielland forceps:
   - It has a sliding lock
   - Little or no pelvic curve
   - On each handle, a knob is present which indicates the direction of the occiput
   - No axis traction device
- **Axis traction device:** It can be applied with advantage in midforceps application especially following manual rotation of head. It provides traction in the correct axis and less force is needed, e.g. Tarnier forceps, Milne Murray forceps.

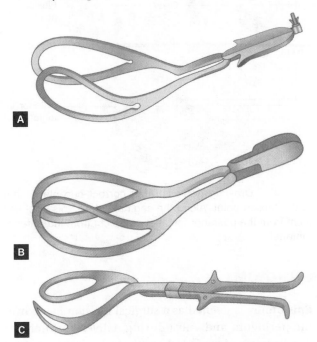

Figs. 13.2A to C: Different types of obstetric forceps currently used—(A) Long-curved with axis traction device; (B) Wrigley's; (C) Kielland's

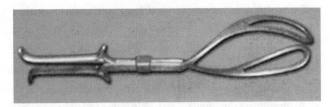

Fig. 13.3: Kielland's forcep

Vacuum

Vacuum or ventouse consists of 2 parts:

1. Suction machine
2. Suction cups

They can be metallic (best suited for rotating head) or sialistic cup (for outlet application when no rotation is needed). Cup size can be:

6 cm: First choice in occipito anterior

5 cm: Best for occipito posterior positions.

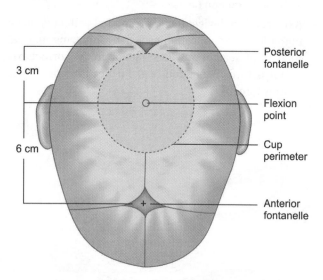

Fig. 13.4: Drawing demonstrates correct cup placement at the flexion point. Along the sagittal suture, this spot lies 3 cm from the posterior fontanel and 6 cm from the anterior fontanel.

EPISIOTOMY

Episiotomy is defined as a surgical incision made over the perineum and vulva during delivery to increase the diameter of the vulval outlet (and not the whole of birth canal) during childbirth and to prevent perineal tears. Thus episiotomy is surgically given perineal tear of second degree.

Episiotomy is recommended in selective cases rather than as a routine.

Indications of Episiotomy

- In elastic (rigid) perineum: Elderly primigravidae.
- Anticipating perineal tear: (a) Big baby, (b) Face to pubis delivery, (c) Breech delivery, (d) Shoulder dystocia.

- Operative delivery: Forceps delivery, ventouse delivery.
- Previous perineal surgery: Pelvic floor repair, perineal reconstructive surgery.

Timing of the episiotomy: Bulging thinned perineum during contraction just prior to crowning (when 3–4 cm of head is visible) is the ideal time to give episiotomy.

Types of Episiotomy:

- Median
- Mediolateral
- Lateral
- 'J' shaped

> Mediolateral and median episiotomy are most common types.
>
> Commonly a right mediolateral episiotomy is performed, angled at 45° from the vulvar rim.

Comparison between Midline (median) and Mediolateral episiotomy	
Median	**Mediolateral**
• Muscles are not cut	• Muscles are cut
• Blood loss is less	• Blood loss is more
• Repair is easy	• Repair is difficult
• Healing is superior	• Healing is less superior
• Dyspareunia is rare	• Dyspareunia is more
• Extension, if occurs, leads to 3rd perineal tear or 4th degree	• Relative safety from rectal involvement from extension
• Incision cannot be extended	• Incision can be extended

Since median episiotomy, if extended can lead to 3rd or 4th degree perineal tear, it is a very big disadvantage and hence this episiotomy is not routinely used.

 Extra Edge

Structures cut in Mediolateral episiotomy (Very important) (Fig. 13.5)

- Posterior vaginal wall
- Superficial and deep transverse perineal muscles, bulbospongiosus (bulbocavernosus) and part of levator ani
- Fascia covering those muscles
- Transverse perineal branches of pudendal vessels and nerves
- Subcutaneous tissue and skin.

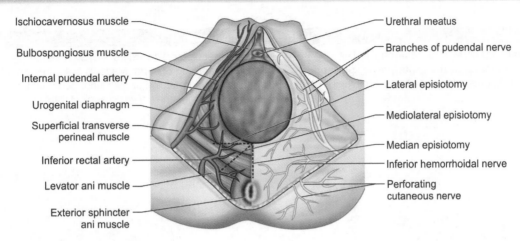

Fig. 13.5: Structures cut in mediolateral episiotomy

CESAREAN SECTION

It is an operative procedure whereby the fetus after the end of 28th week is delivered through an incision on the abdominal and uterine wall. This excludes delivery through an abdominal incision of a fetus, lying free in the abdominal cavity following uterine rupture or in secondary abdominal pregnancy.

The first cesarean done on a patient is referred to as a **primary cesarean section.** When the operation is performed in subsequent pregnancies, it is called **repeat cesarean section.**

Historical Background

This operation derives its name from the notification "lex Cesarea" – a Roman law promulgated in 715 BC which was continued even during Caesar's reign. The law provided either an abdominal delivery in a dying woman with a hope to get a live baby or to perform postmortem abdominal delivery for separate burial. The operation does not derive its name from the birth of Caesar, as his mother lived long time after his birth.

Incidence

The incidence of cesarean section is steadily rising. During the last decade there has been two to three fold rise in the incidence from the initial rate of about 10%.

Important Considerations in Cesarean Section

Skin Incision

The two commonly used incision techniques during cesarean for skin are:

- **Pfannenstiel incision (Fig. 13.6)**
- **Joel-Cohen incision (Fig. 13.7)**

Absolute indications	Relative indications
Vaginal delivery is not possible. Cesarean is needed even with a dead fetus. Indications are few 1. **Central placenta previa** 2. **Contracted pelvis or cephalopelvic** disproportion (absolute) 3. **Pelvic mass** causing obstruction (cervical or broad ligament fibroid) 4. **Advanced carcinoma cervix** 5. **Vaginal obstruction** (atresia, stenosis) **Common indications** **Primigravidae:** (1) Failed indication (2) Fetal distress (non-reassuring fetal FHR) (3) Cephalopelvic disproportion (CPD) (4) Dystocia (dysfunctional labor) nonprogress of labor (5) Malposition and malpresentation (occipitoposterior, breech).	**Vaginal delivery may be possible but risks to the mother and/or to the baby are high** More often multiple factors may be responsible 1. **Cephalopelvic disproportion** (relative) 2. **Previous cesarean delivery**—(a) when primary CS was due to recurrent indication (contracted pelvis). (b) Previous two CS (c) Features of scar dehiscence. (d) Previous classical CS 3. **Non-reassuring FHR** (fetal distress) 4. **Dystocia** may be due to **(three Ps) relatively** large fetus **(passenger)**, small pelvis **(passage)** or inefficient uterine contractions **(power)** 5. **Antepartum hemorrhage** (a) Placenta previa and (b) Abruptio placenta 6. **Malpresentation**—Breech, shoulder (transverse lie), brow 7. **Failed surgical induction** of labor, Failure to progress in labor 8. **Bad obstetric history**—with recurrent fetal wastage 9. **Hpertensive disorders**—(a) Severe pre-eclampsia, (b) Eclampsia—uncontrolled fits even with antiseizure therapy

Contd...

Contd...

Absolute indications	Relative indications
Mutigravidae: (1) Previous cesarean delivery (2) Antepartum hemorrhage (placenta previa, placental abruption) (3) Malpresentation (breech, transverse lie).	10. **Medical-gynecological disorders**—(a) Diabetes (uncontrolled), heart disease (coarctation of aorta, Marfan's syndrome. (b) Mechanical obstruction (due to benign or malignant pelvic tumors (carcinoma cervix), or following repair of vesicovaginal fistula

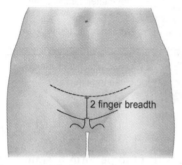

Fig. 13.6: Pfannenstiel incision. It is a suprapubic curvilinear incision, 2 finger breadth above pubic symphysis with lateral displacement using sharp dissection. Also called **sharp technique.**

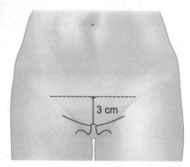

Fig. 13.7: **Joel-Cohen incision**. It is a suprapubic transverse incision above the level of Pfannenstiel incision with lateral displacement of sheath by fingers, i.e. **Blunt technique.**

Uterine Incision

The uterine incision can be given on either: (i) **Upper uterine segment called as classical cesaren section;** or (ii) lower uterine segment called lower segment cesarean section (LSCS).

The actions of upper and lower uterine segments are different during labor:

Upper uterine segment	Lower uterine segment
• Contracts and relaxes actively during labor. Hence, if any incision is given on upper uterine segment, then next time when patient conceives and goes into labor, the upper uterine segment will contract and retract actively at the time of labor. This increases the chances of rupture uterus (4–9%) • A classical cesarean section is always followed by cesarean section in next pregnancy	• Passively dilates during labor. • Hence, if any incision is given on lower uterine segment, then next time when patient conceives and goes into labor, the lower uterine segment will passively dilate. Thus, chances of rupture uterus will be less (0.2–1.5%) • If LSCS was done due to nonrecurring indications like fetal distress, then in next pregnancy, vaginal delivery can be tried. This is called as **vaginal birth after cesarean (VBAC)**

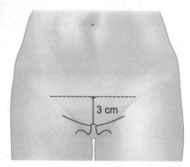

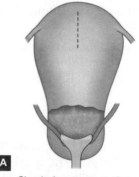

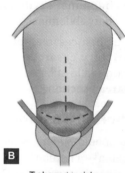

Classical cesarean section: Sangers incision (incision on upper uterine segment) Rupture risk= 4-9%

T shaped incision Rupture risk= 4-9%

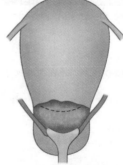

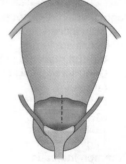

LSCS Kerr incision (low transverse incision) Rupture risk-0.2 to 1.5%

LSCS Kroning incision/ De lee incision (vertical incision on lower uterine segment) Rupture risk=1-7%

Figs. 13.8A to D: Incisions in cesarean section.

Hence, lower segment cesarean section is always preferred.

Current Indications for Classical Cesarean Section

1. Cancer cervix (**absolute indication**)
2. Dense adhesions between bladder and lower uterine segment
3. Post-mortem cesarean section
4. Impacted shoulder (transverse lie) of a large fetus
5. Very small fetus with breech
6. Major degree of placenta previa with placenta attached to anterior uterine wall
7. A very preterm cesarean section (because lower segment is not formed)
8. Previous classical cesarean section

Also Know:

Kronig Incision (Fig. 13.8D)
- It is a vertical incision given on lower uterine segment
- **Indication:** Formation of constriction ring
- Chances of rupture = 1 to 7%
- **Danger:** It can extend to cervix

 Important One Liners

- Level of anesthesia in cesarean section = T4
- Ideal time to conceive after cesarean = 18 months
- Minimum time to conceive after cesarean = 6 months
- **Best time to do cesarean (Primary) for elective reason or cesarean delivery on maternal request is done at = 39 weeks**
- Lower segment scars do not rupture before the onset of labor. Elective repeat cesarean section is done at 39 weeks
- Upper segment cesarean section (classical cesarean section) scars can rupture before the onset of labor. Therefore, repeat classical cesarean section is done at 36-37 weeks.

Also Know:

- **Antibiotic prophylaxis before cesarean**
  ACOG 2009 recommends single preoperative dose of 1 gm IV injection cefazolin half-an-hour prior to cesarean section or 3 doses, 8 hourly can be given for the high-risk cases or suspected infection
- At the time of delivery of fetus in cesarean first part delivered is head. Wrigley's forceps/Barton forceps can be used for delivering fetal head during cesarean
- In deeply impacted head of fetus, shoulders are delivered first and head last. This is called **Patwardhan technique**
- Uterine closure can be done in single layer or double layer. The second layer is hemostatic. But single layer closure does not affect the integrity of scar and chances of rupture are not increased, if uterus was closed in a single layer.

Misgav Ladach method of cesarean delivery:

- This is a very fast technique and is suited for fetal distress patients. It involves following steps:
  - Abdomen is opened by transverse cohen incision at a higher level than Pfannenstiel incision
  - The rectus sheath is cut by a small transverse incision and then the incision is extended on both sides using fingers
  - The peritoneum is then opened by fingers
  - Uterus is opened by a 1 cm stab in center and extended by fingers.
  - The closure of uterus is done in single layer and visceral and parietal peritoneum are not closed
  - Only rectus sheath and skin are closed.

VBAC: VAGINAL BIRTH AFTER CESAREAN/ TRIAL OF SCAR

Favorable Conditions for Vaginal Birth after Cesarean (VBAC) Section

- The mode of delivery should be decided at 37 weeks.
- In developing countries, VBAC is allowed only for women with one previous cesarean section.
- **The best predictor for successful VBAC is the history of a previous vaginal birth before or after the cesarean section**
- There should be no contraindications for vaginal delivery such as placenta previa
- The indication for the previous cesarean section should be non-recurrent
- The previous operation should be an uncomplicated lower segment cesarean section without T-extension or postpartum infection
- The previous child should be alive and healthy.
- The woman should be under 40 years of age
- The interdelivery interval should be more than 2 years
- The present pregnancy should be an uncomplicated, singleton pregnancy without malpresentations or malpositions
- The estimated birth weight should be less than 4 kg
- The pelvis should be adequate with no cephalopelvic disproportion
- There should be no indications for induction of labor
- Spontaneous onset of labor should occur at or before 41 weeks
- Facilities for anesthesia and cesarean should be present

Contraindications of VBAC	
Absolute contraindications	**Relative contraindications**

• Types of incision on uterus
  – Classical cesarean
  – T-shaped incision
  – Kroning incision
• H/O previous uterine rupture
  – Recurrence rate of rupture in classical cesarean **section is 32%**
  – **In LSCS it is –6%**
• Any surgery where uterine cavity was opened like hysterotomy, myomectomy
• Previous ≥ 2 LSCS without previous H/o vaginal delivery
• If any contraindication to vaginal delivery is present
OR
	• Macrosomia in current pregnancy
	• Breech in current pregnancy
	• Post-term pregnancy

Predictors for successful VBAC
1. Prior non-recurring indication for cesarean (breech/fetal distress) 2. Woman having prior vaginal delivery (best predictor) 3. Fetal birth weight-higher birth weight, lower chances 4. Spontaneous onset of labor in present pregnancy-higher success 5. Cervical dilatation (on admission) > 4 cm has higher success. 6. Women who are obese and elderly-lower success rate

Management of Vaginal Birth after Cesarean Trial of Scar

- Vaginal birth after cesarean (VBAC) section should be conducted in a well-equipped hospital, with facilities for continuous intrapartum care and monitoring and resources for immediate cesarean section, blood transfusion and advanced neonatal resuscitation.
- Intravenous access should be obtained and blood should be reserved.
- Amniotomy alone can be used to augment labor
- Oxytocin infusion for induction or augmentation is best avoided as strong contractions produced by oxytocin can cause 2-3-fold increase of uterine rupture. If oxytocin is used, it should be done under the direct supervision of the consultant and continuous fetal heart rate monitoring and one-to-one care should be available. The frequency of contractions should not exceed 4 per 10 minutes
- Vaginal prostaglandin E2 tablets (dinoprostone) should not be used to ripen the cervix or induce labor because of the high risk of uterine rupture
- **Epidural anesthesia is not contraindicated**
- **Misoprost is contraindicated in previous cesarean patients**
- Continuous electronic fetal heart rate monitoring should be carried out for the duration of labor **as fetal distress is one of the earliest signs of scar dehiscence.**

New Pattern Questions

N1. With regards to flexion point, which is correct?
a. Flexion point is located 3 cm anterior to posterior fontanelle
b. Located 6 cm posterior to anterior fontanelle
c. Both a and b are correct
d. Both a and b are incorrect

N2. Traction force required for forceps delivery in primigravida is:
a. 15 kg
b. 18 to 20 kg
c. 13 kg
d. 25 kg

N3. Prerequisite for outlet forceps application are all *except*:
a. Engaged head
b. Fully dilated cervix
c. Uterus contracting
d. Station 0 or +1

N4. An elderly multigravida female presents in labor. She has multiple fibroids in lower uterine segment. Management is:
a. Vaginal delivery
b. Trial of labor
c. LSCS
d. Classical cesarean followed by hysterectomy

N5. Trial of scar is not attempted in:
a. CPD
b. Polyhydramnios
c. Previous LSCS
d. IUGR

N6. Optimum interval between uterine incision and delivery of fetal head during cesarean section should be:
a. < 90 secs
b. 90-150 secs
c. 150-200 secs
d. ≥ 200 secs

N7. All are the contraindications for vaginal birth after previous cesarean *except*:
a. Previous classical uterine incision
b. Previous lower segment transverse cesarean
c. Presence of inverted 'T'-shaped uterine incision
d. Where facilities for emergency cesareans are not available

N8. A forceps rotation of 30° from left occiput anterior (LOA) to occiput anterior (OA) with extraction of the fetus from +2 station is described as which type of forceps delivery?
a. High forceps
b. Midforceps
c. Low forceps
d. Outlet forceps

N9. Indications for cesarean hysterectomy are all *except*:
a. Placenta accreta
b. Couvelaire uterus
c. Atonic uterus with uncontrolled PPH
d. Rupture uterus

N10. A 32-year-old second gravida who had an LSCS in her first pregnancy is admitted in labor. The fetus is in the cephalic presentation. The head is engaged. This estimated fetal weight is 3 kg. Uterine contractions are 2 per 10 minutes. The fetal heart rate is 140 bpm. The cervical dilation is 5 cm. The vertex is felt 1 cm above the ischial spines. The posterior fontanelle is felt. Pelvis is adequate. The membranes are intact. What is the best management option?
a. Do an amniotomy and allow labor to progress
b. Do an amniotomy and commence an infusion of oxytocin
c. Perform a cesarean section
d. Perform a ventous delivery in the second stage

N11. A second para who has had an uncomplicated lower segment cesarean section in her first pregnancy is in labor. She is allowed a trial of vaginal delivery. What is the earliest warning sign of scar rupture?
a. Severe continuous abdominal pain
b. Fetal distress
c. Fresh vaginal bleeding
d. Maternal tachycardia

N12. The following statements are related to symphysiotomy *except*:
a. The operation should be done only when obstruction is anticipated
b. Isolated outlet contraction is the ideal case
c. FHS must be present
d. Ventouse is preferable to forceps for extraction

N13. Symphysiotomy is indicated in:
a. Contraction of brim
b. Contraction of cavity
c. Contraction of outlet
d. All of these
e. None of the above

N14. Cesarean delivery on maternal request should be done at:
a. 37 weeks
b. 38 weeks
c. 39 weeks
d. 40 weeks

N15. All of the following are indications of classical cesarean section except:
a. Small breech baby
b. Large baby with transverse lie
c. Leiomyoma in lower pole of uterus
d. Cancer endometrium

Previous Year Questions

VENTOUSE/FORCEPS

1. **Ventouse in 2nd stage of labor is contraindicated in:**
   a. Persistent occipitoposterior position   **[AI 00]**
   b. Heart disease
   c. Uterine inertia
   d. Preterm labor

2. **Contraindication of vacuum extraction:**   **[PGI June 04]**
   a. Prematurity   b. Brow presentation
   c. Fetal distress   d. Floating head
   e. Undilated cervix

3. **All are complications of vacuum assisted delivery over forceps delivery** *except*:   **[AIIMS Nov 13]**
   a. Cephalohematoma
   b. Subgaleal hematoma
   c. Intracranial hemorrhage
   d. Transient lateral rectus palsy

4. **Which statement is true regarding Ventouse (vacuum extractor)?**   **[AIIMS May 03]**
   a. Minor scalp abrasions and subgaleal hematomas in newborn are more frequent than forceps
   b. Can be applied when fetal head is above the level of ischial spine
   c. Maternal trauma is more frequent than forceps
   d. Cannot be used when fetal head is not fully rotated

5. **True about vacuum extraction of fetus:**
                                                   [PGI May 2010]
   a. Can be used in nondilated cervix
   b. Can be used in incompletely dilated cervix
   c. Used in face presentation
   d. Applied 3 cm posterior to anterior fontanel
   e. Applied 3 cm anterior to posterior fontanel

6. **True about instrumental vaginal delivery:**   **[AI 02]**
   a. Full cervical dilatation is the only prerequisite
   b. Forceps are used in all cases of breech delivery
   c. Forceps may be used, if ventouse fails
   d. Ventouse cannot be used in rotational occipito-transverse/posterior delivery

7. **Outlet forceps means:**   **[PGI Dec 09]**
   a. Head at station "0"
   b. Full cervical dilatation
   c. Rupture of membrane
   d. Rotation > 45°

8. **In the criteria for outlet forceps application, all are incorrect** *except*:   **[AIIMS Nov 2011]**
   a. Fetus should be in vertex presentation or face with mentoanterior

   b. Sagittal suture should be less than 15 degrees from anteroposterior plane
   c. There should be no caput succedaneum
   d. Head should be at zero station

9. **Least complication in outlet forceps is:** **[AIIMS Dec 98]**
   a. Complete perineal tear
   b. Vulval hematoma
   c. Extension of episiotomy
   d. Cervical tear

10. **In heart disease, prophylactic forceps is applied at head station of:**   **[PGI Dec 98]**
    a. −1   b. +1
    c. 0   d. +2

11. **Forceps should not be used in:**   **[UP 01]**
    a. Twin delivery
    b. Hydrocephalus
    c. Postmaturity
    d. Aftercoming head of breech

12. **Forceps delivery is done in all** *except*:   **[PGI 89]**
    a. Mentoposterior
    b. Deep transverse arrest
    c. Aftercoming head
    d. Maternal heart disease

13. **All of the following are true regarding forceps and vacuum delivery** *except*:   **[AIIMS Nov 12]**
    a. Vacuum requires more clinical skills than forceps
    b. Vacuum is preferred more in HIV patients than forceps
    c. Forceps is more associated with fetal facial injury
    d. Vacuum has more chance of formation of cephalo-hematoma

14. **True statement about vacuum extraction of baby:**
                                                   [PGI May 2017]
    a. Pressure is maintained b/w 5 kg/cm^2 to 8 kg/cm^2
    b. Done when cervix is fully dilated
    c. Center of cup should be placed 1 cm in front of posterior fontanelle
    d. Cup rim should be placed 3 cm from the anterior fontanelle

EPISIOTOMY

15. **All of the following statements are true for episiotomies** *except*:   **[AI 02]**
    a. Allows widening of birth canal
    b. Can be either mid-line or mediolateral
    c. Involvement of anal sphincter is classified 3rd–4th degree perineal tear
    d. Mid-line episiotomies bleed less, are easier to repair and heal more quickly

16. An episiotomy is to be performed in a primigravida in labor. Which of these is an advantage of mediolateral episiotomy over midline episiotomy?
    a. Less chance of extension   [AIIMS May 2016]
    b. Can be repaired at ease
    c. Fewer breakdown
    d. Lesser blood loss

CESAREAN SECTION

17. The following is always an indication of cesarean section *except*:   [AI 02]
    a. Abruption placentae
    b. Untreated stage of Ib Ca cervix
    c. Active primary genital herpes
    d. Type IV placenta previa (major previa)

18. An absolute indication for LSCS in case of a heart disease is: [AIIMS Nov 00]
    a. Coarctation of aorta
    b. Eisenmenger syndrome
    c. Ebstein's anomaly
    d. Pulmonary stenosis

19. Indication of classical cesarean section:
                                        [PGI Dec 03]
    a. Ca cervix   b. Kyphoscoliosis
    c. Previous 2 LSCS d. HSV infection
    e. Contracted pelvis

20. Which of the following is not a contraindication of vaginal delivery after previous cesarean?   [AI 08]
    a. Previous classical C/S
    b. No history of vaginal delivery in the past
    c. Breech presentation in previous pregnancy
    d. Puerperial infection in previous pregnancy

21. Vaginal birth after cesarean section (VBAC) is contraindicated in: [PGI Nov 12]
    a. Previous classical section
    b. Suspected CPD
    c. NO vaginal birth previously
    d. Previous uterine rupture

22. In a woman having a previous history of cesarean section all of the following are indications VBAC *except*:   [AIIMS May 01]
    a. Occipito posterior position
    b. Fetal distress
    c. Breech presentation
    d. Midpelvic contraction

23. Trial of scar is contraindicated in all *except*:
                                        [AIIMS Nov 12]
    a. History of previous classical cesarean section
    b. History of previous CS due to contracted pelvis
    c. Previous 3 LSCS
    d. Previous history of LSCS (Indication malpresentation)

24. Best level of anesthesia for LSCS: [AIIMS Nov 13]
    a. T8   b. T10
    c. T6   d. T4

OTHERS

25. A cesarean section was done in the previous pregnancy. All of the following would be indications for elective cesarean section except:
                                        [AIIMS May 14]
    a. Breech
    b. Macrosomia
    c. Polyhydramnios
    d. Post-term

Answers with Explanations to New Pattern Questions

N1. **Ans. is c, i.e. Both a and b are correct**   *Ref. Dutta Obs. 9/e, p 540*

Vacuum cup should be applied at flexion point which is situated—at 3 cm anterior to posterior fontanelle or 6 cm posterior to anterior fontanelle. See figure in text.

N2. **Ans. is b, i.e. 18 to 20 kg**   *Ref. Dutta Obs. 9/e, p 533*

> **Traction force required by forceps is:**
> Primigravida = 18–20 kg
> Multigravida = 13 kg
> Vacuum = Initial pressure is 0.2 kg/cm² induced over 2 minutes. The pressure is gradually increased at the rate of 0.1 kg/cm² to a maximum of 0.8 kg/cm² (600 mm Hg).

N3. **Ans. is d, i.e. Station 0 or +1**

The outlet forceps are applied when station of fetal head is ≥ +3 station and not at 0 or +1.

Rest all options are prerequisites of forceps application in general

N4. **Ans. is d, i.e. Classical cesarean section followed by hysterectomy**

Since this female is multigravida with multiple fibroids in lower uterine segments - vaginal delivery is not possible as multiple fibroids are present in lower uterine segment. We will have to do cesarean - but LSCS is also not feasible due to fibroids in lower segment (a lot of bleeding will occur if we cut through fibroid). Hence classical cesarean section should be done. The treatment of multiple fibroids in a multipara is hysterectomy, so classical cesarean section should be followed by hysterectomy).

N5. **Ans. is a, i.e. CPD**

Trial of scar/VBAC should not be attempted in case of CPD

N6. **Ans. is a, i.e. < 90 secs**

N7. **Ans. is b, i.e. Previous lower segment transverse cesarean**   *Ref. JB Sharma Obs, p 595*

Previous 2 LSCS without any vaginal delivery in the past and not a single one is a C/I for VBAC

N8. **Ans. is c, i.e. Low forceps**   *Ref. Dutta Obs. 9/e p 533, Table 37.2*

Presence of fetal head at +2 station indicates low forceps delivery.

> High forceps   =   Head not engaged
> Mid cavity forceps =   Head engaged, presenting part above +2 station
> Low forceps   =   Head at +2 or below it but not yet reached pelvic flow
> Outtet   =   Head at or on perineum

N9. **Ans. is b, i.e. Couvelaire uterus**   *Ref. Dutta Obs. 7/e, p 598 Williams 24/e, p 599*

Cesarean hysterectomy refers to an operation where cesarean section is followed by removal of the uterus. Peripartum hysterectomy is the surgical removal of the uterus either at the time of cesarean delivery or in the immediate postpartum period (even following vaginal delivery).

Some indications for peripartum hysterectomy

- Uterine atony
- Abnormal placentation
  - Bleeding
  - Accreta syndromes
- Uterine extension
- Uterine rupture
- Cervical laceration
- Postpartum uterine infection
- Leiomyoma
- Invasive cervical cancer
- Ovarian neoplasia

M/C cause of cesarean/peripartum hysterectomy is abnormal placentation.

 Point to Remember

Couvelaire uterus (as seen after abruptio placenta) is not an indication for hysterectomy.

N10. Ans. is a, i.e. Do an amniotomy and allow progress of labor

In this case, all findings are suitable to allow VBAC. This patient is 5 cm dilated. Contractions are 2 in 10 minutes i.e. inadequate. Adequate contractions are 3 in 10 minutes. Hence logically augmentation of labor should be done. In previous LSCS patients augmentation should be done by doing ARM i.e. amniotomy and oxytocin should best be avoided.

N11. Ans. is b, i.e. Fetal distress

Earliest sign of scar rupture is fetal bradycardia i.e. change in FHR i.e. fetal distress.

N12. Ans. is a, i.e. The operation should be done only when obstruction is anticipated

N13. Ans. is c, i.e. Contraction of outlet   *Ref. Dutta Obs. 9/e, p 554*

- **Symphysiotomy is the operation designed to enlarge the pelvic capacity by dividing the symphysis pubis.**
- It can be done as an alternative to risky cesarean section when there is a likelihood of scar rupture in subsequent labors. Moreover, symphysiotomy produces permanent enlargement of the pelvis, as such future dystocia will be unlikely.
- The operation should be done in established obstruction and not when it is only anticipated.
- The conditions to be fulfilled before doing symphysiotomy are:
  - The pelvis should not be severely contracted; isolated outlet contraction is ideal
  - Vertex must be the presenting part
  - The FHS must be present.
- The operation consists of dividing the symphysis pubis strictly in the midline from above downwards until the arcuate ligament is cut.
- The baby is delivered spontaneously with liberal episiotomy or by traction—ventouse (preferable) or forceps.
- **Complications:** Retropubic pain, osteitis pubis, stress urinary incontinence and rarely vesicovaginal fistula.

N14. Ans. is c, i.e. 39 weeks   *Ref. Williams Obs. 25/e, p 568*

Cesarean delivery on maternal request (CDMR) should be done at 39 weeks.

N15. Ans. is d, i.e. Cancer endometrium   *Ref. Williams Obs. 25/e, p 578-579*

As discussed in text

(i)   Large baby with transverse lie necessitates classical cesarean

(ii) In small fetus with breech, the poorly developed lower uterine segment provides inadequate space for manipulation needed for breech delivery.

(iii) Fibroid is lower uterine segment are all indications of classical cesarean section. Cancer cervix but not cancer endometrium is an indication classical cesarean.

Answers with Explanations to Previous Year Questions

1. **Ans. is d, i.e. Preterm labor** *Ref. Dutta Obs. 9/e, p 539*

2. **Ans. is a, b, c, d and e, i.e. Prematurity, Brow presentation, Fetal distress, Floating head and Undilated cervix**
   Ref. Dutta Obs. 7/e, p 580; COGDT 10/e, p 466-467, Williams Obs 24/e

   Ventouse/Vacuum extraction: Ventouse is an instrument which assists in delivery by creating a vacuum between it and fetal scalp.

   Vacuum can be used when cervix is **at least 6 cm dilated (i.e. ventouse can be applied in incompletely dilated cervix)** but not undilated cervix

   Contraindications for vacuum:

   > **Mnemonic**
   >
   > **PCM not demanded in common public**
   > **P** = **P**rematurity (< 34 weeks or weight < 2 kg) as chances of scalp avulsion or subperiosteal hemorrhage are more
   > **C** = Fetal **c**oagulopathy
   > **M** = Fetal **m**acrosomia (weight ≥ 4 kg)
   > **N**ot = **N**onengaged fetal head
   > **D**emanded = Fetal **d**istress where urgent delivery is needed
   > **In** = **In**fection = HIV
   > **C**ommon = **C**PD (Cephalopelvic disproportion)
   > **P**ublic = **P**resentation other than vertex (including face presentation)

   Relative contraindication–Recent scalp blood sampling *Ref. Williams Obs 23/e, p 523*

3. **Ans. is None** *Ref. Williams Obs. 23/e, p 524*
   Ref. JB Sharma TB of Obs. p 637
   Complications of vacuum

Maternal	Fetal
• (In ventouse maternal complications are less than with forceps)	• MC is retinal hemorrhage (COGDT 10/e, p 468)
• Soft tissue injuries to the vagina, cervix and perineum	• Scalp injury
• Annular detachment of the cervix	• **Cephalhematoma** (More common with vacuum)
• Traumatic PPH	• **Intracranial hemorrhage**
	• **Subgaleal hemorrhage** (More common with vacuum)
	• Neonatal jaundice (More common with vacuum)
	• Asphyxia in difficult vacuum
	• Shoulder dystocia (More common with vacuum)
	• Erb's palsy, **6th and 7th nerve palsy.**

   Comparison of vacuum extractor with forceps:

Complications seen more with forceps:
• Maternal trauma
• Blood loss
• Episiotomy extension
• 3rd and 4th degree perineal lacerations
• Anal sphincter dysfunction

Fetal complications:

More with forceps	More with vacuum
• Intracranial hemorrhage • Facial N palsy • Brachial plexus palsy	• Sixth nerve palsy • Retinal injury • Cephalohematoma • Subgaleal hematoma

6th nerve palsy is a complication of vacuum extraction (Williams 23/e, p. 524) and fetal complications are more with vacuum than forceps. So, ideally the answer to this question should be none.

4. **Ans. is a, i.e. Minor scalp abrasions and subgaleal hematomas in newborn are more frequent than forceps**
   Ref. Dutta Obs. 9/e, p 539; Sheila Balakrishnan, p 545; COGDT 10/e, p 468
   Maternal trauma is less in vacuum than in forceps *(Option "c" is incorrect)*
   Vacuum promotes autorotation. So, it can be used in unrotated or malrotated occipitoposterior position of the head *(Option "d" is incorrect).*

    Point to Remember

   The two main advantages of vacuum over forceps are:
   i. *It can be used in unrotated or malrotated occipitoposterior position of the head, e.g. in deep transverse arrest with adequate pelvis.*
   ii. *It can be applied even through incompletely dilated cervix.*
      As far as **option "b"** is concerned: *Ref. Dennen's Forcep's Deliveries 3/e, p 178*
      "Although Malmstrom originally described application of the Ventouse to a scalp prior to full dilatation of the cervix and at any station of the head, the reported subsequent higher incidence of fetal injury has altered the indication."
   Currently, use at high stations and with incomplete cervical dilatation is discouraged.
   So, ventouse should not be applied when fetal head is above the level of ischial spine *(Option "b" incorrect).*
   COGDT 10/e, p 468 says about subgaleal hematomas:
   "Subgaleal hematoma, a more serious complication, occurs in 50 out of 10,000 vacuum deliveries.
   Subgaleal hematoma is mentioned as a complication of ventouse and not of forceps in all the books *(i.e. option "a" is correct).*

5. **Ans. is b and e, i.e. Can be used in incompletely dilated cervix and Applied 3 cm anterior to posterior fontanel.**
   Ref: Dutta Obs 9/e, p 539, Williams Obs 23/e, p 552-524, John Hopkins Manual of Obs. and Gynae 4/e, p 84
   Vacuum can be applied if cervix is atleast 6 cm dilated i.e. **option 'b' –'can be used in incompletely dilated cervix'** is correct but **option 'a' – can be used in nondilated cervix** is incorrect.
   Vacuum cannot be applied in presentation other than vertex. Hence, it cannot be applied in face presentation. **Option 'c' –'used in face presentation'** is incorrect.
   Proper cup placement is the most important determinant of success in vacuum extraction.
   "The center of the cup should be over the sagittal suture and about 3 cm in front of the posterior fontanel towards the face. Anterior placement on the fetal cranium – near the anterior fontanel rather than over the occiput–will result in cervical spine extension unless the fetus is small". *Ref. Williams Obs. 23/e, p 523*
   "The suction cup is applied in the midline on the sagittal suture about 1 to 3 cm anterior to the posterior fontanel (the flexion point)". *Ref. John Hopkins Manual of Obs and Gynae 4/e, p 84*
   i.e. option e – applied 3 cm anterior to posterior fontanel is correct.

6. **Ans. is b, i.e. Forceps are used in all cases of breech delivery** *Ref. Dutta Obs. 9/e, p 533; COGDT 10/e. p 468*

   Conditions (Criteria) to be fulfilled prior to forceps operation

Fetal and uteroplacental criteria	Maternal criteria
• The fetal head must be engaged • The cervix must be fully dilated • The membranes must be ruptured • The position and station of the fetal head must be known with certainty	• No major cephalopelvic disproportion by clinical pelvimetry • Bladder must be emptied • Adequate analgesia

Thus, fully dilated cervix is not the only prerequisite *(Option "a" is incorrect).*

Option "b" i.e. Forceps are used in all cases of breech delivery
The most commonly used method in breech presentation is the **assisted breech delivery** where Burns Marshall technique is used for the aftercoming head which does not involve the use of forceps but,
*Dutta 9/e, p 360 **says "Forceps can be used as a routine".***
Sheila Balakrishnan p 454 says "Forceps for the aftercoming head, Piper's forceps or any straight forceps can be used. This is the best method of delivery of the head."
*COGDT 10/e, p 347 **says "Piper forceps may be used electively or when the Mauriceau-Smellie-Veit maneuver fails to deliver the aftercoming head".***
So, forceps can be used routinely in breech deliveries but it is not a common practice. *So, option 'b' can be kept in +/– status.*
Earlier we have studied that ventouse is used in unrotated/malrotated occipitotransverse/posterior deliveries *(option 'd' incorrect).*
As far as *option 'c'* is concerned, i.e. Forceps may be used if ventouse fails.
*COGDT 10/e, p 468 **says "Under no circumstances should the operator switch from vacuum to forceps or vice versa. An excellent study examining neonatal injury clearly demonstrated that the greatest incidence of neonatal injury occurred in babies in whom both vacuum and forceps were used."***
So, amongst all the options given, option 'b' is partially correct. We are taking it as the answer of choice here.

7. **Ans. is b and c, i.e. Full cervical dilatation and Rupture of membrane**

8. **Ans. is a, i.e. Fetus should be in vertex presentation or face with mentoanterior**

Ref: Dutta Obs. 9/e, p 533, Williams 23/e, p 513

Outlet forceps are a variety of low forceps. So, the basic criteria to be fulfilled before any forceps application should be fulfilled here also.

Mnemonic

Criteria to be fulfilled before forceps application.

F	=	**F**avorable head position and station
O	=	**O**pen OS (fully dilated)
R	=	**R**uptured membranes
C	=	**C**ontractions present and consent taken
E	=	**E**ngaged head, empty bladder
P	=	No major C**P**D/pelvis should not be contracted

Classification of forceps delivery according to station and rotation

Type of procedure	Criteria	Forceps used
A. High forceps	• Vertex not engaged • No longer used	Kielland forceps
B. Mid forceps	• Head is engaged but presenting part/station is between 0 to +2	Anderson's or Simpson's forceps
C. Low forceps	• Station is ≥2 but has not yet reached the pelvic floor. Rotation can be more or less than 45°	
D. Outlet forceps	• Station is more than +2 and fetal skull has reached the level of pelvic floor (i.e. station ≥ + 3) • Scalp is visible at the introitus without separating the labia • Fetal head is at or on the perineum • Sagittal suture is AP diameter or Right or left occipitoanterior or posterior position • Rotation is < 45°	Wrigley's forceps

---

Note:
- The most important point of reference in the use of forceps is the station of biparietal diameter.
- These days forceps are not applied at station < + 2.
- When correctly applied, the long axis of the blades should correspond to occipitomental diameter.

Coming to Q7.

Option a: Head at 0 station–Incorrect as in outlet forcep, head is at the perineum

Option b: Full cervical dilatation–correct

Option c: Membrane should be ruptured–correct

Option d: Rotation >45 degrees–incorrect as rotation should be less than 45 degrees

Coming to Q8.

Option a: Fetus should be in vertex or mentoanterior position is correct

Option b: Sagittal suture should be less than 15° from anteroposterior plane is incorrect

Forceps can be applied till maximum 45° rotation

Option c: There should be no caput succedaneum – again incorrect as presence of caput succedaneum is not a contraindication for forceps application

Option d: Head should be at zero station—also incorrect as outlet forceps is applied when head reaches the perineum

9. **Ans. is d, i.e. Cervical tear**   *Ref. COGDT 10/e, p 463; Sheila Balakrishnan, p 463*

In case of outlet forceps, all the complications given in the options may occur but cervical tear is unlikely, as outlet forceps is applied at the level of introitus and does not reach the cervix.

10. **Ans. is d, i.e. +2**   *Ref. COGDT 10/e, p 463; Sheila Balakrishnan, p 463*

- In heart disease, forceps are applied prophylactically to cut down the second stage of labour and usually low or outlet forceps applied.
    - *Low forceps:* Applied when leading point of fetal scalp is at station + 2 and not on pelvic floor.
    - *Outlet forceps:* Applied when fetal skull has reached pelvic floor and scalp is visible at the introitus even without separating the labia, i.e. station ≥ + 3

> *Note:* "0" station means the level of ischial spine.
>
> Although outlet forceps was traditionally preferred over ventouse as maternal efforts are not needed with forceps but, ventouse is preferred these days as it obviates the need of lithotomy position, which may be hazardous for heart disease women.

11. **Ans. is b, i.e. Hydrocephalus**   *Ref. Dutta Obs. 9/e, p 533*

As discussed previously, one of the criteria to be fulfilled before applying forceps is—there should be no major cephalopelvic disproportion (CPD) by clinical pelvimetry and hydrocephalus is an important cause of CPD.

Ref. Dutta Obs. 7/e, p 352

12. **Ans. is a, i.e. Mentoposterior**   *Ref. Dutta Obs. 9/e, p 537*

As discussed previously, forceps can be applied in all those conditions where vaginal delivery can be done and cesarean section is not mandatory. In mentoposterior, vaginal delivery is not possible and hence cesarean has to be done.

So forceps cannot be applied.

'Forceps delivery is only reserved for mentoanterior position'.   *Ref. Dutta Obs. 9/e, p 537*

13. **Ans is a, i.e. Vacuum requires more clinical skills than forceps**   *Ref Dutta Obs. 7/e*

- Forceps require more skills than vacuum.
- Ventouse: It is comfortable and has lower rates of maternal trauma and genital tract lacerations.
    - Reduced maternal pelvic floor injuries.
    - Perineal injuries are less.

Due to these reasons, vacuum is preferred more than forceps in HIV patients to decrease the mother-to-child transmission.

14. **Ans. is b and d, i.e. Done when cervix is fully dilated, Cup rim should be placed 3 cm from the anterior fontanelle**

Ref. Williams 24/e, pg 584

An important step in vacuum extraction is proper cup placement over the flexion point. This pivot point maximizes traction, minimizes cup detachment, flexes but averts diameter through the pelvic outlet. This improves success rates, lowers fetal scalp injury rates, and lessens perineal trauma because the smallest fetal head diameter distends the vulva

- The flexion point is found along the sagittal suture, approximately 3 cm in front of the posterior fontanel and approximately 6 cm from the anterior fontanel. Because cup diameters range from 5 to 6 cm, when properly placed, the cup rim lies 3 cm from the anterior fontanel (i.e **option d is correct**).

Operative vaginal delivery –vacuum and forceps are done when cervix is fully dilated. Although vacuum can be applied in incompletely dilated cervix but it is better used in completely dilated cervix (**option b is correct**).

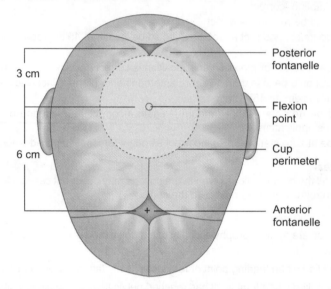

Fig. (William): Drawing demonstrates correct cup placement at the flexion point. Along the sagittal suture, this spot lies 3 cm from the posterior fontanel and 6 cm from the anterior fontanel.

Indications for vacuum delivery

1. Prolonged second stage of labor
2. Nonreassuring fetal heart rates
3. To cut short second stage of labor e.g. in heart disease , preeclampsia , post caesarean delivery

Absolute Contraindications for vacuum delivery:

1. Underlying fetal disorder
   i. Fetal bleeding disorders(haemophilia etc)
   ii. Fetal demineralizing diseases (osteogenesis imperfect)
2. Failure to fulfill all the requirements for operative vaginal delivery
   i. Incomplete dilatation of the cervix
   ii. Intact fetal membranes
   iii. Unengaged vertex
3. Abnormalities of labor
   i. Fetal malpresentations—breech, transverse lie
   ii. Suspected CPD
4. Estimated gestational age <34 weeks or weight of fetus <2500 g

Relative contraindications

   i. Suspected fetal macrosomia >/= 4500 g
   ii. Uncertainty about fetal position
   iii. Prior scalp sampling.

15. **Ans. is a, i.e. Allows widening of birth canal**   *Ref. Dutta Obs. 7/e, p 568, 569; Dewhurst 6/e, p 307*
   - **Episiotomy:** It is defined as a surgical incision made over the perineum and vulva during delivery to increase the diameter of the vulval outlet (and not the whole of birth canal) during childbirth and to prevent perineal tears. Thus, episiotomy is a surgically given perineal tear of second degree.
   - As discussed in the text, episiotomy can be either mediolateral or median (option b) although median episiotomy has many advantages like less bleeding, easy to repair, quick to heal (option d) but if it extends it can involve anal sphincter so this episiotomy is not preferred.
   - Commonly a right mediolateral episiotomy is performed, angled at 45° from the vulvar rim.
   - Anal sphincter involvement is equivalent to 3 degree, perineal tear (perineal tears are dealt with in detail in Chapter 8).

16. Ans. is a, i.e. Less chance of extension   *Ref. Dutta Obs. 9/e, p 537*

See the text for explanation

17. Ans. is a, i.e. Abruptio placentae   *Ref. Dutta Obs. 9/e, p 242; COGDT 10/e, p 334*

Cesarean Section is not indicated in all cases of abruptio placentae.

"An attempt at vaginal delivery is indicated if the degree of separation appears to be limited and if continuous FHR tracing is reassuring. When the placental separation is extensive but the fetus is dead or of dubious viability, vaginal delivery is indicated".   *Ref. COGDT 10/e, p 334*

- In carcinoma cervix, classical cesarean section should be done. Vaginal delivery should not be allowed because of cervical dystocia and injuries.   *Ref. Dutta Obs. 9/e, p 288*
- Cesarean section is indicated in an active primary genital HSV infection where the membranes are intact or recently ruptured.   *Ref. Dutta Obs. 9/e, p 282'*
- In severe degree of placenta previa (Type II posterior, Type III or Type IV), cesarean section is indicated for maternal interest even if the baby is dead. During the recent years there has been a wider use of cesaren section, so in an attempt to reduce maternal risk and improve fetal salvage.   *Ref. Dutta Obs. 9/e, p 235*

18. Ans. is a, i.e. Coarctation of Aorta   *Ref. Dutta Obs. 9/e, p 260*

- *Heart disease during pregnancy in itself is not an indication for cesarean section.*
- Cesarean section in heart disease is done in cases where aorta is involved, like coarctation of aorta, aortic aneurysm or aortopathy with aortic root > 4 cm or recent MI or if patient is on Warfarin therapy as discussed in Chapter 16.

"In coarctation of aorta, elective cesarean section is preferred to minimize dissection associated with labor."
                                                      Ref. Dutta Obs. 9/e, p 26

19. Ans. is a and e, i.e. Ca cervix; and Contracted pelvis
                         Ref. Dutta Obs. 7/e, p 590, 591; Williams Obs. 22/e, p 597, 598, 23/e, p 555
                                                  Ref. JB Sharma TB of Obs. p 659

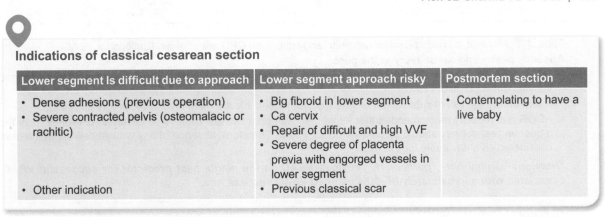

Indications of classical cesarean section

Lower segment Is difficult due to approach	Lower segment approach risky	Postmortem section
• Dense adhesions (previous operation) • Severe contracted pelvis (osteomalacic or rachitic) • Other indication	• Big fibroid in lower segment • Ca cervix • Repair of difficult and high VVF • Severe degree of placenta previa with engorged vessels in lower segment • Previous classical scar	• Contemplating to have a live baby

Also Know:

Classical cesarean section:

- It is associated with maximum incidence of rupture uterus[Q] (4–9%)[Q].
- **Rupture can occur during pregnancy[Q] even prior to onset of labor.**
- Site of rupture – upper segment.

20. Ans. is c, i.e. Breech presentation in previous pregnancy
                   Ref. Williams Obs. 22/e, p 610-613, 23/e, p 567-571; Mudaliar 9/e, p 449

21. Ans. is a, b and d, i.e. Previous classical section, Suspected CPD and Previous uterine rupture

Vaginal birth after cesarean section—VBAC: Or Trial of Scar

Earlier previous cesarean section was considered as an absolute contraindication for vaginal delivery.

—Dutta Obs. 6/e, p 355

But now this statement is considered as an exaggeration.   *—Williams Obs. 22/e, p 608, 23/e, p 565*

Vaginal delivery can be tried in post LSCS cases in institutions equipped to respond to emergencies (i.e. rupture uterus) with physicians immediately available to provide emergency care.

Recommendations of American College of Obstetricians and Gynecologists (ACOG) for vaginal birth after cesarean delivery (VBAC) selection criteria.   *—Williams Obs. 22/e, p 610, 23/e, p 567, Table 26.2*

- One prior low-transverse cesarean delivery.
- Clinically adequate pelvis (No CPD).
- No other uterine scars of previous rupture.
- Physician immediately available throughout active labor who is capable of monitoring labor and performing emergency cesarean delivery.
- Availability of anesthesia and personnel for emergency cesarean delivery.

Contraindications:

- *Prior classical or T- or J-shaped uterine incision* or extensive transfundal uterine surgery (e.g. myomectomy).
- Previous 2 or more LSCS
- Previous history of uterine rupture
- Contracted pelvis or CPD
- Medical or obstetrical complications that preclude vaginal birth (e.g. placenta previa), malpresentations
- Inability to perform emergency CS due to factors related to the facility, surgeon, anesthesia, or nursing staff.

Thus, it is clear that previous classical cesarean and suspected CPD are contraindications for VBAC.

Absence of any vaginal delivery in the past.

- Previous history of vaginal delivery either before or following a cesarean birth significantly improves the prognosis of a subsequent successful VBAC.
- It also lowers the risk of subsequent uterine rupture. Indeed it is the most favourable prognostic factor.
- ACOG has recently recommended that for women with prior two low transverse cesarean deliveries, only those with a prior vaginal delivery should be considered for VBAC. Therefore, absence of any vaginal delivery in the past can be considered as unfavorable for VBAC.

"Previous vaginal birth, particularly previous VBAC, is the single best predictor for successful VBAC and is associated with approximately 87–90% planned VBAC success rate."

—Management of High-risk Pregnancy by SS Trivedi, Manju Puri, p 235

"A history of two or more C sections without any successful vaginal delivery may preclude offering VBAC as well".

Johns Hopkins Manual of Obs and Gynae 4/e, p 86

Thus, no vaginal delivery in the past is also a relative contraindication for VBAC.

This leaves us with two options, i.e. puerperal infection and breech presentation (in Q 16).

- **Puerperal infection in previous pregnancy** may interfere with healing and predisposes to a weak scar. Previous uterine infection is listed as one of the causes of uterine scarring and is considered a risk factor for uterine rupture during trial of labor for VBAC. It is, thus, a relative contraindication for VBAC (ACOG bulletin).
- **As far as breech presentation** in the previous pregnancy is concerned. The success rate for a trial of scar depends to some extent on the indication for the previous cesarean delivery. Generally, about 60–80% of trial after prior cesarean birth result in vaginal delivery, with success being maximum if previous cesarean section was because of breech presentation.

The ideal interdelivery interval after cesarean should be 18 months. But minimum it should be 6 months.

22. Ans. is d, i.e. Midpelvic contraction

Ref. Williams Obs. 22/e, p 610-613, 23/e, p 567, Bedside Obs/Gynae by Richa Saxena 1/e, p 122

As discussed in previous question –VBAC (trial of scar) should be attempted only in patients with clinically adequate pelvis. Hence, if previous cesarean was done for midpelvic contraction, we would not attempt VBAC.

Remember: VBAC and trial of scar are synonyms of each other but VBAC and trial of labor have two different meanings.

Trial of Labor: It means trying vaginal delivery in a pelvis which is mildly contracted at the inlet only, i.e. mild CPD at the level of inlet.

Trial of Labor should not be done in a previous LSCS patient. Let me explain you with examples:

- Suppose there is a G_2P_1, female with previous LSCS due to fetal distress (nonrecurring reason for cesarean section). This time she presents in labor. No fetal distress. Pelvis is adequate.

Management will be: VBAC (i.e. try vaginal delivery)

- Suppose there is a G_2P_1, female with previous vaginal delivery. This time she presents in labor, but there is mild CPD cut the level of inlet. No fetal distress. Management will be: try vaginal delivery – **now this is called trial of labor.**
- Suppose there is a G_2P_1, female with previous LSCS due to fetal distress. This time she presents in labor. No fetal distress. There is mild CPD at the level of inlet. Now management will be: cesarean section, not trial of labor as trial of labor is contraindicated in previous cesarean patients.

23. Ans. is d, i.e. Previous history of LSCS (Indication malpresentation)   *Ref. Williams 24/e, p 611*

As discussed:

- If there is history of previous LSCS due to contracted pelvis next pregnancy, LSCS has to be done. VBAC cannot be tried.
- If there is history of previous classical cesarean section—again VBAC is contraindicated.
- History of previous 3LSCS also means VBAC is contraindicated. But if there is history of previous LSCS done because of fetal distress or malpresentation, next time VBAC can be tried.

24. Ans. is d, i.e. T4   *Ref. Dutta Obs. 7/e, p 519*

Spinal anesthesia:

Spinal anesthesia is done by injection of local anesthetic agent into the subarachnoid space. It has less procedure time and high success rate. Spinal anesthesia can be employed to alleviate the pain of delivery and during the third stage of labor. For normal delivery or for outlet forceps with episiotomy, ventouse delivery, block should extend from T10 (umbilicus) to S1. For cesarean delivery, level of sensory block should be up to T4 dermatome. Hyperbaric bupivacaine (10-12 mg) or lignocaine (50-70 mg) is used.

25. Ans. is c, i.e. Polyhydramnios   *Ref. Williams 24/e, p 611*

Some factors that influence a successful trial of labor in a woman with prior cesarean delivery

Low-risk	Favors success	Increases failure rate	High-risk[a]

• Transverse
• **Incision,**
  prior vaginal
  delivery,
• Appropriate
  counseling,
• Sufficient
  personnel and
  equipment
	• Teaching hospital
	• White race
	• Spontaneous labor
	• Prior, fetal malpresentation
	• 1 prior transverse incisions
	• Nonrecurrent indication
	• Current preterm
	  pregnancy
		• Single mother
		• Increased maternal age
		• Macrosomic fetus
		• Obesity
		• Breech
		• Multifetal pregnancy
		• Preeclampsia
		• EGA > 40 weeks
		• Unknown incision
		• Labor induction
		• Medical disease
		• Multiple prior cesarean deliveries
		• Education < 12 years
		• Short interdelivery interval
		• Liability concerns
			• Classical or T incision, low
			  vertical incision
			• Prior rupture
			• Patient refusal
			• Transfundal surgery
			• Obstetrical
			  contraindication, e.g.
			  previa
			• Inadequate facilities

[a]Most consider these absolute contraindications.
EGA = estimated gestational age.

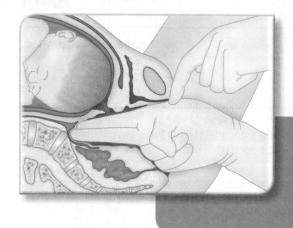

Chapter 14

Preterm Labor, Premature Rupture of Membranes and Post-dated Pregnancy

 Chapter at a Glance

➢ Preterm Labor
➢ PROM

➢ Post-term or Post-dated Pregnancy

PRETERM LABOR

DEFINITION

American College of Obstetricians and Gynecologists (ACOG) has defined preterm labor as the onset of labor (regular painful uterine contractions associated with effacement and dilatation of the cervix) prior to the completion of 37 weeks (259 days) of gestation counting from the first day of the last menstruation period.

- **Preterm (or premature) infant**: Infant born before 37 completed weeks of gestation.
- **Very preterm infant**: Infant both before 32 completed weeks of gestation.
- **Moderately preterm infant**: Infant born between 32 and 34 completed weeks of gestation.
- **Late preterm infant**: Infant born between 34 and 36 weeks of gestation.

Incidence

5-15%.

RISK FACTORS AND CAUSES OF PRETERM LABOR (PTL)

- Most important risk factor for preterm labor (PTL) is previous H/O PTL:
  - If previous PTL occurred at ≥ 35 weeks: Chances of recurrence are 5%.
  - If previous PTL occurred at < 34 weeks: Chances of recurrence are 15%

  - If there is H/O previous 2 PTL at <34 weeks: Chances of recurrence are 40%.
- M/C cause of preterm labor is idiopathic followed by infection.
- Infections which can lead to PTL are:

  - Bacterial vaginosis
  - Gardnerella vaginalis
  - Ureaplasma urealyticum
  - Mycoplasma hominis
  - Fusobacterium

- Other causes are:
  - Low socioeconomic status
  - Smoking
  - Obesity
  - Diabetes
  - Congenital anomalies of uterus
  - Incompetent os
  - Overstretching of uterus like in twins, polyhydramnios.

PROPHYLACTIC MEASURES TO DECREASE PRETERM LABOR

- Stop smoking
- Progesterone: ACOG recommends the use of progesterone—17-OH progesterone intramuscularly—in women with documented history of previous spontaneous preterm delivery. Progesterone decreases uterine activity by suppressing cytokine activity.

Regimes

i. 17α-hydroxyprogesterone caproate 500 mg I/M weekly

ii. Oral dydrogesterone
10-20 mg daily

iii. Vaginal micronized
progesterone 200 mg daily

} given between 16–36 weeks of pregnancy

Progesterone can be given to women with
i. Past H/O preterm labor
ii. Women with cervical cerclage
iii. Uterine malformation
iv. Short cervix (vaginal progesterone)
ACOG (2008) recommends their use only in women with a documented history of a previous spontaneous preterm delivery.

- **Cerclage surgery:** If cervical incompetence is also present.

DIAGNOSIS OF PRETERM LABOR

1. **Symptoms and signs of PTL**
   - Uterine contractions occurring at a frequency of 4 in 20 minutes or 8 in 60 minutes.
   - Lower back pain
   - Passage of blood stained vaginal discharge (show)
   - Sensation of pelvic pressure
   - Bulging membranes/rupture of membranes.

2. **On TVS:**
   - Length of cervix < 2.5 cm **(2.5 cm is the cut off length of cervix to predict PTL)**[Q]
   - Dilatation of cervix > 2 cm
   - Shape of cervix appears 'U' shaped

   Shape of cervix on USG: There is bulging of fetal membranes into a widened internal os in case of preterm labor. **The normal shape of cervix is T shape and it changes to Y shape → V shape and finally to U shape.** *(See "Ans. 4" of this chapter for different shapes of cervix).*

3. Levels of fibronectin protein.

   Fibronectin assay: Presence of fibronectin glycoprotein produced by fetal amnion in the cervico-vaginal discharge between 24 and 34 weeks is a predictor of preterm labor. When the test is negative it reassures that delivery will not occur within the next 7 days.
   Test = ELISA done between = 24-34 weeks of pregnancy
   Value ≥ 50 ng/ml are positive for PTL.

 Note: Alkaline phosphatase if > 90 percentile, is also considered as a predictor of PTL.

MANAGEMENT OF PRETERM LABOR

General Principles

- Most important risk of PTL is, that lungs of fetus are not mature and hence it can lead to respiratory distress syndrome
- Drug to enhance fetal lung maturity is corticosteroids.

Uses of corticosteroid

- Decreases chances of respiratory distress syndrome
- Decreases chances of intraventricular hemorrhage
- Decreases chances of Necrotising enterocolitis

Corticosteroid can lead to neonatal hypoglycemia (more with betamethasone) and development delay. This is more in fetuses ≥ 34 weeks. So although ACOG recommended use of corticosteroids beyond 34 weeks, it has not been universally adopted.

Administration of Corticosteroids

- Corticosteroids cause a significant reduction (40 to 60%) in rates of neonatal death, respiratory distress syndrome and intraventricular hemorrhage and necrotising enterocolitis. They are safe for the mother.
- Two doses of betamethasone (12 mg) is given intra-muscularly 24 hours apart, or 4 doses of 6 mg of dexame-thasone is given intramuscularly 12 hours apart, to enhance lung maturation.
- There is some concern that Betamethasone available in India has only one component of Betamethasone that is betamethasone sodium phosphate and does not have Betamethasone sodium acetate, which may not be very effective. Hence currently dexamethasone is becoming drug of choice in india and is economical also.
- Minimum duration needed for corticosteroid to act is 24 hours after the last dose.
- Maximum benefit occurs between 2 to 7 days of injection
- **ACOG-August 2017 guidelines for use of corticosteroid**
  - **In pregnancy of < 24 weeks:** corticosteroid is not recommended
  - **In pregnancy between 24 weeks to 33 weeks** *+6* days corticosteroids should be given to all patients of preterm labour including those with ruptured membrances and twin pregnancy
- If labor does not occur within 14 days of giving corticosteroid, rescue dose of steroid is given
- **Maximum number of rescue which can be given is one.** If given more times, it results in cerebral palsy of the fetus
  - **In pregnancy between 34 weeks and 36 weeks and 6/7 days:** Give corticosteroid if earlier no steroid was given

- No rescue dose is given after 34 weeks.
- Corticosteroids are most effective if delivery occurs 24 hours to 48 hours after and up to 7 days of administration of the second dose. They reduce the neonatal death rate even within the first 24 hours.
- Weekly repeat courses are not recommended as it can lead to cerebral palsy in the fetus.
- **Contraindication for** corticosteroid is chorioamnionitis.

 Note: ACOG says a first dose of antenatal corticosteroid is administered regardless of ability to complete additional dose before delivery.

Corticosteroid can lead to neonatal hypoglycemia (more with betamethasone) and development delay. This is more in fetuses ≥ 34 weeks. So although ACOG recommends use of corticosteroid beyond 34 weeks. It has not been universally adopted.

Tocolytic Therapy

 Note: Since the best effect of corticosteroid occurs after 24-48 hours of administration, at least for this time uterine activity should be stopped, hence short term tocolytic therapy should be given.

- ACOG 2016 has concluded that tocolytic agents donot markedly prolong gestation but may delay delivery in some women till 48 hours.
- Tocolytic drugs do not cause a clear reduction in perinatal or neonatal mortality or neonatal morbidity.
- Tocolysis may be considered for women with suspected **preterm labor before 34 weeks**.
- Tocolysis is contraindicated if prolonging the pregnancy carries a risk to the mother or the fetus.

 Mnemonic

Drugs used as TOCOLYTICS
P: **P**rostaglandin synthetase inhibitor: Indomethacin
C: **C**alcium channel blocker: Nifedipine
O: **O**xytocin antagonist: Atosiban
S: **M**agnesium **s**ulfate
NO: **N**itric **O**xide donor: Glyceral trinitrate
Bleeding: **B**eta agonist viz Ritodrine, Terbutaline, Isosuprine, Salbutamol

 Important One Liners

- Tocolytic of choice: Nifedipine
- Tocolytic of choice in heart disease patient - Atosiban
- Tocolytic with maximum maternal side effects - β agonist
- Side effects of β agonist -   M/C = Tremors
                              Hyperglycemia
                              Hypokalemia
                              Pulmonary edema
- Tocolytic with maximum fetal side effects: Indomethacin (like premature closure of ductus arteriosus, oligohydramnios, neonatal pulmonary hypertension)

Betamimetics and PTL
- The Betamimetic which is not used in US for protein labor: Ritodrine
- In US, Terbutaline is used for PTL
- **Uses of Terbutaline**
  i. Short-term tocolytics
  ii. For managing tachysystole
  iii. Prior to external cephalic version
- Tocolytic contraindicated in diabetes: β agonist

Dose of Nifedipine as Tocolytic

- 20 mg oral stat (not sublingual) followed by 10 mg oral 4-6 hourly till contractions cease followed by 10 mg 8 hourly for a week.

 Also Know:
- MgSO$_4$ inhibits uterine contractility at serum levels of 8-10 meq/L.
- Long term MgSO$_4$ given for several days for tocolysis is associated with neonatal osteopenia (due to loss of calcium from fetus) due to loss of calcium from fetus).

Contraindications of Tocolytics

- Chorioamniotis
- Advanced labor
- Pregnancy > 34 weeks
- Preeclampsia/eclampsia
- Abruptio placenta
- Congenital anomaly of fetus not compatible with life.

MgSO$_4$ as Neuroprotective in Preterm Labor

- MgSO$_4$ is used by some hospitals in case of preterm labor to prevent cerebral palsy in the fetus born between 24-27, 6/7 weeks.
- Loading dose of 4-6 gm is given over 20-30 minutes followed by infusion of 1-2 gm/hour

Prevention of Group B Streptococci Infection

Benzylpenicillin or ampicillin should be given in established preterm labor as prophylaxis against early onset neonatal sepsis due to Group B Streptococcus in those with a known carrier status. In cases of penicillin allergy, clindamycin can be substituted. Ideally, it should be administered 4 hours prior to delivery.

 Remember: **Following have no role in preterm labor management**

i. *Antibiotics* (do not have any role in PTL unless and until membranes are also ruptured)
ii. *Progesterone* (helps in preventing preterm labor but cannot be used as a tocolytic).
iii. Bed rest
iv. Cervical pessary or arabin pessary to support cervix in females with short cervix

MANAGEMENT OF PRETERM LABOR AT GESTATIONAL AGE ≥ 34 WEEKS

- If corticosteroid was not given earlier, it has to be given single dose. No rescue dose to be given.
- Then Just wait and watch (No induction of Labor)
- Send rectal or vaginal swab for group B streptococcal infection.

MANAGEMENT OF PRETERM LABOR AT < 34 WEEKS

- Corticosteroids (Betamethasone/Dexamethasone)

    +

    Short term tocolytic (Best-nifedipine)

    +

    $MgSO_4$ (for neuroprotection in pregnancy <28 weeks)

Mode of Delivery

The earlier concept was all patients delivering at <34 weeks in both cephalic and breech, preferred mode of delivery is cesarean section

New concept: With cephalic presentation preferred mode is vaginal delivery even if delivery occurs at < 34 weeks. But in breech with delivery at < 34 weeks cesarean section is done.

PROM

Premature rupture of membranes is defined as spontaneous rupture of membranes before the onset of labor.

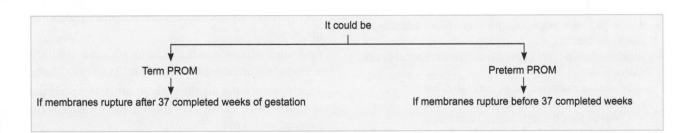

It could be

Term PROM
If membranes rupture after 37 completed weeks of gestation

Preterm PROM
If membranes rupture before 37 completed weeks

Etiology

Etiology of PROM is multifactorial but infection (Chlamydia-trachomatis, group B streptococci and bacterial vaginosis) plays an important role.

Presentation

- Patients present with a typical history of sudden gush of clear or pale yellow fluid leaking from vagina. However many women may present with history of intermittent or constant leaking of small amounts of fluid or just sensation of wetness within the vagina.

Diagnosis

Per speculum examination – First step in the diagnosis of PROM includes **"a sterile per speculum examination** to demonstrate leaking. Pooling of fluid in the posterior fornix or leakage of fluid from the cervical os confirms the diagnosis of PROM.

A per vaginal examination should not be done as it increase the risk of intrauterine infection and preterm labor. If the condition is still doubtful, following tests are done.

Tests for PROM

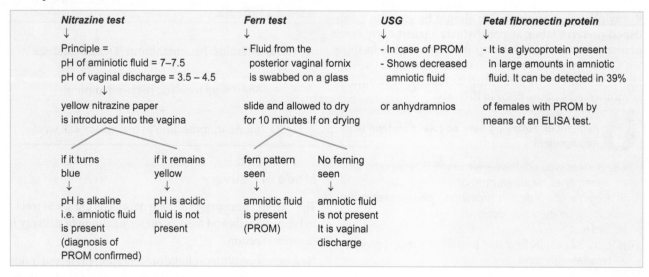

Nitrazine test		Fern test		USG	Fetal fibronectin protein
↓		↓		↓	↓
Principle = pH of aminiotic fluid = 7–7.5 pH of vaginal discharge = 3.5 – 4.5		- Fluid from the posterior vaginal fornix is swabbed on a glass		- In case of PROM - Shows decreased amniotic fluid	- It is a glycoprotein present in large amounts in amniotic fluid. It can be detected in 39%
↓					
yellow nitrazine paper is introduced into the vagina		slide and allowed to dry for 10 minutes If on drying		or anhydramnios	of females with PROM by means of an ELISA test.
if it turns blue	if it remains yellow	fern pattern seen	No ferning seen		
↓	↓	↓	↓		
pH is alkaline i.e. amniotic fluid is present (diagnosis of PROM confirmed)	pH is acidic fluid is not present	amniotic fluid is present (PROM)	amniotic fluid is not present It is vaginal discharge		

Effects of Preterm Premature Rupture of Membranes (PPROM)

- Preterm labor and birth
- Pulmonary hypoplasia due to severe oligohydramnios
- Skeletal and joint deformities of the fetus due to compression.
- Chorioamnionitis

General Principles of Management

- Bed rest.
- Sterile pads for inspection for meconium staining and signs of infection.
- Women should be observed for signs of clinical chorio-amnionitis.
  - Maintain a temperature chart 4–8 hourly.
  - Auscultate the fetal heart rate 4–8 hourly.
  - Observe for offensive vaginal discharge.
- A high vaginal swab may be performed at the initial speculum examination, but weekly high vaginal swabs need not be performed.

- Maternal full blood count or C-reactive protein is performed initially, but it is not necessary to carry out these tests weekly, because the sensitivity of these test in the detection of intrauterine infection is low.
- Cardiotocography is useful as fetal tachycardia can be due to chorioamnionitis.
- Use of prophylactic antibiotics has been found to reduce chorioamnionitis. Erythromycin is given for 10 days. Penicillin also can be used. Co-amoxiclav increases the risk of necrotising enterocolitis in the neonate and should not be used.
- Antenatal corticosteroids should be administered if the period of gestation is between 28 and 34 weeks.
- Tocolysis does not significantly improve the perinatal outcome and is recommended for 48 hours for corticosteroids to be effective.
- Delivery is considered at 34 weeks after completion of a course of corticosteroids.

Management of PPROM: See Table 14.1

Table 14.1: Management of preterm premature rupture of membranes

Gestational age	Management
34 weeks or more	Plan delivery: labor induction unless contraindicated Group B streptococcal prophylaxis Single corticosteroid course may be considered up to 36⁶ᐟ⁷ weeks
32 weeks to 33 completed weeks	Expectant management Group B streptococcal prophylaxis Single corticosteroid course Antimicrobials to prolong latency

Contd...

Contd...

Gestational age	Management
24 weeks to 31 completed weeks	Expectant management Group B streptococcal prophylaxis Single corticosteroid course Tocolytics: no consensus Antimicrobials to prolong latency Magnesium sulfate for neuroprotection may be considered
<24 weeks	Expectant management or induction of labor Group B streptococcal prophylaxis is not recommended Single corticosteroid course may be considered Tocolytics: no consensus Antimicrobials: may be considered

POST-TERM PREGNANCY

A pregnancy continuing beyond two weeks of the expected date of delivery (> 42 weeks or >294 days) is called postmaturity or post-term pregnancy. Pregnancy between 41-42 weeks is called prolonged pregnancy.

Most common cause of post-term pregnancy is wrong dates so, a careful review of menstrual history is important in all such cases.

Once the menstrual history is confirmed, investigations like USG and amniocentesis are done:

i. To confirm fetal maturity

ii. To detect any evidence of placental insufficiency

Causes of Post-term pregnancy:
- Wrong dates: Due to inaccurate LMP (most common).
- Biologic variability (hereditary) may be seen in the family.
- Maternal factors: Primipara/elderly multipara/H/o previous prolonged pregnancy, sedentary habit.
- Fetal factors: Congenital anomalies: Anencephaly – (abnormal fetal HPA axis), adrenal hypoplasia (Diminished fetal cortisol response).
- Placental factors: Sulphatase deficiency (low estrogen).

In post dated pregnancy perinatal mortality and morbidity is much increased.

Fetal complications in Post-dated pregnancy

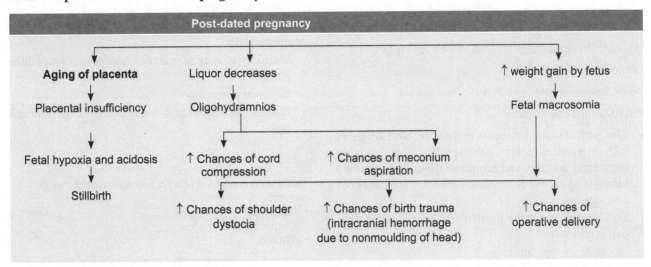

Neonatal complications:

- Chemical pneumonitis, atelectasis and pulmonary hypertension due to meconium aspiration.
- Hypoxia and respiratory failure.
- **Hypoglycemia and Polycythemia.**

Algorithm for management of postterm pregnancy

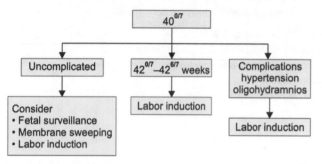

Fig. 14.1: Algorithm for management of postterm pregnancy (summarized from American College of Obstetricians and Gynecologists, 2016d).

When gestational age is uncertain the ACOG (2017) recommends delivery at **41 weeks gestation** using best clinical estimate of gestational age. It also recommends against use of amniocentesis for fetal lung maturity.

Table 14.2: Adverse maternal and perinatal outcomes associated with postterm pregnancy

Maternal	Perinatal
Fetal macrosomia	Stillbirth
Oligohydramnios	Postmaturity syndrome
Preeclampsia	NICU admission
Cesarean delivery Dystocia Fetal jeopardy	Meconium aspiration Neonatal convulsions Hypoxic-ischemic encephalopathy
Shoulder dystocia	Birth injuries
Postpartum hemorrhage	Childhood obesity
Perineal lacerations	

(NICU: Neonatal intensive care unit)

Post Maturity Syndrome

- The postmature newborn is unique, and features include wrinkled, patchy, peeling skin; a long, thin body suggesting wasting; and advanced maturity in that the infant is open-eyed, unusually alert and appears old and worried.
- Skin wrinkling can be particularly prominent on the palms and soles.
- The nails are typically long.

- Most postmature neonates are not technically growth restricted because their birthweight seldom falls below the 10th percentile for gestational age.
- The syndrome complicates 10 to 20 percent of pregnancies at 42 completed weeks (American College of Obstetricians and Gynecologists, 2016).
- Associated oligohydramnios substantially raises the likelihood of postmaturity. It is seen that 88 percent of fetuses were postmature if there was oligohydramnios defined by a sonographic maximal vertical amniotic fluid pocket that measured ≤1 cm at 42 weeks.

Chorioamnionitis

- It is the inflammation of fetal membranes and literally means intrauterine infection.
- The WBC infiltrate the chorion and cells are of maternal origin.
- If cells are found in the amniotic fluid it is called **amnionitis**.
- If cells are found in umbilical cord it is called **funiculitis**. M/C cause of chorioamnionitis is PROM
  - **Others:** Prenatal diagnostic procedures like amniocentesis, CVS
  - Bacterial vaginosis
  - H/O amino acid infusion, cerclage surgery
  - Cases handled by dais

Diagnosis: Is made if there is fever (> 100.4°F) with any of the following signs or investigations
- Maternal tachycardia
- Fetal tachycardia
- Uterine tenderness
- Foul smelling amniotic fluid
- Maternal leukocytosis (≥ 16000/cc)
- Raised C-reactive protein > 2.5
- High vaginal swab culture and stain positive

Management:
- Mainstay of management is Antibiotics-Ampicillin 500 gm 6 hour
- Removal of cerclage
- Delivery as soon as possible regardless of gestational age.

There is no role of following is management of chorioamnionitis:
- Tocolytics
- Corticosteroids
- Waiting

New Pattern Questions

N1. A primipara complains of lower abdominal pain at period of amenorrhea of 32 weeks. The fetus is in cephalic presentation.

P/A = 1-2 contractions/10 minutes

FHR = 138 beats per minute

O/E = Cx = 2 cm dilated

75% effaced

Membranes intact

What is the next step in management?
a. Allow labor to progress normally
b. Commence intramuscular corticosteroid and oral nifedipine
c. Start intramuscular corticosteroid and I/V ritrodrine
d. Start I/V broad spectrum antibiotics

N2. A Primipara complains of sudden onset vaginal discharge at 32 weeks of pregnancy.

P/A = No contractions

Cephalic presentation

Fetal heart sounds = Normal

What is the first step in management?
a. Start broad spectrum antibiotics
b. Start corticosteroid
c. Perform sterile perspeculum examination
d. Perform sterile vaginal examination

N3. A G_2P, female attends antenatal clinic at 31 weeks. She has H/o previous preterm delivery at 20 weeks. Under which of the following circumstances would you do a cervical cerclage?
a. Cervical funneling detected on TVS
b. Occurrence of abdominal pain and uterine contraction
c. Rupture of membranes
d. Cervical length of 22 mm on TVS

N4. Which of the following investigations are essential before cervical cerclage is performed?
a. Estimate C-reactive protein levels
b. Perform a white cell count
c. Perform a transvaginal ultrasound scan to assess the cervical length and exclude funnelling
d. Perform an ultrasound scan for fetal abnormalities and screen for aneuploidy

N5. All are risk factors for preterm delivery *except*:
a. Absence of fetal fibronectin at < 37 weeks
b. Previous history of preterm baby
c. Asymptomatic cervical dilatation
d. Chlamydial infection of genital tract

N6. The following infection is associated with preterm labor:
a. Trichomonas vaginitis
b. Candidiasis
c. Bacterial vaginosis d. HPV

N7. In preterm labor, the risk of fetal complication is highest with the use of following drug:
a. Ritrodrine
b. Nifedipine
c. Indomethacin
d. Isoxsupine

N8. Best tocolytic in a cardiac patient is:
a. Atosiban
b. Isoxsuprine
c. Nifedipine
d. $MgSO_4$

N9. All of the following are contraindications to tocolysis *except*:
a. Chorioamnionitis
b. Fetal distress
c. Anencephaly
d. Placenta previa

N10. AG_2P_1 to female has a history of previous preterm birth at 32 weeks. The percentage chances of preterm birth in this pregnancy are:
a. 5%
b. 10%
c. 15%
d. 25%

N11. A G_2P_1 female at 35 weeks experiences uterine contractions. No fetal distress is seen and membranes are not ruptured. Which of the following is to be done?
a. 12 mg betamethasone injection
b. Vaginal swab culture
c. Tocolytic therapy d. Cervical cerclage

N12. Blood will interfere with the nitrazine test for detecting ruptured membranes because:
a. It is acid
b. It is alkaline
c. It contains increased amounts of sodium chloride
d. It contains decreased amounts of sodium chloride
e. It reacts with the normal flora of vaginal bacteria to give an acid reaction

N13. Post-term labor is seen in:
a. Hydramnios
b. PID
c. Anencephaly
d. Multiple pregnancy

N14. In post-term pregnancy, there is increased risk of all *except*:
a. Postpartum hemorrhage
b. Meconium aspiration syndrome
c. Intracranial hemorrhage
d. Placental insufficiency leading to fetal hypoxia

N15. Saffron colored meconium is seen in:
a. Postmaturity
b. TB
c. Breech
d. Normal in appearance

N16. The following is used for neuro protection in Preterm Labor:
a. Ca
b. Mg^{+2}
c. K^+
d. Na^+

N17. Management of PTL does not include all *except*:
a. Antibiotics
b. Progesterone
c. $MgSO_4$
d. Cervical cerclage

N18. Features of post maternity syndrome are all *except*:
a. Wrinkled skin
b. Macrosomia
c. Long thin body
d. Long nails

Previous Year Questions

1. **All of the following are risk factors for preterm labor** *except*: **[LEP]**
   a. Previous history of preterm birth
   b. Multiple pregnancy
   c. Previous LLETZ
   d. Marfan's syndrome
   e. Punch biopsy of cervix

2. **Risk of preterm delivery is increased if cervical length is:** **[AI 05]**
   a. 2.5 cm   b. 3.0 cm
   c. 3.5 cm   d. 4.0 cm

3. **Cut-off value of cervical length at 24 weeks of gestation for prediction of preterm delivery is:** **[AI 03]**
   a. 0.5 cm   b. 1.5 cm
   c. 2.5 cm   d. 3.5 cm

4. **On TVS which of the following shape of cervix indicates preterm labor:** **[AI 07]**
   a. T   b. Y
   c. U   d. O

5. **All are used in preterm labor to decrease uterine contractility** *except*? **[AIIMS Dec 97]**
   a. Methylalcohol
   b. Ritodrine
   c. Magnesium sulphate
   d. Dexamethasone

6. **Which of the following drugs may be used to arrest premature labor?** **[AI 99]**
   a. Aspirin
   b. α-Methyl dopa
   c. Magnesium sulphate
   d. Diazoxide

7. **All are tocolytics** *except*: **[AI 08]**
   a. Ritodrine   b. Salbutamol
   c. Isoxsuprine   d. Misoprostol

8. **In primi, in preterm labor, all of the following can be used as Tocolytic** *except*: **[PGI Dec 08]**
   a. Ritodrine   b. MgSO$_4$
   c. Dexamethasone   d. Propranolol

9. **Drug used for preventing preterm labor:** **[LEP]**
   a. Estrogen   b. Progesterone
   c. Nifedipine   d. Ritrodrine

10. **A pregnant mother at 32 weeks gestation presents in preterm labor. Therapy with antenatal steroids to induce lung maturity in the fetus may be given in all of the following conditions** *except*: **[AI 04]**
    a. Prolonged rupture of membranes for more than 24 hours
    b. Pregnancy induced hypertension

    c. Diabetes mellitus
    d. Chorioamnionitis

11. **A 32-year-old female with a history of 2 mid-trimester abortions, comes now with 32 weeks of pregnancy and labor pains with Os dilated 2 cm. All are done,** *except*: **[AI 00]**
    a. Immediate circlage
    b. Betamethasone
    c. Antibiotics
    d. Tocolytics

12. **G3 with previous second trimester abortion presents at 22 week of gestation with abdominal pain, USG shows funneling of internal os and cervical length 21 mm. What is the ideal management?** **[AIIMS Nov 07]**
    a. Dinoprost and bed rest
    b. Misoprost and bed rest
    c. Fothergills stitch
    d. McDonald stitch

13. **A woman at 32 weeks of pregnancy, presents with labor pains. On examination, her cervix is dilated and uterine contractions are felt. The management is:** **[AI 00]**
    a. Isoxsuprine hydrochloride
    b. Dilatation and evacuation
    c. Termination of pregnancy
    d. Wait and watch

14. **All of the following are known side effects with the use of tocolytic therapy** *except*: **[AIIMS May 03]**
    a. Tachycardia   b. Hypotension
    c. Hyperglycemia   d. Fever

15. **Adverse effect of tocolytic agonist in pregnancy:**
    a. HTN   b. ↓ glucose
    c. ↓ K$^+$ d. Arrhythmia
    e. Pulmonary edema

16. **The drug that inhibits uterine contractility and cause pulmonary edema is:** **[AIIMS May 01]**
    a. Ritodrine   b. Nifedipine
    c. Indomethacin   d. Atosiban

17. **Drug given to reduce uterine contractions during preterm labor with least side effects:** **[AIIMS Nov 07]**
    a. Ritodrine   b. Nifedipine
    c. Magnesium sulphate d. Progesterone

18. **Rupture of membrane is said to be premature when it occurs at?** **[AI 97]**
    a. 38 weeks of pregnancy
    b. 32 weeks of pregnancy
    c. Prior to Ist stage of labor
    d. II stage of labor

19. A lady presented with features of threatened abortion at 32 weeks of pregnancy. Which of the following statements with regard to antibiotic usage is not correct? [AIIMS May 2010]
    a. Antibiotic prophylaxis even with unruptured membranes
    b. Metronidazole, if asymptomatic but significant bacterial vaginosis
    c. Antibiotics if asymptomatic but significant bacteremia
    d. Antibiotics for preterm premature rupture of membranes

20. All are true about premature rupture of membrane (PROM) except: [PGI May 2010]
    a. Amnioinfusion is done
    b. Amoxiclav antibiotic should be given
    c. Aseptic cervical examination
    d. Steroid is used
    e. Preterm labor

21. A 35-year-old G2P1L1 presents to antenatal clinic at 35 weeks of pregnancy with C/O, leaking pervagina. Sample of pooled liquid turned red litmus paper blue and ferning was present. The temperature of the patient is 102°F and her pulse is 104. What is the next step in management?
    a. Administer betamethasone
    b. Administer tocolytics
    c. Administer antibiotics
    d. Place a cervical cerclage

22. A woman comes with postdated pregnancy at 42 weeks. The initial evaluation would be: [AIIMS May 01]
    a. Induction of labor
    b. Review of previous menstrual history
    c. Cesarean section
    d. USG

23. Anticipated preterm delivery. Dose of dexamethasone given to mother is: [AIIMS May 2015]
    a. 12 mg 12 hourly 2 doses
    b. 12 mg 24 hourly 4 doses
    c. 6 mg 24 hourly 2 doses
    d. 6 mg 12 hourly 4 doses

Answers with Explanations to New Pattern Questions

N1. Ans. is b, i.e. Commence intramuscular corticosteroid and oral nifedipine

Ref. Williams Obs. 22/e, p 503; 23/e, p 471

Since the period of amenorrhea is 32 weeks, administration of corticosteroids will cause significant reduction in neonatal deaths, due to respiratory distress syndrome and intraventricular hemorrhage. Nifedipine has fewer side effects than ritodrine. It is cheap, effective and is given orally and is therefore the preferred tocolytic drug. It should be administered in a dose of 20 mg twice or thrice daily for at least 48 hours till corticosteroids are effective. Therefore, the best management option is to commence intramuscular corticosteroids and oral nifedipine.

N2. Ans. is c, i.e. Perform sterile perspeculum examination

The first step in the management is to perform a sterile speculum examination.

N3. Ans. is d, i.e. Cervical length of 22 mm on TVS

USG indicated cerclage is done in females with history of 1 or more preterm births with cervical length ≤ 25 mm before 24 weeks.

N4. Ans. is d, i.e. Perform an ultrasound scan for fetal abnormalities and screen for aneuploidy

Before answering the question lets discuss a few details on cervical cerclage surgery.

Nomenclature for cerclage application

Old (1999)	New (2007)
Prophylactic, elective	History indicated
Therapeutic, salvage	Ultrasound indicated
Rescue, emergency urgent	Physical examination indicated

Recommendations for history indicated cerclage

- Should be offered to women with 3 or more previous preterm births and/or second trimester losses
- Should not be routinely offered to women with two or fewer previous preterm birth and/or second trimester losses (Level B evidence)

Recommendations for USG indicated cerclage

- Women with history of 1 or more spontaneous preterm births or/mid trimester losses with Y, V or U detected on USG or cervical length < 25 mm before 24 weeks
  - Not recommended for women without a history of spontaneous preterm delivery or second trimester losses with incidentally detected cervical length ≤ 25 mm
  - Not recommended for funneling of cervix in the absence of cervical shortening to ≤ 25 mm

A cervical cerclage should be carried out in her as she has H/O 3 previous preterm deliveries.

An ultrasound scan for fetal abnormalities and screening for aneuploidy should be carried out, before insertion of a history-indicated suture, to ensure both viability and the absence of lethal/major fetal abnormalities. Assessment of cervical length is not indicated before applying a history indicated cerclage. It is not essential to perform a white cell count or C-reactive protein levels before performing a cervical cerclage.

N5. Ans. is a, i.e. Absence of fetal fibronection at < 37 weeks

Ref. Fernando Arias 4/e

Risk factors for preterm labor: have been discussed in Ans. 1

Fetal fibronectin

- It is a fetal glycoprotein found in the cervicovaginal discharge before 22 weeks and again after rupture of membranes.
- Levels of fibronectin > 50 mg/ml indicates preterm delivery (not absence of fibronectin).

N6. Ans. is c, i.e. Bacterial vaginosis

Infections which can lead to preterm labor are

- Gardenella vaginalis (Bacterial vaginosis)
- Fusobacterium
- Ureoplasma ureolyticum
- Mycoplasma hominis

N7. Ans. is c, i.e. Indomethacin

See the text for explanation.

N8. Ans. is a, i.e. Atosiban *Ref. Textbook of Obs.tetrics, Shiela Balakrishnan 1/e, p 231*

Role of Tocolytics in Heart Disease

- Most of the tocolytics are contraindicated in heart disease
- Safest tocolytic is atosiban (oxytocin antagonist)
- Beta agonist is contraindicated in cardiac arrhythmias, valvular disease and cardiac ischemia because of their sympathomimetic side effects such as tachycardia, palpitation and hypotension.
- Nifedipine is contraindicated in conduction defect, left ventricular failure due to side effects as tachycardia, hypotension, etc.

Tocolytics of choice	
• Overall tocolytic of choice	• Nifedipine
• Safest tocolytic agent (as it can be used in heart disease patient)	• Atosiban
• Most efficacious tocolytic agent	• Nifedipine
• Tocolytic preferred in heart disease	• Atosiban

N9. Ans. is d, i.e. Placenta previa *Ref. Dutta Obs. 7/e, p 319*

Contraindications to tocolysis

• Chorioamnionitis	• Preeclampsia/eclampsia
• Advanced labor	• Fetal distress
• Abruption	• IUFD
• Congenital anomalies not compatible with life	• Pregnancy >34 weeks

As far as placenta previa is concerned tocolysis is not contraindicated

Management of patient with placenta previa and preterm labor:

- Tocolytic agent: *"Uterine contractions are common in patients with placenta previa. Since uterine contractions have the potential to, disrupt the placental attachment and aggravate the bleeding, most obstetricians favor the use of tocolytic agents in the expectant management of patient with placenta previa"*.... High risk pregnancy Fernando arias
- **Most commonly used tocolytics in case of placenta previa.**
  - Nifedipine
  - Magnesium sulphate
- **Tocolytics which are not used**
  - Terbutaline and Ritodrine: They cause tachycardia and make the assessment of patient's pulse rate unreliable.
  - Indomethacin: It causes inhibition of platelet cyclo-oxygenase system and prolongs the bleeding time.

N10. Ans. is c, i.e. 15% *Ref. Williams Obs 24/e, p 841*

Recurrent spontaneous preterm births according to prior outcome

Birth outcome	Second birth (< 34 weeks) (%)
First birth ≥ 35 weeks	5
First birth ≤ 34 weeks	16
First and second birth ≤ 34 weeks	41

N11. Ans. is b, i.e. Vaginal swab culture *Ref. Fernando Arias 3/e, p 240; Sheila Balakrishnan, p 233*

The patient is having uterine contractions at 35 weeks of pregnancy.

At 35 weeks:

- There is no role of Betamethasone (corticosteroid). ***"Current evidence supports the administration of a single course of antenatal corticosteroids between 24-34 weeks to enhance fetal lung maturation".***

Ref. Arias 4/e, p 139

Self Assessment & Review: Obstetrics

- **Tocolytic therapy:** It is given for short-time use so that corticosteroids can act. Since at 35 weeks, there is no role of corticosteroid, So therefore, no role of Tocolytic.
- Cervical cerclage – no role at 35 weeks. Done before 32 weeks.

- Vaginal/rectal swab culture should be sent to detect group B streptococcus infection. **ACOG recommends universal screening of all pregnant women at 35–37 weeks for rectovaginal GBS followed by intrapartum antibiotic prophylaxis in GBS positive women.**

N12. Ans. is b, i.e. It is alkaline   *Ref. Fernando Arias 3/e, p 245; COGDT 10/e, p 279*

Nitrazine Test for Diagnosis of Premature Rupture of Membranes:

Principle:	The vaginal pH is normally 4.5 to 5.5, where as amniotic fluid usually has a pH of 7.0 to 7.5.
Test:	Nitrazine paper is smeared with vaginal secretions.
Result:	Nitrazine paper will turn deep blue if amniotic fluid is present in vagina i.e., membranes have ruptured as pH will become alkaline. The membranes probably are intact if the color of the paper remains yellow (pH 5.0 to 5.5).
False result:	Antiseptic solution, urine, blood, and vaginal infections alter the vaginal pH and cause false-positive results.

N13. Ans. is c, i.e. Anencephaly   *Ref. Dutta Obs. 9/e, p 299*

Causes of Post-term pregnancy:

- Wrong dates: Due to inaccurate LMP (most common).
- Biologic variability (Hereditary) may be seen in the family.
- Maternal factors: Primipara/elderly multipara/H/o previous prolonged pregnancy, sedentary habit.
- Fetal factors: Congenital anomalies: Anencephaly – (Abnormal fetal HPA axis), adrenal hypoplasia (Diminished fetal cortisol response).
- Placental factors: Sulphatase deficiency (Low estrogen).

N14. Ans. is a, i.e. Postpartum hemorrhage   *Ref. Dutta Obs. 9/e, p 300*

Post dated/post term/post maturity are pregnancies which have completed 42 weeks or 294 days as calculated from the first day of the LMP, assuring dates are correct.

In post dated pregnancy perinatal mortality and morbidity is much increased.

Fetal complications in Postdated pregnancy:

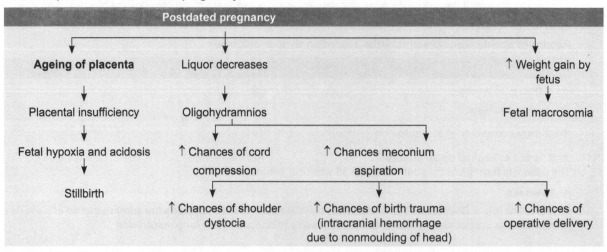

Neonatal complications:
- Chemical pneumonitis, atelectasis and pulmonary hypertension due to meconium aspiration.
- Hypoxia and respiratory failure.
- **Hypoglycemia and Polycythemia.**

N15. Ans. is a, i.e. Postmaturity   *Ref. Dutta Obs. 9/e, p 34*

Color of amniotic fluid
- Pregnancy – Colorless
- Near term – Pale straw colored due to presence of exfoliated lanugo hairs and epidermal cells from the fetal skin.
- Abnormal color
  - *Green* - meconium stained (fetal distress in conditions other than breech or transverse position).
  - *Golden yellow* - Rh-incompatibility.
  - *Greenish yellow (saffron)* - postmaturity.
  - *Dark colored* - in concealed hemorrhage.
  - *Dark brown (tobacco juice)* - in case of IUD.

N16. Ans. is b, i.e. Mg^{+2}.   *(William Obs 25/e, p 824)*

$MgSO_4$ is used for neuro protection in all PTL or PROM cases born before 28 weeks.

N17. Ans. is c, i.e. MgSO$_4$.

See the text for explanation.

N18. Ans. is b, i.e. Macrosomia.   *(William Obs 25/e, p 836-837)*

Macrosomia is seen in post dated/post term pregnancy but if fetus develops post maturity syndrome then it will be long, thin and emaciated so it can not be macrosomic. Postmaturity syndrome is seen in 10–20% of post-term pregnancies, rest all babies are macrosomic.

For more details see text.

Answers with Explanations to Previous Year Questions

1. Ans. is e, i.e. Punch biopsy of cervix   *Ref. Fernando Arias 4/e, p 136, 137*

> **Risk factors for preterm labor:**
> 1. H/O previous preterm labor
> 2. In utero exposure to DES
> 3. Cervical surgery like cone biopsy, LLETZ, laser ablation and trachelectomy.
> ***Note:*** Punch biopsy, laser vaporization and cryotherapy have not been associated with preterm birth.
> 4. Obstetrical trauma to cervix during labor or delivery including spontaneous labor, forceps and vacuum delivery and cesarean section.
> 5. Uterine overdistension as in multifetal pregnancy, polyhydramnios.
> 6. Multiple dilation and evacuation
> 7. Infections like bacterial vaginosis, asymptomatic
> 8. Connective tissue disorders—Ehlers-Danlos syndrome, Marfan's syndrome
> 9. Preterm premature rupture of membranes
> 10. Uterine anomalies – unicornuate uterus.

> ***Note:*** M/C cause of preterm labor – idiopathic followed by infection.

2. Ans. is c, i.e. 3.5 cm   *Ref. Dutta Obs. 9/e, p 294; Fernando Arias 3/e, p 229, 230*

3. Ans. is c, i.e. 2.5 cm.

Preterm labor (PTL): Preterm labor is defined as labor (regular, painful frequent uterine contractions causing progressive effacement and dilatation of cervix) occurring before 37 completed weeks of gestation.

"Risk of preterm birth increases markedly when the cervix is less than 2.5 cm. This measurement has been widely accepted as the threshold to define the risk of premature birth. The possibility of preterm delivery when the cervix is < 25 mm is 17.8%. This risk is significantly greater than the normal risk, and hence these women require additional diagnostic tests and special care."   —*Fernando Arias 3/e, p 229, 230*

> *Also Know:*
> - *Most common cause of preterm labor is idiopathic followed by infection like urinary tract infection, vaginal infections etc*
> - Most common organisms responsible for preterm labor:
> - *Ureoplasma urealyticum and Gardenerella vaginum causing bacterial vaginosis.*
> - **Diagnosis of Preterm labor is by:**   —*Dutta 9/e, p 294*
>   - Regular uterine contractions with or without pain (at least 4 in every 20 min or 8 in 60 min).
>   - Dilatation (> 2 cm) and effacement (80%) of cervix.
>   - ***Length of cervix (measured by TVS) < 2.5 cm and funneling of internal os.***
>   - Pelvic pressure, backache and or vaginal discharge or bleeding.
>
> Thus for detecting preterm labor -TVS should be done and cervical length measured. Besides this fetal fibronectin if present in vaginal/cervical secretions before 37 weeks indicates preterm labor.

> **Fetal fibronectin:**
> - It is a fetal glycoprotein.
> - Normally it is found in the cervicovaginal discharge before 22 weeks and again after rupture of membranes.
> - If detected in cervicovaginal secretions prior to rupture of membranes, it indicates disruption of the maternal-fetal interface and may be predictive of impending preterm labor.
> - It is measured by ELISA and a value equal to or exceeding 50 ng/ml is considered positive and predictive of preterm delivery.
> - When the test is negative it reassures that delivery will not occur within next 14 days.

> *Remember:* Fetal fibronectin equal to or more than 50 ng/ml and cervical length < 2.5 cm on TVS are the best predictors especially in a woman with a prior history of preterm birth.

4. **Ans. is c, i.e. U**

*Ref. USG in Obs. and Gynae. Callens 4/e, p 581, 582;
Donald School Textbook of USG in Obs., p 342; Fernando Aris 3/e, p 265*

Shape of cervix	Seen in
T shaped	Normal
Y shaped	Suspicious of preterm labor
U shaped	Funneling of os–seen in incompetent os, preterm labor

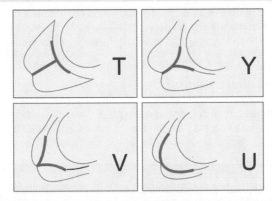

Extra Edge

Ultrasound of cervix during pregnancy *—USG in Obs. and Gynae. Callens 4/e, p 581*
* Cervical (endocervical) length is the distance between the internal os and external os.
* There are three ways to measure cervical length by sonography: transabdominal, transvaginal, and translabial (transperineal).
* Transvaginal sonography is the best method for cervical measurement.

5. **Ans. is d, i.e. Dexamethasone**
6. **Ans. is c, i.e. Magnesium sulphate**
7. **Ans. is d, i.e. Misoprostol**
8. **Ans. is a and b, i.e. Ritodrine and MgSO₄.**

Ref. Fernando Arias 3/e, p 227; COGDT 10/e, p 275; Dutta Obs. 7/e, p 508

Tocolytics are drugs to arrest preterm labor.
In case of preterm labor main problem is lungs of the fetus are not mature so the main treatment is antenatal steroid injection to the mother,but steroids require a minimum waiting period of 24 hours to act, so in the meanwhile tocolytics are given to arrest uterine contractions.

Mnemonic

Commonly used tocolytics are:
Mnemonic—
PCOS NO Bleeding
P = Prostaglandin synthetase inhibitors (indomethacin, sulindac)
C = Calcium channel blocker (nifedipine)
O = Oxytocin antagonist, i.e. atosiban
S = Magnesium sulphate
NO = Nitric oxide donor (glyceryltrinitrate)
Bleeding = Betamimetics (ritodrine, terbutaline, salbutamol and isoxsuprine HCl)

Drugs with tocolytic effect but poor efficacy:

- Ethyl alcohol[Q]
- Nitrites[Q]
- Atropine[Q]
- Phenothiazine[Q]
- General anesthetics[Q]

—KDT 6/e, p 319

 Note: Dexamethasone is used for fetal lung maturation in case of preterm labor but has no role as a tocolytic.

Progesterone: *Williams 23/e, p 816, Fernando Arias 2/e, p 87*

- Progesterone is not a tocolytic, it cannot stop pretern labor once contractions begin.
- It is used for prevention of miscarriages and for prevention of preterm labor.
- Progesterone is used only in those females who have risk factors for preterm labor but not in those in whom preterm labor has already begun.

Diazoxide: *Ref. Fernando Arias 3/e, p 227*

- It is a thiazide diuretic used to arrest preterm labor.
- Hypotension, tachycardia, hyperglycemia and decreased utero placental flow are some important maternal side effects.
- Hyperglycemia and fetal distress due to decreased utero placental flow are fetal side effects.
- *Diazoxide has more fetal adverse effect than Magnesium sulphate, so, MgSO$_4$ is a better tocolytic if we have to choose one answer out of these two.*

9. Ans. is b, i.e. Progesterone *Ref. Fernando Arias 4/e, p 138*

Drug used for preventing preterm labor is progesterone.

 Also Know:

- Progesterone is not a tocolytic
- Therapeutic cervical circlage can also be used for preventing preterm labor in pregnant females with gestational age <32 weeks and short cervix.
- MgSO$_4$, 4 g I/V loading dose followed by maintenance dose of 1 g/hr for 24 hours, reduces the risk of cerebral palsy in preterm infants. Thus, MgSO$_4$ should be given to all females having preterm labor between 24-32 weeks for neuroprotection.

10. Ans. is d, i.e. Chorioamnionitis

Ref. Meherban Singh 5/e, p 227; Fernando Arias 3/e, p 220; Sheila Balakrishnan p 230

"Corticosteroids can be given even in presence of maternal hypertension or diabetes mellitus, but should preferably be avoided if PROM is associated with definitive evidence of chorioamnionitis" —Meherban Singh 5/e, p 227

"Steroid treatment is contraindicated in presence of overt infection." —Fernando Arias 3/e, p 220

There are some concerns that betamethasone available in India has only one components of betamethasone that is betamethasone sodium phosphate and does not have betamethasone sodium acetate which may not be very effective. Hence currently dexamethasone is becoming drug of choice and is economical also in India. Ref: JB Sharma pg 461

11. Ans. is c, i.e. Antibiotics *Ref. Williams Obs. 24/e, p 850, 851*

In the question, patient is presenting with history of 2 midtrimester abortions and gestational age is 32 weeks with labor pains and dilatation of cervix 2 cm

The membranes are not ruptured, hence management includes:

- **Betamethasone:** To accelerate lung maturation of the fetus.
- **Tocolysis:** Tocolytics are not given with the aim to arrest preterm labor for a long time, but to prolong the labor for 48 hours.

  This servers the following purposes:
  - The corticosteroids get time to act.
  - Allows time for transport of the woman to better obstetrical centre.

  In this patient G: Age is 32 weeks and cervix is 2 cm dilated so the use of tocolytics is justified along with
- **Rescue cerclage (Williams 24/e, p 857):** There is support for the concept that cervical incompetence and preterm labor lie on a spectrum leading to preterm delivery. If cervical incompetence is recognized with threatened preterm labor, then emergency cerclage can be attempted.

> **Cervical cerclage is done in 3 conditions:**
> 1. Cervical incompetence
> 2. Prophylactically in women identified on USG to have short cervix <25 mm
> 3. Rescue cerclage–as discussed above.

- **Antibiotics: Do not have a role in preterm pregnancy with intact membranes.** In a study (ORACLE 11 trial) antimicrobials were given to patients with preterm labor but without membrane rupture, the results were disappointing. In his review, Goldenberg (2002) also concluded that antimicrobial treatment of women with preterm labor for the sole purpose of preventing delivery is generally not recommended. In a follow-up of the ORACLE II trial, Kenyon and associates (2008 b) reported that fetal exposure to antimicrobials in this clinical setting was associated with an increased cerebral palsy rate at age 7 years compared with that of children without fetal exposure.

12. **Ans. is d, i.e. McDonald stitch** *Ref. JB Sharma p 121*

Patient presenting at 22 weeks with:
- Length of cervix 21 mm on ultrasound examination and history of second trimester abortions indicating cervical incompetence as the cause of preterm labor. In this case Mc Donald stitch will be the ideal treatment as it will prevent preterm labor.

13. **Ans. is a, i.e. Isoxsuprine hydrochloride** *Ref. Fernando Arias 3/e, p 223, 224, 227, 228*

Now, in this case note - patient is presenting at 32 weeks (i.e., third trimester) with cervix dilated and uterine contractions are felt, which indicate it is a case of early preterm labor and should be managed by giving tocolytics i.e. isoxsuprine hydrochloride.

The tocolytic will delay labor by 48 hours, in the mean while we will give corticosteroids, so that the lung of the fetus matures.

14. **Ans. is d, i.e. Fever** *Ref. Dutta Obs. 9/e, p 472*

15. **Ans is c, d and e, i.e. ↓ K⁺; Arrhythmia and Pulmonary edema.**
Ref. Fernando Arias 3/e, p 224-227; COGDT 10/e, p 276, Dutta Obs 7/e, p 508.

Friends I am listing down the side effect of various tocolytics, just go through them. Amongst them, most important are side effects of betamimetics.

Commonly used tocolytics

Drugs	Maternal side effects	Fetal side effects
i. Betamimetics – Ritodrine – Salbutamol – Terbutaline – Isoxsuprine HCl	Tachycardia[Q], hypotension[Q], pulmonary oedema[Q], myocardial ischemia, hyperglycemia[Q] hypokalemia, cardiac arrythmias	Tachycardia, hyperglycemia hypokalemia, ileus, increased risk for intraventircular hemorrhage
ii. Indomethacin/Sulindac	GI side effects, coagulation disturbances thrombocytopenia, hepatitis, renal failure elevated BP only in hypertensive patients	Renal dysfunction, oligohydraminos, premature pulmonary closure of ductus arteriosus in utero[Q], neonatal pulmonary hypertension Increased risk of IVH and necrotising enterocolitis
iii. Glyceryl trinitrate patch	Headache[Q]	
iv. Magnesium sulphate	Diplopia, Respiratory depression[Q], **pulmonary edema[Q]**, cardiac arrest, hypothermia, Neuromuscular toxicity[Q], tetany (i.e. contraindicated in myasthenia gravis and renal failure)	Lethargy, hypotonia, respiratory depression, Intraventricular hemorrhage
v. Atosiban (Oxytocin antagonist)	Nausea, vomiting, arthralgia	
vi. Nifedipine (Calcium channel blocker)	Headache	None

 Remember: Most of the tocolytics lead to tachycardia, hypotension, (and not hypertension except indomethacin and that too only in hypertensive patients), **hyperglycemia** (not hypoglycemia), **hypokalemia**, pulmonary edema, respiratory depression, cardiac arrhythmias and cardiac arrest.

16. **Ans. is a, i.e. Ritodrine** *Ref. Fernando Arias 3/e, p 225; COGDT 10/e, p 276*

- Pulmonary edema is a serious complication of beta-adrenergic therapy (ritodrine) and $MgSO_4$.
- This complication occurs in patients receiving oral or (more common) intravenous treatment.
- It occurs more frequently in patients who have excessive plasma volume expansion, such as those with twins or those who have received generous amounts of intravenous fluids and in patients with chorioamnionitis.
- Patient presents with respiratory distress, bilateral rales on auscultation of the lungs, pink frothy sputum, and typical X-ray picture.
- Patients receiving IV beta-adrenergic drugs should be monitored continuously with pulse oxymeter to anticipate the development of pulmonary edema.

17. **Ans. is b, i.e. Nifedipine** *Ref. Fernando Arias 3/e, p 224*

Well friends - I know most of you will raise your eyebrows on this question. But read for yourself what high risk pregnancy *Ref. Fernando Arias 3/e, p 224 has to say-*

Nifedipine

"Randomized trials have demonstrated that nifedipine is a better tocolytic agent than ritodrine and terbutaline. Nifedipine is the best first line tocolytic agent available at this time.
Headaches are the main maternal side effect but overall the drug is well tolerated and has no apparent fetal effects." *Ref. Fernando Arias 3/e, p 224*

"When tocolysis is indicated for women in preterm labor, calcium channel blockers are preferred to other tocolytic agents compared mainly with betamimetics." *Ref. Mgt of High Risk Pregnancy, SS Trivedi, Manju Puri*

So undoubtedly **nifedipine is the answer of choice as well as the tocolytic of choice.**

IInd choice tocolytics are - Beta adrenergic drugs. *Ref. Fernando Arias 3/e, p 224*

As far as progesterones are concerned, though they are not associated with any significant side effect but they are not used as tocolytics.

They are used mainly for threatened abortion and for preventing preterm labor in patients who have risk factors for preterm labor.

18. **Ans. is c, i.e. Prior to 1st stage of labor** *Ref. Fernando Arias 3/e, p 240; Sheila Balakrishnan, p 233*

> Premature rupture of membranes (PROM) is defined as spontaneous rupture of membranes before the onset of labor. Preterm premature rupture of membranes (PPROM) is defined as premature rupture of membranes before 37 completed weeks.

19. **Ans. is a, i.e. Antibiotic prophylaxis even with unruptured membranes**
Ref. Danforth'sobs and Gynae, 10/e, p 169, 170, 171,172; Williams Obs. 23/e, p 163; COGDT 10/e, p 281, 278; Fernando Arians 3/e, p 234, 235

In the question, patient is presenting at 32 weeks with features of threatened abortion, means she is having warning symptoms and sings of preterm labor viz:

• Menstrual like camps	• Low dull backache
• Pelvic pressure	• Increase or change in vaginal discharge
• Fluid leaking from vagina	• Uterine contractions that are 10 or less than 10 minutes apart
• Lower uterine segment thinned out.	

In such patients (i.e. patients at risk for preterm labor), management should be:

Diagnostic	Therapeutic
• Ultrasound examination of cervical length • ELISA test for detecting Fetal fibronectin Protein in cervicovaginal secretion	• Bed rest • Avoidance of coital activity • Progesterone injection (weekly) or suppository (daily) till 35 weeks of pregnancy

As far as – antibiotics are concerned:

> *"Antibiotic therapy as a treatment of preterm labor and a means of prolonging pregnancy has been studied and for the most part has shown no benefit in delaying preterm birth".* *Ref. COGDT 10/e, p 278*

Thus antibiotics prophyllaxis to prevent preterm birth in pregnant women with intact membranes is not recommended. (**i.e.** option 'a' **is incorrect**)

> " *Antibiotic prophyl axis is given to prevent preterm birth in pregnant women with preterm premature rupture of membranes (for pregnancies between 24 and 32 weeks)*   *Ref. Fenando Arias 3/e, p 252*
> *One of the most important objectives of antibiotic treatment in women with PPROM is the prolongation of the latency period. Prolongation of the latency period is important because fetal lung maturity imporves with advancing gestational age, resulting in fewer days in the ventilator and shorter stay at NICU."*
>   *Ref. Fernando Arias 3/e, p 252*

Thus option 'd' **i.e.** antibiotics are recommended for preterm premature rupture of membranes is correct.

Now it is obvious – if a female is presenting with significant bacteremia, whether she is symptomatic or asymptomatic, we have to give antibiotics – that means option 'c' is also correct

Coming to option 'b' i.e. Metronidazole should be given for asymptomatic bacterial vaginosis, remains controversial

Williams 23/e. p 814 says – studies have found no evidence to support such use of metronidazole for prevention. Some other books like – COGDT say –

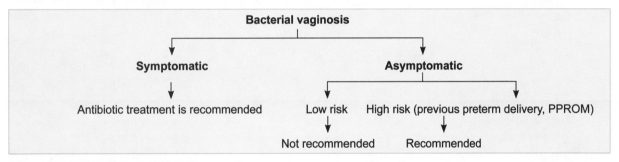

Thus option 'b' can be kept in +/- status

Since option 'a' is absolutely incorrect we are taking it, as the answer of choice.

20. **Ans. is a, i.e. Amnioinfusion is done.** *Ref: Dutta'sobs 7/e, p 317, 318, Williams Obs 23/e, p 163, COGDT 10/e, p 281*
    See the text for explanation.

21. **Ans. is c, i.e Administer antibiotics**   *Ref. Williams 23/e, p 819, Fernando Arias 3/e, p 197, 198*
    The fluid in vagina is amniotic fluid, as it showed in fern pattern on microscopy (presence of sodium chloride in liquor) and the red litmus turned blue (vaginal pH is acidic; amniotic fluid is alkaline).
    This patient with premature rupture of membranes (PROM) has a physical examination consistent with an intrauterine infection or chorioamnionitis.

> Acute Chorioamniotis is diagnosed clinically in presence of fever (100.4°F or 37.8°C) and at least two of the following:
> a. Maternal tachycardia   b. Fetal tachycardia
> c. Uterine tenderness   d. Foul smelling amniotic fluid
> e. Maternal leucocytosis

When chorioamnionitis is diagnosed, fetal and maternal morbidities increase and delivery is indicated regardless of the fetus's gestational age. In the case described, labor should be induced and antibiotics to be given to avoid neonatal group of streptococcal infection. Ampicillin is the drug of choice.

There is no role for tocolysis in the setting of chorioamnionitis and also because gestational age of patient is 35 weeks, since delivery is the goal: There is also no role for the administration of steroids as it is contraindicated in case of chorioamionitis.

 Remember: Management of chorioamnionitis at any age is delivery, regardless of the gestational age.

22. **Ans. is b, i.e. Review of previous menstrual history**   *Ref. Dutta Obs. 9/e, p 299*
    A pregnancy continuing beyond two weeks of the expected date of delivery (> 42 weeks or >294 days) is called postmaturity or post-term pregnancy. Pregnancy between 41-42 weeks is called prolonged pregnancy.
    Most common cause of post term pregnancy is wrong dates so, a careful review of menstrual history is important in all such cases –

"If the patient is sure about her date with previous history of regular cycles, it is a fairly reliable diagnostic aid in the calculation of the period of gestation. But in cases of mistaken maturity or pregnancy occurring during lactational amenorrhea or soon following withdrawal of the pill', confusion arises. In such cases, the previous well documented antenatal records of first visit in first trimester if available, are useful guides."

Ref. Dutta Obs. 9/e, p 399

Once the menstrual history is confirmed, investigations like USG and amniocentesis are done:

i. To confirm fetal maturity

ii. To detect any evidence of placental insufficiency

23. Ans. is d, i.e. 6 mg 12 hourly 4 doses

> Dose of Dexamethasone is 4 injections of 6 mg each, given @ 12 hourly interval intramuscularly.
> Dose of Betamethasone is 2 injections of 12 mg each, given @ 24 hours interval intramuscularly.

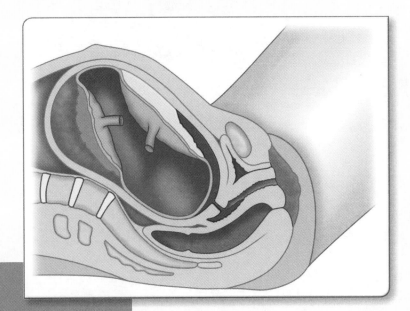

3

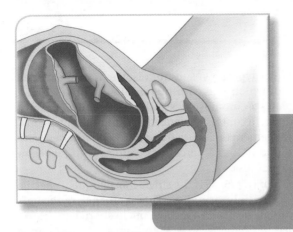

Abortion and MTP

Chapter at a Glance

➢ Spontaneous Abortion
➢ Types of Abortion

➢ Cervical Incompetence
➢ Antiphospholipid Antibody Syndrome

SPONTANEOUS ABORTION

Abortion is the expulsion or extraction from its mother of an embryo or fetus at less than 20 weeks, or weighing 500 g or less when it is not capable of independent survival.
Note: Period of viability is the period of gestation beyond which fetus is capable of independent existence.

Period of viability depends on medical facilities of a country and hence varies.

- As per WHO, Period of viability is 22 weeks.
- As per RCOG, Period of viability is 24 weeks.
- **In India:** beyond 28 weeks, Fetus is 100% viable.
- At <26 weeks—Not viable individualized.
- Between viable 26–28—case should be individualized.

Incidence: 10–20% of all clinical pregnancies end in miscarriage. 75% abortions occur before the 16th week and of those, about 75% occur before the 8th week of pregnancy.

Note:

- At 20 weeks, weight of fetus—300 gm
- Between 22–23 weeks—500 gm.
- At 24 weeks, weight of fetus—630 gm
- At 28 weeks, weight of fetus—1 kg
- 500 g of fetal development is attained approximately at **22 weeks (154 days) of gestation**.

Classification

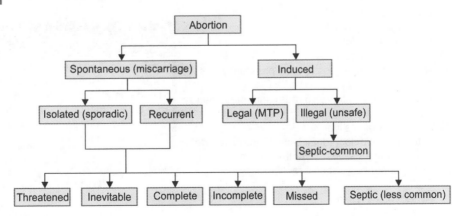

Nomenclature

- **Early Pregnancy Loss:** Currently ACOG (2017) defines this as a non viable intrauterine pregnancy with either an empty gestational sac or gestational sac containing an embryo or fetus without fetal heart activity within first 12 6/7 weeks of gestation.

- **Recurrent abortion:** RPL recurrent pregnancy loss. It is defined as a sequence of three or more consecutive spontaneous abortion before 20 weeks. American society for reproductive medicine (2013) defines RPL as 2 or more failed pregnancies confirmed by USG or histologically.

Common Causes of Abortion (Table 15.1)

- Most common cause of abortion (spontaneous abortion)—Chromosomal defect i.e. aneuploidy (genetic factor/defective germplasm).

It leads to 50% cases of abortion in 1st trimester and 30% in 2nd trimester.

Fetal Factors

- Both abortion and chromosomal anomaly rates decline with advancing gestational age
- It is noted that 75 percent of chromosomally abnormal abortions occurred by 8 weeks; gestation. Of chromosomal abnormalities, 95 percent are caused by maternal gametogenesis errors, and 5 percent by paternal errors. Most common abnormalities are trisomy, found in 50 to 60 percent; monosomy X, in 9 to 13 percent; and triploidy, in 11 to 12 percent.

- Trisomies typically result from isolated nondisjuction, rates of which rise with maternal age (Boué, 1975). Trisomies of chromosomes 13, 16, 18, 21, and 22 are most common. In contrast, balanced structural chromosomal rearrangements may originate from either parent and are found in 2 to 4 percent of couples with recurrent pregnancy loss.

Monosomy X (45, X) is the single most frequent specific chromosomal abnormality. This is *Turner syndrome*, which usually results in abortion, but liveborn females are described in Chapter 13 (p. 259). Conversely, *autosomal monosomy* is rare and incompatible with life.

Maternal Factors

In chromosomally normal pregnancy losses, maternal influences play a role. The cause of euploid abortions are poorly understood, but various medical disorders, environmental conditions, and developmental abnormalities have been implicated.

Euploid pregnancies abort later than aneuploid ones. Specifically, the rate of euploid abortion peaks at approximately 13 weeks (Kajii, 1980). In addition, the incidence of euploid abortion rises dramatically after maternal age exceeds 35 years (Stein, 1980).

Paternal Factors

Increasing paternal age is significantly associated with an greater risk for abortion (de La Rochebrochard, 2003). In the Jerusalem Perinatal Study, this risk was lowest before age 25 years, after which it progressively increased at 5-year intervals (Kleinhaus, 2006). The etiology of this association is not well studied, but chromosomal abnormalities in spermatozoa likely play a role (Sartorius, 2010).

Table 15.1: Causes of abortion

Fetal factors	Maternal factors	Paternal factors

• Chromosomal abnormalities (M/C cause)
• Hydropic degeneration of villi
• Multiple pregnancy
	• *Maternal infections* like: TORCH infections, malaria, ureoplasma, chlamydia, brucella, spirochaetes
	• *Maternal medical disorders like:*
	  • Hypertension
	  • Chronic renal disease
	  • Cyanotic heart disease
	  • Hemoglobinopathies
	• *Environmental factors like:*
	  • Alcohol, smoking (leads to early pregnancy loss) caffeine.
	  • Exposure to radiation (> 5 rads) and anaesthetic gases
	• *Endocrine problems* like:
	  • Luteal phase defect (deficiency of progesterone)
	  • Thyroid abnormalities - hypothyroidism.
	  • Poorly controlled diabetes mellitus
	  • PCOD
	  • Hyperprolactinemia
		• Increased paternal age is associated with increased abortion
		Mnemonic to remember maternal causes of abortion—**TIMED 'O'**
		
		Mnemonic
		
		T = Trauma (Leads to second trimester loss)
		I^2 = Infections/immunological causes
		M = Maternal medical diseases
		E^2 = Environmental factors/endocrine problem
		D = Developmental/anatomical problems
		O = Obesity in mother

Contd...

Contd...

Fetal factors	Maternal factors	Paternal factors

	• *Immunological causes:*
	  ⋄ Antiphospholipid antibody syndrome (APLA syndrome)
	  ⋄ Inherited thrombophilias
	• *Uterine factors like:*
	  ⋄ Cervical incompetence
	  ⋄ Mullerian anomalies (M/C associated with abortions is septate uterus)
	  ⋄ Large and multiple submucous leiomyoma
	  ⋄ Asherman syndrome
	  ⋄ DES exposure in utero
	• *Weight of mother:*
	  ⋄ Under weight or nutritional deficiency does not lead to abortion.
	  ⋄ Obesity leads to abortion
	• *Others:* Trauma; Subchorionic hematoma; Defective placentation	

 Key Concept

- **M/C cause of 1st trimester or 2nd trimester spontaneous abortion**–chromosomal abnormality/genetic factor/Defective Germplasm.
- Of the chromosomal abnormalities 95% are caused by maternal gametogenesis error & 5% by paternal gametogenesis error.
- **M/C chromosomal abnormality causing spontaneous abortion** – Aneuploidy (alteration in number of chromosome) followed by Autosomal trisomy (M/C is Trisomy 16).
- **M/C specific chromosomal anomaly associated with abortions** → Monosomy X (20%) > Trisomy 16 (16%)
  So if in question—it is asked M/C cause of 1st trimester abortion:
  ⋄ Best answer—Aneuploidy
  ⋄ 2nd best answer—Trisomy
  ⋄ 3rd best answer—Monosomy X
  ⋄ 4th best answer—Trisomy 16
- In chromosomally normal pregnancy losses, maternal influences play a role
- Euploid pregnancies abort later than aneuploid ones.
- Specifically, the rate of euploid abortion peaks at approximately 13 weeks (aneuploid abortions M/C time <8 weeks).
- The incidence of euploid abortion rises dramatically after maternal age exceeds 35 years
- M/C cause of 1st trimester recurrent abortion–Idiopathic
- **Common causes of 1st trimester Recurrent abortion** (in decreasing order of frequency):
  – Idiopathic (40–50%)
  – Endocrine
  – Anatomical factors (uterine leiomyomas, Asherman syndrome, Mullerian duct anomalies, Incompetent os)
  – Inherited thrombophilia
  – Immunological cause (APLA)
  – Chromosomal anomaly (4%)
- **M/C chromosomal anomaly associated with recurrent abortion**—Balanced translocation of chromosomes.
- **M/C cause of 2nd trimester recurrent abortion is cervical incompetence**
- Infections can lead to spontaneous abortion but it can never lead to recurrent abortions.
- Hence in workup of a patient with recurrent abortions—TORCH testing is not done.
- Only infection which can lead to recurrent abortions **is syphilis[Q]**.
- The 3 M/C causes of recurrent abortion are:
  1. Parental chromosomal abnormalities
  2. Antiphospholipid antibody syndrome
  3. Chromosomal uterine abnormalities
- Investigative measures useful in the evaluation of recurrent early pregnancy loss:

  —Novak 14/e, p 1302; Leon Speroff, p 1090

  – Parental peripheral blood karyotyping[Q] with banding technique.
  – Assessment of the intrauterine cavity with either office hysteroscopy or hysterosalpingography.
  – Thyroid function tests, serum prolactin levels if indicated.
  – **Note:** Blood sugar levels are not routinely checked in patients of previous recurrent pregnancy loss.

Contd...

Contd...

- – Anticardiolipin antibody and lupus anticoagulant testing (aPTT or Russell Viper venom testing).
- – *Complete blood counts with platelet count.*
- – Thrombophilia testing:
- – *Factor V leiden, prothrombin gene mutation, Protein S activity.*
- – *Serum homocysteine level.*
- – In the presence of a family or personal history of venous thromboembolism, **protein C and antithrombin** activity.
- • The American College of Obstetricians and Gynaecology recognizes only 2 types of tests as having clear value in the investigation of recurrent miscarriages:
  1. Parental cytogenetic analysis
  2. Lupus anticoagulant and anticardiolipin antibodies assay.

—Williams Obs 23/e, p 241

Note: Karyotype of parents is more important in recurrent pregnancy loss whereas karyotype of conceptus is more important in 1st trimester abortion. ACOG does not recommend routine use of chromosomal microarray testing of first trimester fetal tissue.

TYPES OF ABORTION

Table 15.2: Types of abortion

Type of abortion	Complain	P/A	Internal os	Diagnosis	Important points
1. Threatened abortion	Spotting +/– abdominal pain	Height of uterus = period of gestation	Closed	USG–Live intrauterine pregnancy	Management- • Reassurance • Avoid intercourse • Value of Bed rest and progesterone uncertain
2. Inevitable abortion	Bleeding + Pain in abdomen	Height of uterus = period of gestation	Open	USG–Live/Dead fetus	Insert vaginal misoprost to complete the process
3. Incomplete abortion	Pain + bleeding + Product of conception coming out through internal or	Height of uterus is less than period of gestation	Open with product of conception coming out	Always do USG in this case to know the amount of tissue left in uterus	• Oral misoprost 600 mcg or vaginal 800 mcg. I needed curettage can be done.
4. Complete abortion	Patient complains of initial bleeding and pain and product of conception comes, then bleeding stops	Height of uterus is less than period of gestation	Os closed	USG–empty uterus	–
5. Missed abortion	Dirty brown discharge	Height of uterus less than period of gestation	Closed	⦿ Mean sac diameter ≥ 25 mm or crown rump length ≥ 7 mm with no fetal heart beat. For more details see Table 15.4.	• Single 800 mcg vaginal misoprost repeated in 1-2 days if needed.

Table 15.3: Adverse outcomes that are increased in women with threatened abortion

Maternal	Perinatal
Placenta previa	Preterm ruptured membranes
Placental abruption	Preterm birth
Manual removal of placenta	Low-birthweight infant
Cesarean delivery	Fetal-growth restriction
	Fetal and neonatal death

Table 15.4: Guidelines for early pregnancy loss diagnosis

Sonographic Findings
CRL ≥ 7 mm and no heartbeat
MSD ≥ 25 mm and no embryo
An initial US scan shows a gestational sac with yolk sac, and after ≥ 11 days, no embryo with a heartbeat is seen
An initial US scan shows a gestational sac with yolk sac, and after ≥ 2 weeks, no embryo with a heartbeat is seen

Anti D prophylaxis for early bleeding

Indications for giving Anti D

- Ectopic pregnancy
- Following suction evacuation
- All abortions > 12 weeks (including threatened abortion)
- All abortions where uterus is evacuated surgically
- Threatened abortion < 12 weeks if bleeding is heavy, recurrent or associated with pain

Anti D is Not given in
- Threatened abortion < 12 weeks
- Complete abortion < 12 weeks if no medical/surgical management is done.
- Dose of Anti D at < 12 weeks: 50 mcg
- Dose of Anti D at ≥ 12 weeks = 100 mcg

CERVICAL INCOMPETENCE

Cervical incompetence is characterized by painless[Q] cervical dilatation in the second[Q] or early third trimester[Q] with ballooning of the amniotic sac into the vagina[Q], followed by rupture of membranes and expulsion of a usually live fetus. The usual timing is 16 to 24 weeks.

 Note: With every loss, the gestational age at which abortion occurs keeps on decreasing in contrast to syphilis which follows Kassowitz law, i.e. with every loss period of gestation keeps on increasing.

Etiology

- *Congenital*
  - Developmental weakness of cervix.
  - Associated with uterine anomalies like septate uterus.
  - Following in utero exposure to diethyl stilbestrol.
- *Acquired due to previous cervical trauma*
  - Forcible dilatation during MTP and D and C.
  - Conization of cervix.
  - Cauterization of cervix.
  - Amputation of cervix or Fothergill's operation.

Diagnosis

- **History:** The typical history of painless rupture of membranes[Q] followed by the quick delivery of a live fetus in midtrimester is very suggestive.[Q]
- **Nonpregnant state:**
  - The internal os allows the passage of a No. 8 Hegar's cervical dilator or Foley's catheter filled with 1 ml water without resistance.[Q]

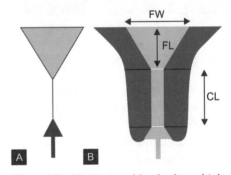

Figs. 15.1A and B: Hysterographic shadow obtained in the premenstrual phase. (A) Competent cervix (B) Incompetent cervix showing funneling. (FW = Funnel width, FL = Funnel length, CL = Cervical length)

- Premenstrual hysterocervicography will show the typical funneling of the internal os[Q] (Figs. 15.1A and B)
- **In Pregnancy:**
  - Transvaginal ultrasound is the ideal method to follow up and detect early incompetence.

	Normal pregnancy	Cervical incompetence
Length of cervix (at 14 weeks)	30–40 mm	< 2.5 mm
Diameter of internal Os	< 8 mm	≥ 8 mm
Shape of cervix	T-shaped, Y-shaped	V or U shaped

Cervix index: Funnel length + 1/endocervical length.
Normal = 0.32
If it is ≥ 0.52, it indicates cervical insufficiency.

- Normal shape of cervix on USG is 'Y' shaped. If it becomes U shaped, it indicates cervical incompetence. (Normal shape = T ⇒ Y ⇒ V ⇒ U is the order of change, as discussed in preterm labor).

Note:
- Funneling is the ultrasound finding of herniation of the fetal membranes into the upper part of the endocervical canal.

Management

*The treatment is surgical by a **cervical circlage**, which can be done prophylactically or in emergency (Rescue cerclage)*

The new nomenclature for cerclage application.

Old (1999)	New (2007)
Prophylactic	History indicated
Therapeutic	Ultrasound indicated
Rescue, emergency	Physical examination indicated

Recommendations for History Indicated cerclage

1. Should be offered to women with ≥ 3 second trimester abortions/Preterm births.
2. Should not be offered to females ≤ 2 second trimester abortion/Preterm births.

Recommendations for USG Indicated Cerclage

1. Women with history of 1 or more second trimester abortion or preterm birth and now USG shows cervical length ≤ 25 mm before 24 weeks.
2. Not recommended for women with cervical length ≤ 25 mm on USG, but no history of previous midtrimester abortion or preterm labor.
3. Not indicated for funneling of cervix in absence of short length of cervix.

Recommendations for Rescue/Emergency Cerclage

- Done in cases where cervical dilatation has started and fetal membranes can be seen in the vagina.
- Chances of failure are high in such cases if cervical dilatation is > 4 cm or if membrane prolapse beyond the external os.

Time of operation: Prophylactic cervical cerclage is usually delayed up to 12–14 weeks (and can be done uptil 24 weeks) so that miscarriage due to other causes can be eliminated or it should be done at least 2 weeks earlier than the lowest period of earlier wastage (but it is never done earlier than 10 weeks).

Note: Sonography should be done prior to circlage to confirm a live fetus and to rule out anomalies.

Procedures

- **Vaginal circlage**

McDonald's operation	Shirodkar's operation
• It has good success rate and less blood loss. • It is the most commonly performed procedure nowadays.	• The Shirodkar operation is technically more involved and takes longer to perform.

- *Abdominal cerclage (Benson and Durfee Cerclage)*

  Indications

  - Women with incompetent cervix due to severe trauma to cervix such as deep laceration, extensive conization or repeated LEEP for treatment of Ca in situ or who have congenitally short cervix.
  - H/O repetitive 2nd trimester loss and failed vaginal circlages.
  - Cervicovaginal fistulas follow abortion.
  - In transabdominal circlage (**Benson and Durfee circlage**) stitches are placed at the level of internal os via pfannenstiel incision and the stitches are permanent.

Disadvantage: In these cases, LSCS has to be done for delivering the fetus.

Removal of Cerclage Stitch: The stitch should be removed at 37 weeks or earlier if labor pain starts or features of abortion appear.

Contraindications	Complications
• Intrauterine infection	• Chorioamnionitis
• Ruptured membranes	• Rupture of membranes
• H/o vaginal bleeding	• Preterm labor
• Severe uterine irritability	• Necrosis of cervix
• Cervical dilatation > 4 cm	• Rupture uterus

Other cerclage operations:
- Wurm's stitch
- Lash and Lash operation
- Laparoscopic cerclage
- Robotic cerclage.

Non-surgical treatment of cervical incompetence: If patient is unwilling for cerclage, progesterone injection or micronized progesterone is given.

ANTIPHOSPHOLIPID ANTIBODY SYNDROME

- It is a treatable, autoimune disorder associated with recurrent *second trimester pregnancy loss.*[Q]
- It accounts for 15% cases of recurrent pregnancy loss.
- Antiphospholipid antibodies are acquired antibodies targeted against a phospholipid β_2 glycoprotein and prothrombin. They can be IgM, IgG or IgA isotopes.
- Most important antiphospholipid antibodies are:

Lupus anticoagulant (LAC)	Anticardiolipin antibody	Anti β2 Glycoprotein antibodies
• It was named so because it was first found in patients with SLE and prolonged partial thromboplastin time • But the name is a misomer as although it increases PTT (i.e., similar to anticoagulant) but functions as a procoagulant and causes thrombosis	• It is most commonly seen in patients with repetitive early pregnancy loss	• i.e. antibody which causes biologically false positive syphilis test

Remember: M/C antiphospholipid antibody is Lupus Anticoagulant.

Most specific is: Anti β2 glycoprotein

Pathogenesis

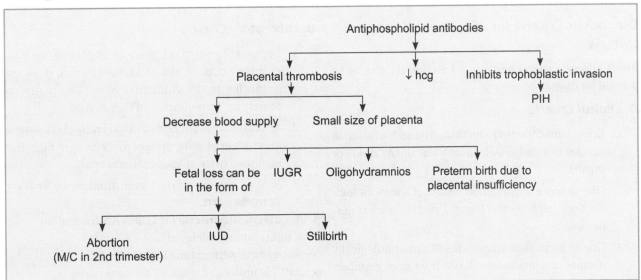

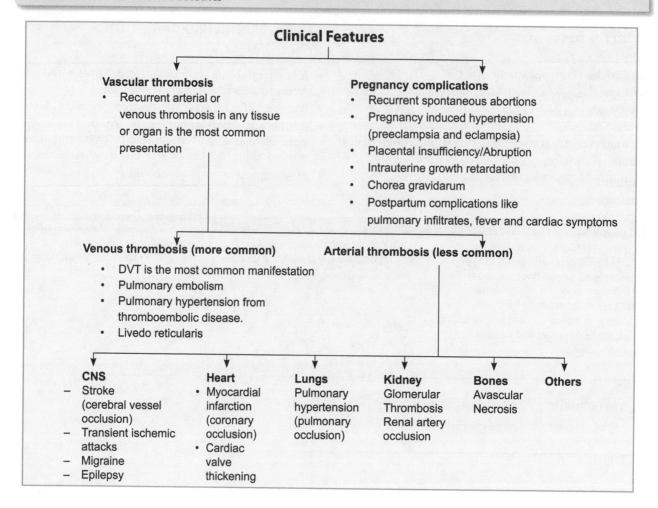

Diagnostic Criteria for APS: Revised Sapporo Criteria

Any 1 clinical criteria and any 1 Lab criteria should be present for diagnosis.

A. Clinical Criteria

1. Unexplained (one or more clinical episode of arterial, venous or small vessel thrombosis, in any tissue or organ).

2. One or more unexplained deaths of a morphologically normal fetus at or beyond the 10th week of gestation.

3. One or more premature births of a morphologically normal neonate before the 34th week of gestation because of (a) eclampsia or severe preeclampsia or because of (b) placental insufficiency.

4. Three or more unexplained consecutive spontaneous abortions before the 10th week of gestation.

B. Laboratory Criteria

1. Lupus anticoagulant present in plasma, on two or more occasion atleast 12 weeks apart, detected according to the guidelines of the International Society on Thrombosis and Hemostasis.

2. Anticardiolipin antibodies of IgG and/or IgM isotype in serum or plasma, present in medium or high titre identified twice at least 12 weeks apart.

3. Anti β_2 glycoprotein–1 identified twice at least 12 weeks apart.

Other diagnostic criteria for Lupus Anticoagulant

- Kaolin clotting is delayed
- Russel viper venom time is prolonged
- APTT is prolonged while PT remains normal.

Management

In females who are known cases of APLA—2 drugs are used for management:

1. Heparin

2. Aspirin

Heparin: Either regular or low molecular weight can be used. It should be started as soon as intrauterine pregnancy is detected on USG without waiting for fetal cardiac activity to appear. The drug has to be continued throughout pregnancy and stopped at the onset of labor.

Aspirin: Should be started as soon as UPT becomes positive. Dose = 40–80 mg. It should be continued throughout pregnancy and stopped 7 days before onset of labor.

2nd line therapy: Immunoglobulin therapy.

MTP: MEDICAL TERMINATION OF PREGNANCY ACT, 1971

In India, the MTP act was passed in August 1971 and came into effect from April 1972 and revised in 1975.

Indications

A. **Therapeutic:** When the continuation of pregnancy endangers the life of woman or may cause serious injury to her physical or mental health.

B. **Eugenic:** When there is risk of the child being born with serious physical or mental abnormalities. This may occur.

- If the pregnant woman in the first three months suffers from:
  - German measles (incidence of congenital defects 10 to 12%).
  - Smallpox or chicken pox.
  - Toxoplasmosis.
  - Viral hepatitis.
  - Any severe viral infection.
- If the pregnant woman is treated with drugs like thalidomide, cortisone, aminopterin, antimitotic drugs, or if she consumes hallucinogens or antidepressants.
- Mother is treated by X-rays or radioisotopes.
- Insanity of the parents.

C. **Humanitarian:** When pregnancy has been caused by rape.[Q]

D. **Social:**

- When pregnancy has resulted from the failure of contraceptive methods in case of a married[Q] woman, which is likely to cause serious injury to her mental health.

- When social or economic environment, actual or reasonably expected can injure the mother's health.

Rules

- Who can do MTP.
  i. Who has degree or diploma in Obs & Gynae
  ii. Who has done 6 months house job in Obs & Gynae.
  iii. Who has assisted in 25 MTP's in an authorized center.

- The pregnancy should be terminated in *Government hospitals*[Q], *or in the hospitals recognised by the Government for this purpose*[Q].

- *Non-governmental institutions* may take up abortion if they obtain *a licence from* Chief Medical Officer of the district.[Q]

- The consent of the woman[Q] is required before conducting abortion. Written consent of the guardian is required if the woman is a minor (<18 years)[Q] or a mentally ill person.[Q] Consent of husband is not necessary.

- Abortion cannot be performed on the request of the husband, if the woman herself is not willing.

- The woman need not produce proof of her age. The statement of the woman that she is over eighteen years of age is accepted.

- It is enough for the woman to state that she was raped, and it is not necessary that a complaint was lodged with the police.

- Professional secrecy has to be maintained. The Admission Register for the termination of pregnancies is secret document, and the information contained therein should not be disclosed to any person.

- If the period of pregnancy is below 12 weeks, it can be terminated on the opinion of a single doctor.[Q]

- *If the period of pregnancy is between 12 and 20 weeks, two doctors must agree that there is an indication.*[Q] *Once the opinion is formed, the termination can be done by any one doctor.*

- Termination is permitted upto 20 weeks of pregnancy.[Q]

- In an emergency, pregnancy can be terminated by a single doctor, even without required training (even after twenty weeks), without consulting a second doctor, in a private hospital which is not recognised.

- The termination of pregnancy by a person who is not registered medical practitioner (person concerned), or in an unrecognised hospital (the administrative head) shall be punished with rigorous imprisonment for *a term which shall not be less than two years, but which may extend to seven years.*

Methods of Performing Medical Termination of Pregnancy

First Trimester (Up to 12 Weeks)	Second Trimester (13–20 Weeks)

Medical
• Mifepristone
• Mifepristone and Misoprostol (PGE₁)
• Methotrexate and Misoprostol
• Tamoxifen and Misoprostol
Surgical
• Menstrual regulation
• Manual Vacuum Aspiration
• Suction evacuation
• Dilatation and curettage
	• **Prostaglandins** PGE₁ (Misoprostol), 15 methyl PGF 2α (Carboprost) and their analogues (used-intravaginally, intramuscularly or intra-amniotically)
	• **Dilatation and evacuation using ovum forceps uptil 15 weeks**
	• **Intrauterine instillation of hyperosmotic solutions**
	  • Intra-amniotic hypertonic urea (40%), saline (20%)
	  • Extra-amniotic—Ethacridine lactate, Prostaglandins (PGE₂, PGF₂α)
	• **Oxytocin infusion** high dose used along with either of the above two methods
	• **Hysterotomy** (abdominal)—less commonly done

 Important One Liners

Best method of abortion uptil 7 weeks–Medical abortion
Best method of abortion between 7–12 weeks–Suction and evacuation
Best method of abortion ≥ 12 weeks Prostaglandin

Important Points to Remember

Medical Abortion

Regimen: Used in India

Medical abortion uptil 7 weeks (A)	Medical abortion uptil 7–9 weeks (B)
Day 1: Mifepristone 200 mg oral. Send her home, come back after 48 hours.	Day 1: Same like (A)
Day 3: Misoprostol 400 mcg (oral or vaginal) Observe 2–3 hours and send her back home.	Day 3: Misoprost 800 mcg (vaginal)
Day 15: Clinical examination done to as certain complete evacuation	Day 15: Same like (A)

 Note: ACOG and WHO recommend medical abortion uptil 9 weeks. In India it is done uptil 7 weeks.
• If on Day 15, abortion has been incomplete, a curettage is done to complete it (Needed in 1–3% cases).
• Success rate = 90–98%

Role of mifepristone in Medical abortion:

• Mifepristone blocks progesterone receptors in the endometrium which leads to disruption of the embryo, production of prostaglandins and a decrease in human chorionic gonadotropin levels.

Contraindications of Medical abortion with mifepristone/misoprostol:

• Ectopic pregnancy[Q]

• Chronic adrenal failure[Q] or concurrent long-term corticosteroid[Q] therapy
• Chronic renal failure

Table 15.5: Various regimens for medical termination of pregnancy *Ref: Williams 25/e p 362*

First trimester
Mifepristone/Misoprostol [a]Mifepristone, 200-600 mg orally; followed in 24-48 hr by: [b]Misoprostol, 200–600 µg orally or 400–800 µg vaginally, buccally, or sublingually
Misoprostol Alone [c]800 µg vaginally or sublingually every 3 hr for 3 doses
Methotrexate/Misoprostol [d]Methotrexate, 50 mg/m² BSA intramuscularly or orally; followed in 3–7 days by; [e]Misoprostol, 800 µg vaginally. Repeat if needed 1 week after methotrexate initially given

Second trimester
Mifepristone/Misoprostol Mifepristone, 200 mg orally; followed in 24–48 hr by: Misoprostol, 400 µg vaginally or buccally every 3 hr up to 5 doses
Misoprostol Alone Misoprostol, 600–800 µg vaginally; followed by 400 µg vaginally or buccally every 3 hr up to 5 doses
Dinoprostone 20 mg vaginal suppository every 4 hr
Concentrated Oxytocin 50 units oxytocin in 500 mL of normal saline infused during 3 hr; then 1-hr diuresis (no oxytocin); then escalate sequentially in a similar fashion through 150, 200, 250, and finally 300 units oxytocin each in 500 mL normal saline

[a]Doses of 200 versus 600 mg similarly effective.
[b]Oral route may be less effective and have more nausea and diarrhea. Sublingual route has more side effects than vaginal route.
[c]Intervals 3–12 hours given vaginally; 3–4 hours given sublingually.
[d]Efficacy similar for routes of administration.
[e]Similar efficacy when given on day 3 versus day 5.
BSA = body surface area.

- History of allergy to mifepristone, misoprostol or other prostaglandins[Q]
- Active liver disease
- Asthma
- Cardiac disease
- Hemorrhagic disease

Relative Contraindication

- Heavy smoker ≥ 35 years, obesity, hypertension > 100 mm of Hg.

- Misoprost is teratogenic when used in first trimester and can lead to **Moebius syndrome** in the fetus. This is due to alteration in transplacental oxygenation.

Suction Evacuation

- It is the most suitable method for Ist trimester abortions from **7 weeks to 15 weeks (In India it is done uptil 12 weeks)**.
- It is done under local anaesthesia/paracervical block.[Q]
- The cervical os is first dilated using Hegar's dilators.[Q]
- Instrument used for evacuation is Karman suction cannula.[Q]
- Diameter of suction cannula should be equal to the weeks of gestation.[Q] **(If even number and in case of odd number 1 less)**.
- Suction pressure is 60–70 cm of Hg **(600 mm of Hg)**.[Q]
- **The end point of suction is denoted by:**
  - No more material sucked out.
  - Gripping of the cannula by the contracting smaller uterus.
  - Grating sensation.
  - Appearance of bubbles in the cannula.

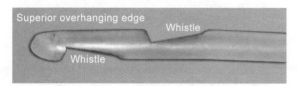

Fig. 15.2: Karman cannula

Advantages of Suction evacuation

- Done as an out patient procedure.
- Low failure rate (< 1%).
- Complications like incomplete evacuation, infection, uterine perforation and excessive bleeding are < 2%.
- Mortality is < 2%.

 Note: Perforation by suction evacuation is more dangerous than by Hegar's dilators.

- If injury is by–dilator–wait and watch.
- If Injury is by–suction evacuation–Laparotomy/ Laparoscopy should be done immediately.

Menstrual Regulation

Consists of aspiration of contents of uterine cavity by means of plastic cannula (Karman's cannula) and a plastic 50 cc syringe.

It is carried out effectively within 3 weeks of missed period (i.e. 7 weeks of pregnancy).

- A paracervical block or preoperative sedative alone suffices but sometimes in apprehensive patient GA is required.
- Blood loss is less.
- It is included in methods of performing MTP.

Manual Vacuum Aspiration

MVA is usually performed upto 7 weeks without cervical dilatation but can be done upto 12 weeks. A 50 mL syringe[Q] is used and 660 mm of Hg, pressure is generated.

It is equivalent to suction evacuation and is used in rural areas where there is no electricity (so suction machines cannot be used).

Second Trimester Abortion

Prostaglandins

Best method–Prostaglandins.

- 15 methyl PGF-2α (carboprost) 250 mcg given I/m. To be repeated after every 3–4 hours. Maximum doses = 10.
- Side effect—diarrhea.
- Misoprost Dose = 200–800 mcg orally, vaginally or sublingually at 3–4 hours interval. Maximum = 5–6 doses.
- In India, misoprost is not approved for MTP beyond 9 weeks.
- Dinoprost = 20 mg suppository every 3–4 hourly. Success rate of prostaglandins = 90%

  Induction-abortion interval = 14–20 hours.

Dilatation and Evacuation

- In 2nd trimester instead of suction evacuation— dilatation & evacuation is done.
- Prior cesarean section is not a risk for dilatation & evacuation.

New Pattern Questions

N1. Blighted ovum is:
a. Synaptic knobs
b. Avascular villi
c. Intervillous hemorrhage
d. None of the above

N2. The most life threatening complications of septic abortion includes:
a. Peritonitis
b. Renal failure
c. Respiratory distress syndrome
d. Septicemia

N3. The method most suitable for MTP in 3rd month of pregnancy is:
a. Dilatation and curettage
b. Extra amniotic ethacridine
c. Hysterectomy
d. Suction and evacuation

N4. The best method of evacuation of a missed abortion in uterus of more than 12 weeks:
a. Oxytocin infusion
b. Intramuscular prostaglandin (15 methyl PGF2α)
c. Prostaglandin E1 vaginal misoprostol followed by evacuation of the uterus
d. Suction evacuation

N5. Pregnancy which continues following threatened abortion is likely to have increased incidence of:
a. Preterm labor   b. Fetal malformation
c. IUGR   d. All of the above

N6. Suction evacuation can be done up to:
a. 6 weeks   b. 10 weeks
c. 15 weeks   d. 18 weeks

N7. A P2 + 1 female comes with amenorrhea of 5 weeks. Her UPT is +ve. On USG, Gestational and yolk sac are seen in uterus. No fetal pole is visible. No fetal cardiac activity is seen. CRL is 8 mm and MSD = 28 mm. What is the next best step?
a. Advise MTP as it is nonviable pregnancy
b. High probability of nonviable pregnancy but still repeat scan after 7 days to confirm
c. Can be ectopic pregnancy – give methotrexate
d. High probability of viable pregnancy-repeat scan after 7 days

N8. The figure shows karman cannula. The number of cannula corresponds to:

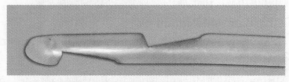

a. Diameter of cannula in mm
b. Diameter of cannula in cm
c. Surface area of cannula
d. Length of cannula

N9. Identify the instrument:

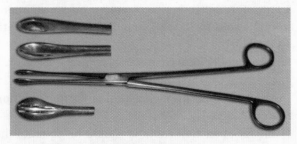

a. Sponge holding forceps
b. Haywood Smiths ovum forceps
c. Allis tissue forceps
d. Lanes tissue forceps

N10. Levels of progesterone indicating unviable pregnancy and viable intrauterine pregnancy are:
a. 5 ng/mL; 20 ng/mL
b. 10 ng/mL; 20 ng/mL
c. 5 ng/mL; 50 ng/mL
d. 10 ng/mL; 50 ng/mL

N11. Best method for MTP in 2nd trimester abortion:
a. Oxytocin
b. Prostaglandin
c. Ethacridil
d. Hypertonic saline

N12. In case of recurrent abortions, M/C uterine malformation seen is:
a. Arcuate uterus
b. Unicornuate uterus
c. Mullerian fusion defects
d. Mullerian agenesis

Previous Year Questions

1. **Most common cause of first trimester abortion is:**
   a. Chromosomal abnormalities [AI 03]
   b. Syphilis
   c. Rhesus isoimmunization
   d. Cervical incompetence

2. **Commonest cause of first trimester abortion is:**
   [PGI June 99]
   a. Monosomy b. Trisomy
   c. Triploidy d. Aneuploidy

3. **A lady has recurrent abortions in Ist trimester with history of autosomal recessive disorder in family. The true statement regarding this is:**
   [AIIMS Nov 99]
   a. Consanguinity may be the cause
   b. Complete penetrance is common
   c. Affected members in the family
   d. All are correct

4. **Spontaneous abortion in 1st trimester is caused by:**
   [PGI June 00]
   a. Trisomy 21 b. Monosomy
   c. Trauma d. Rh-incompatibility

5. **MC cause of abortion in first trimester is, defect in:**
   [PGI June 98]
   a. Placenta b. Uterus
   c. Embryo d. Ovarian

6. **Recurrent abortion in 1st trimester is most often due to:**
   [PGI Dec 97]
   a. Chromosomal abnormalities
   b. Uterine anomaly
   c. Hormonal disturbance
   d. Infection

7. **Recurrent spontaneous abortions are seen in all except:**
   [PGI June 03]
   a. TORCH infection
   b. Uterine pathology
   c. Herpes infection
   d. Balanced paternal translocation
   e. None of the above

8. **All of the following are known causes of recurrent abortion except:**
   [AI 08]
   a. TORCH infection b. SLE
   c. Rhincompatibility d. Syphilis

9. **26 years old lady with H/o recurrent abortion which of the following investigations you will do to confirm the diagnosis?**
   [AIIMS Nov 06]
   a. PT
   b. BT
   c. Anti-Russell viper venom antibodies
   d. Clot solubility test

10. **Recurrent abortion in Ist trimester, investigation to be done:**
    [PGI Dec 06]
    a. Karyotyping b. SLE Ab
    c. HIV d. TORCH infection

11. **In a case of recurrent spontaneous abortion, following investigation is unwanted:**
    a. Hysteroscopy [AIIMS Nov 02]
    b. Testing antiphospholipid antibodies
    c. Testing for TORCH infections
    d. Thyroid function tests

12. **A lady presented to your with a history of recurrent early pregnancy loss. What are the investigations to be ordered:**
    [PGI Dec 09]
    a. VDRL
    b. Toxoplasma serology
    c. Hemogram/blood grouping
    d. Rubella screening
    e. Blood Sugars

13. **A woman with 20 weeks pregnancy presents with bleeding per vaginum. On speculum examination, the os is open but no products have come out. The diagnosis is:**
    [AIIMS Nov 2013]
    a. Missed abortion
    b. Incomplete abortion
    c. Inevitable abortion
    d. Complete abortion

14. **A 25 years old female reports in the casualty with history of amenorrhoea for two and half months and abdominal pain and bleeding per vaginum for one day. On examination, vital parameters and other systems are normal. On speculum examination, bleeding is found to come from Os. On bimanual examination, uterus is of 10 weeks size, soft and Os admits one finger. The most likely diagnosis is:**
    a. Threatened abortion
    b. Missed abortion
    c. Inevitable abortion
    d. Incomplete abortion

15. **A woman with H/o recurrent abortions presents with isolated increase in APTT. Most likely cause is:**
    a. Lupus anticoagulant
    b. Factor VII
    c. Von Willebrand's disease
    d. Hemophilia A

16. **Anti phospholipid syndrome (APS) is associated with all of the following except:** [AI 08/AIIMS May 11]
    a. Pancytopenia
    b. Recurrent abortions
    c. Venous thrombosis
    d. Pulmonary hypertension

17. **All of the following are true about the lupus anti-coagulants** *except*: [AI 09]
    a. ↑ in APTT
    b. Recurrent second trimester abortion in pregnancy females
    c. Can occur without other symptoms of antiphospholipid antibody syndrome
    d. Severe life threatening hemorrhage

18. **Cervical incompetence is characterised by:**
    a. 1st trimester abortion [PGI June 03]
    b. 2nd trimester abortion
    c. Premature rupture of membrane
    d. Circlage operation done

19. **In cervical incompetence, encirclage operation done are:** [PGI Dec 03]
    a. McDonald operation
    b. Shirodkar operation
    c. Purandare's operation
    d. Khanna's sling operation
    e. Abdominal sling operation

20. **A gravida 3 female with H/o 2 previous 2nd trimester abortion presents at 22 weeks of gestation with funneling of cervix and length of cervix 20 mm. Most appropriate management would be:** [AIIMS Nov 07]
    a. Administer dinoprostone and bed rest
    b. Administer misoprostol and bed rest
    c. Apply fothergill stretch
    d. Apply McDonald stitch

21. **McDonald stitch is applied in the following conditions except:**
    a. Incompetent os   b. Septate uterus
    c. Placenta previa   d. Bad obstetrical history

22. **A 28-year-old female with a history of 8 weeks amenorrhoea complains of vaginal bleeding and lower abdominal pain. On USG examination there is gestational sac with absent fetal parts. The diagnosis is:**
    a. Ectopic pregnancy [AIIMS May 01]
    b. Incarcerated abortion
    c. Threatened abortion
    d. Corpus luteum cyst

23. **Antiprogesterone compound RU-486 is effective for inducing abortion, if the duration of pregnancy is:**

a. 63 days   b. 72 days   [AI 04]
c. 88 days   d. 120 days

24. **All of the following drugs have been used for medical abortion** *except*: [AIIMS May 03]
    a. Mifepristone   b. Misoprostol
    c. Methotrexate   d. Atosiban

25. **In extra amniotic 2nd trimester medicolegal termination of pregnancy, which of the following is used?** [PGI June 04]
    a. Ethacrydine lactate b. Prostaglandin
    c. Hypertonic saline   d. Glucose

26. **According to MTP Act, 2 doctor's opinion is required when pregnancy is:** [PGI June 03]
    a. 10 weeks   b. 6 weeks
    c. > 12 weeks   d. > 20 weeks
    e. 8 weeks

27. **For medical termination of pregnancy, consent should be obtained from?** [AI 2012]
    a. The male partner
    b. The male as well as the female partner
    c. The female partner
    d. Consent is not required

28. **Mifepristone is not used in:** [AI 09]
    a. Threatened abortion
    b. Fibroid
    c. Ectopic pregnancy
    d. Molar pregnancy

29. **A G6+0+0 lady h/o recurrent missed abortions at 14–16 weeks comes to you with a missed abortion at 12 weeks. Which of the following tests is not warranted?** [AIIMS May 2015]
    a. Lupus anticoagulant
    b. Anticardiolipin antibodies
    c. VDRL of father and mother
    d. Fetal karyotype

30. **Absolute Contraindications for medical abortion:**
    a. Previous myomectomy [PGI May 2017]
    b. Hypersensitivity to prostaglandin
    c. Previous LSCS
    d. Suspected ectopic pregnancy
    e. Undiagnosed adnexal mass

Answers with Explanations to New Pattern Questions

N1. **Ans. is b, i.e. Avascular villi** *Ref. Dutta Obs. 7/e, p 161; Fernando Arias 2/e, p 56*

According to the clinical and echographic findings, it is possible to separate early pregnancy losses into two groups:

- *Blighted ova:* Those early pregnancy losses in which foetal development is not observed with ultrasound (so that only a gestational sac is present with or without a yolk sac) and fetal tissue is absent on histologic examination of the products of conception.

- *Early Fetal demise:* Those early pregnancy losses in which fetal development is clearly observed by ultrasound and fetal tissue is found on the histologic examination.

The difference between these two types of abortion is of fundamental importance. The lack of development of fetal structures defines a subset of abortions of genetic origin.

In contrast, the early interruption of fetal life is a complex phenomenon with multiple etiologies. Therefore, the patients with blighted ova do not require extensive work up, whereas patients who have aborted cytogenetically normal fetuses need an extensive search for non genetic factors responsible for the pregnancy loss.

N2. **Ans. is c, i.e. Respiratory distress syndrome** *Ref. Dutta Obs. 7/e, p 164, 165; COGDT 10/e, p 987*

> **According to** *COGDT 10/e, p 987*
>
> ***"The most common cause of death in patients with this condition is respiratory insufficiency secondary to ARDS."***
>
> **According to Williams Obs. 23/e, p 222**
>
> ***"With severe sepsis syndrome, acute respiratory distress syndrome or DIC may develop and supportive care is essential".***

N3. **Ans. is d, i.e. Suction and Evacuation**
Ref. Shaw 14/e, p 221; Clinical Obstetrics by Mudaliar and Menon 10/e, p 406; Dutta Obs. 7/e, p 174, 175

Friends, let's first have a second look at the question. The question asks the most suitable method of MTP in the 3rd month, i.e. between 8–12 weeks approximately.

Among the options given – Dilatation and curettage i.e. option a and suction evacuation i.e. option d are the methods of first trimester pregnancy termination.

Between the two:

> *"Vacuum evacuation is the most efficient method of terminating pregnancy up to 12 weeks of gestation. It has gained rapid worldwide acceptance."* ...Shaw Gynae. 14/e, p 221

Point to Remember

Period of pregnancy	Best method of MTP
upto 7 weeks	Medical abortion
7–15 weeks	Suction evacuation
≥15 weeks	Prostaglandin

N4. **Ans. is c, i.e. Prostaglandin E1 vaginal misoprostol followed by evacuation of the uterus** *Ref. Dutta Obs 7/e, p 175*

In all midtrimester abortion, cervical preparation must be done before performing evacuation, to make the process easy and safe.

Intracervical tent, mifeprestone or misoprostol are used as the cervical priming agents. Suction evacuation is not suitable for bigger size of uterus more than 10 weeks as chances of retained products are more.

N5. **Ans. is d, i.e. All of the above** *Ref. Dutta Obs 7/e p161*

Prognosis of threatened abortion

In about two-third, the pregnancy continues beyond 28 weeks. In the rest, it terminates either as inevitable or missed miscarriage. **If the pregnancy continues, there is increased frequency of preterm labor, placenta previa, intrauterine growth restriction of the fetus and fetal anomalies.**

N6. Ans. is c, i.e. 15 weeks *Ref. Dutta Obs. 7/e, p 174; Shaw Gyane. 13/e, p 243, 14/e, p 221*

Suction evacuation can be done uptil 15 weeks. Uptil 12 weeks it is routinely done using Karman cannula. From 13 weeks–15 weeks, it is done using ovum forceps.

N7. Ans. is b, i.e. High probability of nonviable pregnancy but still repeat scan after 7 days to confirm

Ref. Williams 24/e, p 355

First Remember:

- Gestational sac is visible by TVS at ≈ 4.5 weeks when BhCG is 1500 to 2000 mIu/ml
- Yolk sac is visible by TVS at ≈ 5.5 weeks when MSD (mean sac diameter) is 10 mm
- Embryo is visible by TVS at 5–6 weeks when MSD = 15–20 mm
- Fetal cardiac activity can be detected at 6–6.5 weeks with an embryonic length (CRL=) 1–5 mm and MSD of 13–18 mm.

 Point to Remember

An embryonic gestation is diagnosed when the mean gestational sac diameter measures ≥ 20 mm and no embryo is seen. Embryonic death is also diagnosed if an embryo measuring ≥ 10 mm has no cardiac activity. So in the question – MSD is 28 mm and CRL 8 mm and still no cardiac activity or fetal pole is visible. It has to be a nonviable pregnancy. In this case whether we should perform immediate MTP or repeat scan after 7 days is suggested by High Risk Pregnancy 4/e, p 108.

- If fetal pole is not seen and MSD ≥ 25 mm then there is high probability of a non viable pregnancy. Repeat scan with another examiner or after 7 days to confirm.
- If fetal pole is seen then measure CRL. If CRL ≥ 7 mm there is high probability of nonviable pregnancy. Repeat scan should be done after 7 days to confirm.

N8. Ans. is a, i.e. Diameter of cannula in mm

Karman cannula
A long tubular structure made of plastic or metal.
- *Types:* Rigid or flexible
- *Sizes:* 4–12 mm
- Parts
  - *Distal end:* Double whistle at the terminal end.
  - *Proximal end:* Fixes into syringe.
  - Superior overhanging edge acts as a curette.
The number of cannula corresponds to diameter of cannula in millimeters. A plastic cannula is preferred because it is less traumatic, transparent and disposable.

N9. Ans. is b, i.e. Haywood Smiths ovum forceps

Haywood Smiths ovum forceps
Designed by Haywood Smiths.
Parts
Blades
- Blades are spoon-shaped, fenestrated and have blunt ends
- Longitudinal fenestrations can hold good amount of tissue.
Lock
- It is absent.
- Anything held in blades is firmly caught but not nipped and so no crushing.
Haywood Smiths ovum forceps
Designed by Haywood Smiths.

Contd …

Contd …

Parts
Blades
- Blades are spoon-shaped, fenestrated and have blunt ends
- Longitudinal fenestrations can hold good amount of tissue.

Lock
- It is absent.
- Anything held in blades is firmly caught but not nipped and so no crushing.

Ovum forceps is differentiated from sponge holding forceps by following points:
   - It has no lock
   - It has no serrations

Catch lock is absent so less chances of injury to intra-abdominal structures.

Uses
- Evacuation of products of conception in abortion and vesicular mole.
- Evacuation of products of conception in secondary PPH.

N10. Ans. is a, i.e 5 ng/mL; 20 ng/mL   *Ref. Williams 24/e, p 355*

Serum progesterone concentration <5 ng/mL suggest a dying pregnancy and ≥ 20 ng/mL support the diagnosis of a healthy pregnancy.

N11. Ans. is b, i.e Prostaglandin

See the text for explanation.

N12. Ans. is c, i.e Mullerian fusion defects

M/C uterine malformations causing Recurrent abortions is septate and bicornuate uterus, which are Mullerian duct fusion defects.

Answers with Explanations to Previous Year Questions

1. **Ans. is a, i.e. Chromosomal abnormalities** *Ref. Dutta Obs. 7/e, p 159,160; COGDT 10/e, p 259; Williams Obs. 23/e, p 215*

   Abortion is spontaneous termination of pregnancy before 22 weeks or weight of fetus less than 500 gm.

   Incidence: About 15% of all conceptions end up in spontaneous abortions. Out of these 80% occur before 12 weeks i.e. in 1st trimester and among these 50–75% are due to chromosomal anomalies (Germplasm defect).

2. **Ans. is d, i.e. Aneuploidy** *Ref. Williams 24/e, p 351*

   - The M/C cause of early miscarriages is aneuploidy (i.e. chromosomal anomaly).
   - Amongst the aneuploid abortions—autosomal trisomy is the most frequently identified chromosomal anomaly.
   - Trisomies have been identified in abortuses for all except chromosomal number 1 and those with 16, 13, 18, 21 and 22 are most common.
   - **The single most specific chromosomal abnormality in abortions is Monosomy X (45X).**

   As a have discussed Best answer for M/C cause of 1st trimester abortion—Aneuploidy > Trisomy > Monosomy X > Trisomy 16.

3. **Ans. is d, i.e. All are correct** *Ref. Robbin's 7/e, p 151*

   Autosomal recessive inheritance is the single largest category of Mendelian disorders.

   They have following features:
   - *The trait does not usually affect the parents but siblings may show the disease* **(Option "c"** is correct).
   - Siblings have one chance in four of being affected (i.e. recurrence risk is 25% for each birth).
   - *Consanguineous marriage may be the cause* **(Option "a"** is correct).
   - The expression of the defect tends to be more uniform than in autosomal dominant disorders.
   - *Complete penetrance is common* **(Option "b"** is correct).
   - Onset is frequently early in life.

   In the question the lady has recurrent abortions and H/o autosomal recessive disorder in the family, therefore all features of autosomal recessive disorders apply to her.

4. **Ans. is a, b and c, i.e. Trisomy 21; Monosomy; and Trauma** *Ref. Dutta Obs. 7/e, p 160*

   Common causes of abortion

First trimester	Mid trimester
1. Defective germplasm (most common)/ chromosomal anomalies: • ***Trisomy*** (most common overall problem) • Triploidy • ***Monosomy*** X (most specific) • Tetraploidy Structural rearrangements including: *translocation, deletion, inversion* 2. Endocrine disorders: • Luteal phase defect • Thyroid abnormalities (rare) • Diabetes 3. Maternal medical illness including – Cyanotic heart disease – Hemoglobinopathies – Inherited thrombophilia 4. ***Trauma*** 5. Maternal excessive use of alcohol, caffine	1. Anatomical abnormalities • Cervical incompetence • Uterine malformation/mullerian anomalies • Uterine synechiae 2. Autoimmune disorders • Antinuclear antibodies • Antiphospholipid antibodies • Maternal thrombophelia 3. **Rh and blood group incompatibility** 4. Low implantation of placenta 5. Twins/hydramnios 6. Endocrine abnormalities – Progesterone deficiency – Thyroid deficiency – Maternal diabetes – PCOD 7. Genetic abnormalities – Seen in 5–10% of 2nd trimester losses *(Fernando Arias 3/e, p 326)* 8. Sub chorionic bleeding 9. Maternal/uterine infections *(Fernando Arias 3/e, p 329)*

5. **Ans. is c, i.e. Embryo** *Ref. Dutta Obs. 7/e, p 159, 160; Williams Gynae 1/e, p 138*

    As explained earlier most common cause of abortion in first trimester are chromosomal abnormalities involving the zygote or embryo.

6. **Ans. is a and c, i.e. Chromosomal abnormalities and Hormonal disturbance** *Ref. JB Sharma ehs, p 117-118*

    Most common cause of recurrent abortions:

    1st trimester
    1. Idiopathic
    2. Endocrine and metabolic causes like diabetes, thyroid problems, luteal phase defect, PCOD hyperprolactinemia
    3. Inherited thrombophilias
    4. High levels of antiphospholipid antibodies.
    5. **Chromosomal abnormalities.** *Most common type of chromosomal abnormality* is balanced translocation (25%).

    2nd trimester
    - Anatomic abnormalities of uterus $\begin{cases} \text{Congenital} \rightarrow \text{Septate uterus} \\ \text{Acquired} \rightarrow \text{Cervical incompetence} \end{cases}$
    - APLA syndrome
    - Medical disorders of mother-Renal failure, SLE
    - Maternal syphilis

7. **Ans. is a and c, i.e. TORCH infection; and Herpes infection**
    Ref. Williams Obs. 21/e, p 868, 23/e, p 224; Williams Gynae. 1/e, p 144-149; Leon Speroff 7/e, p 1090

    Remember all causes of abortions given earlier in the chapter for spontaneous abortions hold good for recurrent abortions also except for infections be it — TORCH infections or any other infection.

    According to *Williams Gynae 1/e, p 149*—

    "Few infections are firmly associated with early pregnancy loss. Moreover, if any of those infections are associated with miscarriage, they are even less likely to cause recurrent miscarriage because maternal antibodies usually develop with primary infection."

    Leon Speroff says:

    "Overall, data regarding the possibility that cervicovaginal infections might be a cause of early pregnancy loss are relatively scarce. Despite periodic reports that have implicated specific infectious agents as risk factors for miscarriages, there remains no compelling evidence that bacterial or viral infections are a cause of recurrent pregnancy loss."
    —*Leon Speroff*

    It further says on *page 1091*

    "Routine serological tests, cervical cultures and endometrial biopsy to detect genital infections in women with recurrent pregnancy loss can not be justified. Evaluation should be limited to women with clinical cervicitis, chronic or recurrent bacterial vaginosis or other symptoms of pelvic infection."

8. **Ans. is a, i.e TORCH infection** *Ref. 'Pre test' Obstetrics and Gynaecology 11/e, p 68 (Question 77)*

    As discussed in previous question TORCH infection do not lead to recurrent abortion.

    SLE is an established cause for recurrent abortion

    SLE is associated with antiphospholipid syndrome (anti-cardiolipin antibodies) and is known to cause recurrent abortions.

    RH incompatibility is a known cause for spontaneous abortion and may lead to recurrent abortions if it remains unrecognized.

    Syphilis as discussed in the text can lead to recurrent abortion.

9. **Ans. is c, i.e. Anti-Russell viper venom antibodies** *Ref. Dutta Obs. 7/e, p 343*

    As discussed lupus anticoagulant is an important cause of recurrent pregnancy loss.

    Therefore, test for anti-russell viper venom antibodies should be done.

10. **Ans. is a and b, i.e. Karyotyping; and SLE Ab.**

Recurrent abortion in 1st trimester as discussed in Q6 can be due to a number of problems including chromosomal anomaly and metabolic problems.

Amongst the options given–TORCH infection and HIV do not lead to recurrent abortion.

Therefore, we are left with 2 options—Karyotyping and SLE Ab and both should be done.

11. **Ans. is c, i.e. Testing for TORCH infections.** *Williams Gynae 1/e, p 149, Novaks 14/e, p 1302*

Because TORCH infections are not a cause of recurrent abortions:

TORCH profile should not be included in the set of investigations done to find out the cause of recurrent abortion (Ans. 14)

 Investigative measures useful in the evaluation of recurrent early pregnancy loss:

—Novak 14/e, p 1302; Leon Speroff, 1090

- Parental peripheral blood karyotyping^Q with banding technique.
- Assessment of the intrauterine cavity with either office hysteroscopy or hysterosalpingography.
- Thyroid function tests, serum prolactin levels if indicated.
- Anticardiolipin antibody and lupus anticoagulant testing (aPTT or Russell Viper venom testing).
- *Complete blood counts with platelet count.*
- Thrombophilia testing:
  - *Factor V leiden, prothrombin gene mutation, Protein S activity.*
  - *Serum homocysteine level.*
  - In the presence of a family or personal history of venous thromboembolism, ***protein C and antithrombin*** activity.

    The American college of obstetricians and Gynaecology recognizes only 2 types of tests as having clear value in the investigation of recurrent miscarriages:
    1. Parental cytogenetic analysis
    2. Lupus anticoagulant and anticardiolipin antibodies assay. *—Williams Obs 23/e, p 241*

---

12. **Ans. is a and c, i.e. VDRL and Hemogram/blood grouping** *Ref. Novaks 14/e, p 1302, Leon Speroff 7/e, p 1090*

As discussed in previous answer:

Complete blood counts along with platelet count are done in case of recurrent pregnancy loss.

Rubella-virus screening ⎫
Toxoplasma serology ⎭ are not done because as discussed earlier, infections rarely lead to recurrent pregnancy loss except syphilis—so VDRL should be done

"Few infection are firmly associated with early pregnancy loss-moreover, if any of these infections are associated with miscarriage, they are even less likely to cause recurrent miscarriage because maternal antibodies usually develop with primary infection. Thus, there appears no concrete indication to screen for infection in asymptomatic women with recurrent miscarriage" *—Williams Gynae 1/e, p 101*

"Routine serological tests, cervical cultures and endometrial biopsy to detect genital infections in women with recurrent pregnancy loss cannot be justified. Evaluation should be limited to women with clinical cervicits, chronic or recurrent bacterial vaginosis or other symptoms of pelvic infections" *—Leon Speroff 7/e, p 1091*

As far as blood glucose testing is concerned- Neither Novaks, Leon speroff, nor Williams- say that blood glucose levels should be tested in patients with recurrent pregnancy loss.

Leon speroff says:

" In women with recurrent pregnancy loss, evaluation with blood glucose and HbA$_1$C AIC level is indicated for those with known or suspected diabetes, but otherwise it is unwarranted" *—Leon Speroff 7/e, p 1090*

So for our exams purposes we have to learn and remember the list of investigations mentioned in previous question in case of recurrent abortions.

13. **Ans. is c, i.e. Inevitable abortion** *Ref. Dutta Obs 7/e, p 161, 162*

14. **Ans. is c, i.e. Inevitable abortion** *Ref. Dutta Obs 7/e, p 161, 162*

    Clinical features and *diagnosis* of different types of Abortions

Abortion	Clinical picture	Size of uterus	Internal os	Ultrasound
1. Threatened	Slight bleeding	Corresponds	Closed	Live fetus, subchorionic hemorrhage
2. Inevitable	Bleeding and pain, shock	Equal or less	Open with products felt	Dead fetus
3. Incomplete	Bleeding	Smaller	Open	Retained products
4. Complete	Bleeding stopped	Smaller	Closed	Cavity empty
5. Missed	Absent or minimal bleeding	Smaller	Closed	Dead fetus

    In both the question, os is open, size of uterus corresponds to period of amenorrhea and product of conception cannot be seen coming out from os. Thus, it indicates inevitable abortion.

15. **Ans. is a, i.e. Lupus anticoagulant** *Ref. Dutta Obs. 6/e, p 343; Fernando Arias 3/e, p 327; Leon Speroff 7/e, p 1082*

    Isolated increase in APTT is suggestive of lupus anticoagulant.

16. **Ans is a, i.e Pancytopenia** *Ref. API Textbook of Medicine 8/e, p 306, 307; Harrison 17/e, p 732, 1579, 2082*

    Venous thrombosis, recurrent abortions and pulmonary hypertension are all seen in case of antiphospholipid syndrome.

    Antiphospholipid antibody syndrome leads to thrombocytopenia (in 40–50% cases) and hemolytic anemia in 25% cases but leucopenia is not seen in it. Also in causes of pancytopenia - No where is antiphospholipid syndrome mentioned so, it is the best answer.

17. **Ans. is d, i.e. Severe life threatening hemorrhage** *Ref. CMDT 2009, p 735, Williams Obs 23/e, p 151-1154*

    As discussed in the text, Lupus anticoagulant name is a misnomer as it leads to thrombosis and not hemorrhage. Rest all options are true.

18. **Ans. is b, c and d, i.e. 2nd trimester abortion; Premature rupture of membrane; and Circlage operation done**

19. **Ans. is a and b, i.e. McDonald operation and Shirodkar operation**

    Ref. Dutta Obs. 7/e, p 170; Williams Obs. 23/e, p 218, 219

    Read the text for explanation

20. **Ans. is d, i.e. Apply McDonald stitch** *Ref. Dutta Obs. 7/e, p 168-171*
    - In this question: A third gravida female is presenting with 2 previous 2nd trimester losses and with funneling of cervix and length of cervix 20 mm at 22 weeks of gestation which means that the patient has incompetent cervix. This is USG indicated cerclage
    - Management of this condition as discussed in previous question is application of Mc Donald stitch.

21. **Ans. is c, i.e. Placenta previa** *Ref. Dutta Obs. 7/e, p 171*

    Contraindications to Circlage operation:
    - Intra uterine infection
    - Ruptured membranes
    - *H/o vaginal bleeding*
    - Severe uterine irritability
    - Cervical dilatation > 4 cm

22. **Ans. is b, i.e. Incarcerated abortion** *Ref. Dutta Obs. 7/e, p 163*

    Friends, let's consider each option one by one.

    Option 'a': i.e. Ectopic pregnancy

Points in favor	Points against
• Amenorrhea of 8 weeks • C/o vaginal bleeding and lower abdominal pain	• USG examination showing *gestational sac in the uterus* rules out ectopic pregnancy

Option "c" : i.e. Threatened abortion

It is a clinical entity where the process of abortion has started but has not progressed to a state where recovery is impossible.

Points in favor	Points against
• Amenorrhea of 8 weeks. • C/o vaginal bleeding (normally - the bleeding is usually slight but on rare occasion, the bleeding may be brisk and sharp suggestive of low implantation of placenta).	• USG examination showing gestational sac with absent fetal parts. (In threatened abortion USG shows a well formed gestational sac with central echoes from the embryo indicating healthy fetus and observation of fetal cardiac motion).

So, threatened abortion ruled out.

Option "d" : i.e. Corpus luteum cyst   *—Jeffcoate 7/e, p 527*

Points in favor	Points against
• Amenorrhea followed by vaginal bleeding and lower abdominal pain	• USG examination showing gestational sac (in the uterus) with absent fetal parts (rules out corpus luteum cyst, as an adnexal mass should be visible).

So, corpus luteum cyst ruled out.

Option "b" : i.e. Incarcerated abortion, Incarcerated abortion is a variant of missed abortion.

Points in favor	Points against
• Amenorrhea of 8 weeks (incarcerated abortion is seen in fetus before 12 weeks). • USG showing gestational sac with no fetal part. (In incarcerated abortion - small repeated hemorrhage occur in the choriodecidual space, disrupting the villi from its attachment. The clotted blood with the contained ovum in called as blood mole. The ovum is dead and is either absorbed or remains as a rudimentary structure. So on USG - although gestational sac is seen, no fetal parts are seen.	• The only point which goes against incarcerated abortion is that patient does not present with vaginal bleeding and pain but friends, this can be explained on the basis that initially in missed abortion there is no bleeding or pain but later on the uterus itself tries to expel the dead fetus and patient at that time may present with bleeding and pain.

So our answer is incarcerated abortion.

23. Ans. is a, i.e. 63 days   *Ref. Novak 14/e, p 298, Dutta Obs. 7/e, p 174*

Medical abortion using mifepristone and misoprostol can be done for 9 weeks (63 days) but in India, it is done only uptil 7 weeks (49 days).

24. Ans. is d, i.e. Atosiban   *Ref. Dutta Obs. 7/e, p 173*

> **Drugs used for Medical abortion:**
> • Prostaglandins:
>   – Misoprostol
>   – Gemeprost
> • Mifepristone
> • Methotrexate
> • Tamoxifen

25. Ans. is a, i.e. Ethacrydine lactate   *Ref. Dutta Obs. 7/e, p 173*

Ethacridine lactate is drug of choice for extra-amniotic instillation

- Available as injection Emcredil (0.1%)
- Foleys catheter is introduced into extra-amniotic or extraovular space and bulb is inflated by 10–20 ml of Ethacridine solution.
- Dose is calculated as **10 ml/week of gestation upto maximum of 150 ml**
- Catheter is left for 6 hours.
- Uterine action begins in 16–18 hours.

In 30% cases abortion is incomplete and requires oxytocin drip or supplementation with prostaglandin.

26. **Ans. is c, i.e. > 12 weeks** *Ref. Dutta Obs. 7/e, p 173; Reddy 26/e, p 368, 369*

According to MTP act–

If the period of pregnancy is below 12 weeks, it can be terminated on the opinion of a single doctor.[Q]

If the period of pregnancy is between 12 and 20 weeks, two doctors must agree that there is an indication.[Q] Once the opinion is formed, the termination can be done by any one doctor.

27. **Ans. is c, i.e. The female partner** *Ref. Park's Textbook of PSM 21/e, p 468, 469*

For MTP:

Only female's consent is required

Husbands consent is not required. (The confidentiality about name is maintained)

Consent of parent/guardian is required when age of patient is < 18 years and in case of lunatic females

Person who can perform MTP

- RMP with 25 MTPS done in approved institution
- 6 month housemanship in Obstetrics and Gynecology
- Post graduate qualification in Obstetrics and Gynecology
- 3 years practice in Obstetrics and Gynecology who are registered before 1971
- 1 year practice in Obstetrics and Gynecology for those registered on or after the date of commencement of the act.

28. **Ans. is a, i.e. Threatened abortion** *Ref. Read below*

Threatened Abortion is a clinical entity where the process of abortion has started but has not progressed to a state from which recovery is impossible. The treatment of threatened abortion is aimed at preserving pregnancy and not at terminating pregnancy.

Mifepristone is an abortifacient that will cause termination of pregnancy and should not be used in cases of threatened abortion.

Mifepristone may be used for Ectopic pregnancy and for shrinking of Fibroids

"Mifepristone injected into the unruptured ectopic pregnancy causes its resolution" *Ref. Shaws 13/e, p 307*

'Shrinkage of uterine leiomyoma has been observed following Mifepristone therapy' *Ref. Dutta Gynae 5/e, p 911*

29. **Ans. is c, i.e. VDRL of father and mother**

In this question the patient has recurrent abortions at 14–16 weeks normally. This time she has presented with abortion at 12 weeks—this cannot happen in syphilis because **syphilis follows kassowitz law. In syphilis with every loss period of gestation at which the loss occurs, keeps on increasing**.

(Therefore, if 1st time abortion occured in 1st trimester, next time it will be in 2nd trimester and so on). The reverse does not happen. Thus syphilis can lead to recurrent pregnancy loss but not early recurrent pregnancy loss.

Therefore, in this case VDRL test of father and mother is of no use. Rest all the other investigations are needed.

30. **Ans. is b, d and e, i.e. Hypersensitivity to prostaglandin; Suspected ectopic pregnancy; Undiagnosed adnexal mass**
    (Ref: Dutta Obs 8th/204,206; J B Sharma 1st/126; William's Obs 24/368; Novak's Gynae 15th/256-57; Shaw Gynae 4th/435)

    Absolute C/I of medical abortion: J B Sharma 1st/126
    - Suspected ectopic pregnancy
    - or undiagnosed adnexal mass;
    - Allergy to any drug"-

    Relative contraindications to medical abortion- Williams 24e/pg 368
    - **Insitu IUCD device**
    - Severe anemia
    - Coagulopathy or anticoagulants use
    - Liver disease
    - Cardiac disease
    - Seizure disorders
    - Women with diminished glucocorticoid activity
    - In Renal insufficiency patients- dose of methotrexate needs to be modified.

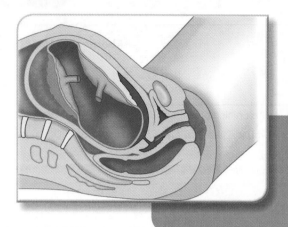

Ectopic Pregnancy

Chapter at a Glance

➢ Ectopic Pregnancy
➢ Ruptured Ectopic

➢ Unruptured Ectopic
➢ Ectopic Pregnancy at other Sites

ECTOPIC PREGNANCY

Definition

It is defined as the implantation and development of the blastocyst at a site other than the endometrial lining of the uterine cavity.

 Important One Liners

- M/C site of ectopic pregnancy—Fallopian tube.
- M/C non tubal site of ectopic pregnancy—ovary
- Least common site of ectopic pregnancy—ectopic in caesarean section scar (< 1%) followed by cervical ectopic (1%).
- In the Fallopian tube—ectopic pregnancy incidence.

⇓

Mnemonic

Ampulla > Is > In > Interstitium
  ↓   ↓   ↓   ↓
Ampulla > Isthmus > Infundibulum > Interstitium
(M/C)   (2nd M/C)

- M/C site of ectopic in Fallopian tube—Ampulla (This is because fertilisation occurs in ampulla)
- Least common site in Fallopian tube—Interstitium
- When ectopic pregnancy occurs in interstitium of Fallopian tube or in rudimentary horn of bicornuate uterus, it is called as **cornual pregnancy** (Therefore cornual pregnancy is a type of ectopic pregnancy).

Contd…

Contd…

- In contrast when intrauterine pregnancy occurs near the cornua of uterus, it is called as Angular Pregnancy. (Thus, angular pregnancy is a type of intrauterine pregnancy).
- **Both cornual and angular pregnancy can be differentiated with the help of round ligament**
  In angular pregnancy, round ligament lies lateral to it (Figs. 16.1A and B).
  In cornual pregnancy, round ligament lies medial to it.
- **Heterotopic pregnancy**—it is an example of twin pregnancy, where one pregnancy is ectopic and other is intrauterine.
  The natural incidence of heterotopic pregnancy is 1 per 30,000 pregnancy, however with ART, it is 9 in 10,000 pregnancy.

 Note: Regardless of location, D-negative women with an ectopic pregnancy who are not sensitized to D-antigen are given IgG anti-D immunoglobulin (American College of Obstetricians and Gynecologists, 2017). In first-trimester pregnancies, a 50-μg is appropriate, whereas a standard 300-μg dose is used for later gestations.

Risk Factors of Ectopic Pregnancy

Factors Related to Genital Tract

1. **Highest risk** of ectopic pregnancy **is with previous history of ectopic pregnancy**.

   - After one episode of ectopic pregnancy, there is 10% risk of having a second ectopic pregnancy.
   - After two ectopics risk increases to 25%.

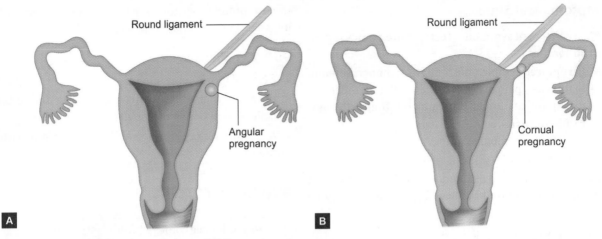

Figs. 16.1A and B: (A) Angular pregnancy; (B) Cornual pregnancy

2. **Previous tubal surgery:** It has the second highest risk of ectopic pregnancy after previous H/O ectopic pregnancy.

3. **Most common risk factor:** Sexually transmitted infections (STIs) and pelvic inflammatory disease especially due to Chlamydia trachomatis and Mycoplasma hominis infection. Each episode of PID increases the risk of ectopic pregnancy by 10%.

Other important causes are:
* Post abortal sepsis
* Puerperal sepsis
* Appendicitis
* Genital TB

4. Congenital factors like tubal tuberosity, accessory ostia, diverticula, etc.

5. **Salpingitis isthmica nodosa of the** tube in which Fallopian tube is constructed at various places due to TB or other infection.

6. **Failed contraception: Use of any method of contraception, decreases the absolute number of ectopic pregnancy.** This is because overall chances of pregnancy are decreased. **But with contraception failure, the relative number of ectopic pregnancies increases.**

7. Endometriosis

8. Assisted reproductive technology

 Important One Liners

* Maximum chances of ectopic pregnancy with contraceptive agents are with **tubectomy failure > IUCD > progesterone only pill**
* Least chances are with –**OCP's, vasectomy**
* Amongst IUCD's: Maximum chances are with **progestasert > Mirena > Cu containing IUCD**

Contd…

Contd…

 Remember: Previous H/O ectopic pregnancy is not an absolute contraindication for IUCD.

Factors Unrelated to Genital Tract

* Multiple partners
* Young age of intercourse
* Low socioeconomic status
* Smokers, IV drug abusers
* In utero exposure to DES (Diethyl stilbestrol)

Fate of Ectopic Pregnancy

Ectopic pregnancy can meet any of the following 2 fates

(i) **Tubal abortion:** Seen when ectopic occurs in ampulla and infundibulum portion of the tube (i.e. if ectopic pregnancy occurs in distal parts of tube)

(ii) **Rupture of the tube:** Seen when ectopic occurs in isthmus and interstitial parts of the tube (i.e. if ectopic pregnancy occurs in proximal part of tube).

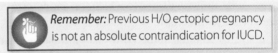 Important One Liners

* M/C site of tubal abortion—ampulla
* M/C site of tubal rupture—isthmus
* Ectopic pregnancy ends earliest in: isthmus (@ 6 weeks)
* In ectopic pregnancy of tubes, in which part ectopic has longest survival: interstitium (@12 weeks)
  This is because uterine myometrium supports ectopic pregnancy at this site
* Hence the most dangerous site for ectopic is: Interstitium
* Overall ectopic pregnancy survives for the longest time in-Abdomen. (here ectopic can continue till term)

Symptoms and Signs

- **Most consistent symptom of ectopic pregnancy is pain in abdomen**
  - **In ruptured ectopic, pain is due to hemoperitoneum.** In this case, pain may be referred to the shoulder due to diaphragmatic irritation by blood (**Danforth Sign**)
  - In **unruptured ectopic** pregnancy pain is due to stretching of Fallopian tube.
- Amenorrhea of 6–10 weeks is seen in 75% patients.
- In 50% patients, triad of amenorrhea (6–10 weeks) pain in abdomen followed by bleeding per vagina may be present.

Signs: In ruptured ectopic, patient will be in shock (BP decreased, HR increased)

- Decidua is endometrium that is hormonally prepared for pregnancy, and the degree to which the endometrium is converted with ectopic pregnancy is variable. Thus, in addition to bleeding, women with ectopic tubal pregnancy may pass a *decidual cast*. This is the entire sloughed endometrium that takes the form of the endometrial cavity (Fig 16.2). Importantly, decidual sloughing may also occur with uterine abortion. Thus, tissue is carefully evaluated visually by the provider and then histologically for evidence of a conceptus. If no clear gestational sac is seen or if no villi are identified histologically within the cast, then the possibility of ectopic pregnancy must still be considered.

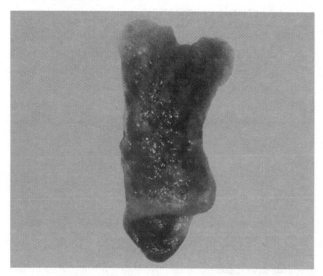

Fig. 16.2: The decidual cast seen in ectopic pregnancy

On P/A examination = Tenderness, tenseness, rigidity and guarding in lower abdomen.

In case of hemoperitoneum-**Cullen sign** (periumbilical bluish discoloration) may be seen.

On P/V examination:

- Cervical movements tender.
- Posterior vaginal fornix may by bulging due to blood collection in pouch of Douglas
- A tender boggy mass may be felt on one side of uterus.

RUPTURED ECTOPIC

> Wherever a female comes with amenorrhea of 6–10 weeks
> +
> Urine pregnancy test is positive
> +
> She is in Shock
> Always think of ectopic pregnancy

Techniques to Identify Hemoperitoneum

1. **TVS:** Sonographically, anechoic or hypoechoic fluid initially collects in the dependent retrouterine cul-de-sac, and then additionally surrounds the uterus as it fills the pelvis. As much as 50 mL of blood can be seen in the cul-de-sac using TVS, and transabdominal imaging then is used to assess the hemoperitoneum extent. With significant intraabdominal haemorrhage, blood will track up the pericolic gutters to fill Morison pouch near the liver. Free fluid in this pouch typically is not seen until accumulated volumes reach 400 to 700 mL.

2. **Culdocentesis:** Culdocentesis is a simple technique used commonly in the past. The cervix is pulled outward and upward toward the symphysis with a tenaculum, and a long 18-gauge needle is inserted through the posterior vaginal fornix into the retrouterine cul-de-sac. If present, fluid can be aspirated. However, a failure to do so is interpreted only as unsatisfactory entry into the cul-de-sac.

> Fluid containing fragments of old clots or bloody fluid that does not clot suggests hemoperitoneum. In contrast, if the blood sample clots, it may have been obtained from an adjacent blood vessel.

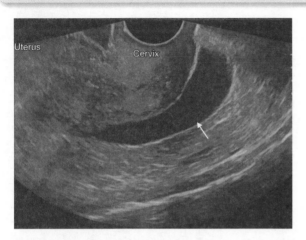

Fig. 16.3: Techniques to identify hemoperitoneum. Transvaginal sonography of an anechoic fluid collection (arrow) in the retrouterine cul-de-sac.

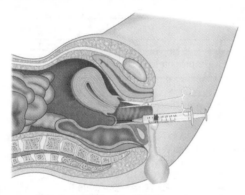

Fig. 16.4: Techniques to identify hemoperitoneum. Culdocentesis: with a 16- to 18-gauge spinal needle attached to a syringe, the cul-de-sac is entered through the posterior vaginal fornix as upward traction is applied to the cervix with a tenaculum

Management

Simultaneous resuscitation and laparotomy

Management of Shock

- Secure 2 IV lines: Start Ringer lactate or dextrose, saline solution immediately.
- Blood sample sent for grouping, cross matching. Arrange 2–4 units of bloods.
- Injection anti-D-50 mcg is given to Rh negative women.

Laparotomy

- In case of ruptured ectopic, laparotomy is preferred.
- Although laparoscopy is not contraindicated unless patient is hemodynamically unstable. Surgeons who have expertise can perform laparoscopy in ruptured ectopic also.

- Abdomen is opened by, transverse incision or midline vertical incision

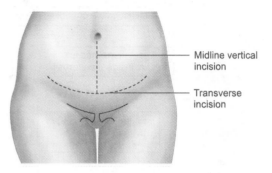

Fig. 16.5: Laparotomy incisions

Surgery of Choice

In all cases of ruptured ectopic whether the female is nulliparous or multiparous—the ruptured tube is removed, i.e. **salpingectomy** is done.

Salpingectomy is the gold standard treatment in ruptured ectopic.

 Note: Expectant management/Medical management/ Any other surgery are not done in ruptured ectopic.

UNRUPTURED ECTOPIC

Diagnosis

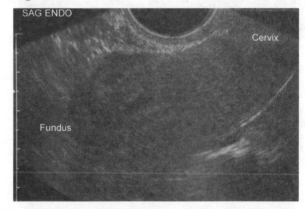

Fig. 16.6: Transvaginal sonography of a pseudogestational sac within the endometrial cavity. Its cavity-conforming shape and central location are characteristic of these anechoic fluid collections. Distal to this fluid, the endometrial stripe has a trilaminar pattern, which is a common finding with ectopic pregnancy. (Reproduced with permission from Gala RB: Ectopic pregnancy. In Hoffman BI, Schorge JO, Bradshaw KD, et al: Williams Gynecology, 3rd ed. New York, McGraw-Hill Education; 2016. Photo contributor: Dr. Elysia moschos.)

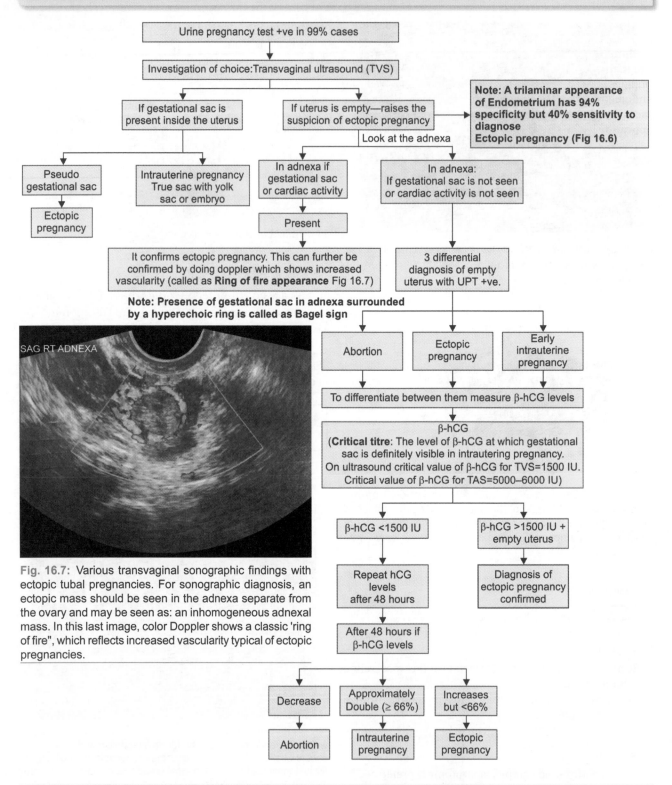

Urine pregnancy test +ve in 99% cases

Investigation of choice: Transvaginal ultrasound (TVS)

Note: A trilaminar appearance of Endometrium has 94% specificity but 40% sensitivity to diagnose Ectopic pregnancy (Fig 16.6)

If gestational sac is present inside the uterus

If uterus is empty—raises the suspicion of ectopic pregnancy

Look at the adnexa

Pseudo gestational sac

Ectopic pregnancy

Intrauterine pregnancy True sac with yolk sac or embryo

In adnexa if gestational sac or cardiac activity

In adnexa: If gestational sac is not seen or cardiac activity is not seen

Present

It confirms ectopic pregnancy. This can further be confirmed by doing doppler which shows increased vascularity (called as **Ring of fire appearance** Fig 16.7)

3 differential diagnosis of empty uterus with UPT +ve.

Note: Presence of gestational sac in adnexa surrounded by a hyperechoic ring is called as Bagel sign

SAG RT ADNEXA

Abortion

Ectopic pregnancy

Early intrauterine pregnancy

To differentiate between them measure β-hCG levels

β-hCG
(**Critical titre:** The level of β-hCG at which gestational sac is definitely visible in intrautering pregnancy. On ultrasound critical value of β-hCG for TVS=1500 IU. Critical value of β-hCG for TAS=5000–6000 IU)

β-hCG <1500 IU

β-hCG >1500 IU + empty uterus

Repeat hCG levels after 48 hours

Diagnosis of ectopic pregnancy confirmed

Fig. 16.7: Various transvaginal sonographic findings with ectopic tubal pregnancies. For sonographic diagnosis, an ectopic mass should be seen in the adnexa separate from the ovary and may be seen as: an inhomogeneous adnexal mass. In this last image, color Doppler shows a classic 'ring of fire", which reflects increased vascularity typical of ectopic pregnancies.

After 48 hours if β-hCG levels

Decrease

Approximately Double (≥ 66%)

Increases but <66%

Abortion

Intrauterine pregnancy

Ectopic pregnancy

Note: An early time gestational sac is seen as an anechoic sac eccentrically located within one of the endometrial stripe layers. The American College of Obstetricians and Gynecologists (2016) advises caution in diagnosing an intrauterine pregnancy in the absence of a definite yolk sac or embryo.

Transvaginal Sonography

Endometrial Findings: In a woman in whom ectopic pregnancy is suspected, TVS is performed to look for findings indicative of uterine or ectopic pregnancy. During endometrial cavity evaluation, an intrauterine gestational sac is usually visible between 4½ and 5 weeks. The yolk sac appears between 5 and 6 weeks and a fetal pole with cardiac activity is first detected at 5½ to 6 weeks. With transabdominal sonography these structures are visualized slightly later.

Key Concept

- **Kadar principle:** During first 48 days of gestation in a normal intrauterine pregnancy, βhCG levels double every 48 hours.
- Sometimes in ectopic pregnancy—**a pseudogestational sac** may be seen in the uterus. The hormonal changes associated with ectopic pregnancy can cause fluid collection in endometrial cavity, which mimic a gestational sac. The pseudogestational sac is seen in 20% cases of ectopic pregnancy.
- **Features of true gestational sac:**
    - The position of a normal gestational sac is in mid to upper uterus. As the sac implants into the decidualized endometrium, it should be adjacent to the linear central cavity echo complex, without initially displacing this hyperechogenic landmark. This is called **intradecidual sign.**

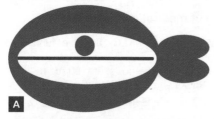

Fig. 16.8A: Diagram of intradecidual sign: The gestational sac (circle) does not displace the central cavity complex (straight black line). The white area represents thickened decidual tissue

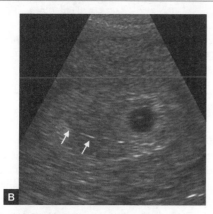

Fig. 16.8B: USG of intradecidual sac sign

- As the true gestational sac enlarges, it gradually impresses and deforms the central cavity echo complex, giving rise to a characteristic appearance **called as double decidual sac. Sign: This sign is present when mean sac diameter is 10 mm or more.** It consists of two concentric echogenic lines surrounding a portion of gestational sac. The line closest to the sac represents the combined smooth chorion-decidual capsularis, whereas the adjacent more peripherally located line represents the decidua parietalis. **This sign is best seen transabdominally by 5–6 weeks.**

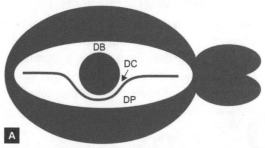

Fig. 16.9A: Diagram of the double decidual sac: The gestational sac (circle) protrudes into and displaces the central cavity echo complex (curved line). The white area represents thickened decidual line. The white area represents thickened decidual tissue. Two concentric lines are due to the echogenic decidua capsularis (DC)—smooth chorion and the peripherally located decidua parietalis (DP in USG)

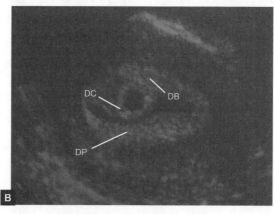

Fig. 16.9B: USG of double decidual sac sign

- In case of pseudogestational sac, both these signs are absent. Other differences between true and pseudogestational sac are given in **Table 16.1**.

Table 16.1: Differences between true and pseudogestational sac

USG finding	True gestational sac	Pseudo gestational sac
Shape	Round	Ovoid
Location with respect to endometrial cavity	Eccentric	Central

Contd...

Contd…

Margins	Well defined	Poorly defined
Decidual reaction	Well defined	Absent
Double decidual sac sign	Present	Absent

> **Gold standard for diagnosis** of ectopic pregnancy is laparoscopy.

Other useful investigations in ectopic pregnancy:

(i) **Serum progesterone levels:** Levels of S progesterone < 5 ng/mL indicate a dying pregnancy and ≥ 25 mg/mL indicate healthy intrauterine pregnancy.

(ii) **Culdocentesis:** This simple technique is used to identify hemoperitoneum, in case of ruptured ectopic.

Remember:
Investigations never done in ectopic
- Hysterosalpingography (hSG)
- Hysteroscopy
  - Colpotomy (done to drain pelvic abscess, but not used in ectopic)

Management of Unruptured Ectopic Pregnancy

In unruptured ectopic pregnancy-management options include:

(i) Expectant management
(ii) Medical management
(iii) Surgical management

A. Expectant Management

Observation of ectopic pregnancy can be done in very early cases, in hope of ectopic pregnancy resolving on its own.

Criteria for Expectant Management: *William obs 25/e page 380*

- Patient should be hemodynamically stable (i.e. done only in unruptured ectopic)
- βhCG levels should be < 1500 mIU/mL (according to ACOG = βhCG levels should be < 200 mIU/mL) and should be falling.
- Size of gestational sac < 3.0 cm
- Done only in case of tubal pregnancies
- Cardiac activity should be absent in ectopic pregnancy.
- The patient should be counselled properly and should be in easy reach of hospital.
  - Monitoring should be done twice weekly with βhCG.

B. Medical Management

- DOC for medical management is **Methotrexate**
- Dose is 50 mg per m² body surface area administered intramuscularly as **a single dose**.

Criteria for Medical Management

William Gynae 3/e pg 120

Absolute requirements	Preferable requirements
• Patient should be hemodynamically stable • No evidence of acute intra-abdominal bleeding • No contraindication to treatment	• Serum βhCG < 5,000 IU/L • Cardiac activity should be absent • Size of ectopic pregnancy should be < 3.5 cm of cardiac activity is present and < 4 cm if cardiac activity is absent • Mild or absent pain

Contraindications of Methotrexate

Methotrexate Contraindications		
Sensitivity to methotrexate	Intrauterine pregnancy	Immunodeficiency
Tubal rupture	Peptic ulcer disease	Hepatic, renal, or hematologic dysfunction
Breastfeeding	Active pulmonary disease	

Procedure of medical management

Day 1 = Measure βhCG, TLC, DLC, liver function test, Renal function test
Day 2 = Single dose methotrexate (50 mg/m² IM)
Day 4 = S βhCG and counts repeated
Day 7 = S βhCG and counts repeated

Now if the decline in serum βhCG between day 7 and day 4 is:

≥ 15% ↓ No further treatment required. βhCG levels are repeated Weekly until they become undetectable	< 15% decrease/cardiac activity is present ↓ Repeat injection. Methotrexate and begin new day 1

Note:
- If after 3 doses of methotrexate, βhCG levels do not decrease or cardiac activity persists—it is a case of Failed Medical Management.
- Management in a case of failed medical management is–Surgery.
- M/C side effect of methotrexate is Liver involvement

C. Surgical Management

In unruptured ectopic – **both laparoscopy and laparotomy can be done. Laparoscopy is the preferred method.**

Indications of laparotomy:
- Hemodynamically unstable patient
- Cornual pregnancy
- Extensive abdominal and pelvic adhesions

Surgery of choice

- **If patient has completed her family-Salpingectomy**
- If patient has not completed her family
  - Best surgery: **Salpingostomy**
  - Other surgery which can be done:
    - Salpingotomy
    - Segmental resection and anastomosis
    - Milking of tube

Procedure of salpingostomy

- Done to remove a small pregnancy < 2 cm and located at distal third of fallopian tube
- A linear incision is given with cautery on the anti-mesenteric border of the tube over the ectopic pregnancy
- The product of conception is extruded using hydro dissection
- The incision is left unstitched to heal by secondary intention.

 Note: Salpingotomy—here the procedure is same as salpingostomy but incision is closed with delayed absorbable suture. It is not performed these days.

- Incomplete removal of ectopic during salpingostomy results in **persistent trophoblast/persistent ectopic** (seen in 5–20% cases)

 Also Know:

Factors increasing the risk of persistent ectopic pregnancy:
1. Small pregnancies (< 2 cm)
2. Early therapy (before 42 menstrual days)
3. βhCG serum levels exceeding 3000 mIU/mL
4. Implantation medial to the salpingostomy site

Future intrauterine pregnancy chances
Highest: Methotrexate > salpingostomy > expectant management

Future ectopic pregnancy chances
Highest: Expectant > salpingostomy > methotrexate

ECTOPIC PREGNANCY AT OTHER SITES

Abdominal Pregnancy

- Criteria for diagnosis: **Studdiford's criteria**
- M/C symptom = lower abdomen pain and bleeding
- Braxton Hicks contractions are absent
- **Management:** Surgery is the only treatment.

 Note: Abdominal pregnancy can continue upto term. Fetal malformation and deformity rate is 20% **M/C deformities** are facial or cranial asymmetry, joint abnormalities, limb deformity and CNS abnormality.

Ovarian Pregnancy

- Criteria for diagnosis—**Spiegelberg criteria**
- **Management:** Surgical (ovariotomy or ovarian wedge resection) or medical management with methotrexate for unruptured ovarian pregnancy.

Cervical Pregnancy

Criteria for diagnosis—**Rubin's criteria or Palmaan McEllen criteria.** These days USG criteria is used:
- **M/C symptom**—Painless vaginal bleeding
- **Management**— 1st choice: Methotrexate therapy
2nd choice: Surgical management
Luke cerclage followed by curettage or arterial embolization followed by curettage.

Heterotopic Pregnancy

- Here ectopic pregnancy coexists with an intrauterine pregnancy in a twin pregnancy
- Earlier incidence was rare = 1 in 30,000 pregnancies. These days due to IVF-incidence has increased = 1 in 8000 pregnancies.
- **Management:** Surgical for ectopic pregnancy. The intrauterine pregnancy continues normally.

New Pattern Questions

N1. A 20-year-old woman complains of sudden onset of right-sided lower abdominal pain and bleeding per vagina. Her last normal menstrual period was 35 days ago. Her blood pressure is 90/70 mmHg and the pulse rate is 100 bpm. There is tenderness and guarding in the right iliac fossa. She denies any sexual intercourse.

What is the most appropriate next step in the management?
a. Estimate serum beta hCG levels
b. Obtain a surgical opinion to exclude acute appendicitis
c. Perform a laparoscopic examination
d. Perform a transvaginal ultrasound scan

N2. A woman complains of right-sided lower abdominal pain and mild bleeding per vagina for one day after a period of amenorrhoea of 6 weeks. Her general condition is satisfactory. There is tenderness in the right iliac fossa. The urine hCG test is positive. Transvaginal ultrasound scan does not reveal an adnexal mass or an intrauterine pregnancy.

What is the next step in the management?
a. Commence treatment with methotrexate
b. Perform a laparoscopic examination
c. Perform two serum beta hCG tests 48 hours apart
d. Repeat the ultrasound scan after 7 days

N3. A third para is admitted with a history of sudden onset of right-sided lower abdominal pain and bleeding per vagina after a period of amenorrhoea of 5 weeks. Her blood pressure is 80/50 mmHg and the pulse rate is 130 bpm. Transvaginal ultrasound scan reveals the presence of a large amount of free fluid in the pelvis and the absence of an intrauterine pregnancy.

What is the most appropriate management?
a. Perform laparoscopic salpingectomy
b. Perform laparoscopic salpingo-oophorectomy
c. Perform a salpingectomy through a laparotomy
d. Treat with intramuscular methotrexate

N4. A woman complains of right-sided lower abdominal pain and mild bleeding per vagina after a POA of 6 weeks. Her general condition is satisfactory. The urine hCG test is positive. Transvaginal ultrasound scan reveals an adnexal mass 30 mm in diameter without evidence of cardiac activity, but no intrauterine pregnancy.

What is the most appropriate management?
a. Perform laparoscopic salpingectomy
b. Perform laparoscopic salpingo-oophorectomy
c. Perform laparoscopic salpingotomy
d. Treat with intramuscular methotrexate

N5. A woman attends the antenatal clinic at a POA of 5 weeks. She has no complaints. Her periods are regular and she is sure of dates. Urine hCG is positive. Transvaginal scan does not reveal an intrauterine or ectopic pregnancy. Serum beta hCG doubles from 900 to 1800 IU/L after 48 hours.

What is the next step in the management?
a. Give a single dose of methotrexate
b. Perform a laparoscopy
c. Perform a serum beta hCG test after 1 week
d. Repeat the transvaginal scan in 3 days

N6. Arias stella reaction is not seen in:
a. Ovarian pregnancy
b. Molar pregnancy
c. Interstitial pregnancy
d. Salpingitis isthmica nodosa

N7. What is the treatment of choice of unruptured tubal pergnancy with serum β-hCG titre 2000 IU/mL:
a. Single dose of methotrexate
b. Variable dose of methotrexate
c. Expectant management
d. Laparoscopic salpingostomy

N8. Diagnostic criteria for primary abdominal pregnancy:
a. Spiegelberg criteria
b. Rubin's criteria
c. Studdiford criteria   d.   Wrigley criteria

N9. Angular pregnancy refers to:
a. Ectopic pregnancy of interstitial part of FT
b. Intrauterine pregnancy
c. Heterotopic pregnancy
d. Ectopic pregnancy of broad ligament

N10. You are called to the operating room. The general surgeons have operated on a woman to rule out appendicitis and the signs of an abdominal pregnancy with an 18 week fetus and placenta attached to the omentum. The best course of action in the case is:
a. Removal of both fetus and placenta
b. Laparoscopic ligation of umbilical cord
c. Removal of the fetus only
d. Closely follow until viability and then deliver by laparotomy

N11. Highest risk of ectopic pregnancy is with:
a. Intrauterine device
b. Surgery for previous ectopic
c. Salpingitis
d. Salpingitis isthmica nodosa

N12. Most dangerous variety of ectopic:
a. Ampulla   b.   Interstitial
c. Fimbrial   d.   Isthmus

N13. Not an indication of expectant management in ectopic pregnancy:
a. β-hCG < 200 IU
b. Decreasing levels of β-hCG
c. Size of ectopic pregnancy < 5 cm
d. Unruptured ectopic

N14. A G2P1 female with 7 weeks amenorrhea with UPT +ve. On TVS nothing is seen. Next step in management is:
a. β-hCG levels
b. S. progesterone levels
c. Culdocentesis
d. Repeat TVS after 10 days

N15. Methotrexate is best suited when β–hCG concentration is:

a. < 5000 IU
b. < 6000 IU
c. < 7000 IU
d. < 10,000 IU

N16. Dose of methotrexate in single and multi dose protocol for ectopic pregnancy:
a. 50 mg/m^2; 1 mg/kg
b. 100 mg/m^2, 1 mg/kg
c. 50 mg/m^2, 0.1 mg/kg
d. 100 mg/m^2, 0.1 mg/kg

N17. Treatment of choice for heterotopic pregnancy:
a. Medical management
b. Surgical management
c. Expectant
d. Any of above

Previous Year Questions

1. Basanti, a 28 years aged female with a history of 6 weeks of amenorrhoea presents with pain in abdomen; USG shows fluid in pouch of Douglas. Aspiration yields dark color blood that fails to clot. Most probable diagnosis is: [AI 01]
a. Ruptured ovarian cyst
b. Ruptured ectopic pregnancy
c. Red degeneration of fibroid
d. Pelvic abscess

2. A young woman with six weeks amenorrhoea presents with mass abdomen. USG shows empty uterus. Diagnosis is: [AI 01]
a. Ovarian cyst
b. Ectopic pregnancy
c. Complete abortion
d. None of the above

3. A woman presents with amenorrhoea of 2 months duration; lower abdominal pain, facial pallor, fainting and shock. Diagnosis is: [AI 01]
a. Ruptured ovarian cyst
b. Ruptured ectopic pregnancy
c. Threatened abortion
d. Septic abortion

4. A 21-years-old girl with 8 weeks amenorrhoea, now comes in shock. The likely diagnosis is: [AI 00]
a. Ruptured ectopic pregnancy
b. Incarcerated amnion
c. Twisted ovarian cyst
d. Threatened abortion

5. Young lady presents with acute abdominal pain and history of 1½ months amenorrhoea, on USG examination there is collection of fluid in the pouch of Douglas and empty gestational sac. Diagnosis is:

a. Ectopic pregnancy [AIIMS Nov 01]
b. Pelvic hematocele
c. Threatened abortion
d. Twisted ovarian cyst

6. Causes of ectopic pregnancy includes A/E:
a. IUCD [PGI June 97]
b. Tubal ciliary damage
c. Blighted ovum
d. Late fertilization

7. True about tubal pregnancy:
a. Prior h/o tubal surgery [PGI Dec 09, June 09, 07]
b. Prior tubal pregnancy
c. Prior h/o PID/Chlamydia infection
d. IUCD predisposes
e. OCP predisposes

8. Ectopic pregnancy is most commonly associated with: [PGI Dec 01]
a. Endometriosis
b. Congenital tubal anomalies
c. Tuberculosis
d. Tubal inflammatory diseases
e. Retroverted uterus

9. Most common symptom present in undisturbed ectopic: [PGI June 98]
a. Pain in lower abdomen
b. Amenorrhea
c. Bleeding P/V
d. Fainting attack

10. Most common manifestation of ectopic pregnancy is: [PGI June 97]
a. Vomiting   b. Bleeding
c. Pain in abdomen   d. Shock

11. In which part of fallopian tube ectopic pregnancy will have longest survival: [AIIMS Nov 01]
   a. Isthmus
   b. Ampulla
   c. Cornua
   d. Interstitium

12. The cause of fetal death in ectopic pregnancy is postulated as: [AIIMS May 08]
   a. Vascular accident
   b. Nutritional adequacy
   c. Endocrine insufficiency
   d. Immune response to mother

13. In ectopic pregnancy decidua is shed as: [AI 98]
   a. Decidua vera
   b. Decidua basalis
   c. Decidua capsularis
   d. Decidua rubra

14. Modern diagnostic aid to diagnose ectopic pregnancy: [PGI June 06]
   a. hCG
   b. Transvaginal USG
   c. AFP
   d. Gravindex

15. Most important investigation for ectopic pregnancy: [PGI May 2013]
   a. TVS
   b. Serial β-hCG levels
   c. Doppler USG
   d. Progesterone
   e. Culdocentesis

16. Most valuable diagnostic test in case of suspected ectopic pregnancy: [AIIMS Nov 09, May 08]
   a. Serial β-hCG revels
   b. Transvaginal USG
   c. Progesterone measurement
   d. Culdocentesis

17. True statement regarding ectopic pregnancy: [PGI Nov 2012]
   a. Serum progesterone >25 ng/ml exclude ectopic
   b. β-hCG levels should be >1000 mIU/ml for earliest detection by TVS
   c. β-hCG levels should be <1000 mIU/ml for earliest detection by TVS
   d. Methotrexate is used for treatment
   e. β-hCG double in 48 hours

18. True about ectopic pregnancy: [PGI June 08]
   a. Transvaginal USG-first imaging test of choice
   b. Associated with decidual reaction
   c. Doppler is of no significance
   d. In ectopic interstitial ring sign is seen
   e. hCG level is sufficient for diagnosis

19. About ectopic pregnancy true statements are:
   a. Rising titre of hCG [PGI Dec 03]
   b. Negative pregnancy test excludes the diagnosis
   c. Common after tubal surgery
   d. Seen in patients taking GnRH therapy
   e. Common in patients taking OCP

20. Drugs used for treatment of ectopic pregnancy are: [PGI June 03]
   a. MTX
   b. Actinomycin-D
   c. hCG
   d. RU-486
   e. KCl

21. Which of the following drug is not used for medical management of ectopic pregnancy? [AIIMS Nov 03]

   a. Potassium chloride
   b. Methotrexate
   c. Actinomycin D
   d. Misoprostol

22. In which of the following conditions, the medical treatment of ectopic pregnancy is contraindicated:
   a. Sac size is 3 cm [AIIMS May 04]
   b. Blood in pelvis is 70 mL
   c. Presence of fetal heart activity
   d. Previous ectopic pregnancy

23. Indications of medical management in ectopic pregnancy: [PGI June 07]
   a. Presence of fetal heart activity
   b. Size <4 cm
   c. Gestation <6 weeks
   d. β-hCG >15000
   e. β-hCG <1500

24. A hemodynamically stable nulliparous patient with ectopic pregnancy has adnexal mass of 2.5 × 3 cm and Beta hCG titer of 1500 mIU/ml. What modality of treatment is suitable for her? [AI 03]
   a. Conservative management
   b. Medical management
   c. Laparoscopic surgery
   d. Laparotomy

25. A female has history of 6 weeks amenorrhea, USG shows empty sac, serum β-hCG 6500 IU/L. What would be next management? [AIIMS Nov 08]
   a. Medical management
   b. Repeat hCG after 48 hours
   c. Repeat hCG after 1 week
   d. Surgical management

26. A 20-years-old woman has been brought to casualty with BP 70/40 mm Hg, pulse rate 120/min. and a positive urine pregnancy test. She should be managed by: [AIIMS Nov 02]
   a. Immediate laparotomy
   b. Laparoscopy
   c. Culdocentesis
   d. Resuscitation and medical management

27. Which of the following treatment is not done in ectopic pregnancy? [AI 98]
   a. Salpingectomy
   b. Salpingo-oophorectomy
   c. Salpingostomy
   d. Resection of involved segment

28. In a nulliparous woman, the treatment of choice in ruptured ectopic pregnancy is: [PGI June 00]
   a. Salpingectomy and end to end anastomosis
   b. Salpingo-oophorectomy
   c. Wait and watch
   d. Linear salpingostomy

29. Management of unruptured tubal pregnancy includes: [PGI Nov 2010]
   a. Methotrexate
   b. Prostaglandins
   c. Hysterectomy
   d. Laparoscopic salpingostomy
   e. Salpingectomy

30. **Not true about ectopic pregnancy:**   [PGI Nov 2010]
    a. Previous ectopic is greatest risk
    b. Pregesterone only pills doesn't increase risk
    c. Increased risk with pelvic infections
    d. Increased risk with IVF
    e. IUCD use increases the risk

31. **A female presents with 8 weeks amenorrhea with pain left lower abdomen. On USG, there was thick endometrium with mass in lateral adnexa. Most probable diagnosis:**   [AIIMS Nov 2012]

    a. Ectopic pregnancy
    b. Torsion of dermoid cyst
    c. Tubo-ovarian mass
    d. Hydrosalpinx

32. **Test not useful in case of tubal pregnancy:**
    a. Pelvic examination   [AIIMS Nov 2012]
    b. USG
    c. hCG
    d. Hysterosalpingography

Answers with Explanations to New Pattern Questions

N1. **Ans. is d, i.e. Perform a transvaginal ultrasound scan**
In this patient:

Rt sided lower abdominal pain with bleeding per vagina and amenorrhea: Indicate ectopic pregnancy. This is further supported by tenderness and guarding of Rt iliac fossa

B/P = 90/70 mm ⎤
               ⎬ Vitals are stable
P/R = 100 bpm ⎦

∴ Next step is to do TVS, i.e. transvaginal ultrasound scan to confirm the diagnosis.

N2. **Ans. is c, i.e. Perform two serum βhCG tests 48 hours apart**
Now in this question:

Patient has Rt sided abdominal pain + tenderness + Amenorrhea of 6 weeks + Bleeding + UPT is positive + TVS is unconfirmatory

So most probably diagnosis is ectopic but D/D can be:

(i) Abortion

(ii) Early intrauterine pregnancy.

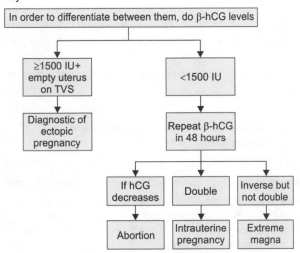

N3. **Ans. is c, i.e. Perform a salpingectomy through a laparotomy**

In this case, the ectopic pregnancy has ruptured as indicated by large amount of free fluid in pelvis on TVS.

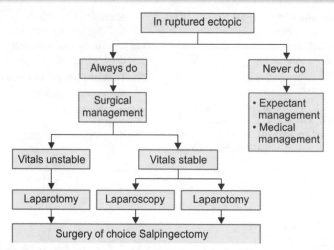

´ The vitals of patient are P/R = 130 bpm and BP = 80/150 mg Hg, i.e. unstable ∴ Management is salpingectomy via laparotomy.

N4. Ans. is d, i.e. Treat with intramuscular methotrexate

In this case, the ectopic is unruptured

Size = 3 cm

No evidence of cardiac activity

All favour medical management with methotrexate.

N5. Ans. is d, i.e. Repeat the transvaginal scan in 3 days

This woman has a positive urine hCG test, but the TVS does not reveal an intrauterine pregnancy (IUP) or an ectopic pregnancy. Therefore, her period of gestation could be less than 5 weeks, or she could be having a pregnancy in an unknown location. Serum βhCG levels doubled up to 1800 IU/L in 48 hours. Accordingly she is likely to have a developing early intrauterine pregnancy with wrong dates, but the possibility of an ectopic pregnancy cannot be excluded, as an IUP was not seen. The next step in the management is to perform a repeat TVS. However the scan should be performed in 3 days, as the serum βhCG is more than 1500 IU/L and there is the risk of rupture if a tubal pregnancy is present.

N6. Ans. is d, i.e. Salpingitis isthmica nodosa *Ref. Novak 14/e, p 608*

Arias stella reaction

- Arias stella reaction is characterized by adenomatous change of the endometrial glands.
- There is intraluminal budding.
- Cells loose their polarity, have hyperchromatic nucleus, vacuolated cytoplasm and occasional mitosis.
- The reaction is seen in ectopic pregnancy *(in 10–15% cases)* and indicates blightening of conceptus either intra or extra uterine.

Arias Stella Reaction is not specific for ectopic pregnancy but for blightening of conceptus either intra uterine or extrauterine.

In the options given:

- Ovarian pregnancy
- Interstitial pregnancy

Are examples of ectopic pregnancy and therefore Arias stella reaction will be seen in them.

Molar pregnancy will lead to blightening of ovum and therefore, Arias stella reaction may be seen.

Salpingitis isthmica nodosa: Salpingitis Isthmica Nodosa (SIN) is a noninflammatory pathologic condition of the tube in which tubal epithelium extends into the myosalpinx and forms a true diverticulum. This condition is found more often in the tubes of women with an ectopic pregnancy than in nonpregnant women. Whether tubal pregnancy is caused by SIN or whether the association is coincidental is unknown.

So by itself in SIN, Arias Stella Reaction is not seen. Only when SIN will lead to Ectopic pregnancy then Arias Stella Reaction will be seen.

N7. **Ans. is a, i.e. Single dose of methotrexate** *Ref. Williams Gyane 1/e, p 166, 167*

The lady in the question is presenting with unruptured ectopic pregnancy with β-hCG levels - 2000 IU/L. So there is no doubt we can manage the patient medically (i.e. option d - ruled out)

Expectant management as explained earlier is not better than medical management as it carries a risk of rupture of ectopic pregnancy (i.e. option C ruled out) and also it is done when β-hCG levels are < 1000 IUL

Now - The question arises whether we should give single dose MTx or multidose methotrexate treatment. In the trials which have been conducted—No difference was found in treatment duration, β-hCG levels and side effects in single dose vs multidose methotrexate therapy.

Single dose therapy is more commonly used because of simplicity. It is less expensive, requires less invasive post therapy monitoring and does not require leucovorin supplementation.

N8. **Ans. is c, i.e. Studdiford's criteria** *Ref. Dutta Obs. 7/e, p 188*

Site of Ectopic pregnancy	Name of criteria	Detailed criteria	Management
Primary Abdominal Pregnancy	Studdiford's criteria	• Both the tubes and ovaries should be normal • (without evidence of recent pregnancy). • Absence of uteroperitoneal fistula. • The pregnancy must be related exclusively to the peritoneal surface.	Surgical management
Ovarian Pregnancy	Spiegelberg's criteria	• The tube on the affected site must be intact. • The gestational sac must occupy the position of ovary. • The gestational sac is connected to the uterus by ovarian ligament. • Definite ovarian tissue must be found in the sac wall.	Surgical management
Cervical Pregnancy	Rubin's criteria (Palmatic's criteria)	• The uterus is smaller than the surrounding distended cervix. • The internal os is not dilated. • Curettage of the endometrial cavity is nonproductive of placental tissue. • The external os opens earlier than in spontaneous abortion.	• Medical management if vitals are stable • Surgical management if vitals are unstable

N9. **Ans. is b, i.e. Intrauterine pregnancy**

Angular pregnancy is defined as a pregnancy implanted in one of the lateral angles of the uterine cavity.

Unlike an interstitial pregnancy, which implants in the intramural part of fallopian tube, an angular pregnancy can progress to term.

N10. **Ans. is c, i.e. Removal of fetus only** *Ref. Dutta Obs. 7/e, p 188; Williams Obs. 23/e, p 250, 251*

Abdominal pregnancy
- Management includes urgent laparotomy irrespective of period of gestation.
- The ideal surgery is to remove the entire sac, fetus, placenta and membrane. This can be done if placenta is attached to a removable organ like uterus or broad ligament.
- If placenta is attached to some vital organs, it is better to take out the fetus and leave behind the placenta and the sac after tying and cutting the cord with its placental attachment.
- Absorption of placenta occurs by aseptic autolysis.
- If placenta is left, its involution is monitored by serum hCG and USG.

Dangers related to leaving placenta attached:
- Infection and abscess
- Adhesions
- Intestinal obstruction
- Wound dehiscence

N11. Ans. is b. i.e. Surgery for previous ectopic *(Ref: William Obs 25/e Pg 371)*

Surgeries for a prior tubal pregnancy for fertility restoration or for sterilization confer highest risk of Ectopic.

William Obs 25/e pg 371

N12. Ans. is b. i.e. Interstitial

In interstitial ectopic, the myometrium of uterus supports the ectopic, hence it goes undetected for a long time and ectopic survives for a long time. So when it ruptures it leads to excessive bleeding and is hence the most dangerous site for ectopic.

N13. Ans. is c, i.e. Size of ectopic pregnancy < 5 cm *(Ref. Williams Obs 25/e pg 380)*

For expectant management

Size of ectopic should be < 3 cm

β-hCG < 1500 mIU/mL.

β-hCG levels should be decreasing

N14. Ans. is a, i.e. β-hCG levels

See the text for explanation.

N15. Ans. is a, i.e. < 5000 IU. *(Ref. Williams Obs 25/e pg 378)*

Failure rate of methotrexate is 3.8%. If β-hCG levels are < 5000 IU but rise to 14% if levels are between 5000-10,000.

N16. Ans. is a, i.e. 50 mg²; 1 mg/kg

Dose of methotrexate in single dose therapy = 50 mg/m²

For multidose therapy = Methotrexate 1 mg/kg day 1, 3, 5 and 7

Folinic acid 0.1 mg/kg day 2, 4, 6, 8

N 17. Ans. is b i.e. Surgical management

Heterotopic pregnancy i.e. where one pregnancy is ectopic and other is intrauterine is never managed medically, as it will kill both ectopic and intrauterine pregnancy. It is always managed surgically.

Answers with Explanations to Previous Year Questions

1. **Ans. is b, i.e. Ruptured ectopic pregnancy** *Ref. Dutta Obs. 7/e, p 182; Williams Obs. 22/e, p 258, 259, 23/e, p 242, 243*

The picture given in the question classically represents a case of ruptured ectopic pregnancy.

The women in the question is presenting with amenorrhea of 6 weeks and pain in abdomen.

On USG - fluid is seen in POD and aspiration of dark coloured blood which fails to clot - all these features leave no doubt of ectopic pregnancy.

"Sonographic absence of uterine pregnancy, a positive pregnancy test (β -hCG), fluid in cul-de-sac and an abnormal pelvic mass, ectopic pregnancy is almost certain."

—*Williams Obs. 22/e p 259*

>
> *Also Know:*
> D/D of fluid in POD:
> 1. Mid cycle   2. PID   3. Tubal abortion (ectopic)

Culdocentesis:

- It is a simple technique used to identify hemoperitoneum.
- Fluid is aspirated from cul-de-sac via posterior fornix with the help of a needle.
- If non clotting blood is obtained, it is indicative of an intraperitoneal bleed and probably a ruptured ectopic.

> *Note:* If the aspirated blood clots, it may have been obtained from an adjacent blood vessel rather than from bleeding ectopic pregnancy.

2. **Ans. is b, i.e. Ectopic pregnancy** *Ref. Dutta Obs 7/e p 182, 183; Shaw 14/e, p 244, 245*
Well friends—a young woman presenting with 6 weeks of amenorrhea and USG showing empty uterus could either mean it is an ectopic pregnancy or abortion. In abortion – patient will give history of bleeding, pain but mass in abdomen does not favour it.

3. **Ans. is b, i.e. Ruptured ectopic pregnancy** *Ref. Dutta Obs 7/e, p 182*
4. **Ans. is a, i.e. Ruptured ectopic pregnancy** *Ref. Dutta Obs. 7/e, p 182*

 Remember: History of acute abdominal catastrophe with fainting attack and collapse i.e. shock following short period of amenorrhea, in a woman of child bearing age always points towards ectopic pregnancy (ruptured) and no other diagnosis.

5. **Ans. is a, i.e. Ectopic pregnancy** *Ref. Dutta Obs. 7/e, p 182, 183*

Young lady presenting with history of:	•	Amenorrhea
	•	Abdominal pain
On USG:	•	Collection of fluid in pouch of Douglas
	•	Empty gestational sac
Indicate:	•	Ectopic pregnancy

6. **Ans. is c and d, i.e. Blighted ovum; and Late fertilisation** *Ref. Dutta Obs 7/e, p 178*

7. **Ans. is a, b, c and d, i.e. Prior H/O tubal surgery; Prior tubal pregnancy; Prior H/O PID/Chlamydia infection and IUCD predisposes** *Ref. Dutta Obs. 7/e, p 178; Novak 14/e, p 605-608; Williams Obs. 22/e, p 254, 23/e, p 239*
Risk factors for ectopic pregnancy
Highest risk: Previous H/O ectopic pregnancy (Recurrence rate after 1 ectopic pregnancy is 15%)
- Tubal surgeries (for prior tubal pregnancy or recanalization surgery)
- **M/C Risk factor—Pelvic infections/*present salpingitis prior STD***
- **Peritubal adhesions subsequent to salpingitis, appendicitis or endometriosis**
- Salpingitis isthmica nodosa. (it is a noninflammatory condition in which tubal epithelium forms a diverticulum in the myosalpinx – in which fertilized ova can lodge)
- Developmental defects of the tube
- In utero DES exposure.
- Infertility treatments: – IVF
  – Ovulation induction using clomiphene and gonadotropin.
- Current cigarette smoking (> 20 cigarettes per day).
- Contraception use:

According to Williams Obs 24/e
- With any form of contraceptive, the absolute number of ectopic pregnancies is decreased because pregnancy occurs less often. However with some contraceptive failures, the relative number of ectopic pregnancies is increased.
- **Examples include tubal sterilization > Progestasert > Mirena > CUT > progesterone only pill.**
- **Least risk is with OCPs**

8. **Ans. is d, i.e. Tubal inflammatory disease**
Ref. Dutta Obs. 7/e, p 178; Shaw 14/e, p 239; Williams Obs. 22/e, p 254, 23/e, p 239
Read the question carefully, it says ectopic pregnancy is most commonly associated with:
"Pelvic inflammatory disease (PID) increases the risk of ectopic pregnancy by 6–10 fold." —Dutta Obs. 7/e, p 178
"The most common cause (of ectopic pregnancy) is previous salpingitis due to sexually transmitted disease such as gonococcal and chlamydial infection or salpingitis that follows septic abortion and puerperal sepsis."
—Shaw 14/e, p 239

- After one episode of PID – 13%
- After two episode of PID – 35%

 Note: M/C cause of ectopic pregnancy is PID but Maximum risk of ectopic pregnancy is after tubal damage, either due to previous ectopic pregnancy or tubal surgery amongst which previous ectopic is more common.
"Prior tubal damage either; from a previous ectopic pregnancy or from tubal surgery to relieve infertility or for sterilization confers the highest risk for ectopic pregnancy."
—Williams Obs 23/e, p 238

9. **Ans. is a, i.e. Pain in lower abdomen** *Ref. Dutta Obs 7/e, p 180*

10. **Ans. is c, i.e. Pain in abdomen** *Ref. Dutta Obs. 7/e, p 180; Shaw 14/e, p 244*
    - Most common and the most consistent symptom of ectopic pregnancy (undisturbed) is *Abdominal pain.*
    - It is seen in 95–100% cases.
    - Pain is located in the lower abdomen/pelvic region.
    - It can be *unilateral* or *bilateral.*
    - *In case of ruptured ectopic pregnancy: pain is due to hemoperitoneum and* when internal hemorrhage floods the peritoneal cavity and irritates the undersurface of diaphragm and phrenic nerve, the patient also complains of shoulder tip and epigastric pain.
    - In case of unruptured ectopic pain is due to stretching of Fallopian tube.

11. **Ans. is d, i.e. Interstitium** *Ref. Dutta Obs. 7/e, p 179; CODGT 10/e, p 267*
    - M/C site of ectopic pregnancy – Fallopian tubes[Q].
    - In Fallopian Tubes – M/C sites in descending order are:

    > Ampulla > isthmus > infundibulum > interstitium

    - Rarest overall site of ectopic pregnancy is cesarean section scar followed by cervix
    - Average period of survival of ectopic pregnancy is 8 weeks.
    - Ectopic pregnancy survives for longest time in abdomen.

12. **Ans. is a, i.e. Vascular accident** *Ref. Williams Gynae 1/e, p 158*
    - Ectopic pregnancy is the leading cause of early pregnancy related deaths.
    - Most common cause of death in ectopic pregnancy is tubal rupture → severe hemorrhage → death.

    Ectopic pregnancy can have 2 outcomes:
    1. Tubal abortion – M/C outcome. It is most common outcome of ectopic pregnancy in ampulla
    2. Tubal rupture–ectopic pregnancy **of isthmus** are the ones which usually rupture.

13. **Ans. is a, i.e. Decidua vera** *Ref. Shaw 14/e, p 244*
    Decidua vera is the parietal layer of decidua, that lines most of the uterine cavity.

    In ectopic pregnancy
    ⇓
    Under the hormonal influence of
    Progesterone and estrogen
    ⇓
    Uterine endometrium is converted to
    ⇓
    Decidua (similar to Intrauterine pregnancy)
    ⇓
    When the ectopic is interrupted
    Levels of progesterone and estrogen decrease
    ⇓
    Withdrawal of support to uterine endometrium
    ⇓
    Endometrium (decidua) Shed off in the form of
    ⇓
    Decidual cast

    > – The passage of decidual cast is pathognomic of ectopic pregnancy.[Q]
    > – Chorionic villi are characteristically absent in the decidua.[Q]
    > – The presence of chorionic villi in the cast however rules out ectopic pregnancy and denotes uterine pregnancy.

 Also Know:

Arias stella Reaction is characterised by typical adenomatous changes of the endometrial glands seen under the influence of progesterone.

"It is not specific for ectopic pregnancy but rather indicates the blightening conceptus, either intrauterine or extrauterine."
—*Dutta Obs 6/e, p 183*

14. **Ans. is a and b, i.e. hCG; and Transvaginal USG** *Ref. Dutta Obs 7/e, p 182, 183*

15. **Ans. is a and b, i.e. TVS and Serial β-hCG levels** *Ref. Dutta Obs. 7/e, p 182, 183; Leon Speroff 7/e, p 1280-1285; Novak 14/e, p 611; Williams Gynae, p 162-163*

Diagnostic Aids in Ectopic Pregnancy

In hemodynamically stable patient presenting with a triad of amenorrhea, abdominal pain and vaginal bleeding

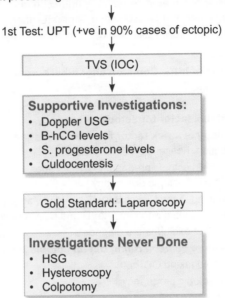

1st Test: UPT (+ve in 90% cases of ectopic)

TVS (IOC)

Supportive Investigations:
- Doppler USG
- B-hCG levels
- S. progesterone levels
- Culdocentesis

Gold Standard: Laparoscopy

Investigations Never Done
- HSG
- Hysteroscopy
- Colpotomy

16. **Ans. is b, i.e. Transvaginal USG** *Ref. Dutta Obs. 7/e, p 182, 183; Williams Gynae 1/e, p 162, 163; Novak 14/e, p 611; Williams Obs. 22/e, p 259, 23/e, p 242, 43*

"As explained earlier transvaginal ultrasound is the best available diagnostic modality for diagnosing ectopic pregnancy. Vaginal sonography yields correct pre-operative diagnosis of ectopic pergnancy in 91% cases. It decreases the need for diagnostic laparoscopy or curettage or both to establish the diagnosis of ectopic pregnancy" —Williams Gynae 1/e, p 163

"Vaginal sonography has become the imaging method of choice." —Williams Obs. 22/e, p 259

17. **Ans. is a, b and d, i.e. Serum progesterone >25 ng/mL exclude ectopic, β-hCG levels should be >1000 mIU/mL for earliest detection by TVS and Methotrexate is used for treatment** *Ref. Dutta Obs. 7/e, p 182*

"Serum progesterone—Level greater than 25 ng/mL is suggestive of viable intrauterine pregnancy whereas level less than 5 ng/mL suggests an ectopic or abnormal intrauterine pregnancy." —Dutta Obs 7/e, p 183

So option a is correct

"The lowest level of serum β-hCG at which a gestational sac is consistently visible using TVS (discriminatory zone) is 1500 IU/L. The corresponding value of serum β-hCG for TAS is 6000 IU/L. When the β-hCG value is greater than 1500 IU/L and there is an empty uterine cavity, ectopic pregnancy is more likely."

So options c is absolutely incorrect, option d can be taken as partial correct\

Methotrexate is the drug of choice for medical management of ectopic pregnancy i.e. option d is correct

"Estimation of β-hCG in ectopic pregnancy: Urine pregnancy test—ELISA is sensitive to 10–50 mIU/ml and are positive in 95% of ectopic pregnancies. A single estimation of β-hCG level either in the serum or in urine confirms pregnancy but cannot determine its location. The suspicious findings are: (1) Lower concentration of β-hCG compared to normal intrauterine pregnancy (2) Doubling time in plasma fails to occur in 2 days."

So option e is incorrect —Dutta Obs 7/e, p 183

18. **Ans. is a, b and d, i.e. Transvaginal USG is the imaging of choice; Associated with decidual reaction; and In ectopic interstitial ring sign seen** *Ref. Dutta Obs. 7/e, p 183; Shaw 14/e, p 247*

- In ectopic pregnancy under the influence of estrogen, progesterone and chorionic gonadotrophin, there is varying amount of enlargement of the uterus with increased vascularity. Decidua develops all the characteristics of intra-uterine pregnancy except that it contains no evidence of chorionic villi. **This is called decidual reaction. (i.e. option b is correct)**
- TVS is the imaging modality of choice in ectopic pregnancy.

- Color Doppler sonography can identify the placental shape (ring of fire pattern) and blood flow pattern outside the urine cavity. It is used to diagnose those cases of ectopic pregnancy which cannot be identified by TVS (**i.e. option c is incorrect**).
- USG findings in ectopic pregnancy include demonstration of an extra uterine gestational sac appearing as fluid containing structure with an echogenic ring, "the tubal ring sign" (**i.e. option d is correct**).
- A single estimation of β-hCG level either in serum or in urine confirms pregnancy but can not determine its location (**i.e. option e is incorrect**). When the β-hCG value is greater than 1500 mIU/ml and there is an empty uterine cavity, ectopic pergnancy is more likely. Failure to double the value by 48 hours along with an empty uterus is very much suggestive.

19. **Ans. is a, c and d, i.e. Rising titre of hCG; Common after tubal surgery; and Seen in patients taking GnRH therapy**
Ref. Dutta Obs. 7/e, p 178-182; Shaw 14/e, p 247 for 'b'; Leon Speroff 7/e, p 1278 for option 'e'
Well friends we have already discussed risk factors for ectopic pregnancy in detail and seen that:

Tubal surgery *(option "c")* **is a risk factor for ectopic pregnancy.**

Assisted reproductive technology is a risk factor for ectopic pregnancy in which ovulation induction is a risk factor. GnRH is used for ovulation induction, hence is a risk factor also.

As far as *option "a"* is concerned – In ectopic pregnancy- β HCG does not double in 48 hours as in intrauterine pregnancy but a slow rise in hCG is suggestive of ectopic pregnancy.

This is the reason why after performing D and C in cases where a non viable and ectopic pregnancy cannot be differentiated, β-HCG is estimated. If β-hCG levels continue to rise after D and C, ectopic pregnancy is confirmed.

Option "b": Negative pregnancy test excludes the diagnosis

"A negative pregnancy test is of no value in ruling out an ectopic pregnancy." —Shaw 14/e, p 247

Option "e": It is common in patients taking OCPs.

OCPs do not increase the risk of ectopic pregnancy.

"Amongst the most common methods of contraception, oral contraceptives and vasectomy are associated with the lowest absolute incidence of ectopic pregnancy." —Leon Speroff 7/e, p 1278

20. **Ans. is a, b, d and e, i.e. MTX; Actinomycin-D; RU-486; and KCl** *Ref. Dutta Obs. 7/e, p 186*

21. **Ans. is d, i.e. Misoprostol** *Ref. Dutta Obs. 7/e, p 186; Shaw 14/e, p 251, Jeffcoates 7/e, p 154*
A number of chemotherapeutic drugs have been used either systemically or directly (surgically administered medical management - SAM under sonographic or laparoscopic guidance) for the medical management of ectopic pregnancy.

Drugs commonly used for medical management:

Mnemonic	Surgically administered medical management	Systemic
Most	Methotrexate[Q] (20%)	Methotrexate (+ leucoverin)
Post	Prostaglandins[Q] (PGF 2α)	
Graduate	Hyperosmolar Glucose[Q]	
Males	Mifepristone (RU486)	
Are	Actinomycin D[Q]	
Very	Vasopressin[Q]	
Knowledgeable	KCl (Potassium Chloride)	

— Jeffcoates 7/e, p 154

22. **Ans. is c, i.e. Presence of fetal heart activity** *Ref. Dutta Obs. 7/e, p 186; Leon Speroff 7/e, p 1287, 1288; Novak 14/e, p 624; Williams Gynae 1/e, p 166*

Methotrexate: It is a folic acid analogue which inhibits dehydrofolate reductase[Q] and prevents synthesis of DNA.[Q]
Candidates for methotrexate *(Williams 24/e, p 384,* **Table 19.2):** —Leon Speroff 7/e, p 1290

Absolute requirements
- Hemodynamic stability[Q]
- No evidence of acute intra-abdominal bleeding[Q]
- Reliable commitment to comply with required follow-up care[Q]
- No contraindications to treatment viz woman should not be breast feeding/renal/hepatic dysfunction.

Preferable requirements
- Absent or mild pain

- Serum beta hCG level less than 5,000 IU/L (best results seen with HCG < 2000 IU/L)[Q]. **It is the single best prognostic indicator of treatment success.**
- Absent embryonic heart activity[Q]
- Ectopic gestational mass less than 4 cm in diameter without cardiac activity and < 3.5 cm with cardiac activity[Q]

Friends, there is no doubt on this issue that presence of cardiac activity is a relative contraindication according to books like *Williams Obs 23/e, Williams Gynae 1/ed and Leon Speroff 7/ed.*

"Fetal cardiac activity – Although this is a relative contraindication to medical therapy, the admention is based on limited evidence."
—*William Obs. 23/e, p 247*

"The presence of embryonic heart activity is not an absolute contraindication for medical management but the likelihood of failure and the risk of tubal rupture are substantially increased (therefore it is a relative contraindication)."
—*Leon Speroff 7/e, p 1287*

As far as **fluid in cul-de-sac is concerned:** Earlier, it was also considered a relative contraindication to medical treatment, but studies have shown that free peritoneal fluid can be seen in almost 40% of women with early unruptured ectopic pregnancy and so it's presence and absence does not accurately predict the success or failure of medical treatment.

Contraindications to methotrexate treatment: (*Williams 24/e, p 384*, **Table 19.2**)
- Breast feeding[Q]
- Immunodeficiency states[Q]
- Alcoholism or evidence of chronic liver disease (elevated transaminases)[Q]
- Renal disease (elevated serum creatinine)[Q]
- Hematological abnormalities (severe anemia, leukopenia or thrombocytopenia)[Q]
- Known sensitivity to methotrexate[Q]
- Active pulmonary disease[Q]
- Peptic ulcer disease.[Q]
- Evidence of tubal rupture

23. **Ans. is b, and e, i.e. Size < 4 cm, β-hcg <1500** *Ref. Dutta Obs. 7/e, p 186; Leon Speroff 7/e, p 1287, 1288; Novak 14/e, p 624; Williams Gynae 1/e, p 166, Williams Obs. 23/e, p 247*

See explanation of previous question.

24. **Ans. is b, i.e. Medical management** *Ref. Dutta Obs. 7/e, p 186; Novak 14/e, p 620-624; Williams Obs. 24/e, p 387, 23/e, 247, 248*

The patient in the question is - Nulliparous.
Her general condition is stable, size of ectopic pregnancy is 2.5–3 cm. β-hCG levels are low, i.e. 1500 mIU/mL. All the criteria required for medical management are being fulfilled, therefore go for medical management.
The question now arises - why not expectant management, i.e. keep her under observation for spontaneous resolution. This is because of 2 reasons-

1. For expectant management, the most important criteria is βhCG should be less than 1000 "falling or decreasing levels of hCG, (hence βhCG = 1500 IU)
2. More importantly - She is a nulliparous woman - We cannot take a chance of rupture of ectopic in her.

If medical and expectant managements are to be compared, medical management is always a better option.

"The potentially grave consequences of tubal rupture, coupled with the established safety of medical and surgical therapy, require that expectant therapy be undertaken only in appropriately selected and counseled women."
—*Williams Obs. 22/e, p 265, 23/e, p 249*

"Minimal side effects of methotrexate make it preferable to avoid the prolonged surveillance (of expectant management) and associated patient anxiety."
—*Williams Gynae 1/e, p 169*

25. **Ans. is a, i.e. Medical management** *Ref. William Obs. 23/e, p 244, Williams Gynae 1/e, p 164*
Now, this is a tricky question.
Patient is presenting with–
- Amenorrhea of 6 weeks

- Absence of gestation at Sac in uterus.
- β-hCG levels 6500 mIU/ml

It is important to note that value of β-hCG is 6500 mIU/ml–much high above the discriminatory zone (1500 mIU/ml) and still gestational sac is not visualised.

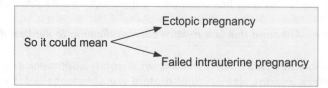

The diagnosis goes more in favour of ectopic pregnancy because values of β-hCG are very high – In case of failed intrauterine pregnancy – at this high level of β-hCG, either the dead fetus or the Yolk Sac etc. would have been visible (if the case was of missed abortion) or patient would have given history of bleeding and passage of product of conception (if it would have been a case of complete abortion → then only the gestational sac can be empty). But here is no such history.

So the chances of ectopic pregnancy are more.

To distinguish between the two – best is do a dilatation and curettage.

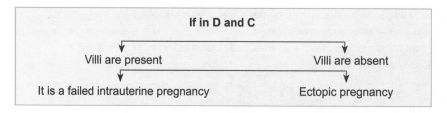

But since, this option is not given so I will directly do medical management in this case.

If in the question βhCG levels would have been < 1500 IU then in that case next step would have been repeat βhCG is 48 hours.

26. **Ans. is a, i.e. Immediate laparotomy**   *Ref. Dutta Obs. 7/e, p 184; Jeffcoates 7/e, p 152*

Patient is being brought to the casualty with - BP = 70/40 mm, P/R = 120/min (i.e. she is in shock).

Her urine pregnancy test is positive i.e. she is a case of ruptured ectopic.

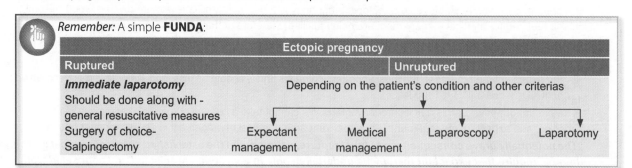

 Also Know:

Even in those cases where there is doubt of ruptured ectopic pregnancy - Laparotomy should be done to "open and see"

"Immediate laparotomy and clamping of the bleeding vessels may be the only means of saving the life of a moribund patient".

—*Jeffcoate 7/e, p 152*

27. **Ans. is b, i.e. Salpingo-oophorectomy**   *Ref. Dutta Obs. 7/e, p 186; Shaw 14/e, p 249*

Surgical management of Ectopic pregnancy (laparoscopy or laparotomy)

Conservative surgery	Radical surgery
Salpingostomy: • It is the procedure of choice when the patient is hemodynamcially stable and wishes to retain her future fertility *Salpingotomy:* • Seldom done nowadays *Segmental resection and anastomosis:* • It is done in case of isthmic pregnancy. *Fimbrial expression of the ectopic pregnancy:* • Risk of recurrence of ectopic pregnancy are high therefore not commonly performed.	*Salpingectomy* **Indications** **Ruptured ectopic** • The patient has completed her family, • The tubes are grossly damaged • Ectopic pregnancy has recurred in a tube already treated conservatively. • Uncontrolled bleeding • Sac size > 5 cm.

Salpingo-oophorectomy i.e. removal of tubes along with the ovaries is not recommended in young patients—

"Presently salpingo-oophorectomy is never recommended unless the ovary itself is grossly diseased or damaged".
                                                                    —*Jeffcoate 7/e, p 154*

"The ipsilateral ovary and its vascular supply is preserved. Oophorectomy is done only if the ovary is damaged beyond salvage or is pathological".   —*Dutta Obs. 6/e, p 188*

28. **Ans. is a, i.e. Salpingectomy and end to end anastomosis**   *Ref. Dutta Obs 7/e, p 185*

In the question the patient is presenting with ruptured ectopic pregnancy therefore surgical management is a must and we have to do laparotomy. (*option "c"* ruled out)

Always remember- In ruptured ectopic, the tube is already damaged so the only surgery which has to be done is Salpingectomy, whether the patient is a young/old or whether she is nulliparous or multiparous. Their is no role of Salpingostomy (i.e. *option "d"* ruled out). As discussed in previous question in case of ectopic pregnancy salpingo oophorectomy is never done (i.e. *option "b"* ruled out).

29. **Ans. is a, b and d, i.e. Methotrexate, Prostaglandins and Laparoscopic salpingostomy.**
                                          Ref. Dutta Obs. 7/e, p 185; Jeffcoates 7/e, p 154 for option b

Repeat

30. **Ans. is b, i.e. Progesterone only pills does not increase risk**
                                          Ref. Williams Gynae 1/e, p 160; Williams Obs. 23/e, p 238, 239

Repeat

31. **Ans. is a, i.e. Ectopic pregnancy**   *Ref. William's Obstetrics 23/e, p 242, 243; Dutta Obs. 7/e, p 181*

A female **with 8 weeks amenorrhea** with **pain left lower abdomen** and on **USG, thick endometrium** with **mass in lateral adnexa** is suggestive of **ectopic pregnancy.**

32. **Ans. is d, i.e. Hysterosalpingography**   *Ref. Dutta Obs. 7/e, p 181*

HSG should never be done in a suspected case of ectopic coz, if by chance it is intrauterine pregnancy, you would be disrupting it.

Investigations not done in ectopic
• HSG • Hysteroscopy • Colpotomy—done to drain pelvic abscess.

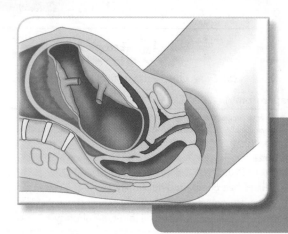

Chapter 17

Trophoblastic Diseases including Choriocarcinoma

 Chapter at a Glance

➢ Hydatidiform Mole
➢ Gestational Trophoblastic Neoplasia

➢ Choriocarcinoma
➢ Placental Site Trophoblastic Tumor

Trophoblastic diseases can be classified as:

Gestational trophoblastic diseases	Gestational trophoblastic neoplasia
• Partial mole • Complete mole	• Invasive mole • Choriocarcinoma • Placental site trophoblastic tumor (PSTT) • Epitheliod trophoblastic tumors (ETT)

Another way of classifying term can be:

Villi seen on HPE	Villi not seen on HPE
• Partial mole • Complete mole • Invasive mole	• Choriocarcinoma • Placentae site trophoblastic tumor (PSTT) • Epitheliod trophoblastic tumor (ETT)

HYDATIDIFORM MOLE

- **Hydatidiform mole is a benign neoplasm of chorion with malignant potential.**
- It is the most common form of gestational trophoblastic disease.
- It is an abnormal condition of the placenta where there are partly degenerative and partly proliferative changes in the young chorionic villi.
- **Grossly:** It is characterised by multiple grape-like vesicles filling and distending the uterus, usually in absence of an intact fetus. The vesicles are filled with interstitial fluid similar to ascitic or edema fluid but is rich in hCG.

- Microscopically it is characterized by :
  - Marked proliferation of the syncytial and cytotrophoblastic epithelium.
  - Thinning of the stromal tissue due to hydropic degeneration (edema of villous stroma).
  - Avascular villi.
  - **Maintenance of villus pattern.**[Q]

Incidence and Risk Factors

- Incidence is maximum in Asia and South America and least in US.
- Maximum incidence is in Philippines (1 in 80). In India it is 1 in 400 pregnancies.
- Risk is more in women too elderly (> *35*) or too younger (< *18 years*) pregnancy.
- Low *socioeconomic status.*
- *History* of molar pregnancy.
- *Diet* deficient in protein, folic acid **and vitamin A.**[Q]
- *Blood group A women* married to group *O men.*

 Note: Maternal age > 35 years and dietary deficiencies are risk factors for complete mole whereas partial mole is linked to the use of oral contraceptive pills and history of irregular menstruation.

Also Know: Familial repetitive hydatidiform mole has been linked to a missense mutation in the **NLRP7 locus on chromosome 19;** in one report, this mutation was present in 60% of patients who had two molar pregnancies.

Concept

Before understanding the differences between partial mole and complete mole, it is important to understand the pathophysiology of H. mole.

In H mole—the problem is marked proliferation of trophoblast. The proliferating trophoblast secrete fluid, which collects in the chorionic villi, distending it to form grape-like vesicles. These undergo hydropic degeneration.

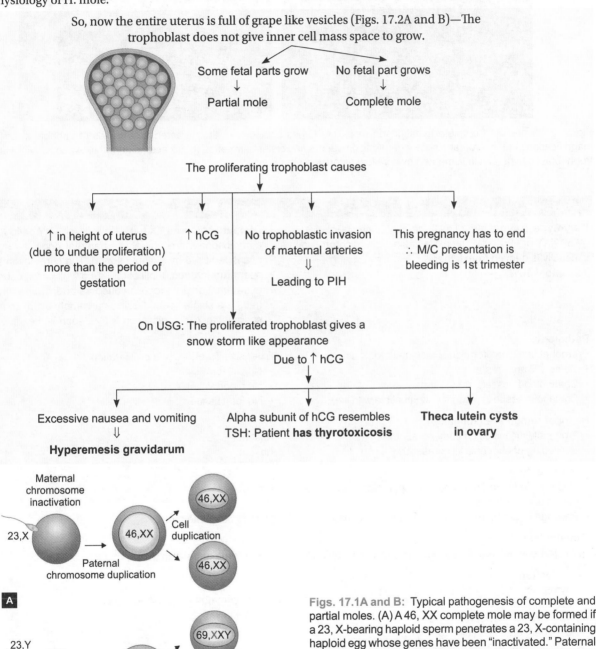

So, now the entire uterus is full of grape like vesicles (Figs. 17.2A and B)—The trophoblast does not give inner cell mass space to grow.

Some fetal parts grow → Partial mole

No fetal part grows → Complete mole

The proliferating trophoblast causes

↑ in height of uterus (due to undue proliferation) more than the period of gestation

↑ hCG

No trophoblastic invasion of maternal arteries ⇓ Leading to PIH

This pregnancy has to end ∴ M/C presentation is bleeding is 1st trimester

On USG: The proliferated trophoblast gives a snow storm like appearance

Due to ↑ hCG

Excessive nausea and vomiting ⇓ **Hyperemesis gravidarum**

Alpha subunit of hCG resembles TSH: Patient **has thyrotoxicosis**

Theca lutein cysts in ovary

Figs. 17.1A and B: Typical pathogenesis of complete and partial moles. (A) A 46, XX complete mole may be formed if a 23, X-bearing haploid sperm penetrates a 23, X-containing haploid egg whose genes have been "inactivated." Paternal chromosomes then duplicate to create a 46, XX diploid complement solely of paternal origin; (B) A partial mole may be formed if two sperm—either 23, X-or 23, Y-bearing—both fertilize (dispermy) a 23, X-containing haploid egg whose genes have not been inactivated. The resulting fertilized egg is triploid with two chromosome sets being donated by the father. This paternal contribution is termed diandry.

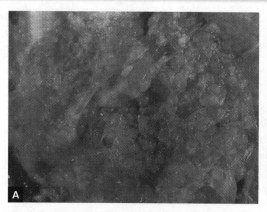 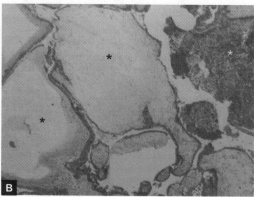

Figs. 17.2A and B: Complete hydatidiform mole. (A) Gross specimen with characteristic vesicles of variable size; (B) Low-magnification photomicrograph shows generalized edema and cistern formation (black asterisks) within avascular villi. Haphazard trophoblastic hyperplasia is marked by a yellow asterisk on the right.

Partial Mole	Complete Mole
Karyotype Triploid 90%: i.e Chromosome number is 69 (69 XXY or 69 XXX). The extra haploid set of chromosomes usually is derived from father. **Tetraploid 10%**	• **Diploid:** (M/C = 46 XX (90%) in 10% – 46 XY or 45 XO). The chromosomes are entirely of paternal origin as an empty ova is fertilised by a single sperm. The chromosomal set of sperm undergoes duplication i.e how all chromosomes are of paternal origin (process **called as androgenesis**). • In 80% a single sperm fertilises an empty ovum i.e monospermic. In 20% fertilisation is by 2 sperms, i.e. dispermic.
Pathology: • Trophoblastic proliferation is less marked. • Some villi are present. • Some blood vessels are present. • Some fetal tissue is present (incompatible with life)	Extensive Trophoblastic proliferation • No villi formation • No blood vessels • No fetal tissue
Histopathological examination: • Trophoblastic inclusion body present. • Scalloping of chorionic villi present.	Absent Absent
Clinical features: • M/C presenting feature is bleeding per vagina following a period of amenorhea. • Passage of grape like vessels—less in partial mole.	Same More in complete mole
Examination: Ht of uterus equal to or less than the period of gestation.	Ht of uterus more than period of gestation.
Complications: • Thyrotoxicosis • Preeclampsia • Hyperemesis gravidarum • Pulmonary emboli leading to ARDS.	All complications are more common in complete mole. Less common in partial mole
IOC: USG • On USG partial mole is often confused with missed abortion (Fig. 17.3).	It gives the typical **'snow storm'** appearance (Fig. 17.4).
Gold standard for diagnosis: • Histopathological examination.	Histopathological examination.

Contd...

Contd...

Partial Mole	Complete Mole
hCG levels: • Raised but not markedly raised.	Markedly raised ($\geq 10^6$ mIU/mL)
Theca lutein cysts Not seen in ovary	B/L cysts, present in ovary.
Persistent Gestational Trophoblastic Disease or (GTN) Chances 3-5%	15-20%
Risk of choriocarcinoma = < 1%	4%

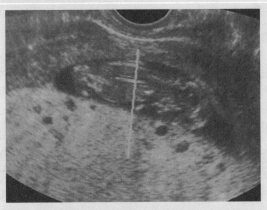

Fig. 17.3: In this image of a partial hydatidiform mole, the fetus is seen above a multicystic placenta.)

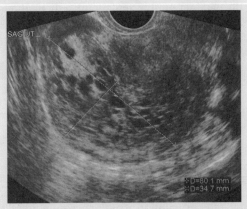

Fig. 17.4: Sagittal view of a uterus with a complete hydatidiform mole. The characteristic "snowstorm" appearance is due to an echogenic uterine mass, marked by calipers, that has numerous anechoic cystic spaces. Notably, a fetus and amnionic sac are absent.

 Note: Whenever hypertension (precelampsia occurs before 24 weeks, it is important to rule out, H mole
- On P/A palpation–uterus has doughy consistency in H. mole.
- Risk of recurrence of H mole in future pregnancy is 1–4%

Management of H Mole

Spontaneous expulsion occurs at around 16 weeks and is rarey delayed beyond 28 weeks.
- **Treatment of choice in H mole**
  - **Suction evacuation (It is the treatment of choice irrespective of uterine size)**
    Suction evacuation is done first. After most of the molar tissue has been removed by aspiration, oxytocin is given. Use of oxytocic drugs prior to completion of the evacuation is not recommended due to risk of tumor embolisation. Once the myometrium has contracted, thorough but gentle curettage with a large curette (10–12 mm)^Q is performed. Intraoperative ultrasonographic examination may help document that the uterine cavity has been emptied. *Ref. Willams 24/e p 401*

Contd...

Contd...

- **Hysterectomy:** It is indicated only in case of:
  - Female has completed her family irrespective of age
  - Age of patient - >40 years (as chances of malignancy are more).
  - Uncontrolled haemorrhage during suction evacuation
  - Perforating mole
  - Placental site trophoblastic tumor
- **Hysterotomy:** Indicated not by ACOG-2012 as it increases chances of persistent trophoblastic disease.

 Remember: After suction evacuation, Anti D is given to all Rh-ve females whether the mole was partial or complete because defective diagnosis of complete vs partial is made cannot be made until HPE is done.
- Theca lutein cysts seen at the time of hysterectomy do not need removal as they spontaneously regress.

Follow-up of Molar Pregnancy

Routine follow-up is mandatory for all cases for at least 6 months following molar pregnancy. Doing hysterectomy does not negate the need for follow-up.

First β-hCG level is obtained 48 hours after evacuation.

- Then monitor serum hCG levels every week till they become normal for three consecutive weeks.
- Once the hCG level falls to a normal level for 3 weeks, test the patient monthly for 6 months; then follow-up is discontinued and pregnancy allowed.
- During the 6 month surveillance period, patient is advised not to become pregnant.

Median time for resolution of partial mole is 7 weeks and for complete mole is 9 weeks.

Prophylactic Chemotherapy

Routine prophylactic chemotherapy is not advocated nowadays after evacuation of molar pregnancy as 80–85% of them regress completely (*Williams 24/e, p 401*).

- **High risk patients needing prophylactic chemotherapy are:**

  - Age of patient ≥ 40 years
  - hCG levels ≥ 10^5 mIU/mL
  - Large uterine size
  - B/L theca lutein cysts (≥ 6 cm).

  Slow decline in β-hCG levels.
  DOC for prophylactic chemotherapy–Methotrexate.

Contraceptive Advice

- Estrogen-progestin contraceptives or depot medroxy-progesterone is usually used to prevent a subsequent pregnancy during the period of surveillance. They should be used after hCG levels come back to normal.
- Contraceptive of choice being combined oral pills.
- **Note:** Earlier the contraceptive of choice was Barrier method.
- Earlier patient was advised not to be pregnant for at least 1 year after H mole evacuation but now it is restricted to 6 months following a negative hCG titre.

Theca Lutein Cyst

- **Theca lutein cysts are seen in H mole due to high circulating levels of hCG (seen in 25–60% cases of complete mole).**

- They vary in size from microscopic to 10 cm size.
- Yellow coloured.
- They are the result of overstimulation of lutein cysts by large amount of hCG.
- Theca lutein cyst are also seen in case of:
  - *Fetal hydrops*
  - *Placental hypertrophy*
  - *Multifetal pregnancy.*

 Remember: Theca lutein cyst regress spontaneously after suction evacuation and do not need any specific management

- It may undergo torsion, infarction and hemorrhage, however oophorectomy is not recommended.
- Patients with theca lutein cysts of > 6 cm, have high risk of developing choriocarcinoma.

GESTATIONAL TROPHOBLASTIC NEOPLASIA

- **Gestational trophoblastic neoplasia** includes invasive mole, choriocarcinoma, placental site trophoblastic tumor and epithelioid trophoblastic tumor.

- Gestational trophoblastic neoplasia almost always develops with or follows some form of pregnancy.

- M/C gestational trophoblastic neoplasia to develop after H mole : Invasive mole
- M/C GTN after full term pregnancy : Choriocarcinoma
- Choriocarcinoma M/C develops after–molar pregnancy.
- High risk choriocarcinoma develops after = full term pregnancy.
- Complete mole has 15–20% chances of developing GTN; partial mole has 3–5% chance of developing GTN.

Risk Factors for Developing GTN

a. Age of female ≥ 40 years
b. β-hCG levels > 10^5 mIU/mL
c. Uterine size larger than gestational age
d. B/L Thecalutein cyst > 6 cm
e. Slow decline in β-hCG levels

Criteria for diagnosis of postmolar gestational tropho-blastic neoplasia.

Criteria for diagnosis of gestational trophoblastic neoplasia (if any 1 of the following is present)

(i) When **4** consecutive hCG values are plateau D_1, D_7, D_{14}, D_{21} (± < 10% of previous value)

(ii) **3** consecutive hCG values are rising (> 10% of previous value) D_1, D_7, D_{14}

(iii) β-hCG level remain above normal even after 6 months of evacuation (Normal value of hCG < 5).

(iv) Histopathological report confirms GTN

Clinical Features Suggesting GTN

- Patients present with continuous bleeding per vagina even after evacuation.
- Uterine subinvolution.
- Invasive mole can lead to myometrium perforation and intraperitoneal haemorrhage and shock.
- Persistence of theca lutein cysts (normally they should disappear in 2 to 4 months after evacuation).
- Metastasis- In choriocarcinoma M/C site of metastasis is lungs.

CHORIOCARCINOMA

- Most malignant tumor of uterus.[Q]
- Among all the cases of choriocarcinoma
  - 50% develop following a hydatidiform mole
  - 25% develop following an abortion
  - 20% develop following a full-term pregnancy and
  - 5% develop following an ectopic pregnancy.
- M/C mode of spread is *hematogenous*
- **Most common sites of metastases in choriocarcinoma are:**
  Lung (80%) > Vagina (30%) > Pelvis (20%) > Liver (10%) and Brain (10%)
- **Symptoms:** Mostly presents as irregular bleeding or uterine hemorrhage following an abortion, a molar pregnancy or a normal delivery.

Metastasis

Lung Metastasis

- It is seen in 80% cases
- Patient presents with respiratory symptoms like dyspnoea, hemoptysis, chest pain, etc.
- On X-ray it may produce the four patterns
  - M/C appearance: Discrete rounded densities or **canon ball appearance**[Q]
  - 2nd M/C appearance: An alveolar **snow storm pattern**[Q] (Remember snowstorm appearance on

USG– means H mole; snowstorm appearance on chest X-ray– means choriocarcinoma)

- Pleural effusion[Q]
  - An embolic pattern caused by pulmonary arterial occlusion.[Q]

Vaginal Metastasis

- It is seen in 30% cases
- Metastasis occurs in suburethra[Q] or in fornices[Q]
- Metastasis appears as purple hemorrhagic projections which are highly vascular and bleed on touch (pathognomic of choriocarcinoma).

Tumor Markers

- Tumor marker for choriocarcinoma is β-hCG.
- Tumor marker for placental site trophoblastic tumor is hPL.

On histopathology

- **Choriocarcinoma:** It is composed of cells of early cytotrophoblast and syncytiotrophoblast. However there are **No villi**. It has ability to metastasic.
- **Invasive mole:** It is characterized by excessive tissue invasion by trophoblast and whole villi.

Staging

FIGO anatomic staging for GTT

Stage I	The lesion is confined to the uterus.
Stage II	The lesion spreads outside the uterus but within pelvis
Stage III	The lesion metastasizes to the lungs.
Stage IV	The lesion metastasizes to sites such as brain, liver or gastrointestinal tract.

WHO prognostic scoring system for gestational trophoblastic disease   *Williams 24/e, p 402*

Score				
Parameter	**0**	**1**	**2**	**3**
• Age (years)	< 40	> 40	–	–
• Antecedent pregnancy	Mole	Abortion	Term	–
• Interval in months from index pregnancy and chemotherapy started within	< 4 months	4–6 months	7–12 months	> 12 months
• Pretreatment β-hCG level	< 10^3	10^3–10^4	10^4–10^5	> 10^5

Contd...

Contd...

Score				
• ABO group (female x male)		O or A	A or AB	
• Largest tumor (cm)	< 3	3–4 cm	> 5	
• Site of metastases	Lungs	Spleen, kidney	Gastro-intestinal	Brain, Liver
• Number of metastases	–	1–4	4–8	> 8
• Prior chemotherapy	–	–	Single	> 2
Total score:				

Patients having a score of 6 or less are considered as having low risk or good prognosis and patient having a score of 7 or more are considered as having high risk or bad prognosis.

In general a patient belonging to good prognosis or low risk group (score 0–6) means that they can be treated by a single agent chemotherapy which is usually successful in them, whereas a patient belonging to poor prognosis/high risk group (score > 7) respond badly to chemotherapy and require prolonged hospitalization with multiple courses of chemotherapy.

Management
Chemotherapy

- Chemotherapy is the treatment of choice for chorio-carcinoma
- **Methotrexate is the drug of choice.**
- In low risk patients-single drug, i.e. methotrexate is given.
- If the patient has **jaundice then actinomycin D** should be given.

Single Drug Regimen in Low-risk Cases			
Methotrexate	1–1.5 mg/kg	IM/IV	Days 1, 3, 5 and 7
Folinic acid	0.1–0.15 mg/kg	IM	Days 2, 4, 6 and 8

The course is to be repeated at interval of 7 days till hCG levels return to normal followed by 3 more cycles of Chemotherapy after the value normalises.

- In high risk patients, i.e. if score ≥ 7 and or Multidrug Chemotherapy is given. Multidrug therapy used most commonly is **Bagshaw regime** consisting of:

  E = etoposide
  M = methotrexate
  A = actinomycin D   **BAGSHAW REGIME**
  C = cyclophosphamide
  O = vincristine (oncovin)

Radiation

Patients with **brain metastases** require whole-brain radiation therapy (3000 cGy over 10 days). Intrathecal high dose methotrexate may be administered to prevent hemorrhage and for tumor shrinkage.

Liver metastasis: Interventional radiology (hepatic artery ligation or embolization) or whole liver radiation (2000 cGy over 10 days) along with chemotherapy may be effective. Hepatic metastasis has a poor prognosis.

Prognosis

The cure rate is almost 100% in low risk and about 70% in high risk metastatic groups.

Follow-up is mandatory for all patients. In low risk patients: period of surveillance is 12 months and in high risk patients, follow up is done for 24 months. Serum hCG is measured weekly until it is negative for three consecutive weeks. Thereafter it is measured monthly for 6 months and then 6 monthly.

 Note: When a female becomes pregnant after H mole or GTN treatment, a β hCG level should be done 6 weeks postpartum in that pregnancy also.

Recurrences

For non-metastatic GTN : 2–3%;
Good prognosis' metastatic disease : 3–5%
Poor prognosis' disease : 21%.
Recurrence following 12 months of normal hCG level is <1%.

PLACENTAL SITE TROPHOBLASTIC TUMOR (PSTT)

Characteristics of PSTT

- The tumor arises from the intermediate trophoblasts of the placental bed and is composed mainly of cytotrophoblastic cells.
- These tumors have been associated with modestly elevated serum β-hCG levels but they produce variant forms of β-hCG. In these tumors identification of a high proportion of free β-hCG (>30%) is considered diagnostic.
- hPL (human placental lactogen) is also a tumor marker for these tumors.
- Patient presents with vaginal bleeding.
- Local invasion into the myometrium and lymphatics occurs.

- PSTT is not responsive to chemotherapy. Hysterectomy is the preferred treatment.

Choriocarcinoma	PSTT
M/C	Rare
• M/C after molar pregnancy	• M/C after full term pregnancy
• Malignant	• Benign
• Tumor marker hCG	• Tumor marker - hPL > placental alkaline phosphatase
• Chemosensitive	• Chemoresistant
• TOC - chemotherapy	• TOC - Hysterectomy

Important Single Liners

 Important One Liners

Invasive mole	Choriocarcinoma
Histological: Villi are present Has monomorphic cells	Villi are absent Has dimorphic cells

- Choriocarcinoma develops M/C after H mole
- High risk choriocarcinoma develops M/C after full term pregnancy
- M/C Gestational trophoblastic neoplasia to develop after full term pregnancy: Choriocarcinoma
- Placental site trophoblastic tumor develops M/C after: Full term pregnancy.

New Pattern Questions

N1. Hydatidiform mole is principally a disease of:
   a. Amnion
   b. Chorion
   c. Uterus
   d. Decidua

N2. Molar pregnancy is diagnosed in:
   a. I trimester
   b. II trimester
   c. III trimester
   d. All of the above

N3. Hydatidiform mole is characterized histologically by:
   a. Hyaline membrane degeneration
   b. Hydropic degeneration of the villous stroma
   c. Nonproliferation of cytotrophoblast
   d. Nonproliferation of syncytiotrophoblast

N4. True regarding partial mole:
   a. It has more chances of malignancy
   b. Cellular atypia seen
   c. Trophoblastic proliferation with no villi
   d. Triploid or tetraploid

N5. The endocrinological condition associated with H mole:
   a. Hypothyroidism
   b. Hyperthyroidism
   c. Diabetes
   d. Hyperprolactinemia

N6. A 36-year-old G1P0 woman presents for her first prenatal visit late in her first trimester of pregnancy; she complains of persistent vaginal bleeding, nausea, and pelvic pain. Physical examination is notable for a gravid uterus larger than expected for gestational age. Fetal heart tones are absent.

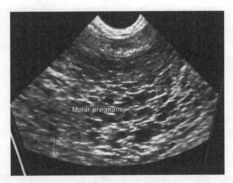

Molar pregnancy

Which of the following is most likely to be true?
   a. β-hCG levels will be higher than normal
   b. β-hCG levels will be lower than normal
   c. Uterus will be of normal levels
   d. TSH levels will be increased

N7. A 30-year-old female complains of vaginal bleeding for 2 weeks. A diagnosis of H mole is made by ultrasound scanning. Suction evacuation is performed and the diagnosis of a complete H mole is confirmed by HPE of curettings.

What is the most appropriate next step in the management?
   a. Give 1/m methotrexate daily for 5 days
   b. Perform hysterectomy
   c. Perform serum β-hCG levels weekly till the test becomes negative
   d. Perform curettage after 2 weeks

N8. Prophylactic chemotherapy in hydatidiform mole should preferably be given:
a. Prior to evacuation as a routine
b. Following evacuation as a routine
c. Selected cases following evacuation
d. As a routine 6 weeks postevacuation

N9. The following are related to prophylactic chemotherapy in molar pregnancy:
a. It may be given in 'at risk' patients
b. Multiple agents are preferred
c. Malignant sequelae becomes nil
d. Follow-up is not required

N10. The advantages of hysterectomy in molar pregnancy are:
a. Chance of choriocarcinoma becomes nil
b. Follow up is not required
c. Enlarged ovaries can be removed during operation
d. Chance of pulmonary embolisation is minimal

N11. Risk of recurrence of H mole in future pregnancy is:
a. 1–4%   b. 4–8%
c. 8–10%   d. 10–12%

N12. A female with H/O trophoblastic has _____% chances of developing trophoblastic disease in next pregnancy:
a. 2%   b. 5%
c. 8–12%   d. 15–20%

N13. Percentage of complete moles progressing to persistent GTN:
a. 1–4%   b. 4–8%
c. 8–12%   d. 15–20%

N14. Choriocarcinoma is differentiated from invasive mole (chorioadenoma destruens) by:
a. Presence of high titre of urinary chorionic gonadotrophin
b. Presence of cannon ball shadow in the lungs
c. Absence of villi structure on histological examination of the lesion
d. All of the above

N15. The criteria for diagnosing GTN are all *except*:
a. Persistently increasing β-hCG for 3 weeks
b. Plateau levels of β-hCG for 4 weeks
c. Theca lutein cyst $\geq$ 6 cm
d. Histological criteria for choriocarcinoma

N16. Most important prognostic marker for Gestational Trophoblastic neoplasia:
a. Number of metastasis
b. Site of metastasis
c. β-hCG levels
d. Stage of Tumor

N17. A woman complains of excessive vomiting and mild vaginal bleeding for two weeks at a POA of 12 weeks. The fundal height corresponds of 16 weeks. The cervical os is closed. Ultrasound scan demonstrates a snowstorm appearance in part of the uterus together with a foetus. The crown-rump length corresponds to 10 weeks. The fetal heart beat is absent. What is the best management option?
a. Carry out medical termination with vaginal misoprostol
b. Carry out medical termination with an oxytocin infusion
c. Perform suction evacuation
d. Perform a total abdominal hysterectomy

N18. A 30-year-old woman with one child underwent suction evacuation of a complete hydatidiform mole, which was confirmed by histology. Her serum beta hCG level is 20000 IU/L 8 weeks after evacuation.

What is the most appropriate management?
a. Commence treatment with combination chemotherapy
b. Commence treatment with intramuscular methotrexate
c. Perform a hysterectomy
d. Perform repeat suction evacuation

N19. A 40-year-old woman complains of irregular bleeding for 7 months after delivery of her fourth baby. Curettage is performed and histology reveals a choriocarcinoma. Her serum beta hCG level is 2 × 10⁵ IU/L.

What is the most appropriate next step in the management?
a. Commence treatment with intramuscular methotrexate
b. Commence treatment with multi-agent combination chemotherapy
c. Perform a hysterectomy
d. Repeat serum hCG after 4 weeks

Previous Year Questions

1. **True about H mole:** [PGI Dec 03]
   a. Complete mole seen in human only
   b. Trophoblastic proliferation
   c. Hydropic degeneration
   d. Villus pattern absent

2. **True about complete hydatidiform mole is:**
   a. Chromosome pattern is XX [PGI Dec 01]
   b. It is of maternal origin
   c. Enlarged ovarian cyst occurs
   d. It is common in developed countries
   e. Associated with preeclampsia

3. **Complete H mole is:** [PGI June 03]
   a. Triploid   b. Diploid
   c. Increased β-hCG
   d. 2% cases may convert to carcinoma
   e. Chance of malignant conversion less than partial mole

4. **False about partial mole:** [AI 10]
   a. Caused by triploidy
   b. Can be diagnosed very early by USG
   c. Can present as missed abortion
   d. Rarely causes persistent GTD

5. **Which of the following is true about partial mole?**
   a. Karyotype is 69 XXY or 69 XXX [PGI May 2015]
   b. High malignant potential
   c. β-hCG level is < 50,000
   d. Thecan lutein cysts common
   e. Immunostaining (p57^{KIP2}) positive

6. **The highest incidence of gestational trophoblastic disease is in:** [AI 05]
   a. Australia   b. Asia
   c. North America   d. Western Europe

7. **Follow-up in a patient of H mole is done by:**
   a. Serum Beta-hCG monitoring [AIIMS Feb 97]
   b. Serum CEA level estimation
   c. Serum amylase level
   d. Serum α-fetoprotein estimation

8. **Snow storm appearance on USG is seen in:**
   [AI 01; PGI Dec 03, PGI Nov 2010]
   a. Hydatidiform mole   b. Ectopic pregnancy
   c. Anencephaly   d. None of the above

9. **True about H mole:** [PGI June 08]
   a. Always associated with raised uterine size for gestational age
   b. Raised hCG
   c. Hysterectomy in selected cases
   d. Chemotherapy is the treatment of choice
   e. Thyrotoxicosis rare

10. **Prophylactic chemotherapy is indicated after evacuation of H mole in all, except:** [AI 00]
    a. Initial level of urine hCG is 40000 IU after 6 week of evacuation
    b. Increase in hCG titre 24000 IU after 10 week of evacuation
    c. Metastasis   d. Nulliparous lady

11. **Indication of methotrexate in molar pregnancy:**
    a. Fetal heart activity present [PGI June 09]
    b. Theca lutein cysts size < 4 cm
    c. β-hCG 4000 MIU/ml
    d. Evidence of metastasis
    e. Age > 50 years

12. **Treatment of the lutein cyst in hydatidiform mole is:**
    a. Ovarian cystectomy [AI 99]
    b. Ovariectomy
    c. Suction evacuation
    d. Ovariotomy

13. **A 40 years old P4+2 female has been diagnosed to have H mole. The treatment would be:** [AI 96]
    a. Radiotherapy   b. Chemotherapy
    c. Total hysterectomy d. Radiochemotherapy

14. **A case of gestational trophoblastic neoplasia belongs to high risk group, if disease develops after:** [AI 03]
    a. Hydatidiform mole
    b. Full term pregnancy
    c. Spontaneous abortion
    d. Ectopic pregnancy

15. **In a case of vesicular mole all of following are high risk factors for the development of choriocarcinoma except:** [AIIMS Nov 02]
    a. Serum hCG levels > 100000 mIU/mL
    b. Uterus size larger than 16 week
    c. Features of thyrotoxicosis
    d. Presence of bilateral theca lutein cysts of ovary

16. **Prognosis of gestational trophoblastic disease depends on all, except:** [AI 00]
    a. Number of living children
    b. Blood group
    c. Age of patient
    d. Previous hCG titre

17. **Bad prognostic markers of choriocarcinoma treatment are:** [PGI June 04]
    a. Liver metastasis   b. Lung metastasis
    c. Previous H mole   d. High hCG titre
    e. Chemotherapy started 12 months after pregnancy

18. A case of gestational trophoblastic neoplasia is detected to have lung metastasis. She should be staged as: [AIIMS May 04]
   a. Stage – I   b. Stage – II
   c. Stage – III   d. Stage – IV

19. Most common site for metastasis in choriocarcinoma is: [AI 07; 98]
   a. Lungs   b. Brain
   c. Liver   d. Spine

20. Choriocarcinoma commonly metastasize to:
   a. Brain   b. Lungs   [PGI June 06]
   c. Vagina   d. Ovary
   e. Cervix

21. A 25-year-old female was diagnosed to have chorio-carcinoma, management is: [PGI June 06]
   a. Chemotherapy
   b. Radiotherapy

   c. Hysterectomy
   d. Hysterectomy and then radiotherapy

22. A 35 years old female with choriocarcinoma treatment of choice is: [AIIMS June 00]
   a. Dilatation and evacuation
   b. Radiotherapy
   c. Hysterectomy   d. Chemotherapy

23. The ideal treatment for metastatic choriocarcinoma in the lungs in a young woman is: [PGI June 99]
   a. Chemotherapy   b. Surgery with radiation
   c. Surgery   d. Wait and watch

24. True about complete mole: [PGI Nov 2010]
   a. Presence of foetal parts and cardiac activity
   b. Normal uterine size
   c. Beta-hCG doubling time is 7–10 days
   d. Preeclampsia at < 24 weeks
   e. Per vaginal bleeding is commonest presentation

Answers with Explanations to New Pattern Questions

N1. **Ans. is b, i.e. Chorion**   *Ref. Dutta 7/e, p 190*

Now don't tell me you want me to explain this—
H mole is a benign neoplasm of chorion with malignant potential

N2. **Ans. is a, i.e. 1st trimester**   *Ref. COGDT 10/e, p 888*

In H mole:
"Abnormal uterine bleeding usually during the first trimester is the most common presenting symptom, occuring in more than 90% of patients with molar pregnancies. Three fourths of these patient present prior to the end of the first trimester."

N3. **Ans. is b, i.e. Hydropic degeneration of the villous stroma**   *Ref. Dutta Obs. 7/e, p 191*

Pathological features of H mole	Naked eye appearance
• Uterus is filled with multiple clusters of grape like cysts.[Q] • No trace of embryo/amniotic sac.	• Marked proliferation of synctio and cyto trophoblast • Marked thinning of stromal tissue due to hydropic degeneration. • Absence of blood vessels • Villous pattern is maintained.[Q]

N4. **Ans. is d, i.e. Triploid or tetraploid**

Partial mole has less chances of malignancy.
In molar pregnancy villi are present and villi pattern is mantained but there are no blood vessels in the villi.
Partial mole is generally (90% cases) triploid but in 10% cases it can be tetraploid or mosaic also.

N5. **Ans. is b, i.e. Hyperthyroidism**

In H mole-hCG levels are high.
The α subunit of hCG is similar to TSH, hence molar pregnancy is associated with hyperthyroidism.

N6. **Ans. is a, i.e β-hCG levels will be higher than normal**

In the given question patient is presenting late in her first trimester of pregnancy with complains of persistent vaginal bleeding, nausea, and pelvic pain. Physical examination is notable for a gravid uterus larger than expected for gestational age. Fetal heart tones are absent.

D/D of height of uterus larger than the period of gestation:

- Wrong dates
- Twin pregnancy
- Molar pregnancy
- Concealed variety of Abruptio placenta
- Polyhydramnios.

- **Twin pregnancy** can be ruled out because it does not explain persistent vaginal bleeding and moreover in twin/multiple pregnancy fetal heart tones are not absent...2 or more FHS are heard depending on the number of fetuses.
- Concealed variety of APH does not occur in late first trimester. APH by definition means any bleeding which occurs after 28 weeks of pregnancy and uptil the birth of the child and hence it can be ruled out although absent fetal tones and Fundal height more than the gestational age are seen.
- Polyhydramnios again can be ruled out since bleeding cannot be explained by it ...so we are left with molar pregnancy which explainds all the findings.

Always remember: Patient complaining of extremes of nausea, vomiting + bleeding in first trimester + size of uterus more than the period of amenorrhea–think of Molar pregnancy.

The USG shown in the plate is typical snow storm appearance. Hence diagnosis is confirmed.

N7. Ans. is c, i.e. Perform serum β-hCG levels weekly till the test becomes negative

Best T/t for H mole is suction evacuation. No need for:
1. Hysterectomy after it to give methotrexate if patient is not high risk.
2. Best is to follow-up with weekly hCG.

N8. Ans. is c, i.e. Selected cases following evacuation

N9. Ans. is a, i.e. It may be given in 'at risk' patients *Ref. Dutta Obs. 7/e, p 196*

Prophylactic chemotherapy in H mole
- Is given only to high risk patients (as discussed earlier) and to not all patients following suction evacuation because these drugs are toxic and can increase the risk of premature ovarian failure and menopause.
- Monotherapy with methotrexate is prefered (not multiple agents).
- The use of prophylactic chemotherapy reduces the chances of developing choriocarcinoma but doest not make it nil.

N10. Ans. is d, i.e. Chances of pulmonary embolisation is minimal *Ref. Dutta Obs. 7/e, p 195*

- Hysterectomy when performed in molar pregnancy significantly decreases the chances of developing choriocarcinoma (by 5 fold times) but does not make it nil and hence follow up is required (so both options a and b are incorrect)

This is supported by following lines from Dutta-

"It should be remembered that following hysterectomy, persistent GTD is observed in 3–5% cases. As such, it does not eliminate the necessity of follow up. The enlarged ovaries (theca lutein cysts) found during operation should be left undisturbed as they will regress following removal of mole. But, if complication arises, like torsion, rupture or infarction, they should be removed." —*Dutta 7/e, p 195*

Thus from above lines it is also clear that ovaries even if they are enlarged should not be removed during hysterectomy for H mole.

As far as pulmonary embolisation in concerned -acute pulmonary insufficiency due to pulmonary embolization of trophoblastic cells, is a complication seen with suction evacuation and not hysterectomy.

N11. Ans. is a, i.e. 1–4% *Ref. Dutta Obs. 7/e, p 194*

N12. Ans. is a, i.e. 2% *Ref. Williams 24/e, p 404, Dutta Obs. 8/e, p 226*

Friends: Remember both the values–specifically–risk of recurrence of trophoblastic disease in future pregnancies is 2% range is 1–4%

N13. Ans. is d, i.e. 15–20% *Ref. Dutta Obs. 7/e, p 194*

N14. Ans. is c, i.e. Absence of villi structure on histological examination of the lesion *Ref. Dutta Gynae 6/e, p 362*

Choriocarcinoma is characterised by absence of villi

High titre of urinary chorionic gonadotrophin and cannon ball shadow in the X-ray lungs are found in both choriocarcinoma and invasive mole.

N15. Ans. is c, i.e Theca lutein cysts ≥ 6 cm *Ref. Williams 24/e, p 402*
Criteria for diagnosis of postmolar gestational trophoblastic neoplasia.

Criteria for diagnosis of gestational trophoblastic neoplasia
1. When **4** consecutive hCG values are plateau D_1, D_7, D_{14}, D_{21} (± 10% of previous value)
2. **3** consecutive hCG values are rising (> 10% of previous value) D_1, D_7, D_{14}
3. β-hCG level remain above normal even after 6 months of evacuation
4. Histological criteria for choriocarcinoma

N16. Ans. is c, i.e. β-hCG levels

Most important prognostic marker for Gestational Trophoblastic neoplasia is β-hCG level.

N17. Ans. is c, i.e. Perform suction evacuation

Suction evacuation is the method of choice, for evacuation of a partial molar pregnancy.

N18. Ans. is b, i.e. Commence treatment with intramuscular methotrexate

Since this women has a high serum hCG level even after 8 weeks of suction evacuation, she is at risk of developing gestational trophoblastic neoplasia. Therefore, the most appropriate management is to commence chemotherapy. Now we have to decide single agent or multi-agent. Since this patient is under 40 years of age and the antecedent pregnancy is a molar pregnancy which was evacuated 8 weeks age, she has a low risk according to the FIGO scoring system. Therefore, she can be commenced on single agent chemotherapy, with methotrexate and leucovorin rescue. Methotrexate 50 mg intramuscularly (or 1 mg/kg) is given every other day for 4 days, with leucovorin 15 mg (or 0.1 mg/kg) 24–30 hours after each dose of methotrexate. The course is repeated after 6 rest days till the serum hCG becomes negative. Treatment is continued for 6 consecutive weeks after the hCG becomes negative. Combination chemotherapy is not necessary as the score is less than 6. Chemotherapy is the most important mode of treatment for choriocarcinoma.

N19. Ans. is b, i.e. Commence treatment with multi-agent combination chemotherapy

This woman is at high risk as she has a prognostic score of 7:
- Antecedent normal pregnancy—2
- Age more than 40 years—1
- Antecedent pregnancy 7 months ago—2
- Serum hCG level 2×10^5—2

Therefore, she needs treatment with multi-agent comnination chemotherapy with EMA-CO.

Answers with Explanations to Previous Year Questions

1. Ans. is b and c, i.e. Trophoblastic proliferation; and Hydropic degeneration *Ref. Dutta Obs. 7/e, p 191*
H mole:

Microscopically: It is characterised by :
- Marked proliferation of the syncytial and cytotrophoblastic epithelium.
- Thinning of the stromal tissue due to hydropic degeneration (edema of villous stroma).
- Avascular villi.
- Maintenance of villus pattern.
Absence of villus pattern is characteristic of choriocarcinoma and not H mole:

2. Ans. is a, c and e, i.e. Chromosome pattern is XX; Enlarged ovarian cyst occurs; and Associated with preeclampsia
Ref. Shaw 14/e, p 227; Dutta Obs. 7/e, p 191 - 193; Novak 14/e, p 1582 - 1584
- The incidence of H mole is maximum in oriental and south east countries (maximum incidence is in Philippines: 1 in 80 pregnancies), i.e., it is more common in developing countries (*option 'd'* ruled out).
- H mole can be categorized as either complete or partial mole on the basis of Gross morphology, histopathology and karyotype.

Complete H mole - shows no evidence of fetal tissue at all.
- Complete hydatiform moles exhibit characteristic swelling and trophoblastic hyperplasia.
- *Most common karyotype is 46XX (10% may have a 46XY karyotype).*
- The molar chromosomes are **entirely of paternal origin,** although mitochondrial DNA is of maternal origin.
- The complete moles arises from an ovum that has been fertilized by a haploid sperm, which then duplicates its own chromosomes called as *Androgenesis.* The ovum nucleus may be either absent or inactivated.

Theca lutein cysts in ovary and preeclampsia (Early onset) are seen in H mole

3. **Ans. is b, c, and d, i.e. Diploid; Increased β-hCG; and 2% cases may convert to carcinoma**

Ref. Dutta Obs. 7/e, p 191, 198; William 24/e, p 397

Differences between complete and partial mole

Features	Complete mole	Partial mole
Karyotype	46XX, (90%) or 46XY (10%) i.e. it is diploid	69 XXX or 69XXY i.e. it is triploid
Pathology		
• Diagnosis	Molar gestation	Missed abortion
• Embryo/fetus	Absent	Present
• Hydropic degeneration of villi	Pronounced and diffuse	Variable and focal
• Trophoblastic hyperplasia	Diffuse	Focal
• Fetal RBC	Absent	Present
• Scalloping of chorionic villi	Absent	Present
• Trophoblastic stromal inclusion	Absent	Present
Clinical features		
• Uterine size	Large for date	Small for date
• Theca lutein cysts	Common (25–30%)	Rare
• Medical complications	Common	Rare
• Initial β-hCG	Very high (>100,000 mlu/ml)	Slight increase (<100,000 mlu/ml)
• Persistent GTD	15–20%	3–5%
• Malignant potential	High (4%)	Low (1%)
• p57k1p2	Negative	Positive

4. **Ans. is b, i.e. Can be diagnosed very early by USG or d. Rarely causes persistent GTD**

Ref. Novac 14/e p 1587, 1588 Willams 23/e p 260, 263

5. **Ans. is a, c and e, i.e. Karyotype is 69 XXY or 69 XXX, β-hCG level is <50,000 and Immunostaining (p57[K1P2]) positive**

Ref. Novac 14/e p 1587, 1588 Willams 23/e p 260, 263

A. Patients with partial mole do not have dramatic clinical features of complete molar pregnancy. In general these patients have signs and symptoms of incomplete or missed abortion and on USG after they are confused with incomplete abortion.

B. Partial mole can cause GTN in 3–5% cases

C. Thus both, option d and b are incorrect, you can choose between the two.

> Presence of focal cystic spaces in the placental tissue and increase in the transverse diameter of the gestational sac has a positive predictive value of 90% for the diagnosis of partial mole.

 Extra Edge

The most significant recent development in the pathological analysis of H mole is the use of **p57[k1p2]** immunostaining to make a definitive diagnosis of androgenetic complete H mole as opposed to an hydropic abortion or a partial mole.

p57[k1p2] is a paternally imprinted gene, which is maternally expressed. The absence of maternal genes in androgenetic complete mole means that the gene cannot be expressed in a complete mole cytotrophoblast.

Hence **p57[k1p2]** staining is negative in complete mole in contrast to partial moles (where it is positive) hydropic abortion and normal placenta. This technique is well validated, easy and inexpensive to perform.

6. **Ans. is b, i.e. Asia** *Ref. Shaw's 14/e, p 226; Devita 7/e, p 1360*

"Incidence of gestational trophoblastic disease varies widely with figures as high as 1 in 120 in some areas of Asia and South America, compared to 1 in 1200 in the united states." —*Devita 7/e, p 1360*

7. **Ans. is a, i.e. Serum Beta hCG monitoring** *Ref. Dutta Obs. 7/e, p 195, 196; Novak 14/e, p 1590*

The chances of persistent trophoblastic disease and choriocarcinoma are high after evacuation of H mole therefore regular follow-up is mandatory.

"After molar evacuation, patients should be monitored with weekly determinations of β-subunit hCG levels until these levels are normal for 3 consecutive weeks, followed by monthly determinations until the levels are nomrmal for 6 consecutive months. The average time to achieve the first normal hCG level after evacuation is about 9 weeks. At the completion of follow-up, pregnancy may be undertaken. After a patient achieves a nondetectable hCG level, the risk of developing tumour relapse is very low and may approach zero." —*Novak 14/e, p 1590*

8. **Ans. is a, i.e. Hydatidiform mole** *Ref. Dutta Obs. 7/e, p 193; Shaw 14/e, p 230*

Ultrasound shows *"Snow storm"* appearance in the uterus: Diagnosis is H mole.

Chest X-ray shows snow storm appearance in lungs–Diagnosis choriocarcinoma.

9. **Ans. is b, c and e, i.e. Raised hCG; Hysterectomy in selected cases; and Thyrotoxicosis rare**
Ref. Dutta Obs. 7/e, p 193 for a and b, 192 for e, 195 for c and 196 for d; COGDT 10/e, p 889

Lets have a look at each option separately-

Option 'a': Always asociated with raised uterine size for gestational age.

This statement is incorrect as:

"The size of the uterus is more than that expected for the period of amenorrhea in 70%, corresponds with the period of amenorrhea in 20% and smaller than the period of amenorrhea in 10%." —*Dutta Obs. 7/e, p 193*

Option 'b': Raised hCG -

H mole is characterised by raised levels of hCG (levels > 10^5 MIU/ml) —*Dutta Obs. 7/e, p 193*

Option 'c': Hysterectomy in selected cases:

> **Management of H mole:**
> - TOC in H mole – Suction evacuation followed by gentle but thorough currettage.
> - Hysterectomy – It is indicated only in case of :
>   – Female has completed her family
> - Hysterotomy – Indicated in cases complicated by haemorrhage.

So, *option 'c'* i.e. hysterectomy is done in selected cases is correct whereas *option 'd'* i.e. chemotherapy is the TOC is incorrect.

Option 'e':

As far as thyrotoxicosis is concerned:

It is seen in only 2% cases of H mole. *It is rare (so, option 'e' is correct).*

"Clinically apparent thyrotoxicosis is unusual." —*William 23/e, p 260*

10. **Ans. is d, i.e. Nulliparous lady** *Ref. Dutta Obs. 7/e, p 196*

11. **Ans. is d and e, i.e. Evidence of metastasis and Age > 50 years**
Ref. Dutta Obs. 7/e, p 200, 196; COGDT 10/e, p 890; Shaw 14/e, p 231

See the text for explanation.

12. **Ans. is c, i.e. Suction evacuation** *Ref. COGDT 10/e, p 889*

Management of theca lutein cysts:

Theca lutein cysts are seen in H. mole due to high circulating levels of hCG.

As such they donot need any separate treatment. Suction evacuation of H mole results in diminishing hCG titre, which leads to spontaneous regression of theca lutein cysts.

"Because theca lutein cysts regress following suction evacuation, expectant management is preferred".
—*William 24/e, p 398*

13. **Ans. is c, i.e. Total hysterectomy** *Ref. Dutta Obs. 7/e, p 195; COGDT 10/e, p 889, William Obs. 23/e, p 261, 24/e, p 401*

"If no further pregnancies are desired, hysterectomy may be preferred to suction curettage. It is a logical procedure in women aged 40 or older because atleast a third of these women will go on to develop gestational trophoblastic neoplasia." —*William Obs 23/e, p 261*

Remember: Hysterectomy only decreases the chances of malignancy in cases of hydatidiform mole and does not eliminate the necessity of follow-up.

14. Ans. is b, i.e. Full term pregnancy *Ref. COGDT 10/e, p 892, 893; Novak 14/e, p 1593, 1594*

Well friends, the question is specifically asking about high risk gestational trophoblastic disease.

FIGO in 2000 devised a staging system for categorisation of gestational trophoblastic neoplasia into good prognostic (low risk) and bad prognostic (high risk) disease.

Good prognosis (Low Risk)	Poor prognosis (High Risk)
• Short duration (< 4 months)	• Long duration (> 4 months)
• Serum β-hCG < 40,000 mIU/ml	• Serum β-hCG > 40,000 mIU/ml
• Metastasis limited to lung and vagina	• Metastasis to brain or liver
• No significant prior chemotherapy	• Unsuccessful prior chemotherapy
No preceeding term pregnancy	*Gestational trophoblastic neoplasia following term pregnancy.*

Also if we have a look at the WHO prognostic scoring system: GTN following a term prgnancy comes under high risk.

 Remember:
* **High risk GTN** occurs after term pregnancy.
* GTN occurs most commonly after H mole.

15. Ans. is c, i.e. Features of thyrotoxicosis *Ref. William 24/e, p 401*

Risk factors for malignant change
• Complete mole (15–20% case)
• Patient's age ≥ 40
• Serum hCG ≥ 100,000 mIU/mL
• Uterine size ≥ **large for gestational age**
• Theca lutein cysts: large (> 6 cm diameter)
• Slow decline in β-hCG

Sonographic appearance of myometrial nodules or hypervascularity postevacuation is also a predictor of subsequent neoplasia.

From the above list it is clear that *option "a"* is correct.

Coming on to *option "d"* i.e. Presence of bilateral theca lutein cyst *Williams Obs. 23/e, p 259*

"Montz and colleagues (1988) reported that gestational trophoblastic neoplasia was more likely in women with theca-lutein cysts, especially if bilateral." (i.e. option "d" is correct).

So that leaves us with 2 options 'b' and 'c'. As far as uterine size larger than 16 weeks is concerned-

According to Dutta p 197 *– Size of uterus > 20 weeks is considered as a risk factor and not > 16 weeks, but according to other books excessive uterine enlargement is one of the risk factor- no specific size hasbeen mentioned.*

As far as thyrotoxicosis is concerned I did not get any literature regarding, it being one of the risk factors.

So, *option 'c'* is the answer of choice.

16. Ans. is a, i.e. Number of living children

17. Ans. is a, d and e, i.e. Liver metastasis; High hCG titre; and Chemotherapy started 12 months after pregnancy
Ref. COGDT 10/e, p 892, 893; Novak 14/e, p 1593, 1594

Again we are referring to the prognostic factors of GTN, i.e. scoring system.

18. Ans. is c, i.e. Stage III *Ref. COGDT 10/e, p 893*

Staging of Gestational trophoblastic disease:

Stage-I   Disease confined to uterus.

Stage-II   Disease extending outside of the uterus but limited to the genital structures (adnexa, vagina, broad ligaments).

Stage-III Disease extending to the lungs, with or without known genital tract involvement.

Stage-IV   Disease at other metastatic sites viz brain, liver, kidney or gastrointestinal tract.

19. **Ans. is a, i.e. Lungs**

20. **Ans. is b and c, i.e. Lungs and vagina**   *Ref. Shaw 14/e, p 233; Novak 14/e, p 1591, 1592; Williams Obs. 23/e, p 262*

Most common sites of metastases in choriocarcinoma are:

Lung (80%) > Vagina (30%) > Pelvis (20%) > Liver (10%) and Brain (10%)

21. **Ans. is a, i.e. Chemotherapy**

22. **Ans. is d, i.e. Chemotherapy**

23. **Ans. is a, i.e. Chemotherapy**   *Ref. Shaw 14/e, p 235; COGDT 10/e, p 892, 893*

"Unlike other malignant lesion, the treatment of choriocarcinoma is mainly chemotherapy, both for local and distant metastasis."   —*Shaw 14/e, p 235*

24. **Ans. is b, d and e, i.e. Normal uterine size; Preeclampsia at < 24 weeks and Per vaginal bleeding is the commonest presentation**   *Ref. Dutta Obs 7/e, p 193 for b, c and e Novak 14/e, p 1582, 1587*

Complete Mole – Is that variety of H mole in which no evidence of fetal tissue is seen (i.e. option 'a' is incorrect)

M/C presenting symptom in H mole is vaginal bleeding.

"Vaginal bleeding is the most-common symptom causing patient to seek treatment for complete mole pregnancy." Novak 14/e, p 1585 (i.e. option 'e' is correct)

Early onset preeclampsia – if features of precampsia are present in < 24 weeks, complete mole should always be suspected (i.e. option 'd' is correct)

• On P/A examination in molar pregnancy –size of the uterus in more than the expected period of amenorrhea in 70%, it corresponds with the period of amenorrhea in 20% and is smaller than the period of amenorrhea in 10% cases. Thus normal size uterus may be seen in case of H mole.

"Excessive uterine enlargement relative to gestational age is one of the classic signs signs of complete mole, although it is present in only about one half of the patients.   —*Novak 14/e, p 1585.*

The clinical presentation of a complete mole has changed considerably over the past few decades.

"More than half of the patients diagnosed in the 1960's and 1970's had anemia and uterine size in excess of that predicted for gestational age. Complete moles, however, present infrequently today with these traditional signs and symptoms."   —*Willimams Gynae 1/e, p757*

So from above lines, it is clear that uterine size more than the period of amenorrhea, was earlier a more common and typical presentation of complete H. moles. These days more common picture is uterine size corresponding of the period of amenorrhea. Thus, I am including option 'b' in correct answers.

As far as hCG levels are concerned:

In case of molar pregnancy, levels of β-hCG are higher than that which are expected for that gestational age (due to trophoblastic proliferation), but the doubling time is same, i.e. 1.4-2 days.

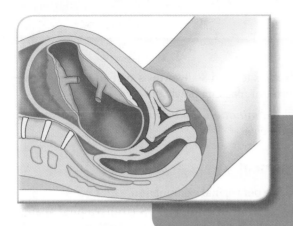

Antepartum Hemorrhage (APH) and DIC

Chapter at a Glance

- Antepartum Hemorrhage
- Placenta Previa
- Abruptio Placenta
- DIC
- Vasa Previa

ANTEPARTUM HEMORRHAGE

Antepartum hemorrhage is defined as bleeding from the genital tract after fetal viability and before delivery. In the past viability was considered to be from 28 weeks onwards, but due to the improvements in neonatal survival, this has been changed. The cut off point for fetal viability is now considered as 22 weeks by the WHO and 24 weeks by IAP.

Causes

Maternal causes
- Placenta previa
- Abruptio placenta
- Local causes like polyp, cancer cervix, varicose veins and local trauma
- Circumvallate placenta

Fetal causes
- Vasa previa
- Unclassified or indeterminate

PLACENTA PREVIA

Definition: Placenta previa is defined as a placenta located partly or completely in the lower uterine segment. The bleeding is called inevitable or unavoidable hemorrhage as dilatation of the internal os inevitably results in hemorrhage.

Note: For localization of placenta ultrasound should be done in third trimester.

Incidence

(1 in 300 pregnancies)

Classification

Older Classification

Table 18.1: Browne's classification for placenta previa

Type 1	Lateral	Placenta dipping into the lower segment but not reaching upto the os.
Type 2	Marginal	Placental edge reaches the internal os
Type 3	Incomplete central	Placenta covers the internal os when closed, but not when fully dilated
Type 4	Central	Placenta covers the internal os even when fully dilated

- Type 1 and 2 are called **minor degrees** and type 3 and 4 called **major degrees** of placenta previa.
- Type 1 and 2 can be anterior or posterior.
- Type 2 posterior placenta is also called the **'dangerous type'** as it is more likely to be compressed producing cord compression. This can cause fetal asphyxia and even death.

- In both the posterior varieties of placenta previa, **Stallworthy sign** is positive
- Stallworthy sign is decreased in fetal heart rate when fetal head is pushed down into the pelvis

Recent Classification

- In a recent Fetal Imaging Workshop sponsored by the National Institutes of Health (Dashe, 2013), the following classification was recommended.
- **Placenta previa:** The internal os is covered partially or completely by placenta. In the past, these were further classified as either total or partial previa.
- **Low-lying placenta:** Implantation in the lower uterine segment is such that the placental edge does not reach the internal os and lies within 2 cm wide perimeter around the os. A previously used term, marginal previa, described a placenta that was at the edge of the internal os but did not overlie it.

Risk Factors

- Previous history of placenta previa-most important risk factor-Recurrence rate = 5%
- Multiparity and increased maternal age
- H/O any previous uterine surgery—like cesarean section (risk increases as number of cesarean increases), myomectomy
- Previous uterine curettage
- Increased placental size as in multifetal pregnancy
- Succenturiate lobe
- Smoking
- Increased maternal serum alpha fetoprotein.

Clinical Features

Symptoms

- In placenta previa hemorrhage/bleeding is
  - Painless
  - Recurrent
  - Causeless

  It is preceded by a small bleeding called as warning hemorrhage.

Signs

- Pallor, if present, will be proportionate to the amount of bleeding.
- Size of the uterus corresponds to the period of amenorrhea.
- Uterus is soft and nontender.
- Malpresentations are common and if it is a cephalic presentation, the head is usually floating.
- Fetal heart sounds will usually be heard (c.f. abruption). Slowing of the fetal heart rate on pressing the head down into the pelvis and prompt recovery on release of the

pressure is termed Stallworthy's sign and is suggestive of posterior placenta previa.[Q]

Vaginal Examination should not be done in Suspected Placenta Previa.

Management

- Never do per vaginal examination
- **Investigation of choice: TVS** (transvaginal scan... surprised don't be- because in placenta previa P/V examination is contraindicated since our finger has to inserted inside the internal os inorder to know the exact location of the placenta, which in turn can lead to torrential hemorrhage but in Transvaginal ultrasound, the probe is never taken beyond the internal os, it is kept in the cervical canal and obviously there are no chance of disturbing the placenta). Read for yourself what Dutt's has to say.
- **"Transvaginal (TVS): Transducer is inserted within the vagina without touching the cervix. The probe is very close to the target area and higher frequencies could be used to get a superior resolution. It is safe, obviates the discomfort of full bladder and is more accurate (virtually 100%) than TAS".**
- **Double set up examination** (i.e Per vaginal examination in the operation theatre with all arrangements of cesarean section) can be done in placenta previa.

Table 18.2: Management options in a Case of Placenta Previa

Expectant management (Called as Macaffee regime) Goal is to carry pregnancy till term without putting mothers life at risk with an aim to achieve fetal lung maturity.	Active management To terminate pregnancy immediately irrespective of gestational age.
Indications	**Indications**
• No active bleeding present • Hemodynamically stable • Gestation age <37 weeks • CTG-should be reactive • No fetal anomaly incompatible with life on USG, e.g. Polydactyly	• If active bleeding is present • Hemodynamically unstable/shock • Gestational age >37 weeks and patient in labor • Fetal distress present/FHS absent • USG shows fetal anomaly incompatible with life like anencephaly or dead fetus

Expectant Management

Called as MaCafee and Johnson regime:

Steps:

1. Hospitalize the patient
2. Arrange for blood
3. If patient is Rh-negative, give her Anti D
4. Give injection corticosteroids to hasten lung maturity of fetus
5. If any contractions are present - given short term tocolytic: Nifedipine

Expectant management should be carried uptil 37 weeks, but if anytime during expectant management patient rebleeds terminate the pregnancy immediately

In active management

Pregnancy is immediately terminated.

Mode of delivery

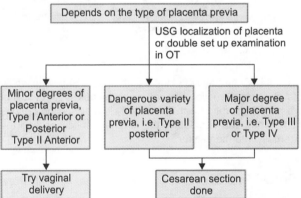

Indications of cesarean section in placenta previa

1. Major degrees of placenta previa
2. Dangerous variety of placenta previa
3. Severe bleeding irrespective of type of placenta previa
4. Fetal age < 32 weeks
5. Fetal distress.

 Note: Practically all patients of placenta previa undergo cesarean delivery *(Williams OBS 25/e pg 777)*

Complication: A major problem with placenta previa, is that after delivery of fetus, it leads to PPH as bleeding occurs from placenta site. This should be managed like PPH & if all conservative measures fail–hysterectomy is done.

 Remember: **Placenta previa and placenta accreta are M/C causes of peripartum hysterectomy**.
- In all patients of placenta previa with previous cesarean section possibility of placenta accreta should be kept in mind

---

 Also Know:

M/C fetal complication of placenta previa is: Low birth weight baby.

ABRUPTIO PLACENTA

 Abruptio placenta is defined as hemorrhage occurring in pregnancy due to the separation of a normally situated placenta. It is also called *accidental Hemorrhage or premature separation of placenta.*

Abruptio placenta is premature separation of normally situated placenta[Q] resulting in hemorrhage.

Risk Factors (Fig. 18.1)

My –My- I pity all of you out there as you have to memorise so many lists (not only in gynae, obs but in other subjects as well). Even I have gone through the same phase. Friends I had devised a simple method to learn these lists. For some lists, I used to draw diagrams and then at the time of exam that diagram was reproduced in my mind. Try it out for yourself. e.g.

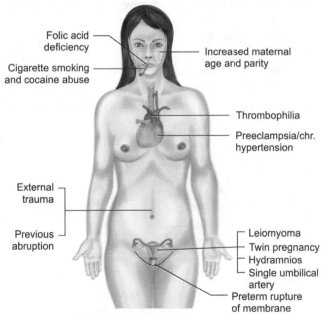

Fig. 18.1: Risk factors for abruptio placentae

Besides these there is a hereditary risk of acquiring abruptio also.

Recurrence rate of abruptio = 12%

Incidence = 1 in 200 pregnancies

Classification

> **Page Classification of abruptio placenta:**
>
> **Grade 0:** Retrospective diagnosis made on the basis of retroplacental clot.
>
> **Grade 1:** Bleeding PV + Pain in abdomen + Fetal heart sounds are normal
>
> **Grade 2:** Bleeding PV + Pain in abdomen + Fetal distress
>
> **Grade 3:** Bleeding PV + Pain in abdomen + Fetal death ± shock ± coagulopathy

Table 18.3: Sher's classification of abruptio: Clinical grading

Grade	Retroplacental clot	Fetal heart rate
I	150 ml or less	Present. It is diagnosed after delivery
II	150–500 ml	Abnormal in 92% cases
III	As above IIIA without coagulopathy IIIB with coagulopathy	Absent fetal heart

Types of Abruptio Placenta

i. **Concealed variety:** In this variety placenta separates in such a manner that, blood collects behind the placenta and does not come outside (Fig. 18.2).

The collected blood may intravasate in between the uterine muscle bundle causing muscular dissociation in the middle and outer muscle layer.

This gives uterus a patchy or diffuse port wine color. Such a uterus is called as **COUVELAIRE uterus** (Uteroplacental apoplexy).

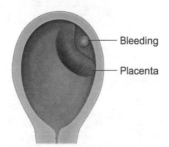

Fig. 18.2: Concealed variety of abruptio

> - **Couvelaire uterus** is seen in concealed variety of APH (Fig. 18.5)
> - Couvelaire uterus is not an indication for doing hysterectomy.

ii. **Revealed variety:** In this variety, placenta separates in such a manner that, bleeding comes out. (Fig. 18.3)

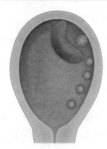

Fig. 18.3: Revealed variety of abruptio

iii.**Mixed variety:** M/C type.

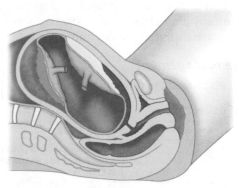

Fig. 18.4: Schematic of placental abruption. Shown to left is a total placental abruption with concealed hemorrhage. To the right is a partial abruption with blood and clots dissecting between membranes and decidua to the internal cervical os and then externally into the vagina.

Clinical Features

Symptoms

- Severe and constant abdominal pain (more in the concealed and less in the revealed types).
- Bleeding is present in the revealed and mixed types, but may be absent in the concealed type.
- Bleeding can be preceded by trauma
- There is no warning Hemorrhage
- Bleeding is not recurrent

Bleeding of Abruptio is different from placenta previa:

1. It is associated with pain in abdomen
2. Non-recurrent in same pregnancy
3. No warning hemorrhage
4. It is never without any reason

Signs

- General condition of the patients is usually out of proportion to the extent of bleeding
- Hypertension may be present (if there is associated pre-eclampsia)

- The uterus will be larger than expected for the period of amenorrhoea (in concealed variety)
- Uterus may be tense, tender and even rigid (woody hard)
- Difficulty in palpating the underlying fetal parts easily
- Fetal distress or absent fetal heart sounds

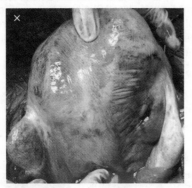

Fig. 18.5: Couvelaire uterus

Management

Principle of management
- Once Abruptio is diagnosed you have to manage it actively irrespective of the gestational age.
- Never wait and watch in abruptio
- Never give tocolytics

- **In case of abruption:** The abruptio delivery interval is important.
- Do not prolong this interval as complications like DIC/ Renal failure (acute cortical necrosis) can occur.
- Pritchard rule for management of abruption is keep hematocrit at least 30% and maintain urine output- 30 mL/hour

Mode of Delivery:

Cesarean Delivery
- The compromised fetus is usually best served by cesarean delivery, and the speed of response is an important factor in perinatal outcomes.
- A major hazard to cesarean delivery is imposed by clinically significant consumptive coagulopathy. Preparations include plans for blood and component replacement and assessment of coagulation— especially fibrinogen levels.

Vaginal Delivery
- If the fetus has died, then vaginal delivery is usually preferred. Hemostasis at the placental implantation site depends primarily on myometrial contraction and not blood coagulability. Thus, after vaginal delivery, uterotonic agents and uterine massage are used to stimulate myometrial contractions.

- In some instances, vaginal delivery may not be preferable, even with a dead fetus. One e.g. is brisk hemorrhage that cannot be successfully managed by vigorous blood replacement.
- In some women with extensive placental abruption, labor tends to be rapid because the uterus is usually persistently hypertonic.
- Evidence supporting this theory is lacking, membrane rupture may hasten delivery.
- No data indicate that oxytocin augments thromboplastin escape into the maternal circulation to worsen coagulopathy
- In light of hypertonus associated with abruption, misoprostol may by a less favored induction agent due to its association with uterine tachysystole

M/C fetal complication of abruptio is prematurity.

DIC

- Release of thromboplastin in placental abruption leads to DIC in abruptio placenta.
- **M/C cause of DIC in obstetrics is abruption.**

Other obstetrical causes of DIC are:
- IUD
- Sepsis
- Amniotic fluid embolism
- Severe PIH/HELLP syndrome/eclampsia

Normal Values of DIC Profile
- Fibrinogen 150–600 mg/dL
- PT-11-16 sec
- PTT 22–37 sec
- Platelet – 1.5 to 3.5 lac D dimer/mm³
- D dimer – <0.5 mg/l
- Fibrin degradation products (FD) <10 µg/dL

In case of DIC: All clotting factors are consumed so levels of fibrinogen decrease; PT and PTT and FDP, D dimer all increase.

- **Management of DIC**
- **Fresh frozen plasma-1** unit of FFP raises – 5–10 mg/dL of fibrinogen.

Note: A fibrinogen level less than 100 mg/dL or sufficiently prolonged PT/PTT in a woman with surgical bleeding is an indication for FFP in doses of 10–15 mL/kg

- **Cryoprecipitate** – also increase fibrinogen but volume of blood lost is not replenished
- **Platelet** should be given may if count < 50,000/ ml. Single unit transfusion raises platelet by 5000-10,000/ml.
- If female is Rh-negative give 300 µg of anti D after platelet transfusion
- **Recombinant factor VII** can be used

- Epsilon aminocaproic acid (EACA) and Tranexemic acid are now abandoned for managing DIC by ACOG (2017).
- Recombinant factor VIIa has been used to help control severe obstetrics haemorrhage from other causes. However to comment on its use in DIC, is too early (ACOG 2017)

- Wherever DIC occurs–First DIC should be managed and then vaginal delivery should be done
- Caesarean is not done in DIC.

Table 18.4: Distinguishing features of placenta previa and Abruptio Placentae

	Placenta previa	Abruptio placenta
Symptoms		
Bleeding and pain	**Sudden, painless and recurrent Always revealed Bright red in colour**	Severe abdominal pain Revealed or concealed
Signs		
Pallor	Proportionate to loss	May be out of proportion
Fundal height	Corresponds to gestation	May be more
Palpation	Soft and relaxed uterus	Tense, tender and rigid
Fetal parts	Easily palpated	Difficult to palpate
Head	High and floating head	Head usually fixed
Malpresentations	Common (M/C being transverse lie)	Uncommon
Fetal heart sounds	Usually normal	Distress or absent
Pre-eclampsia	Normal incidence	Increased
Coagulopathy	Rare	Frequent
IUGR	Not seen	May be seen as it is associated with PIH

VASA PREVIA

- It occurs due to velamentous insertion of the cord (i.e. cord inserted onto the fetal membranes) (Fig. 18.6)

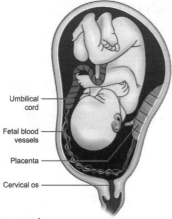
Umbilical cord
Fetal blood vessels
Placenta
Cervical os

Fig. 18.6: Vasa previa

- **Risk factors:**
  - Bilobate or succenturiate placenta
  - Placenta previa.
- Here as the cord is inserted velamentously, so when membranes rupture, cord also gets ruptured and bleeding occurs.
- Blood loss which occurs is fetal in origin and so there is increased fetal mortality – (75 to 90%), maternal mortality is not increased.
- Can be diagnosed antenatally by Doppler study
- When bleeding occurs: Sinusoidal fetal heart rate pattern is seen
- Diagnosis can be made at the time of bleeding by-**Singers alkali denaturation test/Apt test**
- **Management:** Emergency Cesarean section.

Apt test/Singers alkali denaturation test

Principle: Fetal blood has fetal hemoglobin (HbF) and maternal blood has adult hemoglobin (HbA). HbF is resistant to acid and alkali denaturation (not HbA). **Procedure:** Whatever blood is coming out of mothers vagina is taken in a test tube. Reagent NaOH/KOH is added to it.

- If color of blood remains Red/Pink, it means it is not denatured i.e. HbF is present which means fetal blood. So the condition is Vasa previa.

  Thus negative apt test means HbF i.e. Vasa previa

- If color of blood turns yellow brown—it means it is maternal blood (HbA, as it is denatured easily), i.e. condition is placenta previa

  Thus **positive apt test** means HbA, i.e. placenta previa

New Pattern Questions

N1. All of the following are true of placenta previa except:
  a. Postpartum hemorrhage infrequent
  b. First trimester bleeding is not uncommon
  c. Premature labor is common
  d. Higher incidence in women with lower segment cesarean section
  e. Malposition and malpresentation are common

N2. A 29-year-old G3P2 woman at 34 weeks' gestation is involved in a serious car accident in which she lost consciousness briefly. In the emergency department she is awake and alert and complains of a severe headache and intense abdominal and pelvic pain. Her blood pressure is 150/90 mm Hg, heart rate is 120/min, temperature is 37.4°C (99.3°F), and respiratory rate is 22/min. Fetal heart rate is 155/min. Physical examination reveals several minor bruises on her abdomen and limbs, and vaginal inspection reveals blood in the vault. Strong, frequent uterine contractions are palpable. Which of the following is most likely a complication of this pts present condition:
  a. DIC   b. IUGR
  c. Subarachnoid hemorrhage
  d. Vasa previa

N3. A 27-year-old G2P1 woman at 34 weeks' gestation presents to the emergency department following a motor vehicle collision. In the trauma bay her heart rate is 130/min and blood pressure is 150/90 mm Hg. She is alert and oriented to person, place, and time. She complains of severe abdominal pain that began immediately after the collision. Physical examination reveals bruising over her abdomen, along with a hypertonic uterus and dark vaginal bleeding. A sonogram reveals a placental abruption, and the fetal heart tracing reveals some decelerations. Emergency laboratory tests reveal an International Normalized Ratio of 2.5, with elevated fibrin degradation products. Which of the following is the most appropriate first step in management?
  a. Administer a tocolytic
  b. Administer a corticosteroid
  c. Administer fresh frozen plasma
  d. Deliver the fetus immediately by LSCS
  e. Observe closely

N4. Which of the following is true about vasa previa except?
  a. Incidence is 1 : 1500
  b. Mortality rate of 20% with undiagnosed case
  c. Associated with low lying placenta
  d. Cesarean section is indicated

N5. A 29-year-old G3 P2 female at 32 weeks of gestation presents to the emergency dept. with a small amount of vaginal bleeding. She doesn't have any pain.
  a. On examination   b. Her PR: 66/min
  c. B/P: 100/70 mm of Hg
  d. RR: 10/min

FHS tracings show fetal distress and shows late decelerations. What is the best course of action?
  a. Emergent cesarean section
  b. Fetal umbilical blood transfusion
  c. Expectant management
  d. Induction of labor with prost aglandins

N6. IOC to detect abnormally located placenta:
  a. TVS   b. TAS
  c. Doppler   d. MRI

N7. At 28 weeks on USG-(TVS) a G2P1 female was detected as having major placenta previa. A confirmatory scan should be performed:
 a. At 32 weeks   b. At 34 weeks
 c. At 36 weeks   d. At onset of labor

N8. M/C cause of APH is:
 a. Placenta previa   b. Abruptio placenta
 c. Vasa previa   d. Placenta accreta

N9. Rani (G2P1) presents to labor room in labor at 34 weeks of pregnancy with dilatation of cervix 3 cm and minimal uterine contractions. On ARM, fresh bleeding is seen with late decelerations. LSCS was done but fetus could not be saved. No abruptio or placenta previa was noted. Most likely diagnosis is:
 a. Concealed abruptio   b. Battledore placenta
 c. Vasa previa   d. Placenta accreta

N10. Amniotic fluid embolism cause:
 a. Shock   b. DIC
 c. Bleeding tendency   d. All of the above

N11. An elderly multiparous woman with intrauterine foetal death was admitted with strong labor pains.

The patient suddenly goes in shock with cyanosis respiratory disturbances and pulmonary oedema. The most likely clinical diagnosis is:
 a. Rupture of uterus
 b. Congestive heart failure
 c. Amniotic fluid embolism
 d. Concealed accidental hemorrhage

N12. The following tests are related to blood coagulation disorders in obstetrics *except*:
 a. Thrombocytopenia is a feature of fibrinolytic process and not of DIC
 b. In DIC, RBC will be 'helmet' shaped or fragmented but in fibrinolytic process, the cell morphology is normal
 c. Weiner clot observation test gives a rough estimate of total blood fibrinogen level
 d. Thrombocytopenia can be diagnosed from the peripheral smear **N7.** At 28 weeks on USG-(TVS) a G2P1 female was detected as having major placenta previa. A confirmatory scan should be performed:
 a. At 32 weeks   b. At 34 weeks
 c. At 36 weeks   d. At onset of labor

Previous Year Questions

1. All are causes of Antepartum hemorrhage (APH) *except*: [AI 04]
 a. Placenta previa   b. Abruptio placenta
 c. Circumvallate placenta
 d. Battledore placenta

2. Placenta previa mouth is associated with all of the following *except*: [AI 98]
 a. Large placenta   b. Previous C. S. scar
 c. Primigravida   d. Previous placenta previa

3. Placenta previa is characterized by all *except*:
 a. Painless bleeding   b. Causeless bleeding
 c. Recurrent bleeding   d. Presents after first trimester

4. Placenta previa true are: [PGI Nov 07]
 a. Incidence increases by two fold after LSCS
 b. More common in primipara
 c. Most common in developed countries
 d. 1 per 1000 pregnancies
 e. Most common cause of PPH

5. A positive "Stallworthy's sign" is suggestive of which of the following conditions: [AI 06]
 a. Twin pregnancy   b. Breech presentation
 c. Vesicular mole   d. Low lying placenta
 e. Pregnancy induced hypertension

6. Regimen followed in expectant management of placenta previa: [AIIMS Nov 2010]
 a. Liley's method   b. Crede's method
 c. McAfee and Johnson regime
 d. Brandt-Andrews Method

7. Expectant management of placenta previa includes all *except*: [AI 2011]
 a. Anti-D   b. Cervical encirclage
 c. Blood transfusion   d. Steroids

8. A primigravida at 37 week of gestation reported to labor room with central placenta previa with heavy bleeding per vaginum. The fetal heart rate was normal at the time of examination. The best management option for her is: [AI 03]
 a. Expectant management
 b. Cesarean section
 c. Induction and vaginal delivery
 d. Induction and forceps delivery

9. A lady with 37 weeks pregnancy, presented with bleeding per vagina. Investigation shows severe degree of placenta previa. The treatment is: [AI 01]
 a. Immediate C S   b. Blood transfusion
 c. Conservative   d. Medical induction of labor

10. Conservative management is contraindicated in a case of placenta previa under the following situations, *except*: [AIIMS May 04]
    a. Evidence of fetal distress
    b. Fetal malformations
    c. Mother in a hemodynamically stable condition
    d. Women in labor

11. In placenta previa conservative treatment is not done in case of: [PGI June 06]
    a. Active labor   b. Anencephaly
    c. Dead baby   d. Severe placenta previa
    e. Premature fetus

12. Termination of pregnancy in placenta previa is indicated in: [PGI Dec 03]
    a. Active bleeding   b. Active labor
    c. Gestational age > 34 weeks with live fetus
    d. Fetal malformation   e. Unstable lie

13. All the following are indications for termination of pregnancy in APH patient *except*: [AI 01]
    a. 37 weeks   b. IUD
    c. Transverse lie   d. Continuous bleeding

14. A 21-year-old primigravida is admitted at 39 weeks gestation with painless antepartum hemorrhage. On examination uterus is soft non-tender and head engaged. The management for her would be:
    a. Blood transfusion and sedatives [AIIMS May 03]
    b. A speculum examination
    c. Pelvic examination in OT
    d. Tocolysis and sedatives

15. A 34-year-old G1P0 woman at 29 weeks' gestation presents to the emergency department complaining of 2 hours of vaginal bleeding. The bleeding recently stopped, but she was diagnosed earlier with placenta previa by ultrasound. She denies any abdominal pain, cramping, or contractions associated with the bleeding. Her temperature is 36.8°C (98.2°F), blood pressure is 118/72 mm Hg, pulse is 75/min, and respiratory rate is 13/min. She reports she is Rh-positive, her hemoglobin is 11.1 g/dL, and coagulation tests, fibrinogen, and D-dimer levels are all normal. On examination her gravid abdomen is nontender. Fetal heart monitoring is reassuring, with a heart rate of 155/min, variable accelerations, and no decelerations. Two large-bore peripheral intravenous lines are inserted and two units of blood are typed and crossed. What is the most appropriate next step in management:
    a. Admit to antenatal unit for bed rest and betamethasone
    b. Admit to antenatal unit for bed rest and blood transfusion.
    c. Induction of labor
    d. Perform emergency cesarean section.

16. Savita is 32 weeks pregnant presents in causality and diagnosed as a case of APH. Vitals are unstable with BP 80/60 which of the following is next step in M/n:

    a. Careful observation [AIIMS Nov 00]
    b. Blood transfusion
    c. Medical induction of labor
    d. Immediate cesarean section

17. A 32 weeks pregnant women presents with mild uterine contraction and on examination her vitals are stable and placenta previa type III is present. Best m/n is:
    a. Bed rest + Dexamethasone [AIIMS June 00]
    b. Bed rest + Nifedipine and Dexamethasone
    c. Bed rest + Sedation
    d. Immediate caesarean section

18. A lady with 38 weeks pregnancy and painless vaginal bleeding comes to casualty. On examination head is engaged and uterus is non tender and relaxed. The next line of treatment is: [AIIMS Nov. 99]
    a. Perspeculum examination
    b. Conservative management
    c. Termination of pregnancy
    d. Ultrasonography

19. Abruptio placentae occurs in all *except*:
    [PGI June 97; 89]
    a. Smokers   b. Alcoholics
    c. PET   d. Folic acid deficiency

20. Commonly used grading for abruption placenta:
    a. Page   b. Johnson [AIIMS Nov 2010]
    c. McAfee   d. Apt

21. True about placental abruption: [PGI May 2015]
    a. Pre-eclampsia is a risk factor
    b. Common in multigravida
    c. Common in primigravida
    d. Premature separation of normal implanted placentae
    e. Character of bleeding is bright red blood

22. All of the following is true about Abruptio placentae *except*: [PGI Nov 2014]
    a. Premature separation of normal attached placentae
    b. Bright red blood
    c. Risk of recurrence is about 15% with previous abruption
    d. More common in multigravida
    e. Pre-eclampsia is a risk factor

23. A woman at 8 months of pregnancy complains of abdominal pain and slight vaginal bleed. On examination the uterine size is above the expected date with absent fetal heart sounds. The diagnosis: [AIIMS May 01]
    a. Hydramnios   b. Concealed hemorrhage
    c. Active labor   d. Uterine rupture

24. A hypertensive pregnant woman at 34 weeks comes with history of pain in abdomen, bleeding per vaginum and loss of fetal movements. On examination the uterus is contracted with increased uterine tone. Fetal heart sounds are absent. The most likely diagnosis is: [AI 03]
    a. Placenta previa   b. Hydramnios
    c. Premature labor   d. Abruptio placenta

25. **In accidental hemorrhage, TOC:** [PGI Dec. 98]
    a. Induction of labor
    b. Rx of hypofibrinogenemia then blood transfusion
    c. Simultaneous emptying of uterus and blood transfusion
    d. Wait and watch

26. **A pregnant woman at 34 weeks pregnancy, comes with bleeding P/V, B. P. 80:** [AI 98]
    a. Examination in OT and termination of pregnancy
    b. Blood transfusion
    c. Observation
    d. LSCS

27. **All of the following can cause DIC during pregnancy** *except*: [AIIMS May 05]
    a. Diabetes mellitus
    b. Amniotic fluid embolism
    c. Intrauterine death
    d. Abruptio placentae.

28. **The following test may be abnormal in disseminated intravascular coagulation** *except*: [AIIMS Nov 04]
    a. Prothrombin
    b. Activated partial thromboplastin time
    c. D-timer levels
    d. Clot solubility.

29. **True regarding abruption placentae with DIC is:**

a. Decreased factor V [AIIMS Nov 99]
b. Decreased factor VIII
c. All clotting factor decreased and bleeding time prolongs.
d. Decrease blood flow to nephrons

30. **Which of the following is not used in DIC?** [AIIMS 90]
    a. Heparin   b. Epsilon amino caproic acid
    c. Blood transfusion   d. Intravenous fluids.

31. **26 years old female suffers from PPH on her second postnatal day. Her APTT and PTT are prolonged while BT, PT and platelet counts are normal. Likely diagnosis is:** [AIIMS Nov 01]
    a. Acquired hemophilia
    b. Lupus anticoagulant
    c. DIC
    d. Inherited congenital hemophilia.

32. **Which test differentiates maternal and fetal blood cell?** [AIIMS MAY 2013]
    a. APT test   b. Kleihauer test
    c. Bubble test   d. Lilly's test

33. **Risk factors for abruptio placenta is/are:**
    a. Traumatic separation of the placenta
    b. Multigravida   c. Diabetes
    d. Gestational hypertension [PGI MAY 2017]
    e. Submucous fibroid

Answers with Explanations to New Pattern Questions

N1. **Ans. is a and b, i.e. Postpartum hemorrhage infrequent; and First trimester bleeding is not uncommon.**

Ref. Dutta Obs. 7/e, p 247, 248

Placenta previa is a cause of APH which means bleeding from or into the genital tract after the 28th week of pregnancy i.e. it is not a cause of first trimester bleeding. (i.e. option b is incorrect).

As discussed earlier, previous cesarean section increase the chances of placenta previa in next pregnancy (i.e. option d is correct).

As far as other options are concerned - they are all complications of placenta previa.

Complications of placenta previa

A. Maternal
• Antepartum ⎫
• Intrapartum ⎬ Hemorrhage
• Postpartum ⎭
• Malpresentation
• Cord prolapse
• Retained placenta
• Preterm labor
• Premature rupture of membranes
• Slow dilatation of cervix

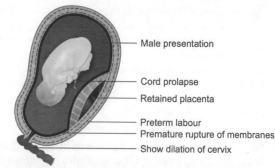

Maternal complications of placenta previa

B. Fetal
- Asphyxia
- Birth injuries
- Low birth weight
- Congenital malformation
- Intrauterine death

N2. Ans. is a, i.e. DIC   *Ref. Dutta Obs. 7/e, p 254*

In the question patient at 34 weeks of gestation is involved in a car accident. (Note: trauma is a risk factor for APH).
Her BP is 150/90 mm (High BP is a Risk factor for abruptio).
On vaginal inspection - bleeding is present along with strong uterine contractions so the diagnosis of abruptio confirmed.
DIC due to release of thromboplastin by damaged placenta is a well known complication of abruptio.

N3. Ans. is c, i.e. Administer fresh frozen plasma   *Ref. Dutta Obs. 7/e, p 258*

In the question again patient at 34 weeks of gestation is involved in a car accident and presented with high B/P and abdominal pain. Her USG shows placental abruption. As discussed in the previous question. DIC is a complication of abruptio. In this patient INR is 2.5 and fibrin degradation products are raised which means she already is in DIC.

> *Remember*: In DIC – Immediate vaginal delivery is contraindicated. Whenever a pregnant patient has DIC - always correct DIC first by giving fresh frozen plasma, then think about vaginal delivery. In DIC, cesarean is not done.

N4. Ans. is b, i.e. Mortality rate of 20% with undiagnosed case   *Ref. Williams Obs 23/e, p 583-584, High risk pregnancy" Fernando Arias 3/e p 348, progress in Obs. and Gynae- John Studd vol. 17/e p 209*

Vasa previa: It is a condition in which the fetal blood vessels unsupported by either umbical cord or placental tissue, overlies the internal os and is vulnerable to rupture when supporting membrane rupture.
Thus bleeding in case of vasa previa is of fetal origin and not maternal origin (unlike placenta previa and abruptio)
- It is rare condition and occurs in 1 in 2000 – 3000 deliveries (i.e. option ais correct).
- Vasa previa should be suspected if any of the following condition exists
  - Velamentous cord insertion
  - Bilobed placenta
  - Succenturiate lobed placenta
  - Placenta previa/low lying placenta in second trimester (option 'c' is correct)
  - Pregnancy resulting from IVF
  - Multiple pregnancies
- Vasa previa is associated with high fetal mortality – (75–100%) because—
  - Wharton's jelly is absent around the fetal vessels, hence they can be easily lacerated at the time of rupture of membranes leading to severe fetal bleeding.
  - Vessels can be easily compressed by the fetal presenting part during uterine contractions leading to fetal exsanguination.

This explains that **option b** i.e. mortality rate is 20% in undiagnosed case is incorrect (mortality is 75-100%)
- Maternal mortality is not increased
- **Diagnosis** of vasa previa – In all cases of antepartum and intrapartum hemorrhage, the possibility of vasa previa should be kept in mind and blood should be tested for fetal hemoglobin characterized by resistance to denaturation by alkaline reagent (Singer alkali denaturation test/Apt test)
- Doppler examination can also reveal fetal blood vessels traversing below the presenting part

Management: In a diagnosed case of vasa previa elective cesarean section should be done or emergency LSCS should be done if it is diagnosed intrapartum.

N5. Ans. is a, i.e. Emergent cesarean section

Now this question can be explained in 2 ways but answer still remains the same:
Expl 1: Patient is presenting at 32 weeks of gestation to the emergency department with a small amount of vaginal bleeding. She doesn't have any pain., This could be a case of placenta previa.. now since there is fetal distress, we will do active management and terminate the pregnancy immediately by doing a cesarean section.

Expl 2: In this question patient has experienced small amount of painless vaginal bleeding…but the fetal distress does not coincide with the amount of blood loss, so probably this small amount of blood loss is fetal in origin this is why it has led to fetal distress i.e it is a case of vasa previa.
Management of vasa previa-Emergency cesarean section.

N6.   Ans. is a, i.e. TVS   *Ref. Willams 24/e, p 802*

TVS is the investigation of choice for detecting abnormally located placenta.

N7.   Ans. is a, i.e. 32 weeks   *Ref. Fernando Arias 4/e, p 154*

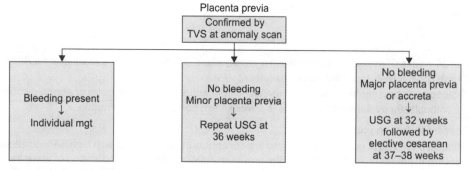

N8.   Ans. is b, i.e. Abruptio placenta   *Ref. Williams 24/e, p 794, 801*

> **Incidence of:**
> Abruptio = 1 in 200 deliveries
> Placenta previa = 1 in 300–400 deliveries
> Vasa previa = 1 in 2000–3000 deliveries
> Placenta accreta = 1 in 533 deliveries.

N9.   Ans. is c, i.e. Vasa previa

Here patient presents to labor room in labor. The moment ARM is done fresh bleeding is seen late declarations are seen (i.e. there is fetal distress) and fetus could not be saved.

There is no placenta previa or abruptio. This points out towards vasa previa as diagnosis because in vasa previa, umbilical cord is attached to membranes. The moment ARM is done, along with membranes, cord is also ruptured which leads to fetal blood loss, fetal distress and ultimately fetal death.

N10. Ans. is d, i.e. All of the above   *Ref. COGDT 10/e, p 992, for a and c, 997, for d; Sheila Balakrishnan, 1/e, p 490, 491*

> **Amniotic fluid embolism:**
> • It is usually fatal and is characterised by an abrupt onset of respiratory distress and coagulopathy.
> • It should be considered in all cases of peripartum collapse.
> • It is diagnosed clinically
> Clinical features: *are due to 2 components:*
>   i. Embolic component causes acute respiratory distress syndrome and ultimately death.
>   ii. Coagulation failure causes hemorrhage, DIC and consumptive coagulopathy.
> • Classically a woman in late labor or immediate postpartium gasps for air, has bronchospasm, becomes cyanotic and undergoes immediate collapse and cardiorespiratory arrest usually accompanied by Hemorrhage.[Q]
> • Sudden death is usual.
> Timing:
> • After ARM and at cesarean section.
> • In labor with strong uterine contractions.
> • Immediate postpartum.

N11. Ans. is c, i.e. Amniotic fluid embolism
Ref. COGDT 10/e, p 991, 992; Sheila Balakrishnan p 490, 491, Dutta Obs. 7/e, p 324, 325

In the question, the female is:
• Multiparous
• Advanced maternal age
• *Fetus is dead*

The patient is having strong uterine contractions and suddenly goes in shock with cyanosis, respiratory disturbance and pulmonary edema. All these favour the diagnosis of amniotic fluid embolism.

Amniotic fluid embolism: It is characterised by an abrupt onset of respiratory distress and coagulopathy.

- Amniotic fluid enters the circulation and sets up a disseminated intravascular coagulation, leading to consumptive coagulopathy.
- Classically a woman in late labor or immediate postpartum gasps for air, has bronchospasm, becomes cyanotic and undergoes immediate collapse and cardiorespiratory arrest, usually accompanied by hemorrhage. Sudden death is usual.
- It is diagnosed clinically.

Risk factors:

• Advanced maternal age	• Multiparity
• Tetanic uterine contraction	• Use of uterine stimulants
• Uterine rupture	• Cesarean section
• Premature separation of placenta	• Intra uterine fetal death.

 Remember: Amniotic fluid enters maternal circulation as a result of breech in the physiological barrier that normally exists between maternal and fetal compartments-so any cause leading to this mixing like cesarean section, premature separation of placenta, rupture uterus etc. Predisposes to amniotic fluid embolism.

Most common timing for:

Amniotic fluid embolism

i. After ARM

ii. At cesarean section

iii. In labor with strong uterine contractions.

iv. Immediate postpartum.

Management: Aimed at minimizing hypoxemia with supplemental oxygen, maintaining blood pressure and managing associated coagulopathy.

N12. **Ans. is a, i.e. Thrombocytopenia is a feature of fibrinolytic process and not of DIC** *Ref. Dutta obs. 7/e, p 628*

In DIC: Thrombocytopenia is seen i.e. on peripheral smear less than 4 platelets per high power field are present. Thrombocytopenia is a feature of DIC but not of fibrinolytic process (i.e. option a is incorrect and option d is correct). In DIC–RBC's are helmet shaped or fragmented but in fibrinolytic process RBC's are normal. As discussed earlier clot observation test is done in DIC.

Answers with Explanations to Previous Year Questions

1. Ans. is d, i.e. Battledore placenta

Ref. Dutta Obs. 7/e, p 214, 216, 217; Textbook of Obs. by Sheila Balakrishnan, p 155

Causes of Antepartum Hemorrhage

• *Placenta previa*
• *Abruptio placenta*
• *Vasa previa*
• *Circumvallate placenta*
• *Local causes like*:
  – Polyp
  – Carcinoma cervix
  – Varicose veins
  – Trauma
  – Unclassified or indeterminate

Circumvallate placenta

- It is an uncommon cause of antepartum hemorrhage.[Q]
- In this condition, the chorionic plate which is on the fetal side of the placenta is smaller than the basal plate on the maternal side.[Q]
- The fetal surface of the placenta presents a central depression surrounded by a thickened grayish white ring.
- These pregnancies may be complicated by IUGR and an increased chance of fetal malformations.
- Bleeding is usually painless[Q].
- Antenatal diagnosis is unlikely and the diagnosis is usually made after examination of the placenta post delivery[Q].

> **Note**: Battledore placenta = It is a condition in which the umbilical cord is attached to the margin of placenta.

2. Ans. is c, i.e Primigravida

Ref. Dutta Obs 7/e, p 242; Fernado Arias 3/e p333

Placenta previa is implantation of the placenta partially or completely over the lower uterine segment. Damage to the endometrium or myometrium due to previous surgery or infection can predispose to low implantation and placenta previa.
Risk factors for placenta previa:

- Prior surgery[Q] (cesarean section/Myomectomy Hysterotomy)
- Previous uterine curettage[Q]
- Endometritis[Q]
- Increasing maternal age (>35 years)[Q]
- Increasing parity[Q]
- Placental size –increased (as in multiple pregnancy)
- Placental abnormality –Succenturiate lobe
- Smoking (due to defective decidual vascularization)
- Elevated prenatal maternal serum alpha fetoprotein levels (unexplained)

> **Note**: The probability of placenta accreta and need for cesarean hysterectomy is increased in patients with prior cesarean section and placenta previa.
> Smoking increases the risk of placenta previa by two fold times.
> Previous cesarean section increases the risk of placenta previa by 4 fold time.

3. Ans. is d, i.e. Present after first trimester

Ref. Dutta Obs. 7/e, p 243

Antepartum hemorrhage is defined as bleeding from or into the genital tract after the period of viability and but before the birth of the baby (the first and second stage of labor included). Hence option d is incorrect.

4. **Ans. is a, i.e. Incidence increaes by two fold after LSCS**

Ref. Fernando Arias 3/e, p 333, 334; Dutta Obs. 7/e, p 242, 243

Chances of placenta previa are increased in case of history of prior cesarean section—

"The probability of placenta previa is four times greater in patients with prior cesareans than in patients without uterine scars." —*Fernando Arias 3/e, p 333, 334*

Therefore, option a is correct (partly though) because the option says two-fold increase

As far as - other options are concerned:

Option 'b' i.e. it is more common in primipara is absolutely wrong as - placenta previa is more common in multipara.

Option 'c' It is more common in developed countries.

Now that is incorrect because -

"Increased family planning acceptance with limitation and spacing of birth, lowers the incidence of placenta previa." —*Dutta obs 6/e, p 243*

Which clearly means it is less common in developed countries than in developing countries.

Option 'd' - Incidence is 1 per 1000 pregnancies:

According to *Dutta Obs 6/e, p 243*

"Incidence of placenta previa ranges from 0.5 to 1% among hospital deliveries."

"According to 2003 birth certificate data in the US, placenta previa complicated almost 1 in 300 deliveries" —*Williams Obs 23/e, p 770*

i.e. *option 'd'* is incorrect.

As far as **option e** is concerned placenta previa is a cause of APH and not PPH.

So, amongst all options - *option 'a'* is partly correct, so it is the answer of choice here

5. **Ans. is d i.e. Low lying placenta** *Ref. Dutta Obs. 7/e, p 244*

Stallworthy's sign: Slowing of the fetal heart rate on pressing the head down into the pelvis and prompt recovery on release of the pressure is termed ***Stallworthy's sign*** and is suggestive of posterior placenta previa.

 Note: Presence of this sign is not always significant because it may be due to fetal head compression even in an otherwise normal case.

6. **Ans. is. c, i.e. McAfee and Johnson regime.** *Ref. Dutta Obs 7/e, p 248*

7. **Ans. is b, i.e. Cervical encirclage.** *Ref. Dutta Obs. 7/e, p 248, 249, Fernando arias 3/e, p 341, 342*

McAfee and Johnson regime is the name given to the expectant management of placenta previa as it was advocated by McAfee and Johnson

Aim of expectant management in case of placenta previa is to continue pregnancy for fetal maturity without compromising the maternal health.

Prerequisites for expectant management:
- Availability of blood for transfusion whenever required
- Facilities for caesarean section should be available throughout 24 hours.

Candidates: Suitable for expectant management are:
- Mother in good health status- Hemoglobin > 10 gm%
- Hematocrit > 30% and she should be hemodynamically stable.
- Duration of pregnancy less than 37 weeks
- Active vaginal bleeding is absent
- Fetal well being is assured by USG and cardiotocography

The expectant management is carried upto 37 weeks of pregnancy until baby matures.

Expectant management includes (i.e. McAfee and Johnson regime includes)
- Hospitalization till active bleeding stops and then readmission at 34 weeks
- Complete bed rest
- Anemia corrected with blood transfusion (if necessary), but blood should always to be kept ready as placenta previa is a recurrent condition.
- Antenatal steroids to promote fetal lung maturity

- Anti D if patient is Rh negative
- If uterine contractions are present - tocolytics (nifedipine) can be given as it leads to more advanced gestational age at delivery, greater birth weight of fetus, less neonatal complications, and decreased cost of hospitalization. Tocolytics should not be used for more than 48 hours.

8   **Ans. is b, i.e. Cesarean section**   *Ref. Dutta Obs 7/e, p 249, 250; Fernando Arias 3/e, p 337, 339*

The patient in the question:

1. Has gestational age = 37 weeks i.e. fetus has attained maturity so immediate termination of pregnancy is recommended.
2. Has central placenta previa Type IV i.e. vaginal delivery is contraindicated, cesarean section has to be done.
3. Patient is having heavy bleeding.

According to   *Fernando Arias 3/e, p 337*

"In patients with heavy bleeding an efficient management plan including life support measures and immediate operative intervention is the only way to avoid a maternal death."

It further says – on *p 339*

"Patients with placenta previa and severe bleeding should be delivered by cesarean section irrespective of the type of placenta previa."

So, from the above discussion, it is very much clear that in this patient, immediate cesarean section is the best resort.

Friends, here I want to point out that earlier it was said that for minor degrees of placenta previa, vaginal delivery can be tried, but now, irrespective of degree of placenta previa, cesarean section is done and recommended.

9.   **Ans. is a, i.e. Immediate C.S.**   *Ref. Dutta Obs 7/e, p 249, 250; Fernando Arias 3/e, p 337, 339*

As Explained in the previous question– Patient presenting with bleeding, at 37 weeks of gestation with central placenta previa, management should be *immediate emergency cesarean section.*

10.   **Ans. is c, i.e. Mother in a hemodynamically stable condition**

Ref. Dutta Obs 7/e, p 248, 249; Fernando Arias 3/e, p 342

All are contraindications for conservative management except hemodynamically stable condition.

11.   **Ans. is a, b, c and d, i.e. Active labor; Anencephaly; Dead baby; and Severe placenta previa**

Ref. Dutta Obs. 7/e, p 249

Well friends, there is no need to **"rattoo"** the conditions where expectant management is required and where active management. For a while - forget all the lists and just think you are a gynae casualty medical officer and a pregnant female with vaginal bleeding in the late months of pregnancy comes to you (suspected case of placenta previa). How will you manage if:

a.	She is in active labor	Obviously you will either do cesarean section or if bleeding is not much and no other adverse circumstances are present, proceed with vaginal delivery but you will never think of arresting her labor and managing conservatively
b.	If the patient is diagnosed of carrying anencephalic fetus.	The aim of conservative management is to continue pregnancy for attaining fetal maturity without compromising the maternal health. But in this case when fetus is anencephalic there is no point in continuing pregnancy i.e active management/ termination should be done.
c.	If fetus is dead	Same is the case with dead fetus, there is no point in continuing pregnancy i.e. active management should be done
d.	Severe placenta previa	In this case patient must be bleeding heavily. Remember always A gynaecologists first aim should be to save the life of mother. If fetus can be saved nothing like it, but in order to save the fetus, mother's life should not be put at risk. So, in this case expectant management (conservative management) should not be done. Immediate termination of pregnancy by cesarean section is the correct management.
e.	Premature fetus	If maternal condition is good, and fetus is premature, patient can be kept under observation. Betamethasone (to hasten fetal lung maturity) and blood transfusion (to raise mother's hematocrit), shoud be given i.e in this case conservative management can be done.

12.   **Ans. is a, b and d, i.e. Active bleeding, Active labor and Fetal malformation**   *Ref. Dutta Obs. 7/e, p 249*

13. Ans. is c, i.e. Transverse lie   *Ref. Dutta Obs. 7/e, p 249*

In these questions, there is no confusion about any option except for 'lie of the fetus'.

As far as lie is concerned:

Friends, why would you terminate pregnancy just because of unstable lie or transverse lie, unless and until there is some other complication associated with it. Transverse lie/unstable lie in a patient of placenta previa simply means that whenever termination of pregnancy is considered cesarean section has to be done.

14 Ans. is c, i.e. Pelvic examination in OT   *Ref. Dutta Obs. 7/e, p 249*

- Patient is presenting with painless vaginal bleeding and uterus is soft and nontender. These findings point towards the diagnosis of placenta previa (In abruptio-bleeding is accompanied by pain, uterus is tense, tender and rigid).
- The gestational age of patient is 39 weeks i.e., fetal maturity is attained so pregnancy has to be terminated, either vaginally or by cesarean section.
- Now to decide the mode of delivery, we need to know which of placenta previa it is. This can be known by USG or pelvic examination in OT. Since USG is not given in options so answer is pelvic examination in OT.

Also Know:

Conditions where vaginal examination should not be done (even in OT):

1. Patient is in exsanguinated stateQ.
2. Diagnosed case of placenta previa on USGQ
3. Associated complicating factors such as ***malpresentation, elderly primigravida, previous cesarean section, contracted pelvis etcQ which prevent vaginal delivery.***

As in all these conditions cesarean section is mandatory (so no point in wasting time to know the type of placenta previa by vaginal examination and taking the risk of occurrence of brisk hemorrhage).

---

15. Ans. is a, i.e Admit to antenatal unit for bed rest and betamethasone.   *Ref. Dutta Obs. 7/e, 248, 249*

G1P0 woman at 29 weeks' gestation presents to the emergency department complaining of 2 hours of vaginal bleeding, the bleeding recently stopped, her vitals are stable (temperature is 36.8°C (98.2°F), blood pressure is 118/72 mm Hg, pulse is 75/min, and respiratory rate is 13/min), FHS are present and reassuring i.e there is no fetal distress.

All this means we will manage this patient expectantly and there is no need to immediately terminate her pregnancy.. ruling out options c and d

- So now we have to choose between option:
  - Admit to antenatal unit for bed rest and betamethasone. And option
  - Admit to antenatal unit for bed rest and blood transfusion.
- The patients Hb is 11.1, there is no need for immediate blood transfusion (ruling out option b), just crossmatch and arrange blood and give betamethasone for hastening lung maturity.

16. Ans. is b, i.e. Blood transfusion   *Ref. Dutta Obs. 6/e, p 259; Fernando Arias 3/e, p 342, fig. 13.2*

Unstable vitals (BP = 80/60) belong most probably to moderate category bleeding.

    In ***Mild cases***   – Vitals remain stable.

    Severe cases   – Patient is in shock with very low or unrecordable B.P.

The gestational age of patient is 32 weeks: As discussed, beyond 36 weeks with moderate bleeding - terminate the pregnancy.

Between 32-36 weeks moderate bleeding - *Management depends on* whether pulmonary maturity is achieved or not.

- If maturity is not achieved, patient is managed conservatively on:
  - *Close monitoring*
  - *Blood transfusions*
  - *Betamethasone (to accelerate lung maturity)*

This is done for 24-48 hours.

- If patients condition improves: expectant management is continued.
- If patients condition does not improve: pregnancy is terminated.

As the patient in the question is 32 weeks pregnant with moderate bleeding, first we will try to improve the general condition of the patient by giving blood transfusion.

17. Ans. is b, i.e. Bed rest, Nifedipine and Dexamethasone *Ref. Fernando Arias 3/e, p 341*

At 32 weeks patient is presenting with uterine contraction which is a warning symptom of preterm labor.

Management of patient with placenta previa and preterm labor:

- **Tocolytic agent**: "Uterine contractions are common in patients with placenta previa. Since uterine contractions have the potential to, disrupt the placental attachment and aggravate the bleeding, most obstetricians favor the use of tocolytic agents in the expectant management of patient with placenta previa".
- Most commonly used tocolytics in case of placenta previa
  - Nifedipine
  - Magnesium sulphate
- Tocolytics which are not used:
  - Terbutaline and Ritodrine: They cause tachycardia and make the assessment of patient's pulse rate unreliable.
  - Indomethacin: It causes inhibition of platelet cyclo oxygenase system and prolongs the bleeding time.
- Besides this - patient should be:
  - Put on bed rest in left lateral position.
  - Glucocorticoids are given to hasten lung maturity.

18. Ans. is c, i.e. Termination of pregnancy *Ref. Dutta 7/e, p 249, 250*

- Painless vaginal bleeding and absence of other significant findings confirm the diagnosis of placenta previa.
- Gestational age of the patient is 38 weeks i.e. fetal maturity is attained so termination should be done.

  In case of severe bleeding pregnancy is terminated by cesarean section irrespective of gestational age.[Q]

 Note: Here I have ruled out option a i.e. per speculum examination because in case of placenta previa a double set up examination (i.e. examination in OT) is done and not simple P/S or P/V.

19. Ans. is b, i.e. Alcoholics *Ref. Dutta Obs. 7/e, p 252, 253; Williams Obs. 22/e, p 813, 814, 23/e, p 763-765*

See the text for explanation

20. Ans. is a, i.e. Page *Ref. Dutta's Obstetric Hemorrhage: Made Easy, p 144, 145*

See the text for explanation.

 Also Know:

Some other named classifications and Regimes

Named classification/Regine	Used in
Macaffee and Johnson Regime	Expectant management of placement previa
Page classification Sher classification	Abruptio plcenta
Clarke's classification	Classification of heart disease based on maternal mortality
Lytic cocktail regime (used 3 drugs - chlorpromazine, Promethazine and pethidine)	Proposed by Menon for management of convulsion in eclampsia
Whites classification	Earlier used for classification of diabetes in pregnancy
Caldwell and Mohoy classification	Types of pelvis

21. Ans. is a, b, and d, i.e Pre-eclampsia is a risk factor, Common in multigravida and Premature separation in a normal implanted placenta *Ref. Dutta, Obs 7/e, p 252, 253*

See the text for explanation.

22. Ans. is b, i.e. Bright red blood *Ref. Dutta Obs 8/e, p 294, 295*

In abruptio placenta—bleeding is dark red in colour and not bright red. Rest see the tex for explanation.

23. Ans. is b, i.e. Concealed hemorrhage *Ref. Dutta Obs. 7/e, p 255, 212, 429*

Let's analyse all options separately to see which suits the best.

Options	Points in favour	Points against
• Option "a" Hydramnios	• Size of uterus > gestational age. • Absent fetal heart sounds (in polyhydramnios fetal heard sound is not distinctly heard) 05	• Abdominal pain and vaginal bleeding (Main complain of patient with hydraminos is difficulty in breathing and swelling over legs **Option "a" ruled out**
• Option "c" Active labor	• Complain of abdominal pain and slight vaginal bleed (Which can be show of active labor)	• Height of uterus > than the period of gestation (Height of uterus = period gestation in normal labor) • Absent fetal heart sound (FHS is present in normal labor
Option "d" **Rupture uterus** Since period of of gestation is 8 month i.e. rupture is occurring during pregnancy and since no H/o scared uterus is given we are taking it as spontaneous rupture during pregnancy	• Height of uterus more than period of gestation • Absent fetal heart sounds	• In rupture patient complains of acute pain in abdomen accompanied by fainting attack/collapse • Acute tenderness on abdominal examination • Palpation of superficial fetal parts Spontaneous rupture during pregnancy of un-scarred uterus occurs in high parous women and is not common
Option "b" Concealed hemorrhage	• Abdominal pain and vaginal bleeding • Height of uterus more than period of gestation • Absent fetal heart sound	

So, concealed hemorrhage is the diagnosis.

24. **Ans. is d, i.e. Abruptio placenta**

    Ref. Dutta Obs. 7/e, p 255

    The patient in the question is hypertensive and presenting with:
    - History of pain in abdomen.
    - Bleeding per vaginum.
    - Loss of fetal movements.
    - O/E = uterus is contracted.
    - Increased uterine tone.
    - Fetal heart sounds are absent.

    All these features confirm the diagnosis of **abruptio placenta**.

    As far as premature labor is concerned – *Complains of abdominal pain and vaginal bleeding will be present but loss of fetal movement, absence of fetal heart sounds and increased uterine tone go against it. (In normal labor - uterus contracts and relaxes intermittently i.e. tone increases and decreases intermittently).*

25. **Ans. is c, i.e. Simultaneous emptying of uterus and blood transfusion**

    Ref: Williams Obs 23/e, p 767; Dutta Obs. 7/e, p 257, 258; COGDT 10/e, p 333

    - The basic principle in the management of abruptio is termination of pregnancy along with correction of hypovolemia and restoration of blood loss.

    "With massive external bleeding, intensive resuscitation with blood plus crystalloids and prompt delivery to control Hemorrhage are life saving for mother and hopefully fetus".
    —*Williams Obs. 23/e, p 767*

    This means option c is correct

    "Expectant management of suspected placental abruption is the exception, not the rule. This management pathway should be attempted only with careful observation of the patient and a clear clinical picture." (Option "d" ruled out)
    —*COGDT 10/e, p 333, 334*

    - Correction of hypofibrinogenemia (i.e. Option "b")

"A rational approach (in abruptio) should be to withhold any specific therapy to rectify the coagulation disorders except in the circumstances such as overt bleeding or clinically evaluated thromboembolic process".

—*Dutta Obs. 6/e, p 260*

26. **Ans. is b, i.e. Blood transfusion**   *Ref. Read Below*

The question is incomplete, we cannot make any diagnosis with this much information only except that – It could be a case of ante partum hemorrhage.

If such a patient comes to the casualty, our first and foremost step will be to save the life of patient as patient's BP is 80 systolic i.e. patient is in shock. Blood transfusion to correct hypovolemia and replenish blood loss should be done.

Extra Edge:

- Guide to adequate blood replacement.[Q]
    - Maintainence of central venous pressure at 10 cm of water.[Q]
    - Hematocrit   =   30%[Q]
    - Urinary output =   30 ml/hour[Q]

27. **Ans. is a, i.e. Diabetes mellitus**   *Ref. Dutta Obs. 7/e, p 628; COGDT 10/e, p 996,997; Harrison 17/e, p 729*

DIC is a pathological condition associated with inappropriate activation of coagulation and fibrinolytic system. It is a secondary phenomenon resulting from an underlying disease state.

Obstetric conditions associated with DIC:

More common	Less common
• Intrauterine fetal death • Amniotic fluid embolism • Pre eclampsia- Eclampsia • HELLP syndrome • Placenta Abruption • Septic Abortion	• Chorioamnionitis • Pyelonephritis in pregnancy • H. mole • Instillation of intraamniotic hypertonic saline • Feto maternal bleed • Incompatible blood transfusion • Viremia –HIV, varicella, CMV hepatitis..COGDT p 997

Pathogenesis:

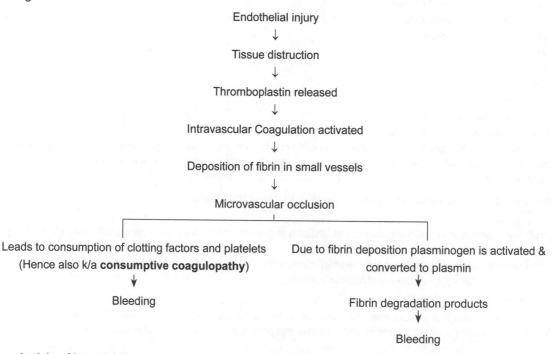

Endothelial injury
↓
Tissue distruction
↓
Thromboplastin released
↓
Intravascular Coagulation activated
↓
Deposition of fibrin in small vessels
↓
Microvascular occlusion

Leads to consumption of clotting factors and platelets
(Hence also k/a **consumptive coagulopathy**)
↓
Bleeding

Due to fibrin deposition plasminogen is activated &
converted to plasmin
↓
Fibrin degradation products
↓
Bleeding

28. **Ans. is d, i.e. Clot solubility**   *Ref. Harsh Mohan 5/e, p 437; Dutta Obs. 7/e, p 628, 629*

Laboratory findings in case of DIC are:

- The platelet count is low
- Blood film shows the features of microangiopathic hemolytic anaemia. There is presence of schistocytes and fragmented red cells (helmet shaped) due to damage caused by trapping and passage through the fibrin thrombi.
- **Prothrombin time, thrombin time and activated partial thromboplastin time, are all prolonged.**
- Plasma fibrinogen levels are reduced due to consumption in microvascular coagulation.
- Fibrin degradation products (FDPs) are raised due to secondary fibrinolysis.
- **D-dimer levels are raised in DIC.**

Clot observation test (Weiner)—It is an useful bed side test. It can be repeated at 2–4 hours intervals. 5 ml of venous blood is placed in a 15 ml dry test tube and kept at 37°C. Usually, blood clot forms within 6-12 minutes. This test provides a rough idea of blood fibrinogen level. If the clotting time is less than 6 minutes, fibrinogen level is more than 150 mg percent. If no clot forms within 30 minutes, the fibrinogen level is probably less than 100 mg percent.

Clot stability test/Clot lysis test: It is gross way of observing the fibrinolytic system.

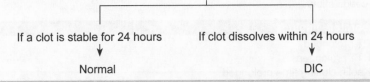

If a clot is stable for 24 hours → Normal

If clot dissolves within 24 hours → DIC

In DIC clot stability test and not clot solubility test is abnormal. Clot solubility test is to estimate factor XIII & will not be increased in DIC.

29. **Ans. is c, i.e. All clotting factor decreased and bleeding time prolongs** *Ref. Dutta Obs. 7/e, p 629*

In abruption placentae leading to DIC due to a massive retroplacental clot-not only fibrinogen but other clotting factors are also decreased and bleeding time prolonged.

DIC is called as consumptive coagulopathy.

30. **Ans. is b, i.e. Epsilon amino caproic acid** *Ref. COGDT 10/e, p 999; Williams Obs. 23/e, p 787*

Well friends, we have discussed the causes and investigations of DIC. Now here let's take a look at its management.

Management of DIC

- The most important step is to terminate the pregnancy- vaginal delivery without episiotomy is preferred to cesarean section
- Volume replacement by crystalloids or colloids will reduce the amount of whole blood needed to restore the blood volume.
- 500 ml of fresh blood raises the fibrinogen level approximately by 12.5 mg/100 ml and platelets by 10,000–15,000 cu mm. Fresh blood- helps in flushing out fibrin degradation product and improving the micro circulation.
- To replace fibrinogen- Fresh frozen plasma should be given:

  Fresh frozen plasma (FFP) is extracted from whole blood. It contains fibrinogen, anti-thrombin III, clotting factors V, XI, XII. FFP transfusion provides both volume replacement and coagulation factors. One unit of FFP (250 ml) raises the fibrinogen by 5-10 mg/dl. FFP does not need to be ABO or Rh compatible.

- Cryoprecipitate is obtained from thawed FFP. It is rich in fibrinogen, factor VIII, Von Willebrand's factor, and XIII. Cryoprecipitate provides less volume (40 ml) compared to FFP (250 ml). So it should not be used for volume replacement. One unit of cryoprecipitate increases the fibrinogen level by 5-10 mg/dl.
- In case of active bleeding with platelet counts < 50,000/μl or prophylactically with platelet count 20–30,000/μl – platelet replacement should be done. Platelet should ABO and Rh specific. 1 units (50 ml) raises the platelet count by 7500/ml
- **Recombinant activated factors VIIA:** (60-100 μg/kg IV) can reverse DIC within 10 minute as it is a precursor for extrinsic clotting cascade which is replaced.

- *Role of Heparin*

According to Williams Obs. **"Heparin is not used in DIC."**

According to *COGDT 10/e, p 999*

"Heparin acts as an anticoagulant by activating antithrombin III but has little effect on activated coagulation factors. Anticoagulation is contraindicated in patients with fulminant DIC and central nervous system insults, fulminant liver failure, or obstetric accidents. The one instance, however, in which heparin has been demonstrated to benefit pregnancy-related DIC is in the case of the retained dead fetus with intact vascular system, where heparin may be administered to

interrupt the coagulation process and thrombocytopenia for several days until delivery may be implemented."

As far as EACA is concerned

-Williams Obs. 22/e, p 844 says –

"EACA is not recommended in case of DIC."

According to *Williams Obs 23/e, p 787*

"It use in most types of obstetric coagulopathy has not been efficacious & not recommended"

31. Ans. is a, i.e. Acquired hemophilia

Ref. Ghai 6/e, p 322, 323; Harrison 16/e, p 342, 685

Test	Significance	Abnormal in
• Bleeding time	Indicates abnormality in number and function of platelets	Idiopathic thrombocytopenic purpura, anaphylactoid purpura, leukemia
• Clotting time viz π Prothrombin time	Indicator of extrinsic and common pathway of coagulation	Factor VII deficiency
• Activated partial thromboplastin time (APTT) or partial thromboplastin (PTT)	Indicator of intrinsic and common pathway of coagulation	Factor VIII, IX, XI and XIII deficiency, von Willebrand's disease

Both PT and APTT are prolonged in case of vitamin K deficiency, severe liver disease, factor V, X, and Fibrinogen deficiency and disseminated intravascular coagulation.

Disorder	Laboratory findings	
Lupus anticoagulant ...*Leon speroff 7/e, p 1082*	• PT prolonged • PTT prolonged • Kaolin clotting time prolonged • Dilute Russel's Viper venom time prolonged	Not corrected by addition of plasma but by addition of excess phospholipid
DIC	• Platelet count decrease • PT prolonged • PTT prolonged • Thrombin time prolonged • Fibrinogen decreased • Fibrin degradation products increased	
Hemophilia	• PTT prolonged (due to deficiency of factor VIII) • PT normal • BT normal • Platelet count normal	

This means the patient is suffering from hemophilia. The question now arises whether it is acquired or inherited/congenital hemophilia.

Inherited congenital hemophilia:

• Is extremely rare in females.
• It is an x linked disorder seen mainly in males.

Acquired hemophilia

• It is a disorder in which antibodies develop against coagulation factors.
• Antibodies can develop against one coagulation factor or several factors.
• The most common target protein is factor VIII.
• Anti-factor VIII antibodies are seen in:
    – Hemophiliacs (apart from the congenital factor VIII or IX deficiency)
    – Post partum females
    – Due to drugs
    – SLE
    – Normal elderly individuals
• The patient in the question is a post-partum female who has developed antibodies against factor VIII (i.e. she is a case of Acquired hemophilia).
• The patients coagulation profile matches exactly with that of acquired hemophilia confirming our diagnosis.

32. Ans. is b, i.e. Kleihauer test   *Ref. Willams 24/e, p 617, 618; Dutta 7/e, p 234, 651*

Both Apt test and Kleihauer-Betke test can be used to detect the presence of fetal blood within a sample.

Apt Test/Singers Alkali Denaturation Test:

- Used to detect the **presence or absence of fetal blood (qualitative)** in a **vaginal discharge to rule out vasa previa late in pregnancy** or to detect the **origin of a neonatal blood vomiting,** whether iti s a genuine upper GI hemorrhage/ hemoptysis or simply swallowed maternal blood during delivery or from cracked nipple.

Kleihauer-Betke Test:

- The sample is **maternal peripheral smear** and is **used to see how much of fetal blood (quantitative)** has been transfused into the maternal serum in order to **assess the risk of isoimmunization** and then the **risk of hemolytic disease of newborn**

Both of them rely on the fact that **HbF is resistant to alkali (Apt)** and **acids (Kleihauer-Betke)** and so the **HbA containing RBCs (Maternal) will be hemolyzed but not the fetal RBCs** as they have the **HbF**.

When **fetal blood needs to be differentiated from Maternal blood—Apt test is used (Qualitative estimation)**
When the **amount of fetal bleeding needs to be estimated—Kleihauer-Betke test is used** (Quantitative estimation)
When **fetal RBC (blood cell)** is to be differentiated from **maternal RBC (blood cell)**–Kleihauer betke test is used

	APT test	Kleihauer-Betke test
• Source of sample	• **Maternal**	• Maternal
• Reagent used	• NaOH	• Citric acid phosphate buffer
• Principle	• Adding 1% NaOH destroys adult HbA but not fetal HbF	• Adding acid destroys adult HbA but not fetal HbF
• Assessment type	• **Qualitative**	• **Quantitative**

33. Ans. is a, b, d and e, i.e. Traumatic separation of the placenta; Multigravida; Gestational hypertension and Submucous fibroid.

See the text for explanation.

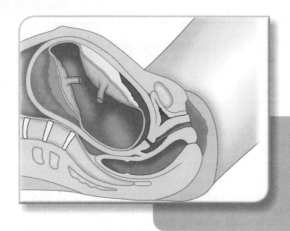

Chapter 19

Multifetal Pregnancy

Chapter at a Glance

- Zygosity
  - Dizygous Twins
  - Monozygous Twins
- Chorionicity
- All Types of Twin Pregnancy at a Glance
- Antenatal Screening of Twins

- USG in Twins
- Vascular Anastomosis in Twins
- Complications Specific to Twins
- Complications of Twins in General
- Management in Labor

ZYGOSITY

Twins can be Monozygotic or Dizygotic

Zygosity - refers to the type of conception.

Twins can be:

Dizygotic (75%)	Monozygotic (25%)
• Arisine from fertilisation of two ova by 2 different spermatozoas • 2 zygotes formed	They arise from splitting of single fertilized ovum and hence are always of the same sex and look like.

Dizygous Twins

- More common (70%)
- Incidence of dizygotic twins changes from country to country and is responsible for worldwide variation in incidence
- Incidence of dizygotic twins increases with:
  - Increased maternal age
  - Increased parity
  - Maternal family history of twining
  - Ovulation induction drugs like clomiphene or gonadotropins
- Sex of the baby can be same or different in dizygous twins
- Dizygous twins always have 2 chorion and 2 amnion i.e. may always are dichorionic and diamniotic
- They have different genetic features, different fingerprints, and their skin grafts are rejected.

Monozygous Twins

- Less Common (30%)
- Incidence remain constant—**1 in 250 deliveries**, throughout the word (i.e. 4 in 1000 deliveries)
- Sex of babies is always same
- They have different fingerprints.
- They have same genetic features, same DNA imprints and their skin grafting is accepted
- The number of chorion and amnion depend at the time which differentiation occurs

> *Also Know:*
> - The incidence of twins is highest in Nigeria (1 in 20)[Q]
> - It is lowest in Japan
> - Incidence in India - 1 in 80[Q]
> - Incidence of twins is increasing in India because of the use of ovulation inducing drugs like clomiphene, gonadotropins[Q] and procedures like IVF.

Hellin's Rule

According to Hellin's Rule

The mathematical frequency of multiple pregnancy is:
- Twins   1 in 80
- Triplets   1 in $(80)^2$
- Quadruplets   1 in $(80)^3$ and so on
- Study of twins is called Gemellology

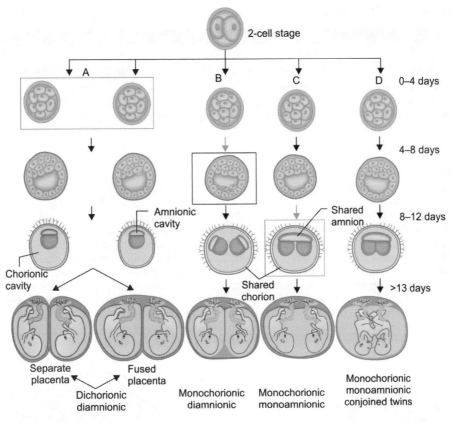

Fig. 19.1: Mechanic of monozygotic twinning.

CHORIONICITY

Chorionicity - denotes the type of placentation:

1. In dizygotic twins - each twin has its own placenta, chorion and amnion, i.e. dizygotic twins are always dichorionic diamniotic. (i.e. 2 chorions and 2 amnions).

2. In monozygous twins, the time at which the fertilized ovum divides - decides the chorionicity. (See flowchart)

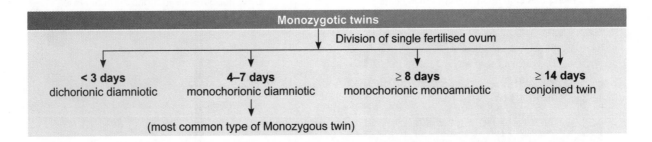

3. Chorionicity is of clinical significance as dichorionic twins, whether monozygous or dizygous, develop as two distinct individuals and are hence not at increased risk of complications. Whereas monochorionic twins are at increased risk because of the vascular anastomosis between the two circulations.

Remember:
- Prognosis depends on chorionicity not zygosity
- Dichorionic twins always have better prognosis than monochorionic twins.
- IOC to determine chronicity = TVS
- Time to do USG to detect chorionicity = 11-14 weeks

Ultrasound Differentiation of Chorionicity

Criterion	Monochorionic	Dichorionic
• Placenta	Single	Double
• Fetal sex	Concordant	Discordant/Concordant
• Membrane	< 2 mm thick	> 2 mm thick
• Number of layers in membrane CT	Two (2 amnion) (Fig. 19.3)	Four (2 amnion, 2 chorion) (Fig. 19.2)
• Twin peak sign	• Absent	• Present

Ultrasound Determination of Chorionicity
- **Number of sacs:** This is applicable only before 10 weeks when 2 sacs indicate dichorionic and single sac indicates monochorionic pregnancy.
- **Placenta:** Two placentae indicate a dichorionic pregnancy.
- **Sex:** Discordant sex indicates dichorionicity but concordant sex does not imply monochorionicity.
- **Intertwin membrane:** It is thicker (>2 μm) and more echogenic in dichorionic twins, whereas it is thin (>2 μm) in monochorionic.
- **Twin peak or lambda sign a delta sign:** It is characteristic of dichorionic pregnancies and is due to the chorionic tissue between the two layers of the intertwin membrane at the placental origin. A potential space exists in the intertwin membrane which is filled by proliferating placental villi, giving rise to a twin peak sign. Twin peak appears as a triangle with base at chorionic surface and apex in intertwin membrane. In monochorionic twins there is no chorionic tissue, and intertwin membrane is composed of 2 amnion only giving rise to the "T" sign on ultrasound (Figs. 19.2 to 19.5).

It is best examined between 10–14 weeks, near the placental insertion of membranes.

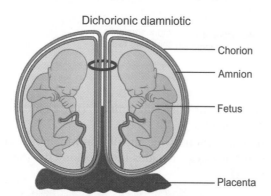

Fig. 19.2: Twin peak sign seen in dichorionic twins

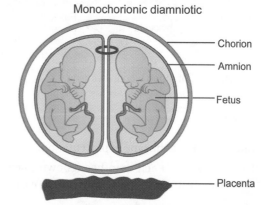

Fig. 19.3: USG appearance in monochorionic twins

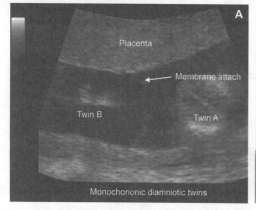

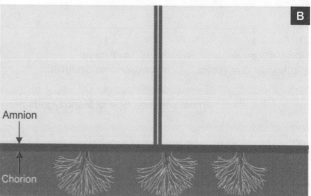

Figs. 19.4A and B: (A) Sonographic image of the "T" sign in a monochorionic diamnionic gestation at 30 weeks. (B) Schematic diagram of the "T" sign. Twins are separated only by a membrane created by the juxtaposed amnion of each twin. A "T" is formed at the point at which amnions meet the placenta.

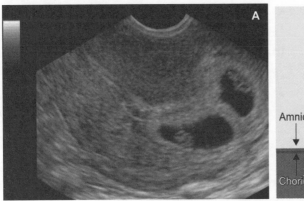
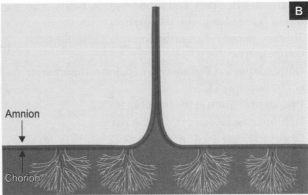

Figs. 19.5A and B: (A) Sonographic image of the "twin-peak" sign, also termed the "lambda sign," in a 24- week gestation. At the top of this sonogram, tissue from the anterior placenta is seen extending downward between the amnion layers. This sign confirms dichorionic twinning. (B) The triangular portion of placenta insinuates between the amniochorion layers.

 Remember:
- All monochorionic pregnancies are monozygotic
- Dichorionic pregnancies can be monozygotic or dizygotic
- Monozygotic twins can be monochorionic or dichorionic
- If the twins are of different sexes, they are always dizygotic.
- Same sex twins can be monozygotic or dizygotic..

All Types of Twin Pregnancy at a Glance

1 Dichorionic Diamniotic twins (DCDA)
- M/c variety of twin pregnancy over all
- Have good prognosis
- Twin peak sign is positive on ultrasound
- Time of delivery = **38 weeks**
- There are 4 layers of membranes between twins

2 Monochorionic Diamniotic twins (MCDA)
- M/C variety of monozygositic twins
- There are 2 layers of membranes between twins (i.e membranes are thin
- Have bad prognosis
- Complication specific to then: Twin to Twin Transfusion syndrome.
- Time of delivery 34 to 37 6/7 weeks (generally 37 weeks)

3. Monochorionic Monoamniotic twins (MCMA) (1% cases)

- No layers of membranes between twin
- A specific complication which can occur in these twins is cord enlargement
- Have increased incidence of congenital anomalies (18-28%). M/C being cardiac – anomaly hence Echocardiography should always be done
- Have bad prognosis
- Always be delivered by caesarean section between 32-34 weeks after giving corticosteroid injection.

Conjoint Twins (Fig. 19.6)
- **Conjoined twins, also called Siamese twins, after Chang and Eng Bunker of Siam** (Thailand)

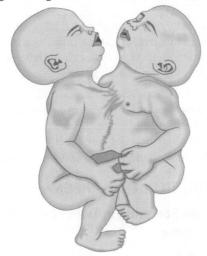

Fig. 19.6 Conjoint twin

- **They affect 1 in every 200 monozygotic twins. The different types of conjoined twins are:**
  a. **Thoracopagus:** Fusion at the chest (40%). It is the most common type
  b. **Omphalopagus (Xiphopagus):** Fusion at the anterior abdominal wall (33%)
  c. **Pyopagus:** Fusion at the buttocks (18%)
  d. **Ischiopagus:** Fusion at the ischium (6%)
  e. **Craniopagus:** Fusion of heads (2%). It is least common.

> **On USG** both twins facing each other or on repeated examination heads are at same level and plane.
> - The thoracic cages are in unusual proximity.
> - There is no change in relative fetal positions with time or manipulation.
> - The outcome of conjoined twins is poor and is dependent largely on the feasibility of surgical separation.
> **Mode of delivery of conjoint twins:** Cesarean section.

ANTENATAL SCREENING OF TWINS FOR FETAL ABNORMALITIES

- Biochemical screening tests are unreliable in twin pregnancy, as the values tend to be elevated. Therefore, biochemical tests are not used for second trimester screening.
- Ultrasound scanning for nuchal translucency between 11 and 13 weeks, can be performed as a screening test for trisomies.
- Occurrence of a trisomy and other genetic and chromosomal diseases is confirmed, by chorionic villous sampling in the first trimester and amniocentesis in the second trimester.

> - Monochorionic twins are monozygotic and only one sample is needed for karyotyping, as chromosomal and genetic defects will affect both fetuses or none. In dichorionic twins both fetuses should be sampled separately.

- The optimal method of diagnosing structural abnormalities is ultrasound scanning of each twin at 20 weeks. Structural abnormalities can affect either one or both twins, in both monochorionic and dichorionic twins.

ULTRASOUND IN TWIN PREGNANCY

Ultrasound Scanning in Twin Pregnancy in the First Trimester

- To confirm twins.
- To confirm dates measuring the crown rump length

- To determine chronicity.
- To assess nuchal translucency

In the Second Trimester

- For structural fetal abnormalities at 20 weeks.
- Scanning is done once in two weeks from 16–24 weeks, in monochorionic twins, for early identification of TTTS.
- Scanning is done once in 3–4 weeks from 20 weeks onwards, for growth and fetal weight discordance.

Complications Specific to Monochorionic Twins
- Twin-twin transfusion syndrome[Q]
- Conjoined twinning[Q]
- Acardiac fetus
- Selective IUGR
- Single fetus demise.

Complications Specific to Monoamniotic Twins
- Cord entanglement

VASCULAR ANASTOMOSIS IN TWIN

Vascular Anastomosis in twins can be of 2 types:-

1. Superficial vascular Anastomosis

- M/c variety of vascular anastomosis seen in twins
- The M/C type is artery to artery anastomosis
- This anastomosis has bidirectional flow of blood i.e. blood can flow in either direction i.e. none of the twin is a permanent donor and none is a permanent recipient.
- Thus it does not lead to development of Twin to Twin transfusion syndrome (TTTS)
- It is M/c seen in **monochorionic monoamniotic twins.**
- Since in MCMA twins, superficial vascular anastomosis occurs therefore TTTS does not occur in this type of twin pregnancy.

2 Deep vascular anastomosis

- It occurs at the level of capillary bed.
- M/C variety is anastomosis between a Deep artery and deep vein
- Here the flow of blood is undirectional i.e. one twin is a **permanent donor** and other a **permanent recipient**
- Thus Twins to Twin transfusion syndrome occurs in this type of anastomosis.
- This type of anastomosis is commonly seen in monochorionic diamniotic twins.
- This is the reason why TTTS is seen in **MCDA twins**.

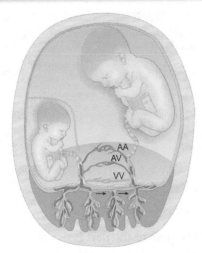

Fig. 19.7: Anastomoses between twins may be artery-to-vein (AV), artery-to-artery (AA), or vein-to-vein (VV). Schematic representation of an AV anastomosis in twin-twin transfusion syndrome that forms a "common villous district" or "third circulation" deep within the villous tissue. Blood from a donor twin may be transferred to a recipient twin through this shared circulation. This transfer leads to a growth-restricted discordant donor twin with markedly reduced amnionic fluid, causing it to be "stuck".

Twin to Twin Transfusion Syndrome

- In this syndrome, blood is transfused from a donor twin to its recipient sibling such that the donor may eventually become anemic and its growth may be restricted.
- In contrast, the recipient becomes polycythemic and may develop circulatory overload manifest as hydrops. The Hb difference between twins is ≥ 5 gm %. **It is also called TAPS Twin anemia polycythemia sequence.** Classically, the donor twin is pale, and its recipient sibling is plethoric.
- Similarly, one portion of the placenta often appears pale compared with the remainder.
- The recipient neonate may also have circulatory overload from heart failure and severe hypervolemia and hyperviscosity. Occlusive thrombosis is another concern.
- Finally, polycythemia in the recipient twin may lead to severe hyperbilirubinemia and kernicterus.
- TTTS typically presents in midpregnancy when the donor fetus becomes oliguric from decreased renal perfusion. This fetus develops oligohydramnios, and the recipient fetus develops severe hydramnios, presumably due to increased urine production.
- Virtual absence of amnionic fluid in the donor sac prevents fetal twins, giving rise to the descriptive term *stuck twin or oligohydramnios polyhydramnios syndrome (TOPS).*

- This amnionic fluid imbalance is associated with growth restrictions contractures, and pulmonary hypoplasia in the donor twin, and premature rupture of the membranes and heart failure in the recipient.

TTTS	
Complications in diamniotic twin	**Complications in Recipient twin**
Anemia	Polycythemia Thrombosis
Less weight (growth restriction)	More weight
Oliguria	Polyuria
Oligohydramnios	Polyhydramnios
⇓	Preterm labor
Pulmonary hypoplasia Limb contracture Renal failure	Fluid overload
	Circulatory heart failure
	Hypervolemia
	Hyperviscosity

Diagnosis of TTTS

According to the **Society for Maternal-Fetal Medicine (2013)**, TTTS is diagnosed based on two criteria:

- Presence of a monochorionic diamnionic pregnancy, and
- Hydramnios defined if the largest vertical pocket is > 8 cm in one twin and oligohydramnios defined if the largest vertical pocket is < 2 cm in the other twin.

Once identified, TTTS is typically staged by the Quintero (1999) staging system:

- Stage I—discordant amnionic fluid volumes as described above, but urine is still visible sonographically within the bladder of the donor twin.
- Stage II—criteria of stage I, but urine is not visible within the donor bladder.
- Stage III—criteria of stage II and **abnormal Doppler studies of the umbilical artery, ductus venosus, or umbilical vein**.
- Stage IV—ascites or frank hydrops in either twin.
- Stage V—demise of either fetus.

Note: In all TTTS – USG surveillance to assess volume of amniotic fluid should began at 16 weeks & repeated 2 weeks after that.

Prognosis

The prognosis for multifetal gestations complicated by TTTS is related to Quintero stage and gestational age at presentation. More than three-fourths of stage I cases remain stable or regress without intervention. Conversely, outcomes in those identified at stage III or higher are much worse, and the perinatal loss rate is 70 to 100 percent.

Management

- The preferred management these days for pregnancy less than 20 weeks is **fetoscopic laser ablation of the anastomosis.** Selective reduction can be considered if severe amniotic fluid and growth disturbances develop before 20 weeks.
- For TTTS in pregnancy more than 20 weeks after serial amniocentesis is done in recipient twin or septostomy is done.

Twin Reversed Arterial Perfusion Sequence and Acardia

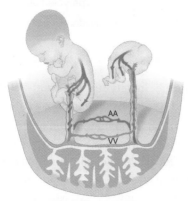

Fig. 19.8: Twin reversed-arterial-perfusion sequence. In the TRAP sequence, there is usually a normally formed donor twin that has features of heart failure, and a recipient twin that lacks a heart. It has been hypothesized that the TRAP sequence is caused by a large artery-to artery placental shunt, often also accompanied by a vein-to vein shunt. Within the single, shared placenta, perfusion pressure of the donor twin overpowers that in the recipient twin, who thus receives reverse blood flow from its twin sibling. The "used" arterial blood that reaches the recipient twin preferentially goes to its iliac vessels and thus perfuses only the lower body. This disrupts growth and development of the upper body.

- Seen in 1% of monochorionic pregnancies.
- It is characterized by a acardiac twin, which receives its blood supply via a large arterio-arterial anastomosis from a normal 'pump' co-twin.
- This results in absent or rudimentary development of the upper body structures like head or neck. This is called **acardiac acephalus** (Fig. 19.9).

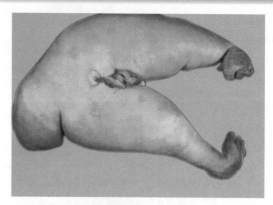

Fig. 19.9 Acardius acephalus

- Sometimes none of the part is developed in acardiac twin it appears just like a mass of flesh. This is acardiac amorphous (Fig. 19.10).

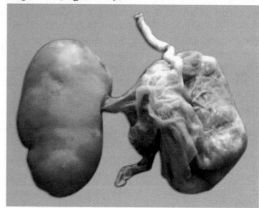

Fig. 19.10 Acardius amorphous

- The mortality of the pump twin is high with death usually occurring from cardiac failure.
- In cases of TRAP, disruption of the acardiac twins cord is the treatment of choice.

Discordant Growth

Unequal sizes of twin fetuses with a difference of 20% (larger twin being used as the index), is called as Discordant growth.

- It is a sign of pathological growth restriction in the smaller fetus.
- As the weight difference within a twin pair increases and the earlier the growth discordance is evident, perinatal mortality increases.
- Most common cause of discordance:
  In dichorionic twins – unequal placental mass.
  In monochorionic twins – Twin-twin transfusion syndrome/genetic syndrome.

- Hazards of discordant growth.
  The smaller fetus is at increased risk of perinatal mortality due to:
  - Respiratory distress
  - Intraventricular hemorrhage
  - Seizure
  - Sepsis
  - Periventricular leukomalacia
  - Necrotising enterocolitis.

  At a difference of more than 30%—Risk of fetal death increases.

- Besides weight—other ultrasonographic parameters indicating discordance:
  - Difference in biparietal diameter is 8 mm or more.
  - Difference in head circumference is 5% or more.
  - Difference in abdominal circumference is 20 mm or more.
  - On color Doppler ultrasound in umbilical arteries systolic to diastolic (S/D) ratio difference is 15% or more.

  But amongst all criterians the best is fetal weight difference i.e. more than equal to 20%.

- Route of delivery: In case of discordant growth vaginal delivery is indicated if:
  - Cervix is ripe
  - Presentation is vertex/vertex
  - Weight of smaller twin is > 1500 gm.

Vanishing Twin

- In a twin pregnancy, if one of the fetuses aborts or gets reabsorbed with 10 weeks of pregnancy, it is called vanishing twin.
- It is seen in up to 20–60% of spontaneous twin conception.
- Bleeding is less.
- It is diagnosed on ultrasound examination by observing a viable pregnancy accompanied by a non-viable one.

- The vanishing twin can cause problems in screening for neural tube defects (elevated levels of alpha fetoprotein).

Note: When fetal death occurs during the second trimester, the remains of the baby get compressed and become paper like and flattened by pressure from the other term called as fetus compressus or papyraceous.

Complications of Twins Pregnancy in General

1. **Maternal complications**
   (1) Anemia
   (2) D/t enlarged uterus: Increased pressure symptoms like odema and respiratory difficulty
   (3) D/t big placenta
       (i) Increased chances of PIH (as mother is exposed to more placental tissue)
       (ii) Increased chances of placenta previa
       (iii) Increased hCG production leading to hyperemesis gravidarum, Theca lutein cyst in ovary.
       (iv) Increased HPL production leading to increased insulin resistance & diabetes
   (4) Increased urine production by fetus leading to polyhydramnios and all its complications like PPH, PROM, abruption placenta.

2. **Fetal complications:**

• Prematurity	• PROM
• IVGR	• Cord prolapse
• Single fetal demise	• Interlocking of twins
• Chromosomal anomaly	• Malpresentation
• Congenital structural anomalies	

Methods to Prevent Preterm Labor in Twins

Do's	Don't DO
1. Frequent antenatal visit	1. Bed rest
2. Frequent USG examination. In monochorionic twins = every 2 weekly. In Dichorionic every 6 weekly	2. I/m progesterone (Ever if there is H/O preterm labor then also I/M progesterone does not lower the risk of PTL)
3. Limited physical activity	3. Prophylactic cervical cerclage
	4. Prophylactic tocolytic

Malpresentations

- In twins most common lie of both the fetus at term is longitudinal.[Q]
- Rarest lie is both the twins transverse.[Q]

Presentations

- Both vertex (Most common)   60%
- Vertex (Ist) – Breech (IInd)   20%
- Breech (Ist) – Vertex (IInd)   10%
- Both Breech   8–10%

Note: Interlocking of twins is a rare complication seen in twins with Ist Breech presentation and IInd vertex presentation..

MANAGEMENT OF LABOR

Time of Delivery

- **Monochorionic monoamniotic twins:** Cesarean section at 32–34 weeks after giving corticosteroid
- Monochorionic diamniotic, elective delivery at 34 to 37$^{6/7}$ weeks (preferred 37 weeks).
- Dichorionic twins elective delivery 38 weeks.
- Triplet pregnancies elective cesarean at 35 weeks after giving corticosteroid.

Mode of Delivery

- **If 1st twin is cephalic–then vaginal delivery is possible**
- **If 1st twin is breech or transverse lie–then cesarean section should be done**

Condition 1

- **If 1st twin is cephalic**
- **If 2nd twin is cephalic** ⎤ **Both vaginal deliveries**

Delivery of First Twin

- Do not give injection methylergometrine after delivery of first twin.

Delivery of the Second Twin

- Soon after delivery of the first twin perform an abdominal examination to determine the lie of the second twin.
- If the second twin is in the longitudinal lie, wait a few minutes for the descent of the presenting part.
- Do a vaginal examination, exclude cord presentation, rupture the membranes and release the liquor carefully to prevent cord prolapse.
- Commence an oxytocin infusion, if contractions do not return in 5–10 minutes.
- Deliver the second twin as soon as possible after the first twin.
- Give a bolus of 5 units of oxytocin after the delivery of the anterior shoulder and conduct active management of the third stage.

Condition 2

If 1st twin cephalic → normal vaginal delivery

2nd twin breech → assisted breech delivery

Condition 3

If 1st twin cephalic - normal vaginal delivery

2nd twin transverse lie = Internal podalic version
under GA in OT
⇓
Make it breech
⇓
Do breech extraction

Internal Podalic Version

- OT procedure
- Done under general anesthesia
- It consists of turning the lie of the fetus by inserting hand into the uterine cavity holding the foot/feet of baby and making them breech
- This should be followed by Breech extraction
- Carries a risk of uterine rupture
- Only indication is: **If 2nd twin is transverse lie**

Condition 4

If 1st twin breech/transverse lie—always cesarean section.

 Note: There is no fixed time interval between the delivery of first or second twin. However, delivery is expedited by forceps or vacuum after a lapse of ≥ 30 minutes.

Indication of cesarean section in twins.

Table 19.1 Indications of cesarean section in twin pregnancy

Indications of elective cesarean delivery
• Conjoined twins.
• Monoamniotic twins (high risk of cord prolapse or entanglement and fetal deaths)
• Twin-twin transfusion syndrome in monochorionic twins
• First baby not cephalic
• Fetal growth restriction in dichorionic twin
• Placenta previa
• Contracted pelvis
• Previous cesarean section
• Severe pre-eclampsia
Indications of emergency cesarean delivery
• Fetal distress
• Cord prolapse in first baby
• Non-progress of labor
• Collision of both twins
Indications of cesarean for second twin
• Second twins transverse, and internal podalic version failed after delivery of first twin
• For a large second twin weighing more than 3.5 kg
• Cord prolapse in 2nd twin
• Prompt closure of cervix after delivery

New Pattern Questions

N1. Which of the following statements about twinning is true?
  a. The frequencies of monozygosity and dizygosity are the same
  b. Division after formation of the embryonic disk result in conjoined twins
  c. The incidence of monozygotic twinning varies with race
  d. A dichorionic twin pregnancy always denotes dizygosity
  e. Twinning causes no appreciable increase in maternal morbidity and mortality over singleton pregnancies

N2. Twin pregnancy predisposes to:
  a. Hydramnios   **[New Pattern Question]**
  b. Pregnancy induced hypertension
  c. Malpresentation
  d. All of the above

N3. Complication specific to monoamniotic twins is:
  a. TTTS   b. Cord entanglement
  c. TRAP   d. Acardiac twin

N4. Absolute proof of monozygosity is determined by:
  a. DNA finger printing
  b. Intervening membrane layers
  c. Sex of the babies
  d. Reciprocal skin grafting

N5. Best time for detecting chorionicity twin pregnancy on USG is:
  a. 8–12 weeks   b. 10–14 weeks
  c. 14–18 weeks   d. 16–24 weeks

N6. The placenta of twins can be:
  a. Dichorionic and monoamniotic in dizygotic twins
  b. Dichorionic and monoamniotic in monozygotic twins
  c. Monochorionic and monoamniotic in dizygotic twins
  d. Dichorionic and diamniotic in monozygotic twins

N7a. A 26-year-old primigravida with a twin gestation at 30 weeks presents for a USG. The sonogram indicates that the fetuses are both male and the placenta appears to be diamniotic and monochorionic. Twin B is noted to have oligohydramnios and to be much smaller than twin A. In this clinical scenario, all of the following are concerns for twin A *except*:
  a. CHF
  b. Anemia
  c. Hydramnios
  d. Widespread thromboses

N7b. If in the same scenario the twins did not show difference in amniotic fluid but PSV of MCA of one twin is > 1.5 MOM and other twin is < 1.0 MOM, the condition could be called as:
  a. TTTS   b. TAPS
  c. TRAPS   d. Any of the above

N8. Indications of urgent delivery of the second baby in twin are all *except*:
  a. Abruptio placentae
  b. Cord prolapse of the second baby
  c. Inadvertent use of IV ergometrine with the delivery of the anterior shoulder of the first baby
  d. Breech presentation of the second baby

N9. In superfecundation which of the following is seen?
  a. Fertilization of 2 ova released at same time, by sperms released at intercourse on 2 different occasions
  b. Fertilization of 2 ova released at same time by sperms released at single intercourse
  c. Both of the above
  d. None of the above

N10. A double headed monster is known as a:
  a. Diplopagus   b. Dicephalus
  c. Craniopagus   d. Heteropagus

N11. Embryo reduction of multiple pregnancy is done at:
  a. 8–10 weeks   b. 11–13 weeks
  c. 13–15 weeks   d. 16–18 weeks

N12. Lowest frequency of twin pregnancy is seen in:
  a. Nigeria   b. Philippines
  c. India   d. Japan

N13. Uncomplicated triplet should be delivered by:
  a. 34 weeks   b. 35 weeks
  c. 37 weeks   d. 38 weeks

N14. Identify the type of twin pregnancy as seen in the USG–plate:

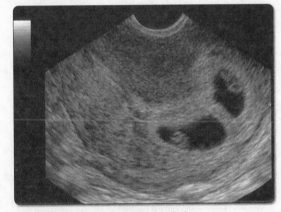

  a. Monochorionic monoamniotic
  b. Monochorionic diamniotic
  c. Dichorionic diamniotic
  d. Conjoint twin

N15. A woman with a dichorionic diamniotic twin pregnancy attends the antenatal clinic at 36 weeks. The first twin is in breech presentation and the second is in cephalic presentation. She has no other pregnancy complications.

What is the best management option?
a. Await spontaneous onset of labor
b. Induce labor at 37 weeks
c. Perform an elective cesarean section at 37 weeks
d. Perform an elective cesarean section at 40 weeks

N16. A woman with a monochorionic monoamniotic twin pregnancy attends the antenatal clinic at 33 weeks. She has no other pregnancy complications.

What is the most appropriate management?
a. Await spontaneous onset of labor till 38 weeks
b. Perform a cesarean section at 33 weeks after administering a course of corticosteroids
c. Perform a cesarean section at 37 weeks
d. Perform a cardiotocograph daily till 37 weeks

Previous Year Questions

1. According to Hellin's law chances of twins in pregnancy are: [PGI Dec 00]
   a. 1 in 60   b. 1 in 70
   c. 1 in 80   d. 1 in 90
   e. 1 in 100

2. Monochorionic monoamniotic twin occurs if division occurs:
   a. Before 24 hours   b. 1–4 days
   c. 4–8 days   d. > 8 days

3. Twin peak sign seen in: [PGI Dec 05]
   a. Monochorionic diamniotic
   b. Dichorionic monoamniotic
   c. Conjoined twins
   d. Diamniotic dichorionic
   e. None of the above

4. Correct statement about establishing the chorionicity in twin pregnancy is: [AI 10]
   a. Same sex rule out dichorionicity
   b. Twin peak in dichorionicity
   c. Thick membrane is present in monochorionic
   d. Best detected after 16 weeks

5. Most common type of twin pregnancy is: [PGI June 97, MP 08]
   a. Vertex + transverse b. Both vertex
   c. Vertex + breech   d. Both breech

6. True statement regarding twin delivery is: [AI 12]
   a. First twin has more chances of asphyxia
   b. Second twin has more chances of developing polycythemia
   c. Second twin has more chances of developing hyaline membrane disease
   d. Increased mortality in first twin

7. Vaginal delivery is allowed in all *except*: [AI 09/AIIMS May 11]
   a. Monochorionic monoamniotic twins
   b. First twin cephalic and second breech
   c. Extended breech
   d. Mento anterior

8. Blood chimerism is maintained by: [AI 11]
   a. Monochorionic dizygotic twins
   b. Dichorionic dizygotic twins
   c. Vanishing twins
   d. Singleton pregnancy

9. To say twin discordance the differences in the two twins should be: [AIIMS May 02]
   a. 15% with the larger twin as index
   b. 15% with the smaller twin as index
   c. 25% with the larger twin as index
   d. 25% with the smaller twin as index

10. In multiple pregnancy, fetal reduction is done by: [AIIMS June 98]
    a. KCl
    b. Mifepristone
    c. PGF2-alpha
    d. Methotrexate

11. Which of the following is part true about monozygotic twin formation. [PGI Nov 2016]
    a. If division occurs after embryonic disc formation it results in conjoint twin.
    b. If division occurs before 72 hrs, it results in formation of diamniotic dichorionic twins.
    c. If division occurs b/w 4-8 days, it results in formation of monochorionic monoamniotic twin
    d. If division occurs after 8 days, it results in formation of monochorionic monoamniotic

Answers with Explanations to New Pattern Questions

N1. **Ans. is b, i.e Division after formation of the embryonic disk result in conjoined twins**

Ref. Dutta Obs 7/e, p 200,202, 204, 205

- As discussed in text–frequency of monozygotic and dizygotic twins is not same. Dizygotic twins are more common.
- The incidence of MZ remains same throughout the wound (1 in 250 pregnancies) whereas incidence of DZ twins varies with race.
- As discussed in the text: DZ twins are always dichorionic but MZ twins can either be monochorionic on dichorionic
- ∴ It is incorrect to say dichorionic twins are always dizygotic (i.e. option d is incorrect).
- In twin pregnancies: there is a higher risk of low birth weight babies and preterm labor. Multiple pregnancies are commonly associated with moderate to severe anemia, gestational hypertension, malpresentation, polyhydramnios, cord prolapse, abruption or placenta previa in mother (i.e. option e is incorrect).

N2. **Ans. is d, i.e. All of the above** *Ref. Dutta Obs. 7/e, p 206*

See the text for explanation

N3. **Ans. is b, i.e. Cord entanglement** *Ref. Williams 24/e, p 902*

Monochorionic twin pregnancy is associated with a specific complication i.e. cord entanglement because both twins lie in the same sac.

Remember: In monoamniotic twins, detailed fetal heart rate monitoring should begin from 26–28 weeks.
- They should be delivered between **32–34 weeks by cesarean section**.

Note: Acardiac twin, Twin to Twin Transfusion Syndrome (TTTS) and Twin Reversed Arterial Perfusion (TRAP–another name for acardiac twin) are complications seen in monochorionic diamniotic twins

N4. **Ans. is a, i.e. DNA finger printing** *Ref. Dutta Obs. 7/e, p 201*

The most definite proof of monozygosity is DNA finger printing by DNA microprobe technique.

Summary of Determination of Zygosity

	Placenta	Communicating vessels	Intervening membranes	Sex	Genetic features (dominant blood group) DNA finger printing	Skin grafting (Reciprocal)	Follow-up
Monozygotic	One	Present	2 (amnions)	Always identical	Same	Acceptance	Usually identical
Dizygotic	Two (most often fused)	Absent	4 (2 amnions 2 chorions)	May differ	Differ	Rejection	Not identical

Ref. Dutta Obs. 7/e, p 207

N5. **Ans. is b, i.e. 10–14 weeks** *Ref. High risk pregnancy areas 4/e, p 177*

Best time to detect chorionicity by USG is between 11–14 weeks, although twin peak sign can be seen until 20 weeks.

N6. **Ans. is d, i.e Dichorionic and diamniotic in monozygotic twins**

Ref. Dutta Obs. 7/e, p 200, 201, Williams 23/e, p 861 figure 39.2

- As discussed in text dizygotic twins always have dichorionic and diamniotic placentas (i.e option a and c are incorrect).
- Monozygotic twins can have monochorionic/monoamniotic placentas depending upon the time of division... but always remember- Amnion develops after the chorion, so dichorionicity implies diamnionicity... it can never be that a twin is dichorionic but monoamniotic (i.e. option b is incorrect).

N7a. Ans. is b, i.e Anemia *Ref. Dutta Obs. 7/e, p 206-207, Williams Obs. 23/e, p 874*

This scenario represents a typical case of twin to twin transfusion syndrome.

N7b. Ans. is b, i.e. TAPS

There is no oligopolyhydramnios but there is difference in PSV of middle cerebral artery.

It means one twin has anemia: so viscosity of blood is less, so Flow in Middle cerebral artery is more hence PSV (peak systolic velocity) will be more In the other twin, PSV is less i.e. polycythemia is seen. This condition in which there is significant Hb difference in twins without discrepency in amniotic fluid volume, of both the twins is called as **twin anemia polycythemia sequelae (TAPS).**

It is diagnosed antenatally by a difference in PSV of MCA of both the twins.

N8. Ans. is d, i.e. Breech presentation of the second baby *Ref. Dutta Obs. 7/e, p 208*

The interval between delivery of twins should be less than 30 minutes. If there is a delay of more than 30 minutes, interference should be done.

But there are some conditions in which urgent delivery of the second baby is required.

Indications of urgent delivery of the second baby: (1) Severe (intrapartum) vaginal bleeding (2) Cord prolapse of the second baby (3) Inadvertent use of intravenous ergometrine with the delivery of the anterior shoulder of the first baby (4) First baby delivered under general anesthesia (5) Appearance of fetal distress.

Management: In all these conditions, the baby should be delivered quickly. A rational scheme is given below which depends on the lie, presentation and station of the head.

- Head
- If low down, delivery by forceps
- If high up, delivery by internal version under general anesthesia.
  - Breech should be delivered by breech extraction
  - Transverse lie—internal podalic version followed by breech extraction under general anesthesia.

If, however, the patient bleeds heavily following the birth of the first baby, immediate low rupture of the membranes usually succeeds in controlling the blood loss.

 Remember: The only indication for internal podalic version these days is:
- Second twin transverse lie

N9. Ans. is a, i.e. Fertilization of 2 ova released at same time, by sperms released at intercourse on 2 different occasions

Ref. Dutta Obs. 7/e, p 202

Superfecundation

It is the fertilization of two different ova released in the same cycle, by separate acts of coitus within a short period of time.

Superfetation

- It is the fertilization of two ova released in different menstrual cycles.
- This is theoretically possible until the decidual space is obliterated by 12 weeks of pregnancy.

N10. Ans. is b, i.e. Dicephalus *Ref. Munro Kerr's 10/e, p 115*

Twin related terminology	Feature
Dicephalus[Q]	Double headed monsters in which the lower parts are more or less fused into one
Syncephalus[Q]	Single headed monster which show duplication of the lower limb and sometimes of the lower part of the trunk
Fetal papyraceous or compressus[Q]	It is a state which occurs if one of the fetus dies early The dead fetus is compressed between the membranes of the living fetus and the uterine wall It can occur in dizygotic as well as monozygotic twins (*most common*)
Fetal acardiacus[Q]	Here one fetus does not possess a heart and the development of upper part of the body almost absent. The normal twin is called "pump twin". It occurs only in monozygotic twin.

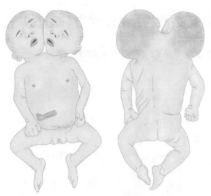

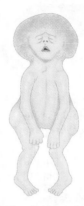

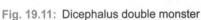

Fig. 19.11: Dicephalus double monster

Fig. 19.12: Syncephalus double monster

N11. **Ans. is b, i.e. 11–13 weeks** *Ref. Dutta Obs. 7/e, p 211*

Selective reduction: If there are 4 or more fetuses, selective reduction of the fetuses leaving behind only two is done to improve outcome of the cofetuses. This can be done by intracardiac injection of **potassium chloride between 11 and 13 weeks under ultrasonic guidance using a 22 gauge needle**. It is done transabdominally. Umbilical cord of the targeted twin is occluded by fetoscopic ligation or by laser or by bipolar coagulation, to protect the cotwin from adverse drug effect. Multiple pregnancy reduction improves perinatal outcome in women with triplets or more.

Risk of miscarriage = 5–7%.

Selective termination of a fetus with structural or genetic abnormality may be done in a dichorionic multiple pregnancy in the second trimester.

N12. **Ans. is d, i.e. Japan** *Ref. High Risk Pregnancy Areas 4/e, p 170*

Highest incidence of twin pregnancy is in Nigeria, lowest incidence of twin pregnancy is in Japan.

N13. **Ans. is b, i.e. 35 weeks** *Ref. Fernando Arias 4/e, p 180*

Uncomplicated dichorionic twin are delivered by 37–38 weeks

Uncomplicated monochorionic twin are delivered by 36–37 weeks

Uncomplicated triplets are delivered by 35 weeks.

N14. **Ans. is c, i.e. Dichorionic diamniotic** *Ref. High Risk Pregnancy Areas 4/e, p 170*

The USG shown in the figure–if you see it carefully you can see placental tissue between the 2 sacs–this means twin peak sign is positive, i.e. it is an example of dichorionic diamniotic pregnancy.

N15. **Ans. is c, i.e. perform an elective cesarean section at 37 weeks**

N16. **Ans. is b, i.e. perform a cesarean section at 33 weeks after administering a course of corticosteroids**

See the text explanation

Answers with Explanations to Previous Year Questions

1. **Ans. is c, i.e. 1 in 80**   *Ref. Dutta Obs. 7/e, p 202*

   According to Hellin's rule

   The mathematical frequency of multiple pregnancy is:

   - Twins   1 in 80
   - Triplets   1 in (80)^2
   - Quadruplets   1 in (80)^3 and so on

2. **Ans. is d, i.e. >8 days**   *Ref. Dutta Obs. 7/e, p 200*

Monozygotic Twins			
		↓ Division of single fertilised ovum	
<3 days	4–8 days	>8 days	>14 days
dichorionic diamniotic	monochorionic diamniotic	monochorionic monoamniotic	conjoined twin

3. **Ans. is d, i.e. Diamniotic dichorionic**   *Ref. Dutta Obs. 7/e, p 203; Williams Obs. 23/e, p 864, 865*

   - **Twin peak or lambda sign:** It is characteristic of dichorionic pregnancies and is due to the chorionic tissue between the two layers of the intertwin membrane at the placental origin. A potential space exists in the intertwin membrane which is filled by proliferating placental villi, giving rise to a twin peak sign. Twin peak appears as a triangle with base at chorionic surface and apex in inter twin membrane. In monochorionic twins there is no chorionic tissue, and inter twin membrane is composed of 2 amnion only giving rise to the "T" sign on ultrasound.
   - Best time to detect chorionicity on USG: 11–14 weeks.

4. **Ans. is b, i.e. Twin peak in dichorionicity**   *Ref: Dutta Obs. 7/e, p 204, Williams Obs 23/e, p 864, 865*

   "Chorionicity of the placenta is best diagnosed by ultrasound at 6 to 9 weeks of gestation. In dichorionic twins there is a thick septum between the chorionic sacs. It is best identified at the base of the membrane, where a triangular projection is seen. This is known as lambda or twin peak sign. Presence of lambda or twin peak sign indicates dichorionic placenta"
   Ref. Dutta Obs. 7/e, p 207

   So it is clear that lambda/Twin peak sign clearly indicates dichorionic placenta and is hence the correct **option 'b'**.

   As far as other options are concerned.

   Option a – Same sex rules out dichorionicity, this is incorrect because:

   Twins of opposite sex are almost always dizygotic dichorionic but same sex does not rule out dichorionicity.

   Option c – Thick membrane is present in monochorionic twins:

   This is also incorrect because monochorionic means there is a single chorion whereas dichorionic means there are 2 chorions so obviously dichorionic membrane will be thick.

   "Monochorionic pregnancies have a dividing membrane that is so thin, it may not be seen until the second trimester. The membrane is generally less than 2 mm thick and magnification reveals only 2 layers (of amnion)"
   Ref. Williams Obs. 23/e p 864

   Option d – Chorionicity is best detected after 16 weeks:

   Again this statement is incorrect because the best time to detect chorionicity by USG is between 6 to 9 weeks.

5. **Ans. is b, i.e. Both vertex**   *Ref. Dutta Obs. 7/e, p 202, 203*
   - In twins most common lie of both the fetus at term is longitudinal.[Q]
   - Rarest lie is both the twins transverse.[Q]

Presentations

• Both vertex (Most common)	60%
• Vertex (Ist) – Breech (IInd)	20%
• Breech (Ist) – Vertex (IInd)	10%
• Both Breech	8–10%

 Note: **Interlocking of twins is a rare complication seen in twins with Ist breech presentation and IInd vertex presentation.**

6. **Ans. is b, i.e Second twin has more chances of developing polycythemia**

Ref. Fernando Arias 3/e, p 312, Dutta Obs. 7/e, p 206

- Twin pregnancy in general is associated with higher incidence of perinatal morbidity and mortality.
- Perinatal mortality in twins is 5 times greater than in singleton pregnancies.
- Perinatal mortality in twins varies with birth order and the type of placentation.
- "Second twins do not do as well as the first twin…perinatal mortality being 9% for the first twin and 14% for the second twin". —*Fernando Arias 3/e, p 297*
- Also monochorionic—monoamniotic twins have a poor prognosis, perinatal mortality being 50%.
- Now with this background lets see each option separately.

Option a: *First twin has more chances of asphyxia—***incorrect as:**

- "*Asphyxia and stillbirth are more common (in twin pregnancy) due to increased prevalence of pre-eclampsia, malpresentations, placental abruption and increased operative interferences. The second baby is more at risk.* —*Dutta Obs. 7/e, p 206*

Option b: Second twin has more chances of developing polycythemia:

- This statement can be true as second baby has more chances of asphyxia which can stimulate erythropoiesis in the second twin. Also there are chances of bleeding from the first twin into the second twin in case of monochorionic twins which can cause polycythemia.

Option c: Second twin has more chances of developing hyaline membrane disease—this is incorrect as is evident from the following lines of Williams:

- "*As measured by determination of the lecithin and sphingomyelin ratio, pulmonary maturation is usually synchronous in twins.*" —*Williams 23/e, p 880*
- Hence second twin does not have increased chances of developing hyaline membrane disease.
- **Remember:** This does not apply to discordant twins, in discordant twins the growth retarded fetus usually has a more advanced degree of lung maturity than the other, therefore timing of delivery of the discordant twin should be based on the testing of amniotic fluid surrounding the larger twin. —*Fernando Arias 3/e, p 312*
- Coming to the last option—Increased mortality in first twin (option d)
  As discussed in the beginning:
- "*Second twins do not do as well as the first twin…perinatal mortality being 9% for the first twin and 14% for the second twin*" —*Fernando Arias 3/e, p 297*
- Thus **option d** is also incorrect.

7. **Ans. is a, i.e. Monochorionic monoamniotic twins** *Ref. Fernando Arias 3/e, p 314; Dutta Obs. 7/e, p 210*

- In face presentation the best presentation is mentoanterior, especially left mentoanterior and delivery is possible. (i.e. option a is correct)
- In twins, the chances of vaginal delivery are high if the first twin or presenting twin is cephalic. (i.e. option b is correct)
- Extended breech is the most common breech presentation and is also the best possible presentation for a normal vaginal delivery in breech (option c is correct)
- In monochorionic monoamniotic presentations the twins share a single amniotic sac and placenta so there is almost a 50% incidence of cord accidents and that is one reason which even prompts to do a preterm cesarean to many practioners to avoid a sudden fetal cord entrapment and fetal death.

"A situation requiring cesarean delivery in twin pregnancy is a monoamniotic placentation. The fetal mortality in these pregnancies is greater than 50% and the overwhelming cause is cord accidents such as cord prolapse or entanglement."
Ref: Fernando Arias 3/e, p 314

Also Know:

Indications of Cesarean in Twins and Malpresentations.

Twins	Malpresentations
a. Twins with bad prognosis viz—Conjoint twins and Monochorionic and monoamniotic twins b. Twin to twin transfusion syndrome (seen in monochorionic twins) c. Discordant twin with weight of smaller twin less than 1500 gm d. Severe IUGR of one or both twins e. First twin non vertex *Obstetrical factors like-contracted pelvis, fetal distress*	a. Transverse lie b. Brow presentation c. Face-mentoposterior presentation d. Breech-Footling/Knee presentation

 Note: There is no valid reason to perform LSCS in all cases of second twins for noncephalic presentation.

8. **Ans. is a, i.e. Monochorionic dizygotic twins**

   Ref. Placental Chimerism in Early Human Pregnancy. Indian Journal of Human Genetics, Year 2005 Vol 11, Issue 2, p 84, 85

   In biology, the word chimerism is used when an organism contains cell population from two or more zygote.

   This may be:

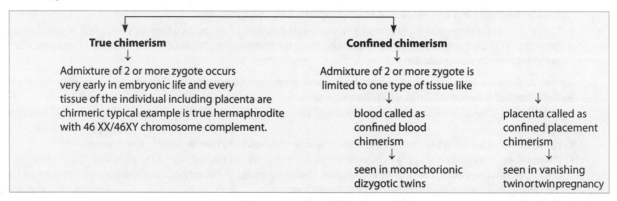

   From the above text, the answer to our question is quite obvious that blood chimerism is seen in monochorionic dizygotic twins.

   But here I would like to point out that in the chapter on multifetal pregnancy we have read dizygotic twins are dichorionic so how do we explain the phenomenon of monochorionic dizygotic twinning.

   Monochorionic Dizygotic Twins

   Monochorionic diamniotic placenta is rare in dizygotic twins. All cases which have been documented are observed by induction of ovulation along or during IVF cycle.

   The most possible cause explaining this phenomenon is formation of 2 placentas originating from two zygotes early in pregnancy which unite to form an architecturally single placenta. The newly formed blood vessels create an anastomosis between the dizygotic twins and allow reciprocal blood chimerism. Since the incidence of IVF is on increase, cases of monochorionic dizygotic twins is also increasing recently.

9. **Ans. is c, i.e. 25% with the larger twin as index**   *Ref. Williams Obs. 23/e, p 876, 877*

   Unequal sizes of twin fetuses with a difference of 25% (larger twin being used as the index), is called as Discordant growth.

10. **Ans. is a, i.e. KCl**   *Ref. Dutta Obs. 7/e, p 211*

Multifetal pregnancy reduction is done in high order pregnancies (> 4 fetus) to minimize complications like:

- Preterm delivery
- Fetal growth retardation
- Anemia   Associated with high
- PPH   fetal numbers
- Pre-eclampsia
- Increased neonatal mortality

Procedure : It is done by intracardiac injection of potassium chloride,[Q] under ultrasound guidance.

Time   : Between 10–12 weeks of gestation.

Usually, two fetuses are left undisturbed and rest reduced.

Complications of Reduction

- Preterm labor
- Amnionitis
- Chances of losing all fetuses.

 Also Know:

Selective fetal reduction **is done when one fetus in a multiple gestation is abnormal. It is done similar to** *multifetal reduction.*

11. **Ans. is a, b, & d i.e. (a) If division occurs after embryonic disc formation it results in conjoint twin; (b) If division occurs before 72 hrs, it results in formation of diamniotic dichorionic twins; and (d) If division occurs after 8 days, it results in formation of monochorionic monoamniotic**   *Ref. Williams Obs. 23/e*

See the text for Explanation

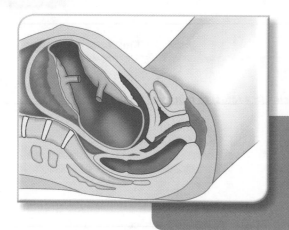

Chapter 20

Pregnancy in Rh-Negative Women

Chapter at a Glance

- Rh-Antigen
- Rh-negative Pregnancy: An Overview
- Rh-negative Female with ICT Negative
- Rh-negative Female with ICT Positive
- Women with Previous Affected Pregnancy
- Anti D Prophylaxis

Rh-ANTIGEN

- The Rh-system was discovered by **Landsteiner in 1940**. The rhesus blood group antigens comprise of 5 antigens C, c, D, E and e. These antigens are located on short arm of chromosome 1.

- Most immunogenic among them is the Rh (D). Its presence or absence (D) designates a person as Rh-positive or negative.

- Lewis and I antigen do not cause erythroblastosis fetalis and differ from all of the other red cell antigens in that they are not synthesized in the red cells membrane but are absorbed into it.

- Fetal Rh-antigen are present by 38th day after conception.

- Although incompatibility for the major blood group antigens A and B is the most common cause of hemolytic disease in the newborn, the resulting anemia is usually very mild. About 20% of all infants have an ABO maternal blood group incompatibility, but only 5% are clinically affected.

- Most species of anti-A and anti-B antibodies are immunoglobulin **M (IgM)**, **which cannot cross** the **placenta** and therefore cannot gain access to fetal erythrocytes. In addition, fetal red cells have fewer A and B antigenic sites than adult cells and are thus less immunogenic. The disease is invariably milder than D-isoimmunization and rarely results in significant anemia.

Rh-NEGATIVE PREGNANCY: AN OVERVIEW

Rh-isoimmunization occurs when a Rh-negative woman bears a Rh-positive fetus. Normally, the fetal red cells containing the Rh-antigen enter the maternal circulation during first trimester in 5% cases, during third trimester in 46% cases. Maximum occurs at the time of delivery. There are a few conditions which predispose to fetomaternal hemorrhage.

Conditions predisposing to isoimmunization in Rh –ve female/fetomaternal hemorrhage/Indications of giving Anti D	
• Abortion[Q], ectopic pregnancy, molar pregnancy	• Trauma
• Cordocentesis	• Antepartum hemorrhage
• Amniocentesis[Q]	• Vaginal delivery
• Chorionic villous sampling[Q]	• Cesarean section
• Attempted version[Q]	• Forceps delivery
• Manual removal of placenta	• Placental abruption
	• Blood transfusion

Fetal Problems in Rh-Negative Pregnancy

As a result of above conditions, fetal blood carrying Rh-antigen enters maternal circulation and stimulates production of antibodies.

Immunization is unlikely to occur unless at least 0.1 mL of fetal blood enters the maternal circulation.

Detectable antibodies usually develop after 6 months following larger volume of fetomaternal bleed.

Antibodies once formed remain throughout life:

Types of Antibodies—Two types of antibodies are formed:

- **IgM**—This type of antibody is the first to appear in the maternal circulation and agglutinates red cells containing D when suspended in saline. **IgM being larger molecules cannot pass through the placental barrier and is not harmful to the fetus**.
- **IgG**—It is also called incomplete or blocking antibody. **Because of its small molecule, it can cross the placental barrier and cause damage to the fetus. It appears at a later period than does the IgM antibody.** This is the reason why first pregnancy is not affected in Rh-negative females.

Fetal Affection by the Rh-Antibody

The antibody formed in the maternal system (IgG) crosses the placental barrier and enters into the fetal circulation. **The antibody will not have any effect on Rh-negative fetus**. If the fetus is Rh-positive, the antibody becomes attached to the antigen sites on the surface of the fetal erythrocytes. The affected cells are rapidly removed from the circulation by the reticuloendothelial system. **Depending upon the degree of agglutination and destruction of the fetal red cells, various types of fetal hemolytic diseases appear.**

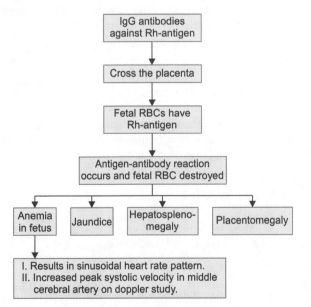

Clinical manifestations of the hemolytic disease of the fetus and neonate are:

- **Hydrops fetalis**
- **Icterus gravis neonatorum**
- **Congenital anemia of the newborn**

Hydrops Fetalis

This is the most serious form of Rh-hemolytic disease. Excessive destruction of the fetal red cells leads to severe anemia, tissue anoxemia and metabolic acidosis.

These have adverse effects on the fetal heart and brain and on the placenta.

Hyperplasia of the placental tissue occurs in an effort to increase the transfer of oxygen but the available fetal red cells (oxygen carrying cells) are progressively diminished due to hemolysis.

Ultimately this leads to **hypoproteinemia** which is responsible for generalized edema **(hydrops fetalis)**, ascites and hydrothorax.

Fetal death occurs sooner or later due to cardiac failure.

Congenital Anemia of the Newborn: This is the mildest form of the disease where the hemolysis is going on slowly. Although the anemia develops slowly within first few weeks of life, the jaundice is not usually evident.

The destruction of the red cells continues up to 6 weeks after which the antibodies are not available for hemolysis.

The liver and spleen are enlarged, as they are sites of extramedullary erythropoiesis.

Thus in Rh-negative pregnancy antibodies formed in mother eventually harm the fetus, so it becomes important to know whether antibodies are present in pregnant female or not.

 Important One Liners

- Rh antigen develops in fetus 30–40 days after fertilisation i.e (7.5 weeks of pregnancy)
- Maximum chances of feto maternal hemorrhage are beyond 28 weeks
- Minimum fetal blood needed to stimulate maternal immune system 0.1 mL

CATEGORY 1

Rh negative female with negative ICT: If the woman is found Rh-negative, Rh-grouping of the husband is to be done. If the husband is also Rh-negative, there is no problem so far as Rh-factor is concerned. If the husband is found to be Rh-positive, further investigation is to be carried out which aim at:

- To detect whether the woman has already been immunized to Rh-antigen by doing **Indirect Coomb's test**

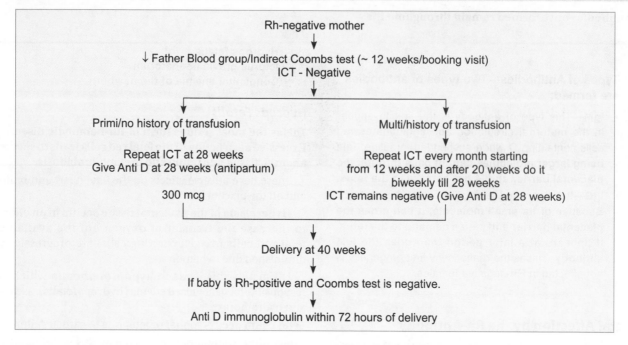

Rh-negative mother
↓
↓ Father Blood group/Indirect Coombs test (~ 12 weeks/booking visit)
ICT - Negative
↓

Primi/no history of transfusion
↓
Repeat ICT at 28 weeks
Give Anti D at 28 weeks (antipartum)
300 mcg

Multi/history of transfusion
↓
Repeat ICT every month starting
from 12 weeks and after 20 weeks do it
biweekly till 28 weeks
ICT remains negative (Give Anti D at 28 weeks)

↓
Delivery at 40 weeks
↓
If baby is Rh-positive and Coombs test is negative.
↓
Anti D immunoglobulin within 72 hours of delivery

Method to know whether antibodies have been formed or not:

- **Indirect Coombs test:** It is done on maternal blood and if it is positive it indicates, Rh-antibodies are formed in mother whereas a negative test indicates that Rh-antibodies are not formed, i.e. isoimmunization has not occurred.

- If the test is found negative at 12th week, it is to be repeated at 20 weeks and 28 weeks in primigravida. In multigravida, the test is to be repeated at monthly intervals from 24 weeks onwards. The need for 4 weekly antibody screening in nonimmunized Rh-negative women is not unusually accepted because Rh-autoimmunization rarely happens during antenatal period and the first immunized pregnancy rarely produces severe fetal hemolytic disease.

- If the test is found positive. Patient should be followed up as a case of Rh-negative immunized pregnancy.

Now here it is very important to understand one very important concept:

Anti D is given to a pregnant Rh-negative mother: (Called as **Antepartum Prophylaxis**)

Principle behind giving Anti D is, that if anti D is given to a Rh-negative mother and if due to any reason fetal blood with Rh antigen enters mothers circulation, this Anti D will lead to an antigen antibody reaction and fetal RBC will be destroyed before it could **stimulate mothers immune system to produce** Rh antibodies.

- Thus the usefulness of administering Anti D is only before maternal Rh-antibodies are formed. If maternal antibodies are already formed then there is no point in giving Anti D.

- *In other words Anti D should only be give if Indirect Coombs test is negative.*

- *If Indirect Coombs test is positive then do not give Anti D.*

CATEGORY 2

Includes those Ph negative females in whom Indirect Coombs Test is positive i.e. Isoimmunized females.

- ICT positive means that already mothers immune system is stimulated and producing antibodies hence no use of giving Anti D

- In these females, it becomes important to know how many antibodies are produced so we Do anti body titre: We take mothers blood & dilute it to 1:2 then 1:4 then 1:8, 1:16, 1:32 etc. Now if antibodies are detected on dilution to 1:16 or more, it means significant number of antibodies are present i.e. critical titre is 1:16:

1. If antibody titre remains below critical titre
⇓
Follow up patient by doing antibody titre every 4 weekly till the 24 weeks and then 2 weekly after that
⇓
If values remains below critical titre then deliver patient between **37-38 weeks of pregnancy**.

2. If antibody titre is more than critical titre at any time- This means significant member of antibodies are present which can cross placenta and lead to fetal hemolysis
   - Now in this case, it becomes important to know how much hemolysis has occurred.
   - This can be known by 2 methods:
     - Amniocentesis (done in past)
     - Peak systolic velocity of middle cerebal artery (Done nowadays)

- **Amniotic fluid evaluation**
  Basis of test: When fetal blood cells undergo hemolysis, breakdown pigments, mostly bilirubin, are present in the amniotic fluid via urine of fetus. The amount of bilirubin in amniotic fluid correlates roughly with the degree of hemolysis and thus indirectly predicts the severity of the fetal anemia.

- Now the amniotic fluid which due to hemolysis will have bilirubin is sent in a dark colored bottle to lab.
- There spectrophotometric analysis of fluid is done between 350 nm & 750 nm
- Normal Amniotic fluid spectrophotometric analysis shows straight line (Green in Figs. 20.1A and B)
- When bilirubin is present in amniotic fluid – a bulge is seen at 450 nm (Red in Fig. 20.1). This difference is called as delta optical density (DOD 450 nm) and plotted on a Liley's graph (Figs. 20.2A and B).
- The more the bilirubin, more is the bulge i.e. more is DOD 450 nm

Also Know:
- Meconium causes a bulge @ 410 nm
- Blood causes a bulge @ 412 nm

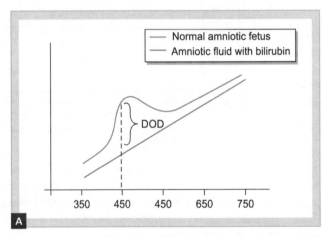

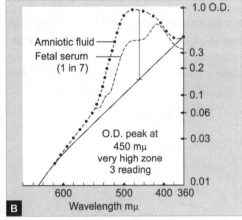

Figs. 20.1A and B: (A) — = Normal amniotic fluid; — = Amniotic fluid with bilirubin; (B) The deviation at 450 nm from a normal optical density cure. The fetal serum bilirubin levels mirror those of liquor amnii.

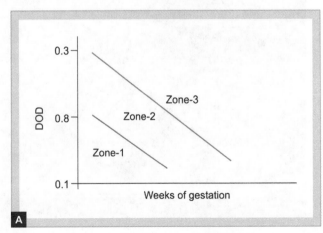

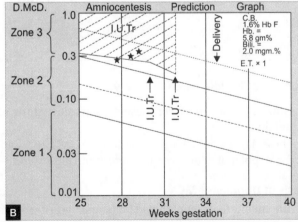

Figs. 20.2A and B: (A) Lileys graph; (B) Liley Zones.)

In zone 1: If DOD comes in Zone 1: fetus is mildly affected

In zone 2: In upper part of zone 2: it means Hb of fetus is 8–10 g/dL. If DOD comes in lower part of zone: Fetal Hb is between 11 to 13.9 g/dL

In zone 3: If DOD comes in zone 3 then fetal Hb is < 8 g/dL

Now upper part of zone 2 and zone 3 come under severe disease.

Management as Per Delta optical density

If DOD comes in zone 1	Repeat amniocentesis every 4 weeks
If DOD comes in lower zone 2	Repeat amniocentesis every 2 weeks
If DOD comes in upper zone 2 or zone 3	In that case if pregnancy is < 34 weeks do In utero blood transfusion If pregnancy is ≥ 34 weeks deliver the patient.

- The **main limitation of the Liley's curve is** that it starts at 27 weeks of gestation and is uptill 42 weeks and extrapolation of the lines to earlier gestational ages is inaccurate.
- Queenan have developed a curve for fetal assessment from 14 to 42 weeks, divided into 4 zones.

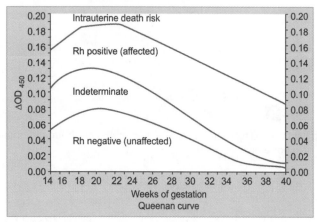

Fig. 20.3: Queenan curve

Doppler of Middle Cerebral Artery

- Now as discussed earlier these days amniocentesis is not done
- These days when ICT is positive and titre is ≥ 1:16 we go for Doppler of middle cerebral artery and ultrasound

Basis of Doppler of MCA

- The anemic fetus shunts blood preferentially to the brain to maintain oxygenation. The velocity rises because of increased cardiac output and decreased velocity.

- Hence peak systolic velocity increases in MCA.(≥ 1.5 multiple of meridian).
- *So there can be 2 situations:*
  - PSV of MCA < 1.5 MOM: In this case, nothing needs to be done

    Just follow up every 2 weekly and deliver patient between 37–38 weeks
  - If PSV is ≥ 1.5 MOM: It means severe hemolysis has occurred leading to fetal anemia. Now if Gestational age is ≥ 34 weeks—Deliver immediately

If gestatinal age is < 34 weeks – do a cordocentesis & if hematocrit is < 30% give Inutero blood transfusion

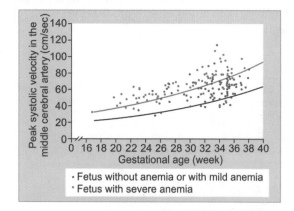

Fig. 20.4: Doppler measurements of the peak systolic velocity in the middle cerebral artery (MCA) in 165 fetuses at risk for severe anemia. The blue line indicates the median peak systolic velocity in normal pregnancies, and the red line shows 1.5 multiples of the median.

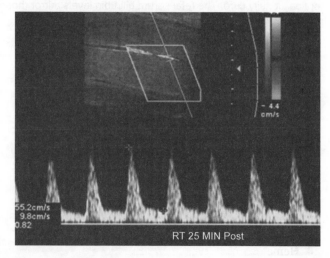

Fig. 20.5:

- **IUT:** Fresh (< 7 days old) **O-negative** blood is given to the fetus by doing a cordocentesis. The amount of blood required to be transfused is calculated by various formulas depending upon fetal Hct and donor Hct.
- Nicolaides and coworkers recommend that transfusions be commenced when the hemoglobin is at least 2g/dL below the mean for normal fetuses of corresponding gestational age. Other clinicians perform transfusion when the **fetal Hct is below 30%**, (Hb < 8 gm/dL).
- Therefore, if PSV-MCA is above 1.5 MOM and period of gestation is <34 weeks, then next step is cordocentesis to determine hematocrit. If hematocrit is < 30% then IUT is done.
- **Note:** M/C complication of cordocentesis is bleeding.

 Important One Liners

- **Conditions of Rh negative when pregnancy is terminated between 37-38 weeks**
  i. PSV of MCA is < 1.5 MOM
  ii. If critical titre is < 1:16.
- Conditions of Rh the negative when pregnancy is terminated at 34 weeks.
  i. Hydrops fetalis on ultrasound
  ii. On amniocentesis if Delta optical density is in upper zone 2 or zone 3.
  iii. If peak systolic velocity in MCA ≥ 1.5 MOM.

CATEGORY 3

Women with Previous Affected Pregnancy

After the first affected pregnancy, the ability to predict fetal anemia from the maternal anti-D antibody titers is lost and now these pregnancies should be monitored by MCA-PSV and amniotic fluid bilirubin concentration.

Delivery in Rh Negative Patient
- Mode of delivery—Vaginal delivery
- Injection Methylergometrine is contraindicated
- Early cord clamping is done
- Do following tests on newborn:

Tests Done on newborn blood
- Blood group/Rh status
- Bilirubin level
- Hematocrit
- Direct coombs Test

- If baby is Rh positive and Direct Coomb test is negative then mother is given a repeat dose of Anti D after delivery **called as post partum prophylaxis.**

ANTI D PROPHYLAXIS

- It is an IgG antibody
- It is a poly clonal antibody
- Current preparations of anti-D immune globulin are derived from human plasma donated by individuals with high titer anti-D immunoglobulin i.e. D antibodies. Formulations prepared by cold ethanol fractionation and ultrafiltration must be administered intramuscularly because they contain plasma proteins that could result in anaphylaxis if given intravenously. However, formulations prepared using ion exchange chromatography may be administered either intramuscularly or intravenously. This is important for treatment of significant fetomaternal hemorrhage, which is discussed subsequently
- Depending on the preparation, the half-life of anti-D immune globulin ranges from 16 to 24 days, which is why it is given both in the third trimester and following delivery
- The standard intramuscular dose of anti-D immune globulin—300 µg or 1500 IU— will protect the average-sized mother from a fetal hemorrhage of up to 30 mL of fetal whole blood or 15 mL of fetal red cells
- Anti-D immune globulin is given prophylactically to all D-negative, unsensitized women at approximately 28 weeks' gestation, and a second dose is given after delivery if the newborn is D-positive (American College of Obstetricians and Gynecologists)
- Following delivery, anti-D immune globulin should be given within 72 hours. Recognizing that 40 percent of neonates born to D-negative women are also D-negative, administration of immune globulin is recommended only after the newborn is confirmed to be D positive (American College of Obstetricians)
- If after delivery it is not given within 72 hours, it may be given till 28 days postpartum.
- Anti-D immune globulin is also administered after pregnancy related events that could result in fetomaternal hemorrhage (See Table 20.1)
- Anti-D immune globulin may produce a weakly positive—1:1 to 1:4—indirect Coombs titer in the mother. This is harmless and should not be confused with development of alloimmunization

Dose of Anti D

- Before 12 weeks of pregnancy = 50 mcg (200 IU).
- After 12 weeks of pregnancy = 300 mcg (1500 IU)
- At 28 weeks of pregnancy for Antepartum prophylaxis = 300 mcg (1500 IU)
- After delivery = usually 300 mcg.
- It is estimated that in 2 to 3 per 1000 pregnancies, the volume of fetomaternal hemorrhage exceeds 30 mL of whole blood (American College of Obstetricians and Gynecologists 2017). A single dose of anti-D immune globulin would be insufficient in such situations. For this reason, all D-negative women should be screened at delivery, typically with **a Rosette test**, followed by **quantitative testing** with **kleihauer Betke test** if indicated (American College of Obstetricians and Gynecologists, 2017)
- **The Rosette** test is a qualitative test that identifies whether fetal D-positive cells present in the circulation of a D-negative women. A sample of maternal blood is mixed with anti-D antibodies that coat any D-positive fetal cells present in the sample. Indicator red cells bearing the D-antigen are then added, and rosettes form around the fetal cells as the indicator cells attach to them by the antibodies. Thus, if rosettes are visualized, there are fetal D-positive cells in that sample
- **Rosette test:** Negative means fetal R B C are < 15 mL, then standard dose of anti D is given i.e. 300 mcg.

  Rossette test positive means—fetal RBC are more than 15 mL, then additional dose needs to given which is calculated by **kleihauer Betke test.**

Kleihauer Betke test

- It is based on principle that HbF is resistant to acid and alkali and HbA is sensitive
- **Reagent used:** Citric acid phosphate buffer
- A standard blood smear is prepared from mothers blood and exposed to citric acid. The mothers RBC elute giving an appearance of ghost cells whereas fetal RBC remain intact (Red in color). That is why the test is also called acid elution test
- Fetal cells are counted in 25 low power field

- **Calculation is done as follows:**

$$\text{Packed fetal red cells (in mL)} = \frac{\text{No of fetal cells} \times 240}{\text{No of maternal cells (100 mcg)}}$$

- A standard dose of 500 IU covers fetal cells upto 4 mL, for every mL of fetal cells above it 125 U of Anti D is needed.

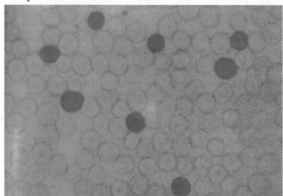

Fig. 20.6: Kleihauer-Betke test demonstrating massive fetal-to-maternal hemorrhage. After acid-elution treatment, fetal red cells rich in hemoglobin F stain darky, whereas maternal red cells with only very small amounts of hemoglobin F stain lightly.

Indication and Recommended Dose of Anti-D

Table 20.1: Conditions predisposing to isoimmunization in Rh –ve female

• Abortion[Q]	• Chorionic villous sampling[Q]
• Ectopic pregnancy	• *Trauma*
• Molar pregnancy	• Antepartum hemorrhage
• Cordocentesis	• Vaginal delivery
• Amniocentesis[Q]	• Cesarean section
• Attempted version[Q]	
• Manual removal of placenta	

 Note:

- In abortions ≥12 weeks: Always give Anti D
- In abortions <12 weeks: Anti D is not given in Threatened abortion or Complete abortion, if no medical or surgical intervention has been done.
- Dose of Anti D: Before 12 weeks = 50 mcg (200 IU) For antenatal prophylaxis or postpartum prophylaxis = 300 mcg (1500 IU)

New Pattern Questions

N1. A 37-year-old primi Rh negative patient is very concerned above her pregnancy at this age. Her pregnancy is 16 weeks and she is HIV negative, hepatitis B surface Ag neg, Rubella nonimmune and has no complain. Her triple test report is normal but still due to her age she insists on getting an amniocentesis done.

Which of the following is the next best step in management?

a. Advise against amniocentesis as it will increase the risk of isoimmunisation

b. Follow Rh titers carefully and give Anti D if evidence of isoimmunisation is present.

c. Give Anti D at 28 weeks of pregnancy and after delivery if baby is Rh negative

d. Give Anti D prior to her amniocentesis

e. Give rubella vaccine as she is Rubella nonimmune

N2. Two weeks later, the results of the patient's prenatal labs come back. Her blood type is A, with an anti D antibody titer of 1:4. What is the most appropriate next step in the management of this patient?

a. Schedule an amniocentesis for amniotic fluid bilirubin at 16 weeks

b. Repeat titer in 4 weeks

c. Repeat titer in 28 weeks

d. Schedule PUBS to determine fetal hematocrit at 20 weeks

e. Schedule PUBS as soon as possible to determine fetal blood type

N3. A Rh-negative second para has an antibody level of 15 IU/ml (IAT 1:32) at a 34 weeks. Her pregnancy is otherwise uncomplicated. The peak systolic velocity in the middle cerebral arteries reaches 1.5 multiples of the median.

What is the most appropriate management?

a. Carry out intrauterine transfusion

b. Induce labor after administration of corticosteroids

c. Deliver the baby by lower segment cesarean section after administration of corticosteroids

d. Perform amniocentesis and estimate the amniotic fluid bilirubin levels

N4. A Rh-negative G2P1 has an antibody level of 6 IU/ml at 8 weeks.

What is the next step in the management?

a. Determine the fetal Rhesus status by amniocentesis at 15 weeks

b. Determine the fetal Rhesus status by cordocentesis at 20 weeks

c. Determine the father's Rhesus genotype

d. Repeat the antibody titer in 4 weeks

N5. Rh-Negative G2P1 who underwent a cesarean section in her first pregnancy has an antibody level of 6 IU/mL at 8 weeks. Her husband is heterozygous Rh-positive.

What is the next step in the management?

a. Assess the amniotic fluid bilirubin levels at 18 weeks

b. Determine the fetal Rhesus status by amniocentesis at 15 weeks

c. Determnine the fetal Rhesus status by analyzing cell free fetal DNA present in the maternal blood at 8 weeks

d. Determine the fetal Rhesus status by cordocentesis at 20 weeks

N6. Rh negative G2P1 has an antibody titer of 4 IU/ml (IAT 1:4) at 8 weeks. Her husband is homozygous Rhesus positive.

What is the next step in the management?

a. Assess middle cerebral artery blood flow from 18 weeks

b. Assess the amniotic fluid bilirubin levels at 18 weeks

c. Determine the fetal Rhesus status by analyzing cell-free fetal DNA present in the maternal blood at 8 weeks

d. Repeat the antibody titer in 4 weeks

N7. A Rh negative G4P3+O has an antibody level of 15 IU/ml (IAT 1:32) at 27 weeks.

What is the most appropriate next step in the management?

a. Estimate the amniotic fluid bilirubin levels

b. Estimate the fetal hemoglobin levels by cordo-centesis

c. Estimate the middle cerebral artery peak systolic velocity

d. Perform intrauterine transfusion

N8. A Rhesus negative third para has an antibody level of 15 IU/mL (IAT 1:32) at 29 weeks. Ultrasound scan reveals features of fetal hydrops and polyhydramnios.

What is the most appropriate next step in the management?

a. Estimate the amniotic fluid bilirubin levels

b. Perform a cesarean section after giving one dose of dexamethasone

c. Perform cordocentesis to estimate the fetal hemoglobin level

d. Estimate the middle cerebral artery peak systolic velocity

N9. A G1+O attends the antenatal clinic for the booking visit at 12 weeks. Her blood group is B Rhesus negative.

What is the next step in the management?
a. Determine the fetal blood group
b. Determine the husband's blood group
c. Perform an ultrasound scan
d. Perform Rhesus antibody titer

N10. Which one of the following does not require treatment with anti-D during the first trimester of pregnancy?
a. Ectopic pregnancy
b. Evacuation of a partial hydatidiform mole
c. Evacuation of retained products of conception
d. Threatened abortion

N11. All of the following are scenarios in which it would have been appropriate to administer RhoGam to this patient in the past *except*:
a. After a spontaneous first trimester abortion
b. After treatment for ectopic pregnancy
c. Within 3 days of delivering an Rh–ve fetus
d. At the time of amniocentesis
e. At the time of external cephalic version

N12. Immediate cord ligation is done in:
a. Pre-term babies
b. Rh incompatibility
c. Both a and b
d. None of the above

N13. The dose of anti D gamma globulin given after term delivery for a Rh-negative mother and Rh-positive baby is:

a. 50 microgram
b. 200 microgram
c. 300 microgram
d. 100 microgram
e. All of the above doses are incorrect

N14. Dose of anti D for antenatal prophylaxis in Rh-negative nonimmunized females:
a. Single dose of 1000 IU at 28 weeks
b. Single dose of 1500 IU at 28 weeks
c. Single dose of 500 IU at 28 weeks
d. Single dose of 1500 IU at 32 weeks

N15. A Rh-negative primipara is delivered by cesarean section. The baby is Rhesus positive. A Kleihauer test is performed and the fetomaternal transfusion is estimated to be 5 mL.

Which of the following is the exact dose of anti-D needed?
a. 1500 IU
b. 750 IU
c. 500 IU
d. 625 IU

N16. Fetal affection by Rh antibody are all *except*:
a. Nonimmune hydrops fetalis
b. Icterus gravis neonatorum
c. Congenital anemia of the newborn
d. Fetal death

Previous Year Questions

1. The consequences of Rh-incompatibility are not serious during first pregnancy because: [AI 04]
   a. In first pregnancy only IgM antibody is formed
   b. Antibody titer is very low during primary immune response
   c. IgG generated is ineffective against fetal red cells
   d. Massive hemolysis is compensated by increased erythropoiesis

2. All predisposes to isoimmunisation in a Rh-ve female except: [AIIMS Dec 97]
   a. Advanced maternal age
   b. Antepartum hemorrhage
   c. Cesarean section
   d. Post-dated pregnancy

3. Which type of Hb is not affected by Rh isoimmuni-sation: [AIIMS Dec 97]
   a. Anti C   b. Anti E
   c. Anti-Lewis   d. Anti D

4. Correct statement regarding Rh-incompatibility is: [AIIMS Nov 99]
   a. Serial USG can diagnose hydrops early
   b. Antibody titer > 4 IU/ml in mother indicate severe risk of hemolysis
   c. Prognosis does not depend on parity
   d. Increase with ABO incompatibility

5. At 28 weeks gestation, amniocentesis reveals a ∆OD 450 of 0.20 which is at the top of third zone of the liley curve. The most appropriate management of such a case is: [AIIMS May 05, Nov 04]
   a. Immediate delivery
   b. Intrauterine transfusion
   c. Repeat Amniocentesis after 1 week
   d. Plasmapheresis

6. Anti-D prophylaxis should be given in all of the following conditions except: [AI 04]
   a. Medical abortion for 63 days pregnancy
   b. Amniocentesis at 16 weeks
   c. Intrauterine transfusion at 28 weeks
   d. Manual removal of Placenta

7. Indication of anti-D immunoglobulin is/are:
   a. Vaginal bleeding   [PGI Dec 03]
   b. ECV
   c. Mid trimester abortion
   d. After amniocentesis

8. True about Anti-D postpartion prophylaxis: [PGI June 02]
   a. Given to the newborn within 72 hrs of birth
   b. Required when baby is Rh+ and mother Rh-

   c. Can be helpful in ABO incompatibility
   d. Can be given up to one month of age of baby

9. Which is not the complication of Rh incompatibility.
   a. APH   b. PPH   [AIIMS Dec 98]
   c. Oligohydramnios
   d. Pregnancy induced hypertension

10. Mother's blood group is Rh-ve. Indirect Coombs is +ve. The following will be seen in baby:
    a. Anemia   [PGI Dec 09]
    b. Abnormal umbilical artery waveform deceleration
    c. Hydrops fetalis
    d. IUGR   e. Oligohydramnics

11. Nonimmune hydrops fetalis is seen in all of the following conditions except: [AI 99]
    a. α-Thalassemia   b. Parvovirus-19
    c. Rh-incompatibility d. Chromosomal anomaly

12. Hydrops fetalis is seen in following except:
    a. Rh incompatibility b. Syphilis   [PGI Dec 97]
    c. ABO incompatibility
    d. CMV

13. Hydrops fetalis is caused by: [PGI June 08]
    a. Parvovirus infection
    b. HZ virus infection
    c. Down syndrome   d. Toxoplasma

14. In nonimmune hydrops which of the following is NOT seen: [AIIMS 00]
    a. Skin edema   b. Ascites
    c. Large placenta   d. Cardiomegaly

15. How is fetal blood differentiated from maternal blood: [AIIMS Nov 2010]
    a. Kleihauer test   b. Apt test
    c. Bubble test   d. Lilly's test

16. Feto maternal transfusion is detected by:
    a. Kleihauer test   b. Spectrophotometry
    c. Benzidine test   d. None of the above

17. Best time to give Anti-D to a pregnant patient: [AIIMS Nov 2015]
    a. 12 weeks   b. 28 weeks
    c. 36 weeks   d. After delivery

18. A Rh negative, ICT negative mother, received anti-D injection at 28 weeks of gestation. After child birth at 37 weeks, what should be done? [AIIMS May 2017]
    a. Anti-D should be given within 72 hours irrespective of child's blood group
    b. Anti-D should be given if direct coombs test is positive
    c. Anti-D should be given if the child is Rh negative
    d. Anti-D should be given if the child is Rh positive

Answers with Explanations to New Pattern Questions

N1. **Ans. is d, i.e. Give Anti D prior to her amniocentesis**

Points worth noting are:
- Primi patient with Rh negative blood group
- She is 37 years old-elderly primi (>30 years) and has risk of Down syndrome (>35 years)
- She is concerned about the risk of having a down syndrome baby at this age and so insists on having amniocentesis done.

  - **Option a:** Advise against amniocentesis as it will increase the risk of isoimmunisation –although the risk of isoimmunisation will definitely be increased but still I will not advise her against amniocentesis seeing her age and her concern.
  - **Option b:** Follow Rh titers carefully and give Anti D if evidence of isoimmunization is present. Come on in the theory I have explained that Anti d should be given only if evidence of isoimmunizationt is absent. If isoimmunization is present it means antibodies are already formed, hence no need for giving Anti D. Thus this statement is absolutely wrong.
  - **Option c:** Give Anti D at 28 weeks of pregnancy and after delivery if baby is Rh negative. If baby is Rh negative, no need to give Anti D.
  - **Option d: Give Anti D prior to her amniocentesis:** This is the most logical step which should be done in this case.
  - **Option e: Give rubella vaccine as she is Rubella non imm**une: Now I don't need to explain that Rubella vaccine is contraindicated during pregnancy.

N2. **Ans. is b, i.e. Repeat titer in 4 weeks**

In the same patient–blood grouping shows A negative, with an anti D antibody titer of 1:4. Now critical titre is 1:16 so 1:4, 1:8 and 1:12 are all below it. The most appropriate next step in the management –Since this patient is a primi patient and her antibody titer is 1:4 so we should follow it by doing a repeat titer after every 4 weeks till 28 weeks then do it once in 2 weeks.

If this pregnancy would not have been her first affected pregnancy, then amniocentesis i.e. option a would have been the correct response.

N3. **Ans. is b, i.e. Induce labor after administration of corticosteroids**

This patient has high titer of antibodies. The increased blood flow in the middle cerebral arteries indicates that the fetus has developed anemia due to hemolysis. Since pregnancy is 34 weeks the best management option is to deliver. As the fetus is uncompromised, induce labor.

N4. **Ans. is c, i.e. Determine the father's Rhesus genotype**

This woman has been sensitised during the previous pregnancy. The fetus can be affected if it is Rhesus positive. If the father is homozygous Rhesus positive the baby will be Rhesus positive, and the maternal antibody titers should be carefully monitored. If the father is heterozygous the fetal blood group should be checked, as the fetus may be Rhesus positive or negative. So, the next best step in the management is to determine the father's Rhesus genotype.

N5. **Ans. is c, i.e. Determine the fetal Rhesus status by analyzing cell free fetal DNA present in the maternal blood at 8 weeks**

This woman has developed antibodies from a sensitizing event during the previous pregnancy. Since the husband is heterozygous, this foetus can be Rhesus positive or negative. The foetus will not be affected if it is Rhesus negative. Therefore, the next step in the management is to determine the Rhesus status of the foetus. Analysis of cell-free fetal DNA in maternal blood. If the foetus is Rhesus positive the antibody titer has to be repeated in 4 weeks because this her first immunized pregnancy.

N6. **Ans. is d, i.e. Repeat the antibody titer in 4 weeks**

Husband is homozygous Rhesus positive, the foetus will be Rhesus positive. Hence it is not necessary to determine the fetal Rhesus status. The next step in the management is to perform the antibody titer in 4 weeks. After 24 weeks antibody titer is done once in two weeks. Middle cerebral artery blood flow or amniocentesis is done only if the antibody levels reach a critical value.

N7. **Ans. is c, i.e. Estimate the middle cerebral artery peak systolic velocity**

The antibody titer is high the next step is to determine whether the ISO fetus is anaemic due to haemolysis. The middle cerebral artery peak systolic velocity (MCA-PSV) is the best method of assessing the fetal condition. When the fetus has developed anemia due to haemolysis, the blood viscosity decreases and the blood flow velocity will be increases. MCA peak systolic velocity value greater than 1.5 multiples of the median. If gestational age is < 34 weeks, it is an indication for estimation of fetal hemoglobin by cordocentesis. Intrauterine transfusion is performed when the fetal hematocrit is less than 30%.

If gestational age is ≥ 34 weeks termination of pregnancy done.

N8. Ans. is c, i.e. Perform cordocentesis to estimate the fetal hemoglobin level

This baby is severely affected at and it is 29 weeks, so intrauterine transfusion, may be needed, therefore, the next step in the management is to perform cordocentesis to directly estimate the fetal hemoglobin level. Delivery by caesarean section would be the best option once the maturity is more than 34 weeks.

N9. Ans. is b, i.e. Determine the husbands blood group

When a rhesus negative primipara attends the antenatal clinic, the first step is to determine her husband's blood group. If the husband is Rhesus negative no further investigations are necessary, as all babies will be Rhesus negative.

N10. Ans. is d, i.e. Threatened abortion

Threatened abortion in first trimester (at < 12 weeks) doesnot need Anti D.

N11. Ans. is c, i.e Within 3 days of delivering an Rh negative fetus

Anti D should not be given after delivering Rh negative fetus.

N12. Ans. is d, i.e. None of the above *Ref. Dutta Obs. 7/e, p 339, 458; Sheila Balakrishnan, p 148*

In case of Rh isoimmunization:

No prophylactic ergometrine should be given:
- Cord should be kept long (2–3 cm) to enable exchange transfusion if required.
- Cord blood sample should be taken from the placental end for:
    - ABO and Rh grouping[Q]
    - Direct Coombs test[Q]
    - Measurement of serum bilirubin[Q]
    - Hemoglobin estimation[Q]
    - Blood smear for presence of immature RBCs.
    - Earlier in case of preterm infants early cord damping was advocated due to the risk of hypervolemia but now delayed cord clamping is done (~ 30 secs – 60 secs).
    - In Rh negative females also, earlier immediate cord clamping was advocated but now delayed cord clamping is done.

Early cord clamping is advised/practised in case of:

Birth asphyxia if fetus needs resuscitation.

N13. Ans. is c, i.e. 300 microgram *Ref. Dutta Obs. 7/e, p 334*

N14. Ans. is b, i.e. Single dose of 1500 IU at 28 weeks

Postpartum prophylaxis in Rh negative women

Rh anti-D IgG is administered intramuscularly to the mother following child birth or abortion.
Timing:
- It should be administered within 72 hrs or preferably earlier following delivery or abortion.
- Should be given only if the baby born is Rh +ve and Direct Coombs Test done on baby's blood is negative
- In case 72 hrs is over, it can be given upto 28 days after delivery to avoid sensitization.

Dose:
- 300 microgram following delivery.
- 50 microgram following induced abortion, ectopic pregnancy or CVS in 1st trimester.
- In case of pregnancy ≥ 12 weeks 300 mcg should be given

Site of Injection

Anti D–immunoglobulin is best given intramuscularly into the deltoid muscle as injections into the gluteal region often reach the subcutaneous tissues and absorption may be delayed.

Antepartum prophyllaxis in Rh negative mother

- It is given at 28 weeks in all Rh negative pregnant females with indirect Coombs test negative. Dose = 300 µg = 1500 I/U (single injection).

N15. Ans. is d, i.e. 625 IU

500 IU of anti D is needed to neutralize 4 mL of fetomaternal hemorrhage

∴ for 1 ml = 125 IU is needed

∴ for 6 ml = 625 IU is needed

N16. Ans. is a i.e. Nonimmune hydrops fetalis *Ref: Dutta Obs 7/e p333*

Immune hydrops fetalis and not nonimmune hydrops fetalis is a complication of Rh negative pregnancy.

Answers with Explanations to Previous Year Questions

1. Ans. is a, i.e. In first pregnancy only IgM antibody is formed

Ref. High Risk Pregnancy - Fernando Arias 3/e, p 359; Turnbull's Obs., p 248, 249

As discussed is the preceeding text – The initial antibodies which are produced are of IgM variety which cannot cross the placenta and by the time IgG antibodies develop, patient has already delivered. Thus first pregnancy is safe.

Another reason is

In sensitised women, anti-D antibodies are produced at such a low level that they are not detected during or after the index pregnancy. Instead, they are identified early in a subsequent pregnancy when rechallenged by another D-positive fetus.

Also Know:

Grandmother's theory: This theory says that rarely the D (Rh)-negative fetus is exposed to maternal D antigen (if she is Rh-positive) and becomes sensitized. When such a female fetus reaches adulthood, she will produce anti D antibodies even before or early in her first pregnancy. This mechanism of isoimmunization is called the **"grandmother theory"** because the fetus in the current pregnancy is jeopardised by antibodies initially produced by its grandmother's erythrocytes.

2. Ans. is a, i.e. Advanced maternal age *Ref. Dutta Obs. 7/e, p 332; Textbook of Obs. Sheila Balakrishnan 1/e, p 369*

Conditions predisposing to isoimmunization in Rh –ve female

- Abortion[Q], ectopic pregnancy, molar pregnancy
- Cordocentesis
- Amniocentesis[Q]
- Attempted version[Q]
- Manual removal of placenta
- Chorionic villous sampling[Q]
- *Trauma*
- *Antepartum hemorrhage*
- *Vaginal delivery*
- *Cesarean section*

Studies show that there is continuous fetomaternal bleed occurring throughout normal pregnancies. During normal pregnancy, fetal red cells cross the placenta in 5% patients during first trimester and in 40-47% patients by the end of third trimester.

So it is not advisable to go beyond the expected date of pregnancy in Rh negative females carrying Rh +ve fetus. Hence post-dated pregnancy is another risk-factor for isoimmunization.

3. **Ans. is c, i.e. Anti-Lewis**   *Ref. Fernando Arias 3/e, p 359, 360*

"An antigen frequently found in routine antenatal screening is the Lewis group (Lea and Leb).

The Lewis antigens do not cause erythroblastosis fetalis and differ from all of the other red cell antigens in that they are not synthesized in the red cell membrane but are absorbed into it."   —*Fernando Arias 2/e, p 116*

Also Know:

Rare antigenic groups which can cause erythroblastosis fetalis (besides Rh)

... Fernando Arias 3/e, p 360; COGDT 10/e, p 283

• Kell (K)	MSSs
• Duffy (Fy)	Diego P
• Kidd (Jk)	Lutheran
• MNSs	Xg

 Extra Edge

- **Besides lewis antigens, I antigen also does not cause erythroblastosis fetalis**
- Du antigen—it is a "weak D positive" antigen. Women confirmed to be Du positive are considered as D antigen positive i.e. Rh positive and do not need an immunoglobulin. If a D negative woman delivers Du positive infant, she should be given D immunoglobulin   —*William 23/e, p 625*

4. **Ans. is a, i.e. Serial USG can diagnose hydrops early**   *Ref. Dutta Obs. 7/e, p 333*

Lets have a look at each option separately.

Erythroblastosis fetalis/Rh incompatibility leads to immune hydrops which can be diagnosed by serial USG as cardinal signs of hydrops fetalis viz scalp edema, ascites, pleural and pericardial effusion can all be detected on USG (therefore *Option "a"* is correct).

Prognosis depends on both parity and ABO incompatibility:

- Parity - As discussed in answer 1 the risk of Rh incompatibility is negligible in the first baby and increases as the parity of mother increases, therefore option "c" is incorrect.

ABO incompatibility:

- If ABO is present along with Rh incompatibility it protects against Rh isoimmunization.
- ABO blood group compatibility of mother and fetus - ABO incompatibility protects against Rh isoimmunisation. **When ABO incompatible fetal red cells enter the mother's bloodstream, they quickly combine with the naturally occurring anti A and anti B agglutinins and are neutralised by sequestration in the liver. On the other hand, ABO compatible fetal red cells will persist in the mother's circulation and thus stimulate the immune response.**

Antibodies titer:

- Antibody titer can be measured by automated tests.
- A titer of < 4 IU/ml is considered as safe.
- Titer of > 4 IU/ml denotes isoimmunization.
- Titer of > 10 IU/ml (in some countries > 15 IU/mL) denotes severe hemolysis – it is also called as the 'critical titer'
- Time for performing indirect coombs test.

In primigravida – at 12 weeks or at booking visit and if it is negative (i.e. mother is not immunised), it is repeated at 28th.

In multigravida – at 12 weeks or at booking visit and then at monthly interval after 28 weeks.

5. **Ans. is b, i.e. Intrauterine transfusion**   *Ref. Dutta Obs. 7/e, p 337; Fernando Arias 3/e, p 366, 367*

Management of Rh negative females depends on whether the female is immunized/nonimmunized.

The question which says- what should be done in case of the patient with 28 weeks pregnancy if Δ OD lies at the top of Zone 3. As discussed in text in this case. At 28 weeks intrauterine transfusion should be done.

Extra Edge

- Fetal blood transfusion should be done when Hb is at least 2 g/dl below the mean or hematocrit < 30% below the mean for normal fetus at that gestational age
- Intrauterine transfer can be done by:

```
                    Intraperitoneal route          Intravascular transfusion
                           ↓                              ↓
                    Done in smaller fetuses        Done in older and larger fetus
```

- Fresh O negative blood should be given.
- In many centres – peak systolic velocity (PSV) of fetal middle cerebral artery (MCA) has replaced amniocentesis for detection of fetal anemia. The anemic fetus shunts blood preferentially to brain to maintain adequate oxygenation. The peak MCA systolic velocity increases because of increased cardiac output and decreased blood viscosity. If MCA peak systolic velocity is more than 1.5 MOM the fetus is likely to be anemic.

6. **Ans. is c, i.e. Intrauterine transfusion at 28 weeks**   *Ref. Dutta Obs. 7/e, p 344; Sheila Balakrishnan, p 369*

Rh anti D immunoglobulin (IgG) is given to unimmunized Rh negative mothers with Rh positive fetus to prevent active immunization and formation of antibodies against fetal RBC's. The Anti D binds to antigen sites on the fetal red cells so that these cells do not mount an immune response, provided the baby is Rh negative and direct coombs test done on baby is negative. If mother's IUT is positive or fetus has positive direct coombs test, it means mother is already immunised. In such cases there is no point in giving anti D.

Indications for Anti D immunoprophylaxis:

First trimester	Later pregnancy
Miscarriage	Miscarriage
Ectopic (medically or surgically managed)	Amniocentesis
Hydatidiform mole	Fetal blood sampling
Threatened abortion	Antepartum hemorrhage
Medical or surgical MTP	External cephalic version
Chorionic villus sampling	Routine antepartum prophylaxis
	Delivery
	Intrauterine fetal death
	Manual removal of placenta

 Note: As far as intrauterine fetal transfusion is concerned. It is done as a therapy in case Rh isoimmunization has occured prior to 34 weeks so, administration of anti-D at this stage will not help.

Dose:
- Ideally amount of Anti D should be calculated according to the volume of fetomaternal bleed by doing a Kleihauer test.
- Generally:
  - Gestational age < 12 weeks – dose is 50 µg
  - Beyond 12 weeks – dose is 300 mcg

Antepartum prophylaxis: *At 28 weeks gestation in a Rh negative patient:* Indirect coombs test is done and if antibodies are not detected i.e. patient is unimmunised, Anti D 300 µg is given as antepartum prophylaxis.
- 300 µg of Anti D will neutralize about 15 mL of **fetal RBC**.

7. **Ans. is a, b, c, and d, i.e. Vaginal bleeding; ECV; Midtrimester abortion; and After amniocentesis**
          Ref. Dutta Obs. 7/e, p 344 "key points"; Shiela Balakrishnan, p 369

As explained in the previous question: Anti D prophylaxis should be given after all types of abortions (threatened, medical, MTP) molar pregnancy, ectopic pregnancy, delivery (+manual removal of placenta), procedures performed antenatally *(Amniocentesis, Chorionic villous sampling, External cephalic version)* and in cases of antepartum hemorrhage *(Vaginal bleeding in this case).*

8. **Ans. is a, b and d, i.e. Given to a newborn within 72 hours of birth. Required when baby is Rh +ve and Mother Rh–ve; and Can be given up to 1 month of age of baby** *Ref. Dutta Obs. 7/e, p 334; COGDT 10/e, p 284*

Postpartum prophylaxis

- If baby is Rh positive and mother Rh negative, 300 μg of Anti D immunoglobulin (IgG) is given to the mother and not infant (provided maternal antibody screening is negative) therefore Option 'b' is correct and Option 'a' is incorrect.
- Postpartum prophylaxis is best given within 72 hours after delivery but it can be given till 28 days after delivery Option 'd' is correct.

"Although Rh IgG generally should be given within 72 hours after delivery, it has shown to be effective in preventing isoimmunization if given upto 28 days after delivery" *—COGDT 10/e, p 284*

Anti D immunoglobulin is not helpful in case of ABO incompatibility.

> *Also Know:*
>
> **Role of postpartum prophylaxis:**
> - Anti D immunoglobulin given postpartum binds to antigen sites on the fetal red cells so that these cells cannot mount an immune response and thus prevent future sensitization and next pregnancy.
> - If after delivery, fetus has a positive direct Coombs test, it means that the mother is already immunized. In such cases, there is no point in giving anti D.

9. **Ans. is c, i.e. Oligohydramnios** *Ref. Dutta Obs. 7/e, p 333, William Obs. 23/e, p 627*

Rh incompatibility has adverse effect on the baby mainly, but mother may also be affected.

In Rh negative mothers there is increased incidence of:

- Preeclampsia[Q] - due to hydropic placenta in case of hydrops.
- Polyhydramnios[Q]
- Preterm labor
- Big size baby and its hazards
- Hypofibrinogenemia (due to prolonged retention of dead fetus in utero).
- Postpartum hemorrhage due to big placenta and coagulopathy.
- Maternal mirror syndrome - Characterized by generalized edema (similar to fetus), proteinuria and pruritus due to cholestasis. These features are omnious and indicate imminent fetal death in utero.

Antepartum hemorrhage is not a direct complication of Rh-incompatibility but may be the result of hypofibrinogenemia.

10. **Ans. is a and c, i.e. Anemia and Hydrops fetalis.** *Ref. Dutta Obs. 7/e, p 333-334*

As given in the question Mother is Rh -ve and indirect Coombs test is positive i.e. baby is suffering from Rh-incompatibility.[Q]

"In all cases of Rh –ve women irrespective of blood grouping and parity, albumin antibody is detected by indirect Coomb's test" *... Dutta Obs. 6/e, p 335*

- Clinical manifestation of Rh-incompatibility on the fetus can range from mild anemia to full blown hydrops fetalis.
- As discussed earlier polyhydramnios and not oligohydramnios is seen in Rh-negative pregnancy. (i.e. option e is incorrect.
- Option b: Abnormal umbilical artery waveform is incorrect, it should have been middle cerebral artery waveform.

11. **Ans. is c, i.e. Rh incompatibility** *Ref. Dutta Obs. 7/e, p 497*

12. **Ans. is c, i.e. ABO incompatibility** *Ref. Dutta Obs. 7/e, p 497*

13. **Ans. is a, b, c and d, Parvovirus infection; HZ virus infection; Down syndrome and Toxoplasma** *Ref. Dutta Obs. 7/e, p 497; Williams Obs. 22/e, p 674, 23/e, p 626, 27; Fernando Arias 3/e, p 96*

Hydrops fetalis: It is the most severe clinical manifestation of fetus in Rh incompatibility.

- It is characterized by excess fluid in 2 or more body areas such as the thorax, abdomen or skin. It is often associated with hydramnios and a hydropic thickened placenta.
- This condition is characterized on ultrasound by generalized skin edema (skin thickness > 5 mm), ascites, pleural effusion and large placenta (placental thickness > 4 cm). The fetus may be in Buddha position and there may be a halo around the head.

- The main pathology in all cases is severe anemia, hypoproteinemia, increased capillary permeability and cardiac failure.
- Hydrops is of 2 varieties:

Immune hydrops	Nonimmune hydrops
• It is due to Rh isoimmunisation	• It is accumulation of extracellular fluid in tissues and serous cavities without evidence of circulating antibodies against RBC antigens.
• It accounts for 1/3rd cases of hydrops fetalis	• It is due to conditions other than Rh isoimmunisation
	• It accounts for 2/3 cases of hydrops fetalis

Non-immune hydrops: Hydrops occurring due to a cause other than Rh incompatibility is called Nonimmune Hydrops
- It can be caused by a number of conditions (there is an exhaustive list given on p 627 Williams 23/e, Just go through it).

Category	Condition	Category	Condition
Cardiovascular	Tachyarrhythmia Congenital heart block Anatomical defects (ASD/VSD, TOF, hypoplastic left heart, pulmonary valve insufficiency, Ebstein subaortic stenosis, and single ventricle)	Urinary	Urethral stenosis or atresia Posterior neck obstruction Prune belly
Chromosomal	Trisomies, Turner syndrome, and triploidy	Gastrointestinal	Midgut volvulus Jejunal atresia Malrotation of intestines Maconium peritonitis Duplication of intestinal tract
Malformation syndromes	Thanatophoric dwarfism Arthrogryposis multiplex congenital Osteogenesis imperfecta Achondroplasia	Medications	Antepartum indomethacin (taken to stop preterm labor, causing fetal ductus closure and secondary noimmune hydrops fetalis)
Hematological	α-Thalassemia=MC cause of NIHF Arteriovenous shunts (vascular tumors) Kasabach-Merritt syndrome	Infections	Syphilis Parvovirus TORCH Leptospirosis
Twin pregnancy	Twin-twin transfusion syndrome Acardiac twin syndrome		
Respiratory	Diaphragmatic hernia Cystic adenomatous malformation Pulmonary hypoplasia	Miscellaneous	Tuberous sclerosis Cystic hygroma Sacrococcygeal teratoma Congenital neuroblastoma Amniotic band syndrome Congenital lymphedema

- Recurrent hydrops is caused by inborn errors of metabolism like Gaucher disease, GM1 gangliosidosis and sialidosis.

14. Ans. is d, i.e. Cardiomegaly   *Ref. Williams 23/e, p 626*

"Hydrops is characterized by excess fluid in two or more body areas such as thorax, abdomen or skin. It is often associated with hydraminos and a hydropic thickened placenta".
It is characterized by:
- Increased skin thickness (> 5 mm)^Q/skin edema (first sign seen on USG).
- Placental enlargement
- Pleural effusion
- Ascites
- The fetus is in Buddha position with a halo around the head.

15. Ans. is b, i.e. Apt test   *Williams Obs. 23/e, p 617, 618, Dutta Obs. 22/e, p 247, 248;*
Bedside Obs. Gynae Richa Saxena p 69

In the given options:
Option a – Kleihauer test and

Option b – Apt test (also called as singers alkali denaturation test) are used for detecting the presence of fetal blood in maternal blood.

Both are based on the principle that fetal blood with HbF is resistant to acid and alkali, whereas maternal blood with HbA is sensitive to acid and alkali.

Test	Reagent	Used for diagnosis of
Apt test (Singer alkali denaturation test)	KOH	Vasa previa
Kleihauer-Betke test	Citric acid phosphate buffer	Fetomaternal hemorrhage in Rh-negative pregnancies

Now: Remember:
- The test which differentiates fetal blood from maternal blood: Apt test.
- The test which differentiates fetal RBC from maternal RBC–Kleihauer-Betke test.

16. **Ans. is a, i.e. Kleihauer test** *Ref. Dutta Obs. 7/e, p 334, Sheila Balakrishnan Textbook of Obs 1/e, p 368*

Kleihauer-Betke test
- It is performed on maternal blood to assess the amount of fetomaternal bleed. In order to calculate the dose of Anti-D prophylaxis required.
- Principle: HbF is more resistant to acid elution than HbA.[Q]
- The maternal blood is subjected to an acid solution (citric acid phosphate buffer).[Q]
- Acid will elute the adult hemoglobins but not the fetal hemoglobin from the red cells. Hence, the fetal red cells appear stained dark red, unlike the light colored maternal red cells or ghost cells.[Q]
- The number of fetal red cells in 50 low power fields is assessed.
- If there are 80 fetal red cells in 50 low power fields, it represents a fetomaternal bleed of 4 ml of fetal blood.
- 25 µg (125 IU) of anti-D will neutralize 4 ml of fetomaternal bleed.
- If the volume of fetomaternal hemorrhage is > 30 ml of whole blood, the dose of Rh immunoglobulin is calculated as 10 µg for every 1 ml of fetal whole blood.

Also Know:
- Indirect Coombs test – detects antibodies in maternal serum.
- Direct Coombs test – detects antibodies in fetus/neonate.

 Extra Edge
- Kleihauer-Betke test: can detect as little as 0.2 ml of fetal blood diluted in 5L of maternal blood.
- It is not useful and should not be used to assess the need for anti D administration.
- Presence of reticulocytes and adult red cells containing fetal Hb may cause false positive test.

17. **Ans. is b, i.e 28 weeks** *Ref. Williams Obs 24/e, p 312*
Anti-D injection should be given to all Rh-negative pregnant females with indirect coombs test negative at 28 weeks.
Dose = 300 mcg
Injection given intramuscularly.
This will protect her present on going pregnancy.

18. **Ans. is d, i.e. Anti-D should be given if the child is Rh positive** *Ref. Williams Obs 25/e, p 305*
In Rh negative females
Anti D should be given after delivery within 72 hrs only if
   a. **Baby is Rh positive**
   b. **Direct coombs test negative**
Dose: 300 mcg i.e 1500 IU

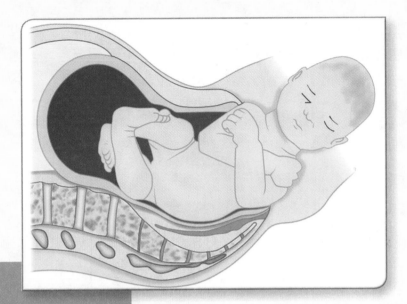

4

Section

Medical Complications in Pregnancy

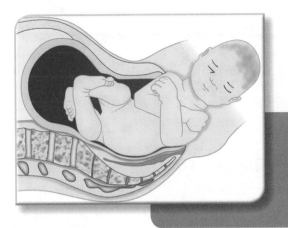

Anemia in Pregnancy

ANEMIA IN PREGNANCY

Definition: World Health Organization (WHO) has defined anemia during pregnancy as hemoglobin concentration of less than 11 gm% and a hematocrit of less than 33%. CDC (Center for Drug Control) proposes a cut off point of 11 gm% in 1st and 3rd trimester and 10.5 gm% during 2nd trimester.

 Note: FOGSI has suggested a cut off of 10 g/dL for India but practically a Hb concentration of <11 g/dL is taken for anemia.

Severity of Anemia

According to ICMR, severity of anemia is graded as:

Mild degree	10–10.9 gm%
Moderate degree	7–10 gm%
Severe degree	Less than 7 gm%
Very severe degree	Less than 4 gm%

PHYSIOLOGICAL ANEMIA DURING PREGNANCY

- The increase in plasma volume (30–40%) is much more than the increase in red cell mass (10–15%) during pregnancy, leading to **hemodilution** and an apparent decrease in hemoglobin level called as **physiological anemia of pregnancy**. This hemodilution during pregnancy serves to reduce maternal blood viscosity, thereby enhancing placental perfusion and facilitating nutrient and oxygen delivery to the fetus.

- **Characteristics of physiological anemia:**
  - Starts at 7th–8th weeks
  - Maximum by 32 weeks
  - Does not go below 11 gm%

Causes of Anemia during Pregnancy (Table 21.1)

Table 21.1: Causes of anemia during pregnancy

Acquired	Hereditary
Iron deficiency anemia	Thalassemias
Dimorphic anemia—anemia due to iron and folic acid deficiency	Sickle-cell hemoglobinopathies
	Other hemoglobinopathies
Anemia caused by acute blood loss	Hereditary hemolytic anemias
Anemia of inflammation or malignancy	
Megaloblastic anemia	
Acquired hemolytic anemia	
Aplastic or hypoplastic anemia	

Diagnosis of Anemia (Flowchart 21.1)

Flowchart 21.1: Diagnosis of anemia

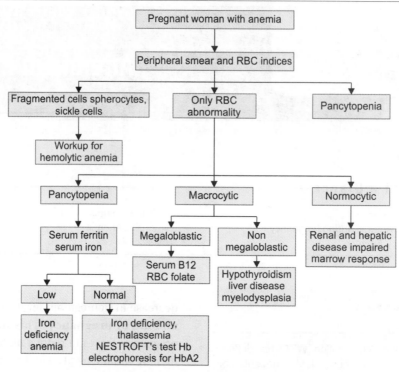

(NESTROFT: Naked eye single tube red cell osmotic fragility test)

Complications of Anemia

Maternal	Fetal
Pre-eclampsia	Low birthweight
Infection	Intrauterine death
Heart failure at 30–32 weeks	
PPH	
Shock	
Subinvolution	
Pulmonary embolism during puerperium	

Prognosis

Maternal: Anemia either directly or indirectly contributes to about 20% of maternal deaths in the third world countries.

Fetal: If detected early and responsive to treatment, the fetal prognosis is not too bad. Baby born at term, to severely anemic mother will not be anemic at birth, but as there is little or no reserve iron, anemia develops in neonatal periods. Mean cord blood levels of serum iron, ferritin, B_{12} and folate are higher than that of mother. However, total iron binding capacity and serum level of vitamin E are lower than that of mother.

IRON DEFICIENCY ANEMIA (IDA): (M/C ANEMIA DURING PREGNANCY)

Iron Requirements during Pregnancy

Total amount of iron required during pregnancy is 1000 mg:

- Fetus and placenta require[Q] – 300 mg
- Growing RBC of the mother require – 500 mg
- Lost through sweat, urine and feces – 200 mg
- Lost at the time of delivery – 200 mg
- Amount of iron saved d/t amenorrhea – 300 mg

So approximately (1200-300 =) 900-1000 mg is required during pregnancy. This means approximately 4–6 mg of iron is needed daily.

 Key Concept

- All parameters of iron metabolism decrease during pregnancy except for the two Ts viz **T**otal iron binding capacity and serum **T**ransferrin levels, which increase.
- No matter in what form iron is being taken–only 10% of it is absorbed, which means in order to fulfill the requirement of 4–6 mg/day, approximately 40–60 mg of iron should be taken in diet daily during pregnancy.

Contd...

Contd...

> This is not possible through diet only, this is the reason why Iron supplementation is absolutely necessary in pregnancy **for at least 6 months.**
> **In National Anemia Control Program under Ministry of Health and Family Welfare**, all pregnant women who are not anemic are given folifer tablet containing 60 mg elemental iron (salt-ferrous sulphate) along with 500 μg folic acid for at least 100 days.
> - **Earliest indicator of iron deficiency:** Decrease in the levels of serum ferritin as ferritin is the storage form of iron. (Normal values are between 50 and 300 mcg/L. Levels < 30 mcg/L show iron deficiency anemia with 90% sensitivity and specificity
> - Most sensitive blood index of iron deficiency is MCHC as MCHC is independent of RBC count.

Diagnosis of Iron Deficiency Anemia (IDA)

- **Peripheral blood smear (Fig. 21.1):** Shows microcytic hypochromic anemia. Reticulocyte count may be slightly raised.
- All indices related to Fe are decreased like MCV, MCH, MCHC, serum ferritin etc.
- TIBC and Red cell distribution width increases in Iron deficiency anemia.
- Most accurate method of measuring Hb is by cyanmethemoglobin method.

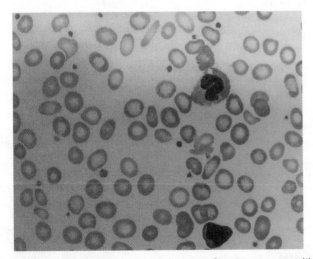

Fig. 21.1: This peripheral blood smear from a women with iron-deficiency anemia contains many scattered microcytic and hypochromic red cells with characteristic central pallor. These exhibit moderate anisopoikilocytosis, namely, varying sizes and shapes including occasional elliptocytes, which can be oval or pencil-shaped.

Management of Iron Deficiency Anemia in Pregnancy

Prophylactic Therapy

- Avoidance of frequent child-births
- Supplementary iron tablets—as discussed above
- Early detection of falling hemoglobin level-hemoglobin level should be estimated at the first antenatal visit, at the 30th week and finally at 36th week.

Curative Therapy

A. Oral Iron Therapy

- Oral iron-180–200 mg elemental iron (approx 3 tablets/day) and 1 mg folic acid is given till blood parameters become normal (the earliest parameter to increase after giving oral iron is reticulocyte count within 7–10 days) followed by one tablet per day as maintenance dose which should be continued throughout pregnancy and for 100 days (3 months) after pregnancy for replenishing the stores.

B. Parenteral Iron Therapy

Important points:

- In patients on hemo/peritoneal dialysis, malabsorption syndrome and in pregnant females with severe anemia, seen for the first time during last 8–10 weeks—parenteral iron is indicated.

> - Rise in hemoglobin concentration after parenteral therapy is same as that with oral iron i.e 0.7 to 1 gm % per week, so remember parenteral iron is not given for rapid rise of Hb.

- The main advantage of **parenteral therapy over oral iron is certainty of administration**.

Parenteral iron

It is available in the market as iron dextran complex, iron sorbitol complex, iron sucrose complex, iron gluconate and iron carboxymaltose.

- Iron dextran and iron sorbitol have been largely replaced by iron sucrose and more recently iron carboxymaltose due to decreased side effects and negligible risk of anaphylactic reactions with it. Cost is the only limiting factor.
- As per ACOG 2017, ferrous sucrose is safer than iron dextran
- **Iron dextran** by intramuscular route is associated with pain at injection site, risk of abscess formation, staining of skin, arthralgia, fever, painful lymphadenopathy, etc. Intravenous administration can result in severe anaphylactic reaction.

- Iron dextran should be administered after a test dose of 50 mg IM 24 hours before the first dose followed by 100 mg OD deep IM by Z technique.
- **Iron sucrose** is administered as intravenous infusion 2–3 times a week in the dose of 200–300 mg per dose to a maximum of 600 mg per week. It can be administered either undiluted 200 mg by slow intravenous injection at the rate of 20 mg/min after a test dose of 20 mg over 1–2 minutes or alternatively as intravenous infusion 200 mg diluted in maximum of 200 mL normal saline over 15–20 minutes. The risk of adverse reactions is only 0.5–1.5% compared to 5% with iron dextran. Anaphylaxis is rare <1/1000.

Overview of Management of Iron Deficiency Anemia in Pregnancy (Flowchart 21.2)

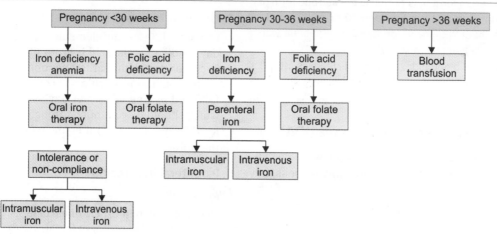

Flowchart 21.2: Management of IDA in pregnancy

- **Iron carboxymaltose can be** administered intravenously either undiluted as slow intravenous push at the rate of 100 mg per minute or as infusion 1000 mg over 15 min. The concentration of infusion should not be less than 2 mg/mL. This does not require any test dose and it should be diluted in normal saline. The risk of adverse reactions is 3% and risk of anaphylactic reaction is <1/100. Both the drugs should be avoided in first trimester. However they are safe during lactation.

Dose of parenteral iron

Total iron requirement is calculated by the following formulae:
a. **4.4 × body weight (kg) × Hb deficit (g/dL)—This formula includes iron needed for replenishment of stores**
b. **0.3 × weight (lb) × (Hb deficit) = iron req in mg. Add 500 mg for stores**
c. **250 mg of elemental iron for each gm% of Hb deficit**
d. **2.21 × body weight (kg) × Hb deficit (g/dL) + 1000 mg (replenishment of stores)**

Note: Weight in kg = wt in lb x 2.2
Normal Hb is taken as 14 g/dL

C. Blood Transfusion

One unit of blood raises the Hb levels by 0.8–1 gm% within 24 hours.

Indications of Blood Transfusion:
- Severe anemia seen beyond 36 weeks of pregnancy
- Anemia due to active blood loss
- Refractory anemia
- Associated infection.

Note: The Hb levels at the time of delivery should be atleast 7 gm%.

Also Know:
- The earliest biochemical evidence of folic acid deficiency is low plasma folic concentration
- In folic acid deficiency—Neutrophils are hypersegmented & macrocytic erythrocytes seen.

DIMORPHIC ANEMIA

- It is due to deficiency of both iron and folic acid or vitamin B_{12}.
- While there is polydeficiency state, the hematological findings or the bone marrow picture usually show predominance of one deficiency. **The red cells** become macrocytic or normocytic and hypochromic or normochromic.
- Bone marrow picture is predominantly megaloblastic as the folic acid is required for the development of the number of red cell precursors.
- The treatment consists of prescribing both the iron and folic acid in therapeutic doses.

SICKLE CELL ANEMIA

- The M/C form of hemolytic anemia seen during pregnancy is the intravascular microangiopathic hemolysis which is a part of HELLP syndrome. Less frequently it is due to sickle cell disease.
- Sickle cell disease is the most common hemoglobinopathy encountered during pregnancy.

Basics of Sickle Cell Anemia

Sickle cell hemoglobinopathies are hereditary disorders. It is caused by a point mutation in the β-globin gene on chromosome II. **This results in substitution of valine for glutamic acid at position 6 of the β-chain of normal hemoglobin.**

- When Gene mutation is **homozygous,** the individual has **sickle cell anemia (Hb-SS).** She has a small quantity of fetal hemoglobin (HbF) but no HbA.
- **Heterozygous** individual for sickle cell hemoglobin has **sickle cell trait (HbAS).** Such an individual has about 55–60% of HbA and 35–40% of HbS. Sickle cells have a life span of 5–10 days compared to normal RBCs of 120 days.

Sickle Cell Trait

- In these patients Hb-S comprises 30–40% of the total hemoglobin, the rest being Hb-A, Hb-A_2 and Hb-F. If the husband is a carrier, there is 25% chance that the infant will be homozygous sickle cell disease and 50%—sickle cell trait. As such, preconceptional counseling should be done to know whether the husband also carries the trait or not.
- There is no special problem so far as reproductive performance is concerned. The patient will require iron supplementation.
- As the concentration of Hb-S is low, crisis is rare but can occur in extreme hypoxia. Hematuria and urinary

infection venous thrombolism pre-eclampsia, are quite common.

Sickle Cell Disease

- Homozygous sickle cell disease (Hb-SS) is transmitted equally by males and females. Partner must be tested. Termination of pregnancy is an option, if fetus is diagnosed to have major hemoglobinopathy on prenatal diagnosis by CVS.

Sickle cell crisis: It is characterised by intense bone pain due to intense sequestration of sickled erythrocytes and infarction in various organs.
- Pregnancy can precipitate sickle cell crisis in both women with sickle cell trait and sickle cell disease.
Management:
- IV fluids
- O_2
- Epidural analgesia
- Antibiotics:
- Thromboprophylaxis
- Red cell transfusion after the onset of pain donot have much benefit but prophylactic transfusions before the crisis, helps in decreasing the pain and shortening the duration of crisis.

Effect of pregnancy on disease	Effect of disease on pregnancy
• Sickle cell crisis	• Preterm labor
• Severe bone pain	• IUGR
• Acute chest syndrome	• Fetal death
• Pulmonary infarction	• Abortion
• Pulmonary embolism	• Increased incidence of
• Pyelonephritis	– Preeclampsia
• Pneumonia	– PPH
• UTI	– Infection

Management during Pregnancy

- Folic acid supplementation 4 mg to 5 mg daily (ACOG 2013) is given to support rapid blood cell turnover.
- Prophylactic penicillin (penicillin V 250 mg twice daily).
- Prophylactic blood transfusions during pregnancy to maintain hematocrit above 25% and Hbs below 60% – are controversial.

> If a transfusion is given, leukocyte depleted packed red cell, pherotyped for major and minor antigens should be used.

- Hydroxyurea is not recommended in pregnancy.
- During every antenatal visit, Hb, hematocrit, platelet count, bilirubin, transaminase and lactose dehydrogenase levels should be checked (fortnightly).
- Vaginal delivery is preferred.

- Epidural analgesia is given during labour to relieve pain.
- Postnatal thromboprophylaxis for upto 6 weeks may be needed.

Contraception:

- Low dose oral progestins or DMPA or progesterone implants are ideal as they prevent painful sickle cell crises.
- OCP's (low dose) and Cu containing IUCDs–earlier considered contraindicated, are now regarded as safe by CDC (2013 b).

THALASSEMIA

- The term **thalassemia** encompasses a group of inherited blood disorders that can cause severe microcytic hypochromic anemia.
  - Alpha (α)-**thalassemia and Beta (β)-thalassemia** result from absent or decreased production of structurally normal α- and β-globulin chains,

respectively, generating an abnormal ratio of α to non-α chains.
  - The excess chains form aggregates that lead to ineffective erythropoiesis and/or hemolysis.
  - A broad spectrum of syndromes is possible, ranging from no symptoms to transfusion-dependent anemia and death.
  - Both diseases are transmitted as autosomal recessive traits.

Alpha-thalassemia

- It is associated with Southeast Asian, African, Caribbean, and Mediterranean origin and results from a delection of one to all α-genes, located on chromosome 16.
  - Excess β-globins then form β-globin tetramers called HbH.
  - A fetus would be affected because fetal Hb also requires α-chains.

Alpha-thalassemias		
Silent carrier	$-\alpha/\alpha\,\alpha$	Normal or slight microcytosis.
α-thalassemia	$--/\alpha\,\alpha$ (Asian) $-\alpha/-\alpha$ (African)	Mild microcytic, hypochromic. Normal Hbg electrophoresis.
HbH disease	$--/-\alpha$	Moderate-severe microcytic, hypochromic anemia. The beta chains in this case are relatively in excess and form an unstable tetramers called **HbH**. **These people can have normal life expectancy. Although multiple transfusions are required.**
Hydrops fetalis "Hb Bart's Disease"	$--/--$	In these individuals the excessive Y-chains form **fetal hemoglobin Bart**. Affected fetus has marked anemia. Hydrops, heart failure, pulmonary edema, transverse limb reduction defects, hypospadias, can also be seen. **This is not compatible with life.**

Beta-thalassemia

- It is associated with Mediterranean, Asian, Middle Eastern, Caribbean, and Hispanic origin.
  - The cause is (mostly point mutations) in β-globin genes, located on chromosome 11.
  - The two consequences of these gene defects are β°, which is the complete absence of the β-chain; and β^{+}, which is decreased synthesis of the β-chain.
  - In both these cases there is excess alpha chain which binds to red cell membrane and causes membrane damage.

Hematological Findings in Thalassemia

- There is **low MCV and MCH but normal MCHC** (Difference from iron deficiency anemia where all are low).
- Serum iron and total iron binding capacity are normal or elevated.

- Hemoglobin electrophoresis shows raised concentration of **HbA2** ($\alpha^2\,\alpha^2$) **to more than 3.5%** with normal or raised Hb-F.
- Serum bilirubin may be raised to about 2–3 mg%.

NESTROFT Test: It is 'naked eye single tube red cell osmotic fragility test'. In this test 2 mL of 0.36 buffered saline solution is taken in one tube and 2 mL of distilled water in another tube. A drop of blood is added to each test tube and both the tubes are left undisturbed for 20 minutes. Both the tubes are then shaken and held against a white paper on which a black line is drawn. Normally, the line is clearly visible through the contents of tube containing distilled water. If the line is clearly visible similarly through the contents of tube with buffered saline, the test is negative.

Contd...

Contd...

> If the line is not clearly visible the test is considered positive. The principle is that normocytic normochromic cells when put in hypotonic solution will undergo lysis whereas in thalassemia trait, the cells are microcytic and hypochromic which are resistant to hemolysis due to decreased fragility. It has 91% sensitivity and 95% specificity and the negative predictive value is 99%.
>
> *Note*: NESTROFT test is only a screening test for thalassemia. The definite test is the estimation of HbA2 levels by high liquid performance chromatography. In thalassemia HbA2 levels are > 3.5%.

- An important screening test used for thalassemia trait these days is NESTROFT test (Naked Eye Single Tube Red Cell Osmotic Fragility Test).

Pregnancy and Thalassemia

- Important obstetrical aspects of some α-thalassemia syndromes depend on the number of gene deletions in a given women and has been discussed above.
- Inheritance of all four abnormal α-genes leads to either stillbirth or babies die very soon after birth and have typical features of nonimmune hydrops fetalis NIHF.

 Key Concept

Sonographic measurement of the fetal cardiothoracic ratio at 12 to 13 weeks gestation has 100% sensitivity and specificity for identifying fetuses with NIHF.

Management

- Women with trait status for either thalassemia require no special care.
- Women at high risk for or diagnosed with thalassemia should be offered preconception counseling and chorionic villi sampling should be done to see whether fetus is affected or not.
- Iron supplements should be prescribed only if iron deficiency is present, otherwise hemochromatosis can occur. Parenteral iron is contraindicated.
- Chelation with desferoxamine in later months of pregnancy can be helpful.
- Thalassemia may confer an increased risk of neural tube defects secondary to folic acid deficiency, so up to 4 mg/day periconceptual folic acid supplementation is recommended.
- If asplenic, vaccinations need to be given and penicillin given.
- **Antepartum fetal testing** should be undertaken in anemic thalassemia patients.
  - Periodic fetal sonography to asses fetal growth as well as nostress testing to evaluate fetal well-being is recommended.
  - Ultrasonography is also useful to detect hydrops fetalis but usually at a later gestational age.

New Pattern Questions

N1. Tablets supplied by Government of India contain:
a. 60 mg elemental iron +500 µg of folic acid
b. 200 mg elemental iron +1 mg of folic acid
c. 100 mg elemental iron +500 µg of folic acid
d. 100 mg elemental iron +5 mg of folic acid

N2. Total amount of iron needed by the fetus during entire pregnancy is:
a. 500 mg
b. 1000 mg
c. 800 mg
d. 300 mg

N3. Thirty years old G4P3L3 with 32 weeks pregnancy with single live fetus in cephalic presentation, Patient complains of easy fatigability and weakness since last 3 months which has gradually increased over last 15 days to an extent that she gets tired on doing household activities. Patient also complaints of breathlessness on exertion since last 15 days. Patient gets breathless on climbing 2 flight of stairs. It is not associated with palpitations or any chest pain. There is no history of pedal edema, sudden onset breathlessness, cough or decreased urine output. There is no history of asthma or chronic cough. There is no history of chronic fever with chills or rigors. There is no history of passage of worms in stool nor blood loss from any site. There is no history of easy bruisability or petechiae. There is no history of yellow discoloration of urine, skin or eyes. She did not take iron folate prophylaxis throughout her pregnancy.
- She is suspected to be anemic and her blood sample was ordered for examination which showed.
- Hb 7.4 gm% (12–14 gm%)
- Hct 22% (36–44%)
- MCV 72 fL (80–97 fL)
- MCH 25 pg (27–33 pg)
- MCHC 30% (32–36%)
- Peripheral smear shows microcytic hypochromic RBCs with anisopoikilocytosis
- Naked eye single tube red cell osmotic fragility test (NESTROFT) is negative. What is the most probable diagnosis:
a. Thalassemia
b. Iron deficiency anemia
c. Megaloblastic anemia
d. Vitamin B12 deficiency anemia.

N4. The following statements are related to the therapy of iron deficiency anemia *except*:
a. Oral iron can be given only if anemia is detected before 20 weeks of pregnancy

b. Parenteral iron therapy markedly increases the reticulocytic count within 7–14 days
c. Parenteral therapy is ideal during 30–36 weeks
d. Blood transfusion may be useful in severe anemia beyond 36 weeks

N5. The following are related to the treatment of thalassemia *except*:
a. Fresh (relatively) blood transfusion
b. Folic acid
c. Routine iron therapy
d. Deferoxamine improves pregnancy outcome

N6. All are used for contraception in sickle cell anemia *except*:
a. Oral 'Pill'
b. IUCD
c. Progestin only pill or implant
d. None of the above

N7. With oral iron therapy, rise in Hb% can be seen after:
a. 1 week   b. 3 weeks
c. 4 weeks   d. 6 weeks

N8. Formula used for estimation of the total iron requirement is:
a. 4 × body weight (kg) × Hb deficit (g/dL)
b. 4.4 × body weight (kg) × Hb deficit (g/dL)
c. 0.3 × body weight (kg) × Hb deficit (g/dL)
d. 3.3 × body weight (kg) × Hb deficit (g/dL)

N9. How much iron a patient can tolerate at a time given intravenously?
a. 1000 mg
b. 2000 mg
c. 2500 mg
d. 3000 mg
e. 3500 mg

N10. Not an indicator for blood transfusion:
a. Severe anemia at 36 weeks
b. Moderate anemia at 24–30 weeks
c. Blood loss anemia
d. Refractory anemia

N11. Which of the following hematological criteria remains unchanged in pregnancy?
a. Blood volume
b. TIBC
c. MCHC
d. S. ferritin

N12. Raised MCV in pregnancy can be due to:
a. Megaloblastic anemia
b. Alcohol use
c. Hypothyroidism
d. All of the above

N13. Dose of folic acid per day for treating megaloblastic anemia in pregnancy:
   a. 400 μg   b. 4 mg
   c. 1 mg   d. 2 mg

N14. Blood transfusion is indicated in following conditions associated with sickle cell anemia:
   a. Frequent sickling episodes
   b. Twin pregnancy
   c. Poor obstetrical outcome
   d. All of the above

N15. Most sensitive index for IDA in pregnancy:
   a. Hb
   b. MCV
   c. MCH
   d. MCHC

N16. WHO recommendation for Fe and Folic acid supplementation in pregnancy
   a. 30–60 mg elemental iron + 400 mcg folic acid
   b. 30–60 mg elemental iron + 500 mcg folic acid
   c. 100 mg elemental iron + 400 mcg folic acid
   d. 100 mg elemental iron + 500 mcg folic acid

Previous Year Questions

1. According to WHO, anemia in pregnancy is diagnosed, when hemoglobin is less than?
   a. 10.0 gm%   b. 11.0 gm%   [AIIMS Dec 97]
   c. 12.0 gm%   d. 9.0 gm%

2. Which of the following tests is most sensitive for the detection of iron depletion in pregnancy?
                                                [AI 04; AIIMS Nov 05]
   a. Serum iron
   b. Serum ferritin
   c. Serum transferrin
   d. Serum iron binding capacity

3. A 37 years multipara construction labourer has a blood picture showing hypochromic anisocytosis. This is most likely indicative of: [AI 04]
   a. Iron deficiency
   b. Folic acid deficiency
   c. Malnutrition
   d. Combined iron and folic acid deficiency

4. In pregnancy, which type of anemia is not common in India?   [PGI June 97]
   a. Vitamin B_{12} anemia
   b. Folic acid anemia
   c. Iron + folic acid anemia
   d. Iron deficiency anemia

5. Most common cause of maternal anemia in pregnancy: [PGI Nov 2010]
   a. Acute blood loss   b. Iron deficiency state
   c. GI blood loss   d. Hemolytic anemia
   e. Thalassemia

6. A pregnant female presents with fever. On lab investigation her Hb was decreased (7 mg%), TLC was normal and platelet count was also decreased. Peripheral smear shows fragmented RBCs. Which is least probable diagnosis?   [AIIMS Nov 12]
   a. DIC   b. TTP
   c. HELLP syndrome   d. Evans syndrome

Answers with Explanations to New Pattern Questions

N1. **Ans. is c, i.e. 100 mg elemental iron + 500 μg folic acid** *Ref. JB Sharma obs p 487, Park 21/e, p 594*

Inorder to prevent nutritional anemia among mothers and children, the Govt. of India sponsored a **National Nutritional Anemia Prophylaxis Programme** during the Fourth Fifth Year Plan. As per the programme the vulnerable groups for anemia viz pregnant females and children were given daily supplements of iron and folic acid tablets. The suggested prophylactic doses were initially 60 mg of elemental iron and 500 μg of folic acid for pregnant females. These tablets were distributed free of cost at all PHCs. But survey done during the years 1985-1986 showed poor results and no impact was seen on the prevalence of anemia in pregnant females. So the dosage of elemental iron was increased.

Presently the tablets supplied contain 100 mg of elemental Iron and 500 μg of folic acid.
Routine supplementation of these tablets is recommended daily for all pregnant females in India for atleast 100 days in the second half of pregnancy.

Thus routine daily administration of folic acid = 500 mcg. But minimum amount of folic acid needed to prevent Neural tube defects = 400 mcg

N2. **Ans. is d, i.e. 300 mg** *Ref. Dutta Obs. 7/e, p 55, Shiela Balakrishnan TB of Obstetrics 1/e, p 336*

In a normal pregnancy, the total amount of iron required by a pregnant female is 900–1000 mg. This is because of the following needs—

Total amount of iron required during pregnancy is 1000 mg, i.e 4–6 mg/day which can be calculated as:
- Fetus and placenta require — 300 mg ⎤
- Growing RBC of the mother require — 500 mg ⎥
- Lost through sweat, urine and faeces — 200 mg ⎬ 1200 mg
- Lost at the time of delivery — 200 mg ⎥
- Amount of iron saved d/t amenorrhea — 300 mg ⎦

So approximately (1200-300 =) 900-1000 mg is required during pregnancy.

From the above calculations, it is clear that **amount of iron required by fetus is 300 mg.**

N3. **Ans. is b, i.e. Iron deficiency anemia**
- In the question patient has Hb 7.4 gm%, hematocrit 22% and symptoms of early fatigue, which indicate she is anemic. Her complete blood picture shows MCV and MCH are low indicating microcytic anemia. Thus differential diagnosis could either be Iron deficiency anemia or thalassemia.

Her NESTROFTS test (screening test for thalassemia) is negative, hence thalassemia is ruled out and diagnosis is confirmed as Iron deficiency anemia.

N4. **Ans. is a, i.e. Oral iron can be given only if anemia is detected before 20 weeks of pregnancy**

Ref: Dutta Obs. 7/e, p 266

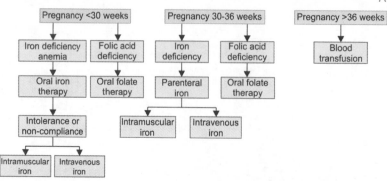

From the chart it is clear that parenteral iron is ideal during 30–36 weeks, blood transfusion is useful in severe anemia beyond 36 weeks (i.e. options c and d are correct). Oral iron is useful in anemias before 30 weeks of pregnancy and not 20 weeks.

N5. **Ans. is c, i.e. Routine iron therapy**

Ref. Williams 23/e, p 1090, 1091; Dutta 7/e, p 274; JH Manual of Obs. and Gynae 4/e, p 225, 226

- As discussed in detail in preceeding text– on thalassemia, routine iron therapy should not be given in patients of thalassemia as it leads to hemochromatosis. Only if there is documented iron deficiency then given iron. Rest all options are correct

N6. **Ans. is d, i.e. None of the above.**

Ref. Williams 24/e, p 1111

Contraception and sterilization (in sickle cell anemia)

"Because of chronic debility, complications caused by pregnancy, and the predictably shortened life span of women with sickle-cell anemia, contraception and possibly sterilization are important considerations. Many clinicians do not recommend combined hormonal pills because of potential adverse vascular and thrombotic effects after a systematic review, however, it was concluded that there was no increase in complications with their use in women with sickle cell syndromes. The CDC (2013b) regards the contraceptive pill, patch, and ring along with the copper intrauterine device (IUD) as having "advantages that generally outweigh theoretical or proven risks".

All progesterone only methods may be used without restrictions. Because progesterone has been long known to prevent painful sickle-cell crises. Low-dose oral progestins or progesterone injections, or implants seem ideal. In one study, de Abood and associates (1997) reported significantly fewer and less intense pain crises in women given depot medroxyprogesterone intramuscularly.
—Williams 24/e, p1111

N7. **Ans. is b, i.e. 3 weeks**

Ref. Dutta Obs. 7/e, p 266

Rise in hemoglobin with oral iron – 0.7 gm-1 gm per week, which is seen after **3 weeks** of initiation of oral therapy.[Q]

(According to COGDT, 10/ed, p 407 — Hemoglobin levels should increase by atleast 0.3 g/dl/week if the patient is responding to therapy)

If there is no significant clinical or hematological improvement within 3 weeks, diagnostic re-evaluation is needed.

N8. **Ans. is b, i.e. 4.4 × body weight (kg) × Hb deficit (g/dL)**

Ref. KDT 6/e, p 585; Dutta Obs. 7/e, p 269

> **Total iron requirement is calculated by the following formulae:**
>
> a. **4.4 × body weight (kg) × Hb deficit (g/dL)**-This formula includes iron needed for replenishment of stores.
>
> b. **0.3 × weight (lb) × (100-Hb%) = iron req in mg. Add 50% of this for stores.**
>
> c. **250 mg of elemental iron for each gm% of Hb deficit**
>
> d. 2.21 × body weight (kg0 × Hb deficit (g/dL) + 100 mg (replenishment of stores)
>
> **Note:** Weight in kg = wt in lb × 2.2
>
> Normal Hb is taken as 14 g/dL

N9. **Ans. is c, i.e. 2500 mg**

Ref. Dutta Obs. 7/e, p 269

The dose of parenteral iron is calculated using formula given in Q. 14. If the dose is more than 50 ml (each ml has 50 mg of iron i.e. 2500 mg iron), then half the dose is given on day one and second half on next day. Thus maximum iron which can be given in a day is 2500 mg.

ACOG recommends the use of iron sorbitol as it is safer than iron dextran.

N10. **Ans. is b, i.e. Moderate anemia at 24–30 weeks**

Ref. Dutta Obs, 7/e, p 267

Indications of Blood transfusion in anemia during pregnancy:

- To correct anemia due to blood loss and to combat PPH
- Severe anemia is seen beyond 36 weeks of pregnancy
- Refractory anemia – i.e. anemia not responding to oral or parenteral iron
- Associated infection.

> *I*
>
> **Important points to remember:**
>
> - In case of severe anemia with cardiac failure, packed cell transfusion is preferred to avoid overload and pulmonary edema.
> - If required blood transfusion should be repeated only after 24 hours.
> - Improvement in Hb after 1 unit of blood transfusion is 1g/dL or 3% in hematocrit

N11. Ans. is c, i.e. MCHC
Ref. High Risk Pregnancy Fernando Arias 4/e, p 234

MCHC (mean corpuscular haemoglobin concentration) remains unchanged during pregnancy.
MCV increases minimally during pregnancy.

N12. Ans. is d, i.e. All of the above
Ref. High Risk Pregnancy, Fernando Arias 4/e, p 236, 237

The first indication of megaloblastic anemia in pregnancy is usually an elevated red cell MCV. This finding is also seen alcohol or azathioprine use, hypothyroidism and in normal pregnancy.

Imp. Points:

- Diagnostic feature of megaloblastic anemia of pregnancy on blood smear is presence of hypersegmented neutrophils.
- Megaloblastic anemia can be either due to deficiency of folic acid or vitamin B_{12}.
- **Diagnostic test for:**
    - Vitamin B12 deficiency—Decreased serum levels of vitamin B12. (< 100 pg/mL)
    - Folic acid deficiency—Red cell folate levels. (< 160 ug/L) and low serum folate levels – < 25 µg/L

Mgt:

- Folic acid deficiency = 1 mg/day Folic acid.
- Vitamin B_{12} deficiency = 1000 µg of parenteral cyanocobalamin every week for 6 weeks, followed by 1000 µg intramuscular injections every month.
- The reticulocyte count shows appropriate response to therapy in 4–6 days and hypersegmentation of neutrophils normally disappears after 2 weeks.

N13. Ans. is c, i.e. 1 mg
Ref. High Risk Pregnancy, Arias 4/e, p 237

Dose of folic acid in Pregnancy: Per day:

- To prevent neural tube defect – 400 µg.
- In pregnant females with previous H/O NTD or in females on anticonvulsants and folate antagonists – 4 mg
- To treat megaloblastic anemia – 1 mg
- In patients with sickle cell disease – 4 mg

N14. Ans. is d, i.e. All of the above
Ref. Fernando Arias 4/e, p 238

Prophylactic blood transfusions are not routinely advocated in all pregnant females with sickle cell anemia.
Indications:

1. Frequent severe sickling episodes.
2. Low haematocrit levels.
3. Twin pregnancy.
4. Poor past obstetrical history.

Target: HbS levels becomes < 20%.

N15. Ans. is d, i.e. MCHC
Ref. JB Sharma obs, p 486

The most sensitive blood index for IDA in pregnancy is MCHC

N16. Ans. is a, i.e. 30–60 mg elemental iron + 400 mcg folic acid
Ref. Williams obs 25/e p 1077

WHO–2012 routinely recommends, daily oral supplementation with 30 to 60 mg elemental iron and 400 mcg folic acid.

Answers with Explanations to Previous Year Questions

1. **Ans. is b, i.e. 11.0 gm%** *Ref. Dutta Obs. 7/e, p 260, Mgt of High Risk Pregnancy-Manju Puri,SS Trivedi, p 274*

"*According to the standards laid by WHO – Anemia in pregnancy is defined as when hemoglobin is 11 gm/100 ml or less or hematocrit is less than 33%*".

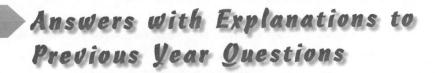

Also Know:

ICMR – Grades of Anemia in Pregnancy	
Mild anemia	10–10.9 gm%
Moderate anemia	7–9.9 gm%
Severe anemia	6.9–4 gm%
Very severe anemia	< 4 gm %

2. **Ans. is b, i.e. Serum ferritin** *Ref. Harrison 17/e, p 630; Fernando Arias 3/e, p 467*

Serum ferritin is the earliest test of iron deficiency anemia and as it correlates best with iron stores in case of iron deficiency.

3. **Ans. is d, i.e. Combined iron and folic acid deficiency** *Ref. Dutta Obs. 7/e, p 270*

Anisocytosis is variation in size of the red blood cells.

The patient in the question has hypochromic anemia along with anisocytosis which can be seen in case of

—*Harshmohan 5/e, p 372*

- Iron deficiency anemia

  Blood picture:
    - Red cells are hypochromic and microcytic
    - There is anisocytosis and poikilocytosis
    - In severe cases target cells, elliptical forms and polychromatic cells are present.
- Dimorphic anemia

  Blood picture:
    - Cells may be normocytic, microcytic or macrocytic (i.e. anisocytosis is seen)
    - Hypochromia or Normochromia.

Therefore in both iron deficiency anemia and dimorphic anemia anisocytosis with hypochromia may be seen.

But since dimorphic anemia is the *commonest type* of anemia seen in tropics so we are taking it as the correct answer.

Dimorphic anemia:

- It is the **commonest type** of anemia seen in the underprivileged sections of society specially in the tropics.
- M/C anemia during pregnancy is iron deficiency anemia.

- It results either from dietary inadequacy or intestinal malabsorption and thus anemia is associated with deficiency of iron as well as vitamin B_{12} **and folic acid.**
- Bone marrow is predominantly megaloblastic (as folic acid is required for the development of the red cell precursors).
- Treatment consists of prescribing both iron and folic acid in the diet.

4. **Ans. is a, i.e. Vitamin B12 anemia**

   Ref. Dutta Obs. 7/e, p 268; Williams Obs. 22/e, p 1147, 23/e, p 1082; Fernando Arias 3/e, p 469

- In countries **like India,** anemia due to iron and folic acid deficiency commonly occur during pregnancy.
- Only Vitamin B_{12} deficiency as a cause of *anemia is rare.*

"*Megaloblastic anemia caused by lack of vitamin B12, that is cyanocobalamin, during pregnancy is exceedingly rare*".

—*Williams Obs. 22/e, p 1147, 23/e, p 1082*

5. **Ans. is b and d, i.e. Iron deficiency state and Hemolytic anemia**

Ref. William's Obstetrics 2/e, p 1080; Dutta Obs. 7/e, p 262; Park 20/e, p 556

"The two most common cause of anemia during pregnancy and puerperium are iron deficiency and acute blood loss[Q]"

6. **Ans is d, i.e. Evans syndrome** *(Read the text below)*

The clinical scenario of the patient shows the following signs and symptoms:
- Fever
- Anemia
- Thrombocytopenia
- Normal total leukocyte count
- Fragmented RBCs (Schistocytes) on peripheral smear.

Now let us review each option one by one

Option (a): DIC   —*Harrison 20/e, p 979*
- DIC may present with sudden onset of **fever** (as the M/c cause of D/c is sepsis)
- Excessive bleeding may lead to **anemia**
- Platelet consumption may lead to **thrombocytopenia**
- Leukocyte count is not affected
- Intravascular microangiopathic hemolysis can lead to **schistocytes on peripheral smear.**

—*Williams Obs 23/e, p 786*

Option (b): TTP i.e Thrombotic thrombocytopenic purpura.

TTP presents with a pentad of:
- Fever
- Microangiopathic hemolytic anemia, leading to **anemia** and **fragmentation of RBCs**
- Thrombocytopenia
- Neurologic symptoms
- Renal failure.

Option (c): HELLP syndrome

HELLP syndrome presents with the combination of:
- **Hemolysis** because of which fragmented RBC's may be seen
- Elevated liver enzymes and
- Low platelet count
- Fever may or may not be present.

Oprion (d): Evans syndrome   —*Hoffman: Hematology: Basic Principle and Practice, 5/e*
- Evans syndrome is an **autoimmune disease** in which an individual's antibodies attack their own red blood cells and platelets.
- Its overall pathology resembles a combination of autoimmune haemolytic anemia and idiopathic thrombocytopenic purpura.
- Autoimmune hemolysis leads to the formation of spherocytes and not schistocytes.
- Schistocytes are fragmented RBCs that are the result of microangiopathic hemolysis.
- Autoimmune destruction of RBCs leads to the formation of spherocytes.

Hence, **Evans syndrome is the least likely possibility in this clinical scenario.**

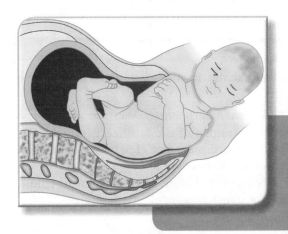

22

Heart Disease in Pregnancy

 Chapter at a Glance

NORMAL FINDINGS IN CVS DURING PREGNANCY

- Pulse rate increases
- Diastolic BP decreases
- First heart sound is prominent and split
- Second heart sound—normal
- Third heart sound—normally not heard but in pregnancy it is prominent
- **Murmurs**
  - Ejection systolic murmur heard normally in aortic or pulmonary area at 10–12 weeks due to expanded intravenous volume heard in 90% cases.
  - A soft diastolic murmur is heard in 10% cases.
  - Continuous murmur heard normally over the tricuspid area in left 2–3rd intercostal space heard in 10% cases.
- Apex beat is heard in the fourth ICS, 2.5 cm left to midclavicular line
- Slight cardiomegaly on X-ray
- ECG- left axis deviation.

HEART DISEASE IN PREGNANCY

Metcalfe's Criteria for Heart Disease in Pregnancy

Indicators of Heart Disease during Pregnancy

Signs	Symptoms
Persistently dilated neck veins (↑ JVP)	Orthopnea
Cyanosis/clubbing	Nocturnal cough

Contd...

Contd...

Signs	Symptoms
Systolic murmur greater than grade 3	Chest pain
Diastolic murmur	Hemoptysis
Marked cardiomegaly	Syncope
Sustained arrhythmia	
Persistent split second heart sound	

Most Common Heart Disease

Most common in pregnancy	Lesion
Acquired valvular disease	Mitral stenosis
Congenital heart disease	Atrial septal defect
Cyanotic congenital heart disease	Fallot's tetralogy

Clark's Classification of Heart Disease in Pregnancy

Group I–Minimal risk (Mortality 0–1%)	Group III (Mortality 25–50%)
• ASD, VSD, PDA (congenital heart diseases)	• Pulmonary hypertension – primary or secondary, an example of secondary being—Eisenmenger syndrome
• Fallot tetralogy (corrected)	• Marfan syndrome with aorta involvement (> 40 mm)

Contd...

Contd...

Group I–Minimal risk (Mortality 0–1%)	Group III (Mortality 25–50%)
• Any disease involving pulmonary and tricuspid valve	• Coarctation of aorta
• Bioprosthetic valve replacement	
• Mitral stenosis belonging to class I, II according to NYHA	

Note: There is no need to remember Class 2 of the Clarkes classification.

Since in group III maternal mortality is high, hence these are also the **indications of termination of pregnancy in heart disease patients** or they are the conditions of **heart diseases in which pregnancy is contraindicated**.

NYHA Classification (Revised 1979)

- **Class I:** No limitation of physical activity
- **Class II:** Slight limitation of physical activity
- **Class III:** Marked limitation of physical activity
- **Class IV:** Severely compromised—Inability to perform any physical activity without discomfort.

WHO Class IV

Heart Diseases in which Termination of Pregnancy is Advised/Pregnancy is Contraindicated
1. Marfans syndrome with aorta involvement (> 40 mm)
2. Coarctation of aorta
3. Eisenmenger syndrome
4. Severe mitral stenosis or severe symptomatic aortic stenosis
5. Any heart disease which belongs to NYHA class 4 or class 3
6. Ejection fraction < 30%.
7. Previous peripartum cardiomyopathy with any residual impairment of LV function.
8. Pulmonary arterial hypertension due to any cause.
9. Severe left heart obstruction

Predictors of Cardiac Event during Pregnancy

Potential for an adverse cardiac event in a pregnant female as pulmonary edema, sustained arrhythmia, stroke, cardiac arrest or cardiac death can be estimated by following parameters.

N New York Heart Association (NYHA) class >2

O Obstructive lesions of the left heart (mitral valve area <2 cm² or aortic valve area <1.5 cm², peak LV outflow tract gradient >30 mm of Hg).

P Prior cardiac event before pregnancy—heart failure, arrhythmia, transient ischemic attack, stroke

E Ejection fraction <40%

The risk of cardiac complications is 5%, 30% and 75% when none, one or more than one of these complications are present.

 Important One Liners

- Heart disease with maximum risk of maternal mortality: Eisenmenger's syndrome.
- M/C cause of maternal mortality in heart disease during pregnancy mitral stenosis
- M/C time of heart failure during pregnancy = immediate postpartum > 2nd stage of labor > late 1st stage of labor > 28–32 weeks of pregnancy > early 1st stage of labor.

Management of Heart Disease in Pregnancy

Antepartum Management

Time of hospitalization:

- Class I of WHO – 36 weeks
- Class II 28 weeks
- Class III and IV – If seen in the first trimester. **MTP should be advised ideally but if patient wants to continue** pregnancy, then the women are hospitalized for the remainder of the pregnancy.

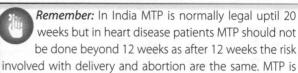

Remember: In India MTP is normally legal uptil 20 weeks but in heart disease patients MTP should not be done beyond 12 weeks as after 12 weeks the risk involved with delivery and abortion are the same. MTP is done using suction and evacuation.

- The most important measure for reducing the impact of pregnancy upon a diseased heart is restricted activity.
- To prevent excessive sodium and water retention, moderate degree of dietary sodium restriction is advised.
- If moderate restriction is sodium intake is insufficient to limit the normal intravascular volume expansion, then diuretics – Furosemide (FDA category C) should be used.

Intrapartum Management

- **Position of Patient:** Semi recumbent
- Patients should be allowed to go into spontaneous labor, if required induction with vaginal PGE2 may be done **(Induction is safe in case of heart disease).**
  —*Williams Obs. 25/e, p 953*
- Trial of labor is contraindicated in patients of heart disease.
- Patients should be advised to lie in propped up position.
- Restrict I/V fluids @ 75 ml/hr.
- Vaginal delivery is preferred. If second stage is more than 30 mins, then use outlet forceps or vacuum. Between the two, vacuum is better (as lithotomy position is not needed).
- Epidural analgesia is given during labor for pain relief.

> **Heart disease where vaginal delivery is contraindicated/ cesarean section is done:** *Williams Obs. 25/e p 953*
> - Aortic aneurysm or dilated aortic root ≥ 4 cm
> - Marfans syndrome with aortic involvement
> - Severe symptomatic aortic stenosis
> - Acute severe congestive heart failure
> - Recent MI
> - Need for emergency valve replacement immediately after delivery
> - A patient who is fully anticoagulated with warfarin at the time of labor needs to be counseled for cesarean section because the baby is also anticoagulated and vaginal delivery carries increase risk to the fetus of intracranial hemorrhage.

- **Anesthesia given during LSCS in heart disese:** Epidural anesthesia.

> **Conditions where general anesthesia is given during cesarean (to prevent hypotension)**
> - Intracardiac shunts
> - Severe aortic stenosis
> - Pulmonary arterial hypertension

Postpartum Management

Prevention of pulmonary edema (as this is the time when cases of heart failure are maximum) by giving I/V furosemide after placental delivery.

After delivery ergometrine or methylergometrine is contraindicated. To control bleeding oxytocin can be given.

> **Conditions where Methylergometrine is Contraindicated.** —*Dutta Obs. 7/e, p 503*
> - **Twin pregnancy:** If given after the delivery of first baby, the second baby will be compromised
> - **Organic cardiac disease:** Can cause overloading of right heart and precipitate heart failure
> - **Severe pre-eclampsia and eclampsia:** Can cause sudden rise in BP
> - **Rh negative mother:** Increased chances of fetomaternal transfusion.

Contraception in Heart Disease

- **Contraception of choice: Temporary** IUCD (earlier IUCD was not recommended but now WHO recommends its use); progesterone only pills, implants or injection, barrier contraceptives (condoms).
- **Contraception to be avoided:**
  – OCPs (can precipitate thromboembolic event)

Contraception of choice—Permanent:

- If the heart is not well—compensated, the patient's husband is advised for vasectomy.[Q]
- If heart is well—compensated–tubal sterilisation can be carried out.

Sterilisation should be considered with the completion of the family at the end of first week in the puerperium under local anesthesia through abdominal route by minilap technique.

Prognosis of Heart Disease in Pregnancy

General Fundae

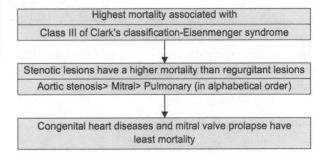

| Highest mortality associated with |
| Class III of Clark's classification-Eisenmenger syndrome |

| Stenotic lesions have a higher mortality than regurgitant lesions |
| Aortic stenosis> Mitral> Pulmonary (in alphabetical order) |

| Congenital heart diseases and mitral valve prolapse have least mortality |

Important One Liners

- Best time for cardiac surgery in mitral stenosis 14–18 weeks
- Surgery of choice (percutaneous transcatheter balloon valvuloplasty–if valves are not calcified
- If valves are calcified–valve replacement is required. This should be done ideally before conception, because during pregnancy it carries a high risk of maternal and perinatal morality.
- Septic abortion–M/C valve affected is tricuspid valve
- M/C fetal complication in heart disease is IUGR
- Best tocolytic in heart disease patient: Atosiban

Mitral stenosis

- Grading
- Normal – Normal mitral valve area is 4–6 cm²
- Mild stenosis – < 4 cm² + to > 1.5 cm²
- Moderate stenosis – 1.5–1 cm²
- Severe stenosis – < 1 cm²

INFECTIVE ENDOCARDITIS

- Bacterial infection of a heart valve involves cardiac endothelium and usually results in valvular vegetations.
- Organisms that cause indolent endocarditis are most often viridans-group streptococci or *Staphylococcus* or *Enterococcus* species.
- Among intravenous drug abusers and those with catheter-related infections, *Staphylococcus aureus* is the predominant organism.
- *Staphylococcus epidermidis* frequently causes prosthetic valve infections.

Diagnosis

Diagnosis is made using the **Duke criteria**, which include positive blood cultures for typical organisms and evidence of endocardial involvement. Echocardiography may be diagnostic, but lesions < 2 mm in diameter or those on the tricuspid valve may be missed. If uncertain, transesophageal echocardiography (TEE) is accurate and informative.

Management

Most streptococci are sensitive to penicillin G, ceftriaxone, or vancomycin given intravenously for 4 to 6 weeks, along with gentamicin for 2 to 4 weeks. Complicated infections are treated longer, and women allergic to penicillin are either desensitized or given intravenous ceftriaxone or vancomycin for 4 weeks.

Antibiotic Prophylaxis against Infective Endocarditis (IE)

Recommendation of American College of Cardiology/ American Heart Association for Endocarditis Prophylaxis Regimens. *(AHA 2007)*

- The American Heart Association recently updated its guidelines regarding which patients should take a precautionary antibiotic to prevent infective endocarditis (IE).
- Prophylactic antibiotics are no longer recommended for gastrointestinal or genitourinary tract procedures. This recommendation follows from the observation that most cases of IE result from bacteremia caused by routine activities such as chewing food, brushing teeth and flossing.

It is recommended that IE prophylaxis may be given during labor in the following subgroups of patients:

- Prosthetic cardiac valve
- Previous endocarditis
- Unrepaired congenital heart disease (including palliative shunts and conduits)
- Completely repaired congenital heart defect with prosthetic material or device, during the first 6 months after the procedure
- Repaired congenital heart disease with residual defects at the site or adjacent to the site of aprosthetic patch or device
- Cardiac transplantation recipients who develop cardiac valvulopathy.

ACOG does not recommend endocarditis prophylaxis for either vaginal or cesarean delivery in absence of pelvic infection.

Antibiotic Regimen for IE Prophylaxis

- Only a few regimens are recommended by the American College of Obstetricians and Gynecologists (2008) for prophylaxis which is given preferably 30–60 minutes before the procedure.

- Either ampicillin, (amoxicillin) 2 gm, or cefazolin or ceftriaxone, 1 gm, is given intravenously.
- For penicillin sensitive patients, cefzolin, ceftriaxone is given or if there is history of anaphylaxis, then clindamycin, 600 mg is given intravenously. If Enterococcus infection is of concern, vancomycin is also given.

HEART FAILURE IN PREGNANCY

M/C time of heart failure corresponds to maximum cardiac output during pregnancy = immediately after delivery > 2nd stage of labor > late 1st stage of labor > 28–32 weeks of pregnancy > early 1st stage of labor.

Risk Factors for Heart Failure

- Respiratory infections
- Anemia
- Obesity
- Corticosteroids
- Tocolytics
- Multiple gestation
- Hypertension
- Arrhythmias
- Pain
- Fluid overload.

Treatment of Cardiac Failure

Cardiac failure is treated in the same way as in non-pregnant patients.

- Digoxin, diuretics, oxygen and morphine are used.
- Arrhythmias require selective beta adrenergic blockers and adenosine for supraventricular tachycardia.
- Metoprolol is preferred.

Fetal Risks

- Premature delivery in cyanotic congenital heart disease.
- In coarctation of the aorta poor placental perfusion can cause growth restriction.
- Risk of developing congenital heart disease.

CARDIOVASCULAR DRUG SAFETY PROFILE IN PREGNANCY

Safe Drugs

- Beta-blockers—metaprolol is the preferred drug for arrhythmias
- Adenosine
- Lidocaine
- Procainamide
- Quinidine
- Digoxin

Drugs which should be used Judiciously

- Diuretics
- Calcium antagonists

Unsafe Drugs

- Angiotensin converting enzyme inhibitors
- Amiodarone

ANTICOAGULATION IN PREGNANCY IN PREGNANCY

During pregnancy, the choice of anticoagulant depends on period of gestation as both the available anticoagulants have their own advantages and disadvantages (Table 22.1)

Table 22.1:

	Warfarin	Heparin
Advantage	Strong anticoagulant	Cannot cross the placenta
Disadvantage	Can cross the placenta and lead to **Chondrodysplasia in fetus**	Weak anticoagulant

Period of gestation	Anticoagulant of choice
≤ 12 weeks	Heparin
12 – 36 weeks	Warfarin
≥ 36 weeks	Heparin

 Note: Stop all anticoagulants before delivery.
- Restart anticoagulants 6 hours after vaginal delivery and 24 hours after cesarean section.
- Warfarin/Heparin both are safe in breastfeeding.

New Pattern Questions

N1. Patients with organic heart disease in pregnancy most commonly die during:
a. 20–24 weeks of pregnancy
b. First stage of labor
c. Soon following delivery
d. Two weeks postpartum

N2. The best method of curtailing the second stage of labor in heart disease is by:
a. Prophylactic forceps
b. Prophylactic ventouse
c. Spontaneous delivery with episiotomy
d. Cesarean section

N3. In severe mitral stenosis during pregnancy area of mitral valve is:
a. 4–6 cm^2 b. 1.5–2.5 cm^2
c. 1–1.5 cm^2 d. 0.8–1 cm^2

N4. A G21, female with mitral stenosis develops dyspnea, chest pain and palpitations. Her period of amenorrhea is 37 weeks. O/E P/R = 120 bpm, RR = 30/min

Basal creps present in both lungs.

Which is the best management option?
a. Induce labor after treating heart failure
b. Do cesarean after treating heart failure
c. Perform cesarean immediately
d. Perform mitral valvotomy

N5. A woman with mitral stenosis but no pulmonary hypertension is in labor at 39 weeks of gestation. She has dyspnea on exertion. Her pulse rate is 80 bpm. There are no basal creps in lungs.

The cervix is 4 cm dilated. She is having 1–2 uterine contractions in 10 minutes. Which of the following steps is best avoided in her?
a. Active management of third stage of labor
b. Augmentation of labor with oxytocin
c. Use of epidural analgesia for pain relief
d. Use of ergometrine in third stage of labor

N6. Cesarean section is mandatory in which cardiac disease?
a. VSD
b. Coarctation of aorta
c. MVP
d. MS

N7. A 35-year-old second para with mitral stenosis has normal vaginal delivery at 40 weeks. The baby is healthy. Her first child is healthy and is 5 year old. Which of the following is the best method of contraception in this woman?

a. Ligation and resection of fallopian tubes after 6 weeks
b. Oral contraceptive pills
c. Postpartum ligation and resection of fallopian tubes
d. Subdermal progesterone implants

N8. Tubectomy in a heart patient who has recently delivered is best done after:
a. 48 hours b. 1 week
c. 2 weeks d. Immediately

N9. A para 2 poorly compensated cardiac patient has delivered 2 days back. You will advice her to:
a. Undergo sterilization (tubectomy) after 1 week
b. Undergo sterilization after 6 weeks
c. Suggest her husband to undergo vasectomy
d. Take oral contraceptive pills after 6 months

N10. A prosthetic valve patient switch to heparin at which time of pregnancy?
a. 28 weeks b. 32 weeks
c. 36 weeks d. Postpartum

N11. Congenital heart disease is most likely in the newborn of mothers suffering from all *except*:
a. Systemic lupus erythematosus
b. Rheumatoid arthritis
c. Diabetes in pregnancy
d. Congenital heart disease of the mother

N12. Chances of adverse outcome in a heart disease patient are increased in all of the following periods *except*:
a. 28–32 weeks of pregnancy
b. At the time of labor
c. 4–5 days after delivery
d. Immediately after delivery
e. None of the above

N13. All of the following rules are increased in infants of heart disease patient *except*:
a. Prematurity
b. IUGR
c. Increased incidence of cardiac disease
d. Neural tube defect

N14. Anticoagulant choice at 24 weeks of pregnancy:
a. LMWH b. Unfractionated heparin
c. Both a + b d. Warfarin

N15. A G2P1 on warfarin presents at 38 weeks in labor: Next step
a. Stop warfarin, proceed with vaginal delivery
b. Stop warfarin, proceed with caesarean section
c. Replace warfarin with heparin and proceed with vaginal delivery
d. Replace warfarin with heparin & proceed with cesarean section

Previous Year Questions

1. **Maximum cardiac output in pregnancy is at:**
   [AIIMS Nov 2013]
   a. 20 weeks   b. 24 weeks
   c. 26 weeks   d. 28 weeks
   e. Nervousness or syncope on exertion

2. **Signs of heart disease in pregnancy:** [PGI June 03]
   a. Diastolic murmur   b. Systolic murmur
   c. Tachycardia   d. Dyspnea on exertion
   e. Nervousness or syncope on exertion

3. **Which of the following features indicates the presence of heart disease in pregnancy and which is not seen in normal pregnancy?**
   a. Exertional dyspnea   **[AIIMS Nov 12, 13]**
   b. Distended neck veins
   c. Systemic hypotension
   d. Pedal edema

4. **Maximum strain of parturient heart occurs during:**
   [AIIMS Nov 07, 06]
   a. At term   b. Immediate postpartum
   c. Ist trimester   d. IInd trimester

5. **In a pregnant woman with heart disease, all of the following are to be done except:**
   [AIIMS June 00; AI 02]
   a. IV methergin after delivery
   b. Prophylactic antibiotic
   c. IV frusemide postpartum
   d. Cut short 2nd stage of labor

6. **In a patient with heart disease, which of the following should not be used to control PPH?**
   [AIIMS Nov 07, AI 11]
   a. Methylergometrine b. Oxytocin
   c. Misoprostol   d. Carboprost

7. **In which of the following heart diseases is maternal mortality during pregnancy found to be the highest:**
   a. Coarctation of aorta   **[AIIMS Nov 07, 06]**
   b. Eisenmenger syndrome
   c. AS
   d. MS

8. **Normal pregnancy can be continued in:**
   [AIIMS May 09/AI 11]
   a. Primary pulmonary hypertension
   b. Wolf-Parkinson-White syndrome
   c. Eisenmenger syndrome
   d. Marfan syndrome with dilated aortic root

9. **Indications for termination of pregnancy include:**
   a. Aortic stenosis   **[PGI May 2013]**
   b. Eisenmengers syndrome
   c. Tricuspid stenosis
   d. Severe mitral stenosis + NYHA grade II
   e. NYHA grade 4 heart disease with history of decompensation in the previous pregnancy

10. **Most common heart disease associated with pregnancy is:** **[AI 97]**
    a. Mitral stenosis
    b. Mitral regurgitation
    c. Patent ductus arteriosus
    d. Tatralogy of Fallot

11. **In which of the following heart diseases maternal mortality is found to be highest?**
    a. Eisenmenger's complex   **[AIIMS May 06; May 07]**
    b. Coarctation of aorta
    c. Mitral stenosis
    d. Aortic stenosis

12. **Indications for cesarean section in pregnancy are all except:** **[AIIMS May 09]**
    a. Eisenmenger syndrome
    b. Aortic stenosis
    c. Aortic aneurysm
    d. Aortic regurgitation

13. **In heart patient the worst prognosis during pregnancy is seen in:** **[AIIMS June 00]**
    a. Mitral regurgitation
    b. Mitral valve prolapse
    c. Aortic stenosis
    d. Pulmonary stenosis

14. **Kalindi 25 years female admitted as a case of septic abortion with tricuspid valve endocarditis. Vegetation from the valve likely to affect is:** **[AIIMS Nov 01]**
    a. Liver   b. Spleen
    c. Brain   d. Lungs

15. **True about is/are:** **[PGI June 06]**
    a. MS surgery better avoided in pregnancy
    b. MR with PHT-definite indication for termination of pregnancy
    c. Aortic stenosis in young age is due to bicuspid valve
    d. Isolated TR always due to infective endocarditis
    e. MS with pressure gradient 10 mm Hg indication for surgery

16. Lady with MS + MR with full term gestation, obstetrician planning to conduct normal delivery, what would be anesthesia of choice?   **[AIIMS May 2012]**
    a. Parenteral opioids
    b. Spinal anesthesia
    c. Inhalational analgesia
    d. Neuraxial analgesia

17. A pregnant woman at 36-weeks of gestation is admitted in your ward. During the morning rounds, she is lying supine as shown in the figure. What syndrome has been depicted below?

        [AIIMS May 2017]

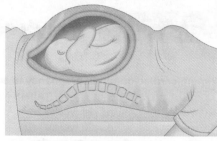

    a. Superior vena cava syndrome
    b. Supine vena cava syndrome
    c. Abdominal aorta syndrome
    d. Inferior vena cava syndrome

Answers with Explanations to New Pattern Questions

N1. **Ans. is c, i.e. Soon following delivery** *Ref. Dutta Obs 7/e, p 225*

This is another way of asking, cardiac failure occurs most common at what time as the M/C cause of death in pregnant females with heart disease is congestive heart failure.

N2. **Ans. is b, i.e. Prophylactic ventouse** *Ref. Dutta Obs 7/e, p 278*

Management of heart disease patient in 2nd stage:

No maternal pushing and the tendency to delay in the second stage of labor is to be curtailed by forceps or ventouse under pudendal and/or perineal block anesthesia. Ventouse is preferable to forceps as it can be applied without putting the patient in lithotomy position (raising the legs increases the cardiac load). —*Dutta Obs 7/e, p 278*

N3. **Ans. is c, i.e. 1–1.5 cm²**

Severe mitral stenosis as per 2014 guidelines is mitral valve area 1.5 cm² or less.

N4. **Ans. is b, i.e. Do cesarean section after treating heart failure**

This patient has developed heart failure which is an emergency and should be treated properly. Since the fetus is mature delivery by cesarean section is the best management as soon as cardiac condition is compensated. Immediate cesarean section is contraindicated because cardiac condition is poor. Oxytocin causes fluid overload, hypotension and arrhythmias and is best avoided for induction and augmentation.

Waiting for spontaneous onset of labor can also worsen her cardiac condition.

Mitral valvotomy can be performed in the second trimester but not in third trimester.

N5. **Ans. is d, i.e. Use of ergometrine in third stage of labor**

Use of Ergometrine/methylergometrine is contraindicated in heart disease patients. Rest all options are correct.

N6. **Ans. is b, i.e. Coarctation of aorta**

See the text for explanation

N7. **Ans. is a, i.e. Ligation and resection of fallopian tubes after 6 weeks**

Permanent sterilization is the best method of contraception for this woman as she has mitral stenosis and has two healthy children. Also she is 35 years of age and eldest child is 5 years of age.

Interval sterilization after 6 weeks is better than immediate postpartum sterilization, to allow time for cardiovascular changes of pregnancy to return to normal. Sterilization by minilaparotomy is safer than the use of laparoscopy for patients with heart disease.

N8. **Ans. is b, i.e. 1 week** *Ref. Dutta Obs. 7/e, p 278*

N9. **Ans. is c, i.e. Suggest her husband to undergo vasectomy** *Ref. Dutta Obs. 7/e, p 278*

Permanent contraception of choice:

- **Best:** Husband should be advised vasectomy especially in patients whose heart is not well-compensated.
- If husband refuses or, if heart of the patient is well-compensated-Tubectomy is advised.

Female sterilisation:

- **Best time**: At the end of first postpartum week.
- Method: Mini laparotomy (never do laproscopic sterilisation in heart disease patient).
- Anesthesia of choice: Local anesthesia.

N10. **Ans. is c, i.e. 36 weeks** *Ref. Williams Obs. 23/e, p 964; Dutta Obs. 7/e Management of High Risk Pregnancy by SS Trivedi, Manju Puri 1/e, p 383*

Pregnancy following valve replacement:

Mechanical valve replacement is not preferred these days as anticoagulation is required throughout pregnancy.

Problem of anticoagulation: During pregnancy, the main problem is of anticoagulation.

Warfarin is safe for the mother but can result in warfarin embryopathy of the fetus, miscarriage, IUGR and stillbirths.

Heparin is safe for the fetus as it does not cross the placenta, but is less effective than warfarin in preventing thromboembolic events.

Low molecular weight heparin is inadequate and ACOG does not recommend its use in pregnant women with prosthetic heart valves.

Period of gestation	Anticoagulant used
Uptil 12 weeks	Unfractionated heparin
12–36 weeks	Warfarin
36 weeks onwards and uptil 6 hours before delivery	IV heparin
For 6 hours after vaginal delivery and 24 hours after casarean	Restart heparin/warfarin

 Note: Warfarin is not contraindicated for breastfeeding.

N11. Ans. is b, i.e. Rheumatoid arthritis *Ref. Dutta Obs 7/e, p 276, 293, 284*

Lets analyse each option separately

"Fetal congenital cardiac disease is increased by 3–10% if either of the parents have congenital heart lessons."

—*Dutta 7/e, p 276. (so option d is correct)*

"Neonatal lupus syndrome is due to crossing of maternal lupus antibodies (anti-Ro or anti-La) to the fetus causing hemolytic anemia, leukopenia and thrombocytopenia. Isolated congenital heart block is present in about one-third of cases. An apparently healthy woman delivering a baby with congenital heart block should be observed for the development of SLE."

—*Dutta 7/e, p 293 (i.e. option a is correct)*

Maternal diabetes we all know leads to fetal heart disease (Dutta 7/e, p 284), so our answer by exclusion is rheumatoid arthritis.

N12. Ans. is e, i.e. None of the above *Ref. Fernando Arias 4/e, p 271, 272*

Period of pregnancy during which a heart disease patient has high chances of adverse outcome are:
1. 12–16 weeks of pregnancy
2. 28–32 weeks of pregnancy
3. At the time of delivery
4. Immediately after delivery
5. 4–5 days after delivery (chances of sudden death due to pulmonary embolization)

N13. Ans. is d, i.e. Neural tube defects *Ref. Fernando Arias 4/e, p 272*

Effect of maternal cardiac disease on fetus:

- Fetal death
- IUGR
- Prematurity
- Increased incidence of heart diseases in fetus (by 4–6%).

N14. Ans. is d, i.e. Warfarin

At 24 weeks of pregnancy, the anticoagulant of choice is warfarin.

N15. Ans. is b i.e. Stop warfarin, proceed with caesarean section

Since the patient is presenting in labor on warfarin, now management is to stop her warfarin and do caesarean section.

 Note: If patient is on warfarin at the time of labor or within 2 weeks of labour, then caesarean section should be done

Answers with Explanations to Previous Year Questions

1. Ans. is d, i.e. 28 weeks *Ref. William 24/e, p 59*

The following graph of Williams shows cardiac output during pregnancy and labor.

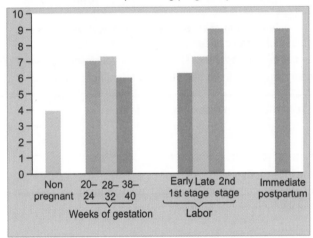

As is clear from the graph cardiac output is maximum at 28–32 weeks of gestation.

Note: At term cardiac output is less in comparison to 28–32 weeks.

2. Ans. is a, d and e, i.e. Diastolic murmur, Dyspnea on exertion and Nervousness or syncope on exertion

3. Ans. is b, i.e. Distended neck veins *Ref. Williams Obs. 22/e, p 1019, 23/e, p 960, Dutta Obs. 7/e, p 275*

- Many of the physiological adaptations of normal pregnancy and physical findings resemble heart disease symptoms and signs, making the diagnosis of heart disease more difficult.
- For example, in normal pregnancy, functional systolic heart murmurs are quite common; respiratory efforts is accentuated, at times suggesting dyspnea and edema in the lower extremities usually develops after midpregnancy.
- It is important not to diagnose heart disease during pregnancy when none exists, and at the same time not to fail to detect and appropriately treat heart disease when it dose exist.

Clinical indicators of Heart disease during Pregnancy: Metcalfes criteria for Heart disease in pregnancy

Symptoms	Clinical findings
• Progressive dyspnea or orthopnea	• Cyanosis
• Nocturnal cough	• Clubbing of fingers
• Hemoptysis	• Persistent neck vein distension
• Syncope with exertion	• Systolic murmur greater than grade 3
• Chest pain related to effort or emotion	• Diastolic murmur
• Symptoms of pulmonary hypertension	• Cardiomegaly
	• Persistent arrhythmia
	• Persistently split second sound
	• Criteria for pulmonary hypertension

 Note: In question 3 – exertional dyspnea, and pedal edema are seen normally during pregnancy and do not indicate heart disease. During pregnancy due to relaxation of the smooth muscles of the arteries by the progesterone, blood pressure decreases (Ref. Dutta 7/e, p 53) i.e. systemic hypotension normally occurs during pregnancy.

- Distended neck veins are suggestive of heart disease in pregnancy and are not a normal physiological condition.

4. Ans. is b, i.e. Immediate postpartum   *Ref. Williams Obs. 22/e, p 1018, 23/e, p 958, 959; Dutta Obs. 7/e, p 53*

"Significant hemodynamic alterations are apparent early in pregnancy, women with severe cardiac dysfunction may experience worsening of heart failure before midpregnancy. In others, heart failure develops after 28 weeks, when pregnancy induced hypervolemia is maximal (32 weeks). In the majority, however heart failure develops peripartum when the physiological capability for rapid changes in cardiac output may be overwhelmed in presence of structural cardiac disease."   —*Williams 22/e, p 1018, 23/e, p 958, 959*

Reading the above text, from *Williams Obs.*, it is clear that maximum chances of heart failure are in the peripartum period. But it is not clear whether maximum chances are during labor or immediate postpartum.

Dutta Obs. 7/e, p 53 provides answer to this:

"The cardiac output starts to increase from 5th week of pregnancy, reaches its peak 40–50% at about 30–34 weeks. Thereafter the cardiac output remains static till term".

"Cardiac output increases further during labor (+50%) and immediately following delivery (+70%) over the prelabor values."

So, maximum chances of heart failure are in immediate postpartum period when cardiac output is maximum.

> *Remember:* **Periods of maximum risk of cardiac failure:**
> Immediate postpartum (best option) > During delivery > at 32 weeks (when hemodynamic changes are maximum).

5. Ans. is a, i.e. IV methergine after delivery   *Ref. Dutta Obs. 7/e, p 278*

As discussed in the chapter overview all the options given in the question are correct except for 'c' i.e. methergine after delivery. Methylergometine is contraindicated in patient of heart desease.

6. Ans. is a, i.e. Methylergometrine

Ref. Dutta Obs. 7/e, p 278; Fernando Arias 3/e, p 511, 512; Williams Obs. 22/e, p 1021, 1022, 23/e, p 962, 963

See the text for explanation

7. Ans. is b, i.e. Eisenmenger syndrome

8. Ans. is b, i.e. Wolf-Parkinson-White syndrome

9. Ans. is b and e, i.e. Eisenmengers syndrome and NYHA grade 4 heart disease with history of decompensation in the previous pregnancy   *Ref. Williams Obs. 23/e, p 980, 981; Fernando Arias 3/e, p 507; Dutta Obs. 7/e, p 276*

Clarkes classification for risk of maternal mortality caused by Various heart disease

Group I- Minimal risk	Group II (Mortality 5–15%)	Group III (Mortality 25–50%)
(Mortality 0–1%) ASD, VSD, PDA Fallot tetralogy (corrected) Any pulmonary and tricuspid disease Bioprosthetic valve replacement MS class I, II (NYHA).	AS Aortic coarctation without valvular involvement, uncorrected fallot tetralogy Marfan syndrome with normal aorta MS class III, IV Previous MI MS with AF Artificial valve	• Primary pulmonary hypertension • Complicated aortic coarctation • Marfan's with aortic involvement • Eisenmenger syndrome

"Maternal mortality may be raised to even 50% in case of Eisenmenger syndrome."   —*Dutta Obs. 6/e, p 278*

"The outcome of pregnancy in patients with Eisenmengers syndrome is very poor maternal mortality is 52% and total fetal wastage is 41.7%."   —*Fernando Arias 3/e, p 520*

10. Ans. is a, i.e. Mitral stenosis   *Ref. Dutta Obs. 7/e, p 275; Fernando Arias 3/e, p 522*

In developing countries like India:

• Most common heart disease in pregnancy is of rheumatic origin, followed by the congenital heart disease.
• Most common rheumatic valvular lesion is mitral stenosis *(in 80%)* followed by mitral regurgitation and aortic stenosis.

In developed countries:

• Most common heart disease is *congenital heart disease.*[Q]
• Most common lesion is *Atrial septal defect.*[Q]

11. **Ans. is a, i.e. Eisenmenger's complex** *Ref. Williams Obs. 22/e, p 1028, 23/e, p 970; Sheila Balakrishnan, p 283*

Eisenmenger's syndrome is the presence of secondary pulmonary hypertension that develops from any cardiac lesion.[Q]

- The syndrome develops when increased pulmonary blood flow due to left to right shunt produces a right side pressure more than left side and hence reversal of shunt occurs and subsequently cyanosis develops.
- It is the heart disease with the worst prognosis during pregnancy with a maternal mortality of 50%.[Q] Hence, pregnancy is contraindicated is patients of Eisenmengers.
- If diagnosis of Eisenmenger is made in the first trimester, termination of pregnancy is advised.
- Most common cause of death in Eisenmenger's syndrome is right ventricular failure with cardiogenic shock.[Q]

12. **Ans. is a, i.e. Eisenmenger's syndrome** *Ref: Williams 24/e, p 978*

> **Cardiac indications for cesarean section:**
> - Aortic aneurysm or dilated aortic root ≥ 4 cm
> - Marfans syndrome with aortic involvement
> - Severe symptomatic aortic stenosis
> - Acute severe congestive heart failure
> - Recent MI
> - Need for emergency valve replacement immediately after delivery
> - A patient who is fully anticoagulated with warfarin at the time of labor needs to be counseled for cesarean section because the baby is also anticoagulated and vaginal delivery carries increase risk to the fetus of intracranial hemorrhage.

13. **Ans. is c, i.e. Aortic stenosis**

   Ref. Williams Obs. 22/e, p 1026, 1027, 1030;23/e, p 966, 967, 968, 971 Sheila Balakrishna, p 281

 Remember: **3 'FUNDAS:** Highest maternal mortality is associated with Class III of Clark's classification, so any of those diseases are given they will have the worst prognosis. Amongst them also Eisenmengers syndrome has the worst prognosis.

2. *Stenotic heart disease have a worse prognosis than regurgitant lesions.*

   > *Among stenotic disease-(in alphabetical order)-Aortic stenosis will have the worst> Mitral stenosis>Pulmonary stenosis.*

3. *Congenital heart disease and Mitral valve prolapse have the best prognosis*

   So now this question becomes very easy—Mitral vave prolapse has the best prognosis, so it is ruled out; Regurgitant lesions have a better prognosis than stenotic lesions so mitral regurgitation is also ruled out.

   Now we are left with 2 options, aortic stenosis and pulmonary stenosis—as I said go alphabetically, aortic stenosis will have a worse prognosis than pulmonary.

Let's consider each of the options one by one and see what Williams has to say about each of them.

Option "a"	**Mitral regurgitation**
	"M R is well-tolerated during pregnancy probably due to decreased systemic vascular resistance which actually results in less regurgitation. Heart failure only rarely develops during pregnancy."
	—*Williams Obs. 22/e, p 1026, 23/e, p 966*
Option "b"	**Mitral valve prolapse**
	"Pregnant women with mitral valve prolapse rarely have cardiac complications. In fact pregnancy induced hypervolemia may improve alignment of mitral valve."
	—*Williams Obs. 22/e, p 1030, 23/e, p 971*
Option "c"	**Aortic stenosis**
	"Although mild to moderate degree of aortic stenosis is well tolerated but severe degree is life threatening." —*Williams Obs. 22/e, p 1026, 23/e, p 967*
Option "d"	**Pulmonary stenosis**
	"It is well tolerated during pregnancy and rarely causes any complication."
	—*Williams Obs. 22/e, p 1027, 23/e, p 968*

14. Ans. is d, i.e. Lungs   *Ref. CMDT '07, p 1447*

"Right sided endocarditis which usually involves the tricuspid valve causes septic pulmonary emboli occasionally with infarction and lung abscesses."

15. Ans. a, b and c, i.e. MS surgery better avoided in pregnancy; MR with PHT- definite indication for termination of pregnancy; and Aortic stenosis in young age is due to Bicuspid valve   *Ref. Harrison 17/e, p 1472, 1473, 1479; Williams Obs. 22/e, p 1023, 23/e, p 964, 965; Sheila Balakrishnan, p 279*

Let us consider each option separately.

Option "a"   **MS surgery better avoided in pregnancy.**
                      Cardiac surgery in pregnancy: *—Williams Obs. 22/e, p 1023, 23/e, p 964, 965; Sheila Balakrishnan p 279*

"Cardiac surgery should usually be postponed until after delivery but if required can be performed safely in the second trimester."
i.e. option 'a' is correct

 Remember: **Indications of performing a surgical procedure in pregnancy:**
- Failure of medical treatment in intractable heart failure.
- Recurrent episodes of acute pulmonary edema.

Procedure of choice: Balloon valvuloplasty (If valves are pliable and noncalcified and regurgitation is minimal).

Option "b"   **MR with PHT-definite indication for termination of pregnancy:**
"Women with pulmonary hypertension from any cause are at increased risk and such women ideally should not become pregnant. If they do, termination is offered in the first trimester". (absolute indications for termination).   *—Sheila Balakrishnan p 275*
Therefore, MR with PHT is a definite indication for termination of pregnancy.

 Remember: Absolute indications for termination of pregnancy:
All, conditions included under Class III of Clarkes classification

Relative indication:
- Any heart disease belonging to Grade III/IV NYHA
- Any heart disease belonging to Grade I/II NYHA with heart failure

Option "c"   **Aortic stenosis in young age is due to Bicuspid valve**
"Aortic stenosis (AS) in adults may be due to degenerative calcification of the Aortic cusps. It may be congenital, or it may be secondary to rheumatic infection."
                                                            —Harrison 17/e, p 1472, 1473
"Aortic stenosis is essentially a disease of aging and hence rare in pregnancy unless associated with a congenital lesion like bicuspid aortic valve".   *—Sheila Balakrishna p 281*

Option "d"   **Isolated TR is always due to infective endocarditis**
Tricuspid regurgitation (TR) is most commonly functional and secondary to marked dilatation of the tricuspid annulus. Isolated TR occurs in:
- Infarction of the right ventricular papillary muscles.
- Tricuspid valve prolapse.
- Carcinoid heart disease.
- Endomyocardial fibrosis.
- Infective endocarditis.
- Trauma.   *—Harrison 17/e, p 1479*
i.e. *option 'd'* is incorrect becasue isolated TR is not just caused by infective endocarditis.

Option "e"   **MS with pressure gradient 10 mm Hg-indication for surgery**
I did not get much information on this one except that valve replacement for MS during pregnancy is done electively.
"When pump flow rate is >2.5 l/min/m², perfusin pressure is >70 mm of Hg and hematocrit is >28%" —Williams 23/e, p 965

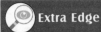 **Extra Edge**

- The normal mitral valve area is about 4 cm^2.
- *Critical or severe stenosis is a valve area less than 1 cm^2, moderate stenosis 1–2.5 cm^2 and mild stenosis 2.5–4 cm^2.*
- **Symptoms** most common–**dyspnea** it develop when stenosis is < 2.5 cm^2.
- Best surgery for MS during pregnancy is Balloon valvuloplasty and best time to do surgery during pregnancy is 14–18 weeks, i.e second trimester.
- M/C fetal complication of heart disease is IUGR.
- **Fetal growth restriction** seen when stenosis is *< 1 cm^2.*

16. **Ans. is d, i.e. Neuraxial analgesia**   *Ref. Williams, 22/e, p 483*

Pain relief is important for heart disease patients as pain can cause tachycardia, which in turn can cause cardiac failure. Epidural and spinal techniques are the most effective means of providing pain relief for labor. These are also known as regional techniques because pain relief is limited to a specific anatomical region. *These modalities are also known as neuraxial techniques, since both the approaches involve administration of drugs that exert their effects in the axial portion of the CNS.*

17. **Ans. is d, i.e. Inferior vena cava syndrome**

Supine Hypotension Syndrome— Mengerts Syndrome

During late pregnancy, the gravid uterus produces a compression effect on the inferior vena cava when the patient is in supine position. This, however, results in opening up of the collateral circulation by means of paravertebral and azygos veins. In some cases (10%), when the collateral circulation fails to open up, the venous return of the heart decreases, co-cardiac output of mother decreases, therefore she experiences tachycardia and hypotension. On the other hand, due to decrease in mothers cardiac output, the fetal blood flow also decreases, so there is fetal distress. That is why all pregnant females are advised not to lie supine in late second and third trimester

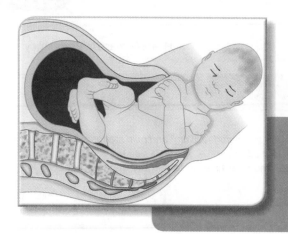

Diabetes and Thyroid in Pregnancy

 Chapter at a Glance

- ➢ Carbohydrate Metabolism in Pregnancy
- ➢ Diabetes in Pregnancy
- ➢ Congenital Malformations in Diabetic Females
- ➢ Gestational Diabetes
- ➢ Management of Diabetes in Pregnancy

- ➢ Complications of Gestational Diabetes
- ➢ Thyroid Disorders in Pregnancy
- ➢ Thyroid Physiology and Pregnancy
- ➢ Hypothyroidism in Pregnancy
- ➢ Hyperthyroidism in Pregnancy

CARBOHYDRATE METABOLISM IN PREGNANCY

- Pregnancy is a diabetogenic state which is associated with hyperinsulinemia as well as insulin resistance
- **Insulin Resistance is due to placental hormones:**
  Human placental lactogen (mainly)
  Estrogen
  Progesterone
  Cortisol
  } All have anti-insulin like action
- Insulin resistance is maximum between **24–28 weeks of pregnancy**.
- Maternal insulin cannot cross the placenta
- Fetus starts secreting insulin **by 12 weeks**.

📝 **Key Concept**

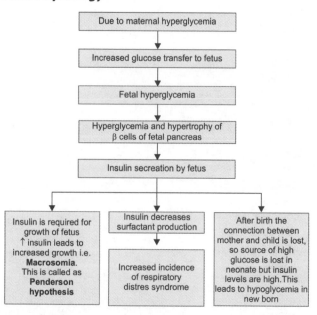

Intervilli space

Villi

Fig. 23.1: Villi and intervillous space in placenta

- We know placenta has villi which has fetal blood and inter-villi spaces which has maternal blood.
- Transfer of nutrients occurs through the placenta

Contd…

Contd…

- The main source of fetal energy is glucose which is transferred by facilitated diffusion using **glucose transport proteins** called **GLUT-1 and GLUT-3**
- This is the reason why, all the mechanisms which increase glucose like insulin resistance, increased lipolysis etc. operate during pregnancy so that fetus has sufficient glucose

Effects of Maternal Hyperglycemia on Fetal Physiology

Due to maternal hyperglycemia

↓

Increased glucose transfer to fetus

↓

Fetal hyperglycemia

↓

Hyperglycemia and hypertrophy of β cells of fetal pancreas

↓

Insulin secreation by fetus

↓

Insulin is required for growth of fetus ↑ insulin leads to increased growth i.e. **Macrosomia**. This is called as **Penderson hypothesis**	Insulin decreases surfactant production	After birth the connection between mother and child is lost, so source of high glucose is lost in neonate but insulin levels are high. This leads to hypoglycemia in new born
	Increased incidence of respiratory distres syndrome	

Also Know:

- Due to maternal hyperglycemia, placenta undergoes hydropic changes (as glucose imbibes water) and so it becomes non-functional at places. This creates a disparity in the demand and supply as demand of oxygen is more by the macrosomic fetus, leading to hypoxia which leads to sudden IUD in diabetic females. This is also the reason for hypertrophic cardiomyopathy seen in infants of diabetic mother.

DIABETES IN PREGNANCY

Diabetes Pregnancy can be Following Two Types

Gestational diabetes	Overt diabetes i.e. Patients of DM type I and type II
• Normoglycemic female develops diabetes in pregnancy due to insulin resistance (insulin resistance in pregnancy is maximum at 24-28 weeks and is mainly due to the effect of hormone human placental lactogen) • These females will thus have high sugar levels at or after approx. 24 weeks of pregnancy	• Overt diabetes means hyperglycemic female becomes pregnant • Switch them from oral hypoglycemic to insulin as oral hypoglycemic can cross the placenta • These females have high sugar levels from Day 1 of pregnancy so free radicals are formed from Day 1 and thus it can lead to congenital malformations in fetus.
Note: In diabetic patients high blood sugar levels lead to formation of free radicals which in turn lead to fetal malformations, now in gestational diabetic patients, free radicals will be formed approx. after 24 weeks (i.e. when blood sugar levels will rise) • By 24 weeks almost the organogenesis is complete in the fetus so it does not lead to congenital malformation in fetus.	• **Diagnostic criteria for diabetes during pregnancy** • According to American Diabetes Association the criteria for diagnosis of overt diabetes during pregnancy is: a. Random plasma glucose > 200 mg/dl + classic symptoms of diabetes b. Fasting blood glucose ≥ 126 mg /dl c. HbA1C > 6.5% d. Two or more abnormal values on 100 gm oral glucose tolerance test during pregnancy.

Important

Gestational diabetes does not lead to congenital malformations in fetus. Overt diabetes leads to congenital malformations in fetus.

CONGENITAL MALFORMATION IN DIABETIC FEMALES

- Best test to predict risk of congenital malformations in overt diabetic females is: Estimation of HbA1C levels
- HbA1C levels: < 6.5%: No greater risk of malformation than non-diabetic mothers
- 6.5–8.5%: risk of anomalies is 5%
- > 10%: risk of anomalies is 22%
- Best Investigation to detect congenital anomalies in fetuses of diabetic mothers – Level II scan / TIFFA (Targeted imaging for fetal anomalies) done at 18–20 weeks
- M/C system involved in congenital malformations = CVS > CNS
- M/C congenital anomaly seen = ventricular septal defect > Neural Tube defect
- Most specific anomaly seen = caudal regression syndrome (Sacral agenesis). But remember this anomaly, in itself is very rare
- Most common cardiac anomaly seen in babes of diabetic mothers = VSD.
- M/C CVS finding seen in babies of diabetic mother = HOCM (hypertrophic cardiomyopathy)
- Most specific cardiac anomaly seen – Transposition of great arteries

Anomalies associated with diabetic females

CNS: NTD, Meningocele, Encephalo cell
CVS: Transposition of great arteries, VSD, ASD, Hypoplastic left heart, coarctation of aorta
Skeletal: Caudal regression syndrome sacral agenesis
Renal: Renal agenesis, cystic kidney, duplex ureter
GIT: Duodenal atresia, anal atresia, rectal atresia

Measures to Decrease the Risk of Congenital Malformation in Overt Diabetic Females

- Strict control of blood sugar in periconceptional period in early pregnancy with insulin

 Note: All oral hypoglycemic agents should be stopped as soon as a diabetic female becomes pregnant except metformin and replaced with rapid acting/ intermediate acting insulin

- Prepregnancy HbA1C levels should be < 6.1% (NICE guideline 2008)
- Folic acid supplementation – dose = 4 mg
  This is called as **therapeutic dose of folic acid**. It should be given 1 month before conception and continued for 3 months after conception.

Protocol for Diagnosis of Congenital Malformation

HbA1C level estimation before 14 weeks

⇓

TVS in 1st trimester to detect anencephaly (11-14 weeks) and levels of PAPPA + βhCG to detect Downs syndrome

⇓

Targeted anomaly scan at 18-20 weeks

⇓

Fetal echocardiography done between 22–24 weeks

GESTATIONAL DIABETES

Any degree of insular intolerance diagnosed for first time during pregnancy irrespective of gestational age and parity is gestational diabetes.

Risk for Gestational Diabetes

Fifth International Workshop on Gestational diabetes: Recommended screening strategy based on risk assessment for detecting GDM.

- **Low Risk**
  - Member of an ethnic group with low prevalence of GDM
  - Age < 25 years
  - BMI= Normal before pregnancy
  - Normal weight at birth
  - No family history of diabetes
  - No H/O poor obstetrical outcome
  - No H/O poor abnormal glucose tolerance.
- **Average Risk**
  - Member of ethnic group with high prevalence of GDM
  - Age > 25 years
  - Overweight before pregnancy
  - High weight at birth of previous baby
- **High Risk**
  - Age > 30 years
  - Marked obesity
  - Previous H/O GDM
  - Strong family history of type 2 DM
  - H/O

- Congenital malformation in previous pregnancies
- ≥ 3 spontaneous abortions
- Still birth / IUD
- Polyhydramnios
- Macrosomia

 Note: ACOG recommends universal screening in Indian population.

Diagnosis of Gestational Diabetes

Can be done by 2 ways:

1. Two step approach as advocated by ACOG
2. One step approach WHO/IAOPSG/DIPSI

Two step approach as advocated by ACOG: As per ACOG, for diagnosis of Gestational diabetes – 2 steps are needed

- **1st step:** Screening Test called as **Glucose Challenge Test** (GCT)
- **2nd step**: Diagnostic Test called as **Glucose Tolerance Test** (GTT)

Earlier ACOG recommended GCT to be done only in females with intermediate or High Risk factors for Gestational Diabetes. But ACOG–2017 recommends universal screening of all pregnant females with GCT.

In Low risk females, screening done only once between 24-28 weeks.

In High risk females or those with intermediate risk – screening done initially on the first antenatal risk & repeated again at 24–28 weeks.

- **1st Step:** Screening test: **Glucose challenge test.**
  - Performed by giving 50 gms of glucose to the female irrespective of previous meals. No fasting is required.
  - Plasma glucose levels are measured after 1 hour.
  - Cut off value is <140 mg%
  - If plasma glucose levels are ≥ 140 mg/dL, and < 180 mg/dL screening is positive and it is followed by confirmatory test (2nd step) i.e. **Glucose Tolerance Test**
  - If plasma glucose values are ≥ 180 mg/dL, no further testing is needed and patient is diagnosed with diabetes.
- **2nd Step:** Confirmatory test: **Glucose Tolerance Test.**
  - GTT as proposed by ACOG, is performed using 100 gm of glucose after overnight fasting (of 8 hrs.)

  - Total 4 blood samples are taken
    Ist sample—FBS sample.
    Then give 100 gm of glucose and collect
        2nd sample—Ist hour PP sample
        3rd sample—2 hour PP sample
        4th sample—3 hour PP sample

Criteria for Diagnosing Gestational Diabetes
Carpenter and Coustan Criteria

Time	100 g Glucose Load	
Fasting	95 mg/dL	5.3 mmol/L
1 hour	180 mg/dL	10.0 mmol/L
2 hour	155 mg/dL	8.6 mmol/L
3 hour	140 mg/dL	7.8 mmol/L

If out of these **any 2 values are abnormal**, it is a confirmed case of Diabetes.

National Diabetes Data group criteria (for Indian Population)

Time	100 g Glucose Load	
Fasting	105 mg/dL	5.8 mmol/L
I hour	190 mg/dL	10.6 mmol/L
2 hour	165 mg/dL	9.2 mmol/L
3 hour	145 mg/dL	8.0 mmol/L

Most of the centres now follow this criteria, as by using Carpenter and Coustan criteria, GDM was detected in more pregnant female, which increases the cost of treatment.

1. One Step Approach as recommended by WHO and IAD PSG

- **It is recommended by American Diabetes Association (ADA) and International Association of Diabetes and Pregnancy study group (IAD PSG) and by WHO**
- It is done only in females with any risk factor @ 24-28 weeks of pregnancy
- It is used both for screening and diagnostic purpose.
- Patient is advised unrestricted diet for 72 hours followed by overnight fasting and then 75 gm of glucose is given
- Total 3 samples are taken:
  - 1st sample = fasting sample
  - 2nd sample = After 1 hour of 75 gm of glucose
  - 3rd sample = After 2 hours of 75 gm glucose

	75 gms OGTT	
	Mg/dl	mmol/litre
Fasting	92	5.1
1 hour	180	10.1
2 hour	153	8.5

Out of these 3 values if any 1 value is abnormal, patient is considered as having gestational diabetes

2. One step approach as recommended by DIPSI (Diabetes in pregnancy study group India).

- Testing done in all pregnant females.
- 75 gms GTT done
- Test done whenever patient comes – not specifically at 24 – 28 weeks.
- No fasting needed

Procedure

Whenever a pregnant female comes for antenatal unit
⇓
Irrespective of her meals
⇓
Give 75 gms glucose
⇓
Check her Blood sugar after 2 hours
⇓

< 120 mg/dL	120-140 mg/dL	≥140 mg/dL	≥ 200 mg/dL
↓	↓	↓	↓
Normal	Glucose Intolerance	Gestational Diabetes	Overt Diabetes

MANAGEMENT OF DIABETES IN PREGNANCY

Antepartum Management

Diet and Exercise

Diet and Exercise are the first line therapy for women with GDM. The total calorie intake varies according to the BMI of the woman

Recommended calories intake as per BMI	
BMI	Recommended calories intake in kcal per day
< 25 kg/m²	3000 Kcal/day
Overweight (BMI 25–30 kg/m²)	2500 Kcal/day
Morbid obese (> 30 kg/m²)	1500 – 1250 Kcal/day

The total calorie requirement should consist of
40% = carbohydrate
20% = Protein
40% = Fat (Unsaturated fats)

This should be accompanied by 30 minutes of mild to moderate exercise.

Glucose Monitoring: Glucose measurement should be done 4 times a day (William Obs 25/e p1112). The first check is done fasting and remainder 1-2 hrs after each meal.

Key Concept

- The diet and exercise should be continued for at least 3 weeks to achieve the following: **Metabolic goals**—
  - Premeal value = < 95 mg/dl
  - Postmeal 1 hr PP = < 140 mg/dl
  - Postmeal 2 hour PP = < 120 mg/dl
  - HbA1C < 6%

If the above metabolic goals are not met within 2 weeks then put the patient on insulin.

Pharmacotherapy: Insulin

- The DOC for diabetes during pregnancy in insulin
- Dose of insulin = 0.7 – 1U kg/day in divided doses
- Short acting and intermediate acting insulin are used
- Oral hypoglycemic agents are not used during pregnancy except for **metformin and glyburide** (starting dose 2.5 mg maxim dose = 20 mg/day)
- These are second line drugs for managing diabetes
- First line being Insulin always

Fetal Surveillance

- According to ACOG, fetal surveillance should begin between 32-34 weeks in stable diabetes and at 28 weeks for growth restricted fetuses
- Overt diabetics and GDM patients on insulin are admitted at 34 weeks and antepartum monitoring done 3 times a week
- Patient should be advised to monitor fetal kick count from 3rd trimester onwards
- Fetal surveillance methods are = kick count, weekly BPP and biweekly NST

Obstetric Management

- **Time and mode of delivery:**

Type of diabetes	Time of delivery
GDM controlled by diet	≥ 39 weeks up to 40 weeks + 6 days
GDM controlled by insulin	≥ 39 weeks to 39 weeks + 6 days
Overt diabetes	37 weeks – 37 weeks + 6 days

- Induction of Labor is safe in diabetic females
- **Preferred mode of delivery** - vaginal delivery

Remember: If weight of fetus ≥ 4.5 kg in diabetics then cesarean section is indicated

- **Follow up:** Women with GDM should have 75 g oral glucose tolerance test at 4–12 weeks puerperium as 50% females develop diabetes mellitus in future life. If it is normal, 3 yearly assessments should be done.

COMPLICATIONS OF GESTATIONAL DIABETES

A. Maternal Complications

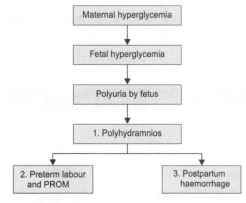

- Increased incidence of infections like UTI, asymptomatic bacteruria, vaginal candidiasis
- In 50% cases, females develop Type 2 diabetes in future life
- Women with gestational diabetes also have increased risk of metabolic syndrome   *(Williams 25/e pg 1114)*

B. Fetal Complications

1. **Fetal hyperglycemia**
2. **Macrosomia**

Macrosomia

The recommended definition is fetal (neonatal) weight exceeding two standard deviations or above 90th centile for the appropriate normal population.

According to ACOG, birth weight of ≥ 4500 g is called macrosomia.

In the Indian context, birth weight of ≥ 4000 g is called macrosomia.

Risk factors associated with macrosomia are:	
• Maternal diabetes	• Maternal obesity (If maternal BMI is > 30 kg/m², it is associated with increased risk)
• Multiparity	• Prolonged gestation
• Increased maternal age	• Male fetus
• Race and ethnicity (Hispanic ethnicity is a/w increased risk)	• Previous infant weight more than 4000 g

Grades of Macrosomia

Grade I	–	4000–4499 g
Grade II	–	4500–4999 g
Grade III	–	≥ 5000 g

- A major concern in the delivery of macrosomic infants is shoulder dystocia and permanent brachial plexus injury (seen in < 10% of all shoulder dystocia cases).
- There are increased chances of operative delivery with macrosomia.
- Some clinicians proposed planed early labor induction when fetal macrosomia is diagnosed in nondiabetic women but it is not supported by ACOG.

> - **ACOG does not support a policy for early delivery of macrosomic babies before 39 weeks of gestation**
> - **Planned LSCS may be done in diabetic women with an estimated fetal weight exceeding 4500 g and in nondiabetics, if expected fetal weight is > 5000.**
> —*Williams Obs, 25/e pg 859*

3. Shoulder Dystocia

- As discussed above, macrosomia can lead to shoulder dystocia.
- Shoulder dystocia is difficulty in delivery of the shoulder after the head is born.

- **Risk factors:**
  D = Maternal diabetes
  O = Maternal obesity/Fetal obesity (Macrosomia)
  P = Post term pregnancy
  A = Anencephaly
- **Diagnosis:** Shoulder dystocia is diagnosed if there is a delay of ≥ 1 min in delivery of shoulder after delivery of head.
- **Turtle sign:** Sudden recoil of fetal head back towards the mother's perineum after it emerges from the vagina.

Management

Shoulder Dystocia Drill

1st line maneuvers:

- Call for help
- Give episiotomy
- Avoid fundal pressure
- Give suprapubic pressure– only one assistant needed for this step (Figs. 23.2 and 23.3)
- **1st/Most effective/Best maneuvre—McRoberts maneuver.** It consists of flexion of maternal legs on the abdomen followed by their abduction. Two assistant are needed for this step. Each assistant grabs a leg. This causes straightening of the sacrum relative to the lumbar vertebral along with relation of the pubic symphysis towards maternal abdomen and a decrease in angle of pelvic inclination.

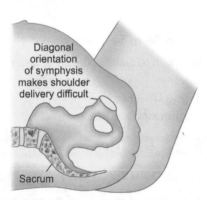

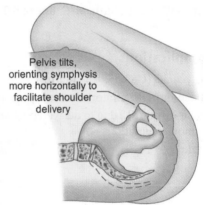
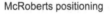

Before McRoberts positioning

Diagonal orientation of symphysis makes shoulder delivery difficult

Sacrum

McRoberts positioning

Pelvis tilts, orienting symphysis more horizontally to facilitate shoulder delivery

Fig. 23.2: Mc Roberts maneuver-mechanism

2nd line measures:

When first line measures fail then second line measures should be adopted.

- Delivery of posterior arm is attempted
- **Woods Cork screw maneuver:**

– In this maneuver, under the pubic symphysis posterior shoulder is progressively rotated anteriorly by 180° in a cork screw manner releasing the impacted arterior shoulder. Simultaneously suprapubic pressure is given.

- **Rubin maneuver**—Not done these days
- **Gaskin maneuver** (All 4 position maneuver) (Fig. 23.4). Here the mother is put on her hands and knees (in all 4 positions) in which gravity aids and there is increased space in the hollow of the sacrum to facilitate delivery of posterior shoulder and arm.

Third line measures: Done only when 2nd line measures fail.

- **Cleidotomy:** Deliberate fracture of one or both clavicles of the fetus.
- **Symphysiotomy:** Dividing the maternal pubic symphysis.
- **Zavanelli maneuver:** It is the last resort. The fetal head is replaced inside the uterus and thereafter delivered by cesarean section.

Complications of shoulder dystocia

Fetal	Maternal
Fetal hypoxia	M/C = PPH
M/C - Brachial plexus injury	Lacerations of cervix and
Fracture of clavicle and	vagina
humerus	Rupture of uterus

Note: Shoulder dystocia poses a greater threat to fetus than mother. Risk of recurrent shoulder dystocia in next pregnancy 1–13%

4. Increased incidence of abortion/IUD and still birth

As discussed earlier in diabetic females there are increased chances of abortion, IUD and stillbirth. M/C time of IUD is last two weeks of pregnancy.

C. Neonatal Complications

1. Neonatal hypoglycemia (Glucose < 45 mg/dL)
2. Prematurity → leading to Respiratory distress syndrome
3. Hypocalcemia (Ca < 8 mg/dL) due to delayed postnatal parathyroid hormone regulation
4. Hypomagnesemia
5. Hypokalemia

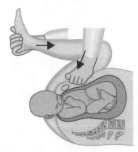
Fig. 23.3: McRoberts maneuver

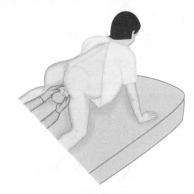
Fig. 23.4: All 4 or Gaskin maneuver

6. Due to imbalance in the demand and supply of oxygen (increased demand is due to macrosomia and fetal hyperglycemia). This causes chronic hypoxia which leads to increase in fetal erythropoietin levels causing Polycythemia and hyperbilirubinemia. Together this is called as Hyperviscosity syndrome.
7. Newborns of diabetic mother may have hypertrophic cardiomyopathy primary affecting intraventricular septum. It is symptomatic & resolves spontaneously.

 Important One Liners

- Anemia is not a complication of diabetes
- Mental retardation is not seen in babies of diabetic mothers
- IUGR may be seen in babies of Type II diabetic females with vasculopathy
- Best investigation to assess lung maturity in fetuses of diabetic mothers:-Presence of phosphatidyl glycerol in amniotic fluid

D. Long Term Sequence

Babies born to diabetic mothers have risk of:

1. Obesity
2. Type 2 Diabetes
3. Cardiovascular disease

THYROID DISORDERS IN PREGNANCY

THYROID PHYSIOLOGY AND PREGNANCY

- Physiological changes of pregnancy cause the thyroid gland to increase production of thyroid hormones by 40 to 100 percent to meet maternal and fetal needs.
- Anatomically, the **thyroid gland undergoes moderate enlargement during** pregnancy caused by glandular hyperplasia and increased vascularity. Such enlargement is not pathological, but normal pregnancy does not typically cause significant thyromegaly. Thus, any goiter should be investigated.

- Early in the first trimester, levels of the principal carrier protein–**thyroxine-binding globulin (TBG)–increase**, reach their zenith at about 20 weeks, and stabilize at approximately double baseline values for the remainder of pregnancy.
- These elevated TBG levels increase **total serum thyroxine (T_4) and triiodothyronine (T_3)** concentrations, but do not affect the physiologically important serum free T_4 and T_3 levels. Specifically, total serum T_4 increases sharply beginning between 6 and 9 weeks and reaches a plateau at 18 weeks.
- **Thyrotropin-releasing hormone (TRH)** is secreted by the hypothalamus and stimulates thyrotrope cells of the anterior pituitary to release thyroid-stimulating-hormone (TSH) or thyrotropin. TRH levels are **not increased** during normal pregnancy.
- *Thyrotropin,* also called *thyroid-stimulating hormone (TSH)*, currently plays a central role in screening and diagnosis of many thyroid disorders. Serum TSH levels in early pregnancy decline because of weak TSH-receptor stimulation from massive quantities of human chorionic gonadotropin (hCG) secreted by placental trophoblast. Because TSH does not **cross the placenta, it has no direct fetal effects**.
- Throughout pregnancy, maternal thyroxine is transferred to the fetus. Maternal thyroxine is important for normal fetal brain development, especially before development of fetal thyroid gland function. And even though the fetal gland begins concentrating iodine and synthesizing thyroid hormone after 12 weeks gestation, maternal thyroxine contribution remains important. In fact, maternal sources account for 30 percent of thyroxine in fetal serum at term.

Autoimmunity and Thyroid Disease

- Most thyroid disorders are inextricably linked to autoantibodies against various cell components.
- *Thyroid-stimulating autoantibodies,* also called *thyroid-stimulating immunoglobulins (TSIs)*, bind to the TSH receptor and activate it, causing thyroid hyperfunction and growth.
- *Thyroid peroxidise* (TPO) is a thyroid gland enzyme that normally functions in the production of thyroid hormones. *Thyroid peroxidase antibodies*, previously called *thyroid microsomal autoantibodies*, are directed against TPO and have been identified in 5 to 15 percent of all pregnant women.

HYPOTHYROIDISM IN PREGNANCY

- It is the commonest thyroid dysfunction in pregnancy.

- The majority of cases of hypothyroidism are due to autoimmune disease[Q] – Hashimoto thyroiditis and are associated with presence of thyroid peroxidase antibodies.

Effect of Pregnancy on Hypothyroidism

- Thyroxine requirements increase in pregnancy.

Effect of Hypothyroidism on Pregnancy

Hypothyroidism can lead to:

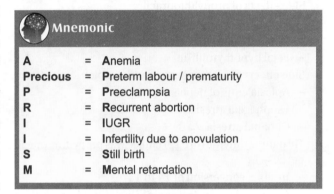

Mnemonic		
A	=	Anemia
Precious	=	Preterm labour / prematurity
P	=	Preeclampsia
R	=	Recurrent abortion
I	=	IUGR
I	=	Infertility due to anovulation
S	=	Still birth
M	=	Mental retardation

Diagnosis and Management

- Diagnosis is made by measuring maternal T3, T4 and TSH levels.
- Treatment is with levothyroxine, beginning in dose of 100 mcg daily. (after 4 to 6 weeks TSH levels are measured again and dose adjusted)

HYPERTHYROIDISM IN PREGNANCY

- Most common cause of hyperthyroidism during pregnancy is autoimmune hyperthyroidism, i.e. Graves' disease
- In Graves disease – Thyroid stimulating antibodies are present.

Complications

- Hyperthyroidism during pregnancy can lead to:

Maternal: Miscarriage, preterm delivery, pre-eclampsia, congestive cardiac failure, placental abruption, thyroid storm and infection.

Fetal/Neonatal: IUGR, prematurity, stillbirth.

A fetus who was exposed to excessive maternal thyroxine can present as:

a. **Goitrous thyrotoxicosis:** Due to placental transfer of maternal thyroid stimulating immunoglobulin.
   Best predictor: is presence of TSH receptor antibodies (>3 times) in mother with Graves disease.

b. **Goitrous hypothyroidism:** Due to fetal exposure to maternally administered thyronamides (antithyroid drugs).

c. **Nongoitrous hypothyroidism:** Due to transplacental passage of maternal TSH receptor blocking antibodies.

Management

- Medical management is the management of choice[Q]

- Both propylthiouracil and methimazole/carbimazole are effective and safe[Q] and are not C/I during lactation also.

- Side effects of propylthiouracil
  - Transient leucopenia
  - Agranulocytosis
  - Fetal hypothyroidism

- Side effects of methimazole/carbimazole:
  - Aplasia cutis of neonate.
  - Esophageal atresia
  - Choanal atresia

- Till date antithyroid drug of choice was propylthiouracil[Q] because it:
  - Inhibits conversion of T4 to T3[Q]
  - Crosses placenta less rapidly than methimazole[Q]

- *The latest edition of williams: 24/e p 1151 says "Until recently, PTU has been the preferred thionamide in the United States (Brent, 2008). In 2009, however, the Food and Drug Administration issued a safety alert on PTU-associated hepatotoxicity. This warning prompted the American Thyroid Association and the American Association of Clinical Endocrinologists (2011) to recommend PTU therapy during the first trimester followed by methimazole beginning in the second*

trimester. The obvious disadvantages is that this might lead to poorly controlled thyroid function."

- Radioactive iodine is an absolute contraindication in the treatment of thyrotoxicosis in pregnancy. In fact, it should not be given to patients even wanting pregnancy within 1 year

- Beta blockers like propranolol are used for management of tremors and tachycardia. They are safe in pregnancy

Surgical Management: Thyroidectomy may be carried out[Q] after thyrotoxicosis has been brought under medical control. Because of increased vascularity of thyroid gland during pregnancy, such surgery is more complicated than in non-pregnant state. It is indicated in women who cannot adhere to medical treatment or in whom drug therapy proves toxic or who develop stridor, respiratory distress because of the disease. Best time to perform thyroid surgery in pregnancy is 2nd trimester.

> **Note:** Cord blood should be collected at the time of delivery for estimation of TSH, T_3, T_4 to detect neonatal thyroid disorders

Fetal thyroid gland is able to synthesize thyroid hormone by 10-12 weeks of gestation.

> *Remember:*
>
> ***Maternal hormones which do not cross placenta***
> - Insulin
> - TSH
> - Erythropoietin
> - Parathyroid Hormone
> - Calcitonin

New Pattern Questions

N1. What happens to insulin secretion during pregnancy?
a. Increases
b. Decreases
c. No change
d. Initially increases then decreases

N2. Insulin resistance is maximum during pregnancy at:
a. 16–20 weeks
b. 20–24 weeks
c. 24–28 weeks
d. 28–32 weeks

N3. Fetus starts secreting insulin by:
a. 8 weeks
b. 10 weeks
c. 12 weeks
d. 16 weeks

N4. Main source of fetal energy is:
a. Amino acids
b. Glucose
c. Fatty acids
d. Electrolytes

N5. Hormone responsible for fetal growth:
a. Growth hormone
b. Insulin and Insulin like growth factors
c. Progesterone
d. Oxytocin

N6. Macrosomia is a result of:
a. Maternal hyperglycemia
b. Fetal hyperglycemia
c. Fetal hyperinsulinemia
d. Maternal hyperinsulinemia

N7. All of the following are seen in case of maternal diabetes *except*:
a. Maternal hyperglycemia
b. Fetal hyperglycemia
c. Neonatal hyperglycemia
d. Neonatal hypoglycemia

N8. M/C time of IUD in diabetic females:
a. 1st trimester
b. 24–28 weeks
c. 32–36 weeks
d. Last 2 weeks of pregnancy

N9. Most common congenital malformation seen in a diabetic pregnant woman amongst the following are:
a. Cardiac defect
b. Renal defect
c. Liver defect
d. Lung defect

N10. Most sensitive screening test in diabetic mothers for congenital malformation is:
a. MS AFP
b. Blood glucose
c. Amniotic fluid AFP
d. HbA1C (Glycosylated haemoglobin)

N11. Caudal regression syndrome is seen in babies of mother having:
a. Diabetes
b. PIH
c. Cardiac disease
d. Anaemia

N12. A 32-year-old female with diabetes visits antenatal clinic at 6 weeks of amenorrhea. She has not been on any treatment. What is the first step in the management?
a. Start Insulin
b. Start diet modification
c. Perform HbA1c
d. Perform PPBs

N13. Fasting Blood sugar should be maintained in a pregnant diabetic female as:
a. 70–100 mg%
b. 100–130 mg%
c. 130–160 mg%
d. 160–190 mg%

N14. A 30-year-old G3P2 obese woman at 26 weeks' gestation with no significant past medical history states that diabetes runs in her family. Her other pregnancies were uncomplicated. The results of a 3-hour glucose tolerance test show the following glucose levels:
- 0 (fasting): 90 mg/dL 1 hour: 195 mg/dL
- 2 hours: 155 mg/dL 3 hours: 145 mg/dL

  As a result, she is diagnosed with gestational diabetes. She is counselled to start diet modification and exercise to control her glycemic levels. 3 weeks after her diagnosis, she presents her values:
- Fasting: 95 mg/dL 1hr pp: 185 mg/dL

What is the best management?
a. Continue diet modification
b. Start insulin
c. Repeat GTT
d. Start metformin

N15. For antenatal fetal monitoring in a diabetic pregnancy all of the following are useful *except*:
a. Non-stress test
b. Biophysical profile
c. Doppler flow study
d. Fetal kick count

N16. A 30-year-old woman with diabetes mellitus presents to her physician at 19 weeks' gestation. She is obese and did not realize that she was pregnant until recently. She also has not been "watching her sugar" lately, but is now motivated to improve her regimen. A dilated ophthalmologic examination shows no retinopathy. An ECG is normal. Urinalysis is negative for proteinuria. Laboratory studies show:
- Hemoglobin A 1c: 10.8%
- Glucose: 222 mg/dL
- Thyroid-stimulating hormone: 1.0 µU/mL
- Free thyroxine: 1.7 ng/dL
- Creatinine: 1.1 mg/dL.

In which of the following condition the risk of developing it is same in diabetics as the general population:

a. Asymptomatic bacteriuria
b. Preeclampsia
c. Congenital adrenal hyperplasia
d. PPH after delivery
e. Shoulder dystocia

N17. 30-year-old G3P2 patient visits an antenatal clinic at 20 weeks. She reveals during history that her first baby was 4.6 kg delivered by cesarean section, second baby was 4–8 kg delivered by c/section. Gynaecologists suspect gestational diabetes and orders a GCT. The blood sugar levels after 50 gms of oral glucose are 206 mg/dl and the patient is thus confirmed as a case of gestational diabetes. All of the following are known complications of this condition *except*:
a. Susceptibility for infection
b. Fetal hyperglycemia
c. Congenital malformations in fetus
d. Neonatal hypoglycemia

N18. Hypothyroidism is associated with the following clinical problems, *except*:
a. Menorrhagia   b. Early abortions
c. Galactorrhoea   d. Thromboembolism

N19. One of the following is an absolute contraindication for treatment of Thyrotoxicosis in pregnancy of 6 months duration:
a. Antithyroid drug   b. I^{131} therapy
c. Telepaque   d. Surgery

N20. Rani a 24-year-old woman presents to her gynaecologist as she has chronic hypothyroidism and wants to conceive now. Her hypothyroidism is well controlled at 75 microgram of Thyroxine. She doesn't smoke or drink and doesn't have any other medical ailment. She would like to know if she should keep taking her Thyroxin. Which of the following is the best advice to give to this patient?
a. Stop taking Thyroxine and switch to methimazole as we would like to control your baby's thyroid levels
b. Thyroxine is safe during pregnancy but it is not absolutely necessary during pregnancy to continue thryoxine.
c. Thyroxine is not safe during pregnancy and it is better for your baby to be hypothyroid than hyperthyroid
d. Thyroxine is absolutely safe and necessary for you in pregnancy but we would like to decrease your dose as pregnancy is accompanied by mild physiological hyperthyroidism
e. Thyroxine is safe in pregnancy and the dose of thyroxine would be increased during pregnancy to avoid hypothyroidism, which may affect the baby adversely

N21. Prolactinoma in pregnancy, all are true *except*:
a. Most common pituitary tumor but rarely symptomatic
b. Increase in prolactin levels worse prognosis
c. Macroadenoma > 1 cm is associated with bad prognosis
d. Regular visual checkup

N22. Neonate of a hyperthyroid mother can present with all *except*:
a. Goitrous thyrotoxicosis
b. Goitrous hypothyroidism
c. Non goitrous hypothyroidism
d. None of the above

N23. The following drug is used in management of thyroid storm during pregnancy:
a. Sodium iodide   b. Dexamethasone
c. Propranolol   d. All of the above

N24. Fasting blood sugar levels to diagnose overt diabetes:
a. 106 mg/dL   b. 116 mg/dL
c. 126 mg/dL   d. 140 mg/dL

N25. Target of Fasting blood sugar & HbA1c in a gestational diabetic patient:
a. < 90 gm/dL, HbA/c < 6
b. < 95 gm/dL, HbA1c < 6
c. < 90 gm/dL, Hb A/c < 6.5
d. 95 gm/dl; Hb A/c < 6.5

N26. Macrosomia is defined as weight of fetus:
a. > 3 kg   b. > 3.5 kg
c. > 4 kg   d. 4.5 kg

N27. GTT recommended by WHO:
a. 75 gm 2 hrs GTT
b. 75 gm 3 hrs GTT
c. 100 gm 2 hrs GTT
d. 100 gm 3 hrs GTT

N28. ACOG recommends cesarean delivery if weight of fetus in diabetes................. & Non diabetics .... respectively:
a. 4.5 kg; 4.5 kg   b. 5 kg; 5 kg
c. 4.5 kg; 5 kg   d. 5 kg; 4.5 kg

N29. All of the following are maternal complications of diabetes *except*:
a. PIH
b. Future Risk of diabetes
c. Future Risk of metabolic syndrome
d. Anemia

N30. Tocolytic which is contraindicated in Diabetic patients:
a. Nifedipine   b. Atosiban
c. MgSO$_4$ d. Ritodrine

Previous Year Questions

1. **A pregnant, diabetic female on oral hypoglycemics is shifted to insulin. All of the following are true regarding this,** *except***:** [AIIMS June 99; Dec 98]
   a. Insulin does not cross placenta
   b. During pregnancy insulin requirement increases and cannot be provided with sulphonylureas
   c. Tolbutamide crosses placenta
   d. Tolbutamide causes PIH

2. **A pregnant diabetic on oral sulphonylureas therapy is shifted to insulin. All of the followings are true regarding this,** *except***:** [AI 01]
   a. Oral hypoglycaemics cause PIH
   b. Insulin does not cross placenta
   c. Cross placenta and deplete foetal insulin
   d. During pregnancy insulin requirement increases and cannot be met with sulphonylureas

3. **A lady with 12 weeks of pregnancy having fasting blood glucose 170 mg/dL, the antidiabetic drug of choice is:** [AIIMS May 01]
   a. Insulin
   b. Metformin
   c. Glipizide
   d. Glibenclamide

4. **True about diabetes in pregnancy are all** *except***:** [AIIMS May 08]
   a. Glucose challenge test is done between 24-28 weeks
   b. 50 gm of sugar is given for screening test
   c. Insulin resistance improves with pregnancy
   d. Diabetes control before conception is important to prevent malformation

5. **Late hyperglycemia in pregnancy is associated with:**
   a. Macrosomia [AIIMS Nov 06; May 06]
   b. IUGR
   c. Postmaturity
   d. Congenital malformation

6. **A G2 P1+0+0 diabetic mother present at 32 weeks pregnancy, there is history of full term fetal demise in last pregnancy. Her vitals are stable, sugar is controlled and fetus is stable. Which among the following will be the most appropriate management?**
   a. To induce at 38 weeks [AIIMS Nov 00]
   b. To induce at 40 weeks
   c. Cesarean section at 38 weeks
   d. To wait for spontaneous delivery

7. **Most sensitive screening test in diabetic mothers for congenital malformation is:** [AIIMS Dec 98]
   a. MS AFP
   b. Blood glucose
   c. Amniotic fluid AFP
   d. Hb A1C (Glycosylated haemoglobin)

8. **Which is best method to assess fetal damage in a diabetes mother in Ist trimester is:**
   a. Blood sugar estimation [AIIMS June 99]
   b. Urine ketone assay
   c. Amniocentesis to see level of sugar in amniotic fluid
   d. Glycosylated Hb

9. **Glucose tolerance test is indicated in pregnancy because of:** [PGI June 06, 03]
   a. Big baby
   b. Eclampsia
   c. Previous GDM
   d. History of diabetes in maternal uncle

10. **Which of the following histories is not an indication to perform oral glucose tolerance test to diagnose gestational diabetes mellitus?** [AIIMS Nov 2011]
    a. Previous eclampsia
    b. Previous congenital anomalies in the fetus
    c. Previous unexplained fetal loss
    d. Polyhydramnios

11. **All are seen in gestational diabetes** *except***:**
    a. Previous macrosomic baby [AIIMS May 2010]
    b. Obesity
    c. Malformations
    d. Polyhydramnios

12. **Commonest congenital malformation in infant of a diabetic mother is:** [AIIMS June 97]
    a. Neural tube defect
    b. Hydrocephalus
    c. Anencephaly
    d. Sacral agenesis

13. **The commonest congenital anomaly seen in pregnancy with diabetes mellitus is:** [AIIMS May 03]
    a. Multicystic kidneys
    b. Oesophageal atresia
    c. Neural tube defect
    d. Duodenal atresia

14. **Most common congenital malformation seen in a diabetic pregnant woman amongst the following are:**
    a. Cardiac defect
    b. Renal defect [AI 97]
    c. Liver defect
    d. Lung defect

15. **Which is the most common congenital abnormality in a baby of a diabetic woman?** [AIIMS May 2016]
    a. Ventricular septal defect
    b. Anencephaly
    c. Meningomyelocele
    d. Sacral agenesis

16. **Infants of diabetic mothers are likely to have the following cardiac anomaly:** [AI 05]
    a. Coarctation of aorta
    b. Fallot's tetralogy
    c. Ebstein's anomaly
    d. Transposition of great arteries

17. Which of the following is seen in the infant of a diabetic mother? [AI 02]
    a. Hyperkalemia   b. Hypercalcemia
    c. Macrocytic anemia d. Polycythemia

18. The effects of diabetic mother on infants is/are:
    a. Brain enlargement as a part of macrosomia
    b. Hyperglycemia in infant   [PGI June 09]
    c. First trimester abortion
    d. Unexplained fetal death
    e. Caudal regression

19. Caudal regression syndrome is seen in babies of mother having:
    a. Diabetes   b. PIH
    c. Cardiac disease   d. Anaemia

20. A diabetic female at 40 weeks of gestation delivered a baby by elective cesarean section. Soon after birth the baby developed respiratory distress. The diagnosis is: [AIIMS May 01]
    a. Transient tachypnea of the newborn
    b. Congenital diaphragmatic hernia
    c. Tracheo oesophageal fistula
    d. Hyaline membrane disease

21. Complication seen in fetus of a diabetic mother is:
    [AIIMS Feb. 97]
    a. B cell hyperplasia b. Hyperglycemia
    c. Small fetus   d. A-cell hyperplasia

22. True about diabetic mother is: [AIIMS Nov. 01]
    a. Hyperglycemia occurs in all infants of diabetic mothers
    b. High incidence of congenital heart anomalies is common
    c. Small baby
    d. Beta agonist drugs are contraindicated during delivery

23. True about diabetes in pregnancy: [PGI Dec. 06]
    a. Macrosomia   b. IUGR
    c. Congenital anomalies
    d. Oligohydramnios   e. Placenta previa

24. Feature of diabetes mellitus in pregnancy:
    a. Postdatism   b. Hydramnios
    c. Neonatal hyperglycemia   [PGI June 06]
    d. Increased congenital defect
    e. PPH

25. Complications of diabetes in pregnancy includes all except: [PGI May 2013]
    a. Macrosomia   b. Shoulder dystocia
    c. Hyperglycemia in newborn
    d. IUGR
    e. Caudal regression

26. Which is/are not fetal complication of uncontrolled diabetes during pregnancy: [PGI Nov 2012]
    a. Stillbirth
    b. Chromosomal anomaly
    c. NTD
    d. Abruptio placenta
    e. Fetal anomalies

27. True about congenital diseases in diabetes mellitus is all except: (AIIMS May 09)
    a. Results due to free radical injury
    b. 6-10% cases are associated with major congenital abnormality
    c. 1-2% of newborns are associated with single umbilical artery
    d. Insulin can be given

28. Best test for fetal maturity in a diabetic mother is:
    a. L:S ratio   [AIIMS June 99]
    b. Lecithin-cephalin ratio
    c. Phosphatidyl choline
    d. Phosphatidyl glycerol

29. The one measurement of fetal maturity that is not affected by a 'bloody tap' during amniocentesis is:
    a. L/S ratio   [AIIMS Nov 05]
    b. Phosphatidyl glycerol
    c. α-fetoprotein
    d. Bilirubin as a measured by DOD 450

30. What are the cut off values in 2 hour oral glucose tolerance test for fasting and at 1 hour and 2 hours after meals respectively: [AIIMS May 15]
    a. 92, 182, 155   b. 92, 180, 153
    c. 95, 180, 155   d. 92, 180, 155

31. Complications of shoulder dystocia is/are:
    a. Humerus fracture   [PGI]
    b. Brachial plexus injury
    c. Birth asphyxia
    d. Sacroiliac joint dislocation of mother

Answers with Explanations to New Pattern Questions

N1. Ans. is a, i.e. Increases

Insulin secretion increases during pregnancy.

N2. Ans. is c, i.e. 24–28 weeks

See the text for explanation.

N3. Ans. is c, i.e. 12 weeks

See the text for explanation.

N4. Ans. is b, i.e. Glucose

See the text for explanation.

N5. Ans. is b, i.e. Insulin and Insulin like growth factors

See the text for explanation .

N6. Ans. is a, i.e. Maternal hyperglycemia   *Ref. High Risk pregnancy, Fernando Arias 4//e, p 259*

The basic cause of macrosomia is maternal hyperglycemia.

N7. Ans. is c, i.e. Neonatal hyperglycemia

Neonatal hypoglycemia is seen in diabetic females and not hyperglycemia.

N8. Ans. is d, i.e. Last 2 weeks of pregnancy

M/C time of IUD in diabetic females is last 2 weeks of pregnancy.

N9. Ans. is a, i.e. Cardiac defect

Ref. Williams Obs. 24/e, p 1128; Fernando Arias 2/e, p 289; COGDT 10/e, p 312; Sheila Balakrishnan, p 288,
—Williams 21/e, p 1369

Cardiac anomalies are the most common single organ anomalies in case of diabetes.

This is supported by 24/e Williams which specifically mention, that cardiovascular anomalies are much common that CNS anomalies in babies of diabetic mothers   *(p 1128)*

Most common cardiac anomalies seen are:

- Ventricular septal defect[Q]
- Atrial septal defect[Q]
- Transposition of the great vessels[Q]
- Aortic coarctation[Q]

N10. Ans. is d, i.e. Hb A1C (Glycosylated haemoglobin)   *Ref. Dutta Obs. 7/e, p 284*

Best screening test for congenital malformations: Hb A1c

Best test to detect congenital malformations: TVS

N11. Ans. is a, i.e. Diabetes   *Ref. Fernando Arias 3/e, p 454; COGDT 10/e, p 312*

"The lesion classically associated with diabetic embryopathy, the 'caudal regression syndrome', is rare, with an incidence of 1.3 per 1000 diabetic pregnancies".   *—Fernando Arias 3/e, p 454*

N12. Ans. is c, i.e. Perform HbA1c

The first step is to do HbA1c to check her glucose status and assess the risk of fetal congenital malformations.

N13. Ans. is a, i.e. 70–100 mg%   *Ref. Dutta Obs. 7/e, p 285*

Metabolic Goals during Pregnancy:

- Fasting <95 mg/dL
- 1 hr PP <140 mg/dL
- 2 hr PP <120 mg/dL (average 100 mg/dl)
- HbA1c-6%
  - If these goals are not achieved patient should be put on Insulin.

N14. Ans. is b, i.e. Start insulin   *Ref. Dutta Obs. 7/e, p 285*

In the question patients GTT showed
- Fasting = 90 mg/dL (upper limit = 95 mg/dL, i.e. normal)
- 1 hour pp = 195 mg/dL (upper limit = 180 mg/dL, i.e. abnormal)
- 2 hour pp = 155 mg/dL (upper limit = 155, i.e. normal)
- 3 hour pp = 145 mg/dL (upper limit = 140, i.e. abnormal)

Thus 2 values are abnormal, i.e. patient is a confirmed case of gestational diabetes.

As indicated, she was put on diet modification for 3 weeks and after 3 weeks, her

Fasting value	= 95 mg/dL
2 hour postprandial	= 180 mg/dL

> **Remember:** Metabolic goals of diabetes are
>
> | | | |
> |---|---|---|
> | Fasting | ≤ | 95 mg/dL |
> | 2 hour PP | ≤ | 120 mg/dL |

If these goals are not achieved by diet alone, **insulin should be started.**

N15. Ans. is c, i.e Doppler flow study   *Ref. Fernando Aris 3/e, p 449; COGDT 10/e, p 315*

Fetal surveillance in gestational diabetes:

"Low risk gestational diabetic patients who achieve adequate control with diet alone and do not develop macrosomia, polyhydramnios or preeclampsia do not require antepartum fetal surveillance testing before 40 weeks. In fact, the risk of fetal distress in those patients is as low as in non diabetics and fetal well being can be assessed by teaching the patients about fetal movements and asking them to fill up a chart for kick counts. On the other hand, high risk gestational diabetics and patients on glyburide and/or insulin should have antepartum fetal surveillance testing starting at 32-34 weeks of gestation. There is no consensus as to what is the best test for these patients.

Weekly or twice weekly NST are the most popular. However biophysical profile (BPP) the modified biophysical profile and CST are also used."
                                                              —Fernando Arias 3/e, p 449

According to *COGDT 10/e, p 315*

"Surveillance for fetal well being often begins at 32 weeks gestation in patients with end organ disease using a twice weekly NST or modified BPP done twice weekly by measuring the fetal heart rate an the amniotic fluid volume. A weekly BPP is similarly useful. Women without end organ disease who require insulin often begin fetal monitoring at 32-34 weeks. Women with diet controlled gestational diabetes usually begin testing at 36-40 weeks until delivered.

Maternal fetal movement monitoring check count using a count to 10 or similar method is recommended for all pregnant women, including those with diabetes to reduce the stillbirth rate.   *—COGDT 10/e, p 315*

So from above 2 texts it is very clear that:
- – Fetal kick count
- – NST – Non stress test
- – CST – Contraction stress test
- – BPP – Biophysical score/profile

are done for anteratal fetal surveillance in diabetes.

As far as Doppler is concerned **"The current evidence suggests the use of Doppler flow studies in patients with diabetes mellitus who have pregnancies complicated by hypertensive disease, fetal growth restriction or vasculopathy. It is not recommended as a routine method of fetal surveillance".**
                        —Management of High Risk Pregnancy, SS Trivedi and Manju Puri, p 338

N16. Ans. is c, i.e. Congenital adrenal hyperplasia   *Ref. Williams Obs. 23/e, p 1113-1115; Dutta Obs. 7/e, p 283*

In the question, patient is presenting with overt diabetes mellitus i.e. she had diabetes before pregnancy also. The question says, in which the following conditions the risk of developing the condition is same in diabetic as well as nondiabetic patients in other words, which of the options is not a complication of diabetes during pregnancy.

Option 'a' – asymptomatic bacteriuria – Diabetes during pregnancy, increases the chances of infections including asymptomatic bacteriuria.
                                                              Dutta Obs. 7/e, p 283

Option 'b' – preeclampsia – In all diabetic patients, there are increased chances of preeclampsia (25%).
                                                              Dutta Obs. 7/e p 283

Option 'c' – Congenital adrenal hyperplasia – It does not have any relation whatsoever with diabetes.

Option 'd' – PPH after delivery – Diabetic pregnancy leads to polyhydramnios which can lead to PPH after delivery.

Option 'e' – Shoulder dystocia is a result of macrosomia during pregnancy.

N17. Ans. is c, i.e. Congenital malformation in fetus

Ref. Textbook of Obs. Shiela Balakrishnan 1/e, p 288; Fernando Arias 3/e, p 445, 441

In the question, patient is presenting to the antenatal clinic at 20 weeks and is diagnosed as a case of gestational diabetes.

Note: Patients blood sugar levels after 50 gms of glucose i.e. after glucose challenge test are 206 mg/dl. Recall that if, after GCT blood sugar values are ≥ 200 mg/dl, there is no need for further testing by GTT and patient is diagnosed as a case of gestational diabetes.

As discussed in the text – in gestational diabetes, blood sugar levels are raised beyond 20-24 weeks of pregnancy, due to insulin resistance and hence free radicals (responsible for causing congenital malformations) are formed after 20-24 weeks and therefore it does not lead to congenital malformation as organogenesis is already complete by this age. Rest all options are complications of diabetes.

N18. Ans. is d, i.e. Thromboembolism *Ref. Dutta Obs. 7/e, p 288; Harrison 17/e p, 2205; Shaws 14/e, p 269*

Untreated hypothyroidism in early pregnancy has a high fetal wastage in the form of abortion, stillbirth and prematurity and deficient intellectual development of the child. However, pregnancy complications like pre-eclampsia and anemia are high. *—Dutta Obs. 7/e, p 288*

"Galactorrhea is caused by hyperprolactinemia of which an important cause is hypothyroidism." *Harrison 17/e, p 2205*
"Hypothyroidism causes menorrhagia." *High Risk Pregnancy, SS Trivedi, Manju Puri, p 413*

N19. Ans. is b, i.e. I¹³¹ therapy *Ref. Dutta Obs. 6/e, p 290; Williams Obs 23/e, p 1130*

Radioactive iodine is an absolute contraindication in the treatment of thyrotoxicosis in pregnancy. In fact, it should not be given to patients even wanting pregnancy within 6 months.

N20. Ans. is e, i.e. Thyroxine is safe in pregnancy and the dose of thyroxine would be increased during pregnancy to avoid hypothyroidism, which may affect the baby adversely

Hypothyroidism in Pregnancy

- M/C cause-Autoimmune cause-Hashimoto thyroiditis
- Hypothyroidism can lead to Mental retardation in baby, abortion, stillbirth, IUGR, prematurity
- Since maternal Hypothyroidism in pregnancy (whether overt or subclinical) may impair fetal neuropsychological development, hypothyroidism should be treated adequately in pregnancy.
- Thyroxine requirement increase during pregnancy and this increased requirement begins as early as 5 weeks (i.e. option e is correct).

N21. Ans. is b, i.e. Increase in prolactin levels worse prognosis *Ref. Leon Speroff 8/e, p 481, Dewhurt's Textbook of Obs. and Gynae, 7/e, p 255, 256; Williams Obs. 23/e, p 1139, 1140*

PROLACTINOMA

- Prolactinoma is a prolactin secreting tumours of the pituitary
- It is a benign tumor
- It is most common type of primary tumour[Q]
- It is more common in women than in men

Prolactinomas are classified according to the size

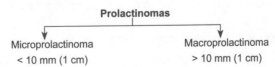

The Clinical features of prolactinomas consists of the endocrine effects due to the hyperprolactinomic state, and local tumor mass effects.

Endocrine effect due to hyperprolactinemia	Local tumour mass effects
• Infertility[Q] • Menstrual irregularity[Q] • Decreased libido • Galactorrhoea	• Visual field defect

Treatment of Prolactinoma

Asymptomatic observation

Symptomatic

Medical therapy
- Initial therapy in all cases
- Dopamine agonists
  DOC = cabergoline followed by Bromocriptine

Surgery
- Resistant cases
- Medical therapy Intolerable

- **Prolactinomas in Pregnancy**

During pregnancy normal pituitary gland doubles in size by third trimester and estrogen levels increase which leads to growth of the prolactinomas during pregnancy.

"The risk for clinically significant growth in women with microadenomas is extremely low-only 1-2%. About 5% will develop asymptomatic tumor enlargement (as determined by imaging), and essentially none will ever require surgical intervention. The risk is significantly higher (15-20%) in those with macroadenomas." —Leon Speroff 8/e, p 481

Thus option 'C' macroadenomas >1 cm is associated with bad prognosis is absolutely correct. (as macroadenoma means only it is ≥ 1 cm)

- It is recommended that pregnant women with microdenomas should be regularly inquired for headache and visual symptoms.

"Those with macroadenomas should have visual field testing during each trimester. CT or MRI is recommended only if symptoms develop" —Williams 23/e, p 1139

Thus option d-regular visual checkup is also correct

As far as option 'b' i.e. increase in prolactin levels means worse prognosis is concerned. In pregnancy prognosis does not depend on the levels of prolactin, this is because during pregnancy the levels of circulating estrogen is very high.

This results in a parallel increase in the circulating levels of prolactin. Prolactin levels begin to rise at 5-8 weeks of gestation period and it parallels the increase in the size and number of lactotrophs. At the end of the first trimester, serum prolactin levels are approximately 20-40 ng/mL. It further increases to 50-150 ng/mL and are 100-400 ng/mL at the end of the second and third trimesters, respectively.

So per increase in prolactin levels does not indicate poor prognosis, as during pregnancy, there is going to be increase in prolactin levels. Thus option b is incorrect.

Also Know:
- Management of prolactinomas during pregnancy *(Leon Speroff 8/e, p 481)*
- Regardless of the size of adenomas there is no indication for treatment with dopamine agonist or for imaging in absence of symptoms, treatment maybe safely discontinued when pregnancy is established.
- In women with microadenomas serum prolaction should be measured approximately 2 months after delivery or the cessation of nursing and if still elevated, treatment with a dopamine agonist can be resumed.
- In women with macroadenomas, an interval of treatment with dopamine agonist before pregnancy is advisable, to shrink the tumor. In those macroadenomas that fail to shrink with treatment, pregnancy should be avoided until after surgical debulking *According to Williams 23/e, p 1139*

If required DOC for Prolactinomas during pregnancy is—Bromocriptine and surgery of choice is– Transnasal transseptal endoscopic resection.

N22. Ans. is d, i.e. None of the above *Ref. Williams Obs. 24/e, p 1150*
Read the preceding text for explanation.

N23. Ans. is d, i.e. All of the above   *Ref. Williams Obs. 24/e, p 1152*

Management of Thyroid Storm in Pregnancy

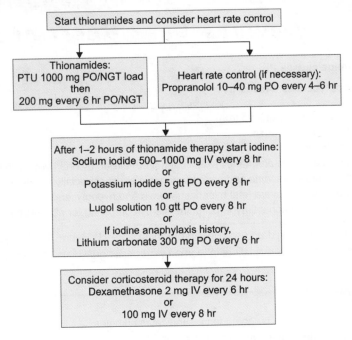

N24. Ans is c, i.e. 126 mg/dL   *(William obs 25/e pg 1099)*

Diagnosis of overt diabetes

- Random plasma glucose level > 200 mg/dL plus classic signs & symptoms like polydipsia, polyuria and unexplained weight loss
- Fasting glucose level > 125 mg/dL

As per ADA (2017) & WHO (2013); even a plasma glucose level > 200 mg/dL measured 2 hours after 75 g of oral glucose lead is diagnostic of overt diabetes

N25. Ans is d, i.e. <95 gm/dL; Hb A/c <6.5   *(Wiliams Obs 25/e pg 1111)*

Metabolic goals in gestational diabetes
Fasting glucose < 95 mg/dL
2 hr PP < 120 mg/dL
HbA1c: < 6.5%

N26. Ans is d, i.e. 4.5 kg   *(Wiliams Obs 25/e pg 857)*

Macrosomia is weight of baby ≥ 4.5 kg

"The ACOG (2016a) Concludes that the term macrosomia was an appropriate appellation for newborns who weigh 4500 gm or a more at birth"

N27. Ans is a, i.e. 75 gm 2 hrs GTT

WHO recommends (IAOPSG & DIPSI)– 75 gm 2 hrs GTT
ACOG recommends – 100 gm 3 hrs GTT

N28. Ans is c, i.e. 4.5 kg < 5 kg

ACOG recommends caesarean section if weight of baby in diabetic patients is ≥ 4.5 kg & in non diabetic ≥ 5 kg

N29. Ans is d, i.e. Anemia

See text for detail

N30. Ans is d, i.e. Ritodrine

Beta mimetics like Ritodrine, Terbutaline, Isoxsuprine and salbutamol lead to Hyperglycemia and are thus contraindicated in diabetic patients.
Tocolytic of choice in diabeters: Nifedipine.

Answers with Explanations to Previous Year Questions

1.   **Ans. is d, i.e. Tolbutamide causes PIH**

2.   **Ans. is a, i.e. Oral hypoglycemics cause PIH**
     Ref. Dutta Obs. 6/e, p 288; Williams Obs. 22/e, p 1182, 23/e, p 1119, 1120; Fernando Arias 2/e, p 288
     A pregnant female with diabetes is switched from.
     Oral hypoglycemics to insulin because:
     - Insulin does not cross placenta[Q].
     - Insulin requirement is increased in pregnancy which cannot be fulfilled by oral hypoglycemics[Q].
     - Oral hypoglycemic drugs cross placenta and have teratogenic effect especially ear defects[Q].
     - Oral hypoglycemic drugs cause severe fetal hyperinsulinemia and hypoglycemia[Q].
     - Oral hypoglycemics aggravate neonatal hyperbilirubinemia by competing for albumin binding sites.

      Note: The only hypoglycemic drug used during pregnancy are: (1) Metformin (2) Glyburide both these drugs are used as a first line therapy for diet failure in woman with gestational diabetics similar to insulin
     (Williams 24/e, p 1142)

3.   **Ans. is a, i.e. Insulin**
     Ref. Dutta Obs. 7/e, p 285

     Fasting blood glucose 170 mg/dl, in a pregnant female indicates diabetes
     In such cases insulin, glyburide or metformin should be started.

4.   **Ans. is c, i.e. Insulin resistance improves with pregnancy**
     Ref. Dutta 7/e, p 282 for option a, b, 283 for option c and 285 for option d; Fernando Arias 3/e, p 440, 442, 443
     - In pregnancy, the insulin sensitivity decreases i.e. insulin resistance increases as the gestation advances mainly due to anti insulin signals produced by placenta (mainly human placental lactogen).
     - Congenital malformations in a diabetic mother occur within first 8 weeks of gestation when most women are just beginning prenatal care. Therefore preconceptional counselling is very essential in a diabetic mother
     - Screening for diabetes during pregnancy is done by glucose challenges test at 24–28 weeks of pregnancy.

5.   **Ans. is a, i.e. Macrosomia**
     Ref. COGDT 10/e, p 316
     "Hyperglycemia at the time of conception results in enhanced rates of spontaneous abortion and major congenital malformations. Hyperglycemia in later pregnancy increases the risk for macrosomia, hypocalcemia, polycythemia, respiratory difficulties, cardiomyopathy, and congestive heart failure."
     COGDT 10/e, p 316

     Macrosomia:
     - Fetal macrosomia is defined by ACOG as fetal birth weight is > 4500 g.
     - Macrosomic fetuses have extensive fat deposits on the shoulder[Q] and trunk[Q] which is associated with increased incidence of shoulder dystocia.[Q]
     - Organ which is not affected in macrosomia is brain.[Q]
     - Control of postprandial blood sugar levels is very important for preventing macrosomia.
     - For diagnosing macrosomia: USG is performed every 4 weeks, starting at 20 weeks of gestation.
     - First sign of developing macrosomia is: increase in abdominal circumference more than other measurements.
     - Management: If wt of fetus is > 4.5 kg in diabetic mothers or > 5 kg in non diabetic mothers c-section is recommended.

6.   **Ans. is a, i.e. To induce at 38 weeks**
     Ref. COGDT 10/e, p 315; Fernando Arias 3/e, p 449
     The most common time of IUD in a diabetic patient is last two weeks of pregnancy, since in this patient there is history of a full term demise as well, so logically speaking we should terminate her pregnancy at 38 weeks. This is what logic says, now let us see what references have to say-

7. **Ans. is d, i.e. Hb AIC (Glycosylated haemoglobin)** *Ref. Dutta Obs. 7/e, p 284*

8. **Ans. is d, i.e. Glycosylated haemoglobin** *Ref. Dutta Obs. 7/e, p 284; Fernando Arias 3/e, p 452; COGDT 10/e, p 312*

   In diabetic patients:
   - Most sensitive test/best test to assess the risk of fetal malformation is maternal HbA1 c levels
   - The best test to detect fetal malformations is USG.

   Now question 8 says - which is the most sensitive screening test to detect congenital malformations.
   Undoubtedly ultrasound should be the first choice but it is not given in the options.

9. **Ans. is a, c and d, i.e. Big baby; Previous GDM; and History of diabetes in maternal uncle**

10. **Ans. is a, i.e Previous eclampsia**
    Ref. Fernando Arias 3/e, p 442; Williams Obs. 24/e, p 1137, Table 52 Dutta Obs. 7/e, p 281

    Indications for performing GCT: All those conditions in which there is risk of having diabetes.

    On the basis of risk factors females are categorised into 3 category:

Low risk	Average risk	High risk
All of the folowing:	*One or more of the following:*	• Marked obesity
• Member of an ethnic group with a low prevalence of GDM	• Member of an ethnic group with a high prevalence of GDM	• Strong family history of type II DM
• No known diabetes in first degree relatives	• *Diabetes in a first degree relative*	• Previous history of GDM impaired glucose metabolism or glucosuria
• Age <25 years	• Age ≥ 25 years	
• Weight normal before pregnancy	• Overweight before pregnancy	• Unexplained stillbirth
• Weight of previous baby normal at birth	• *Weight high at birth (previous baby)*	• H/o previous congenitally malformed baby
• No history of abnormal glucose metabolism		
• No H/o poor obstetrical outcome		

> **Time for performing screening test (glucose challenge test):**
>
> - **In low risk patients:** Blood glucose screening is not routinely required.
> - **In average risk patients:** Blood glucose testing done at 24-28 weeks.
> - **In high risk patients:** Perform glucose testing as soon as feasible.

Thus, average risk and high risk patients are indications for performing screening test and they will also be the indications for performing glucose tolerance test.

11. **Ans. is c, i.e. Malformations** *Ref. Textbook of Obs. Sheila balakrishnan 1/e, p 288; Fenando Arias 3/e, p. 445, p 441*

    As explained in the preceding text, congenital malformations are seen in fetuses of overt diabetics and not gestational diabetics.

12. **Ans. is a and c, i.e. Neural tube defect/Anencephaly**

13. **Ans. is c, i.e. Neural tube defect**
    Ref. Fernando Arias 3/e, p 454; COGDT 10/e, p 312; Sheila Balakrishnan, p 288; Wiilliams Obs. 21/e, p 1369

    Friends, this is one of the most frequently asked and most controversial topic of PGMEE Exams.
    I am giving you all the information I could lay my hands and the rest is up to you.

    Congenital malformation in Diabetes: *—Fernando Arias 3/e, p 454*
    - "The most frequent abnormalities involve the heart and the central nervous system. Most common are anencephaly, spina bifida, transposition of the great vessels, and ventricular septal defects".
    - *"The lesion classically associated with diabetic embryopathy, the 'caudal regression syndrome', is rare, with an incidence of 1.3 per 1000 diabetic pregnancies".* *—Fernando Arias 3/e, p 454*

    Most common Anomalies in Infants of Diabetic mothers:

Central nervous system	Heart and great vessels	Skeletal and spinal system	Genitourinary system	Gastrointestinal system
Anencephaly	Transposition of the great vessels	Caudal regression syndrome	Renal agenesis	Anal atresia
Holoprosencephaly	Ventricular septal defect		Ureteral duplication	
Encephalocele	Aortic coarctation			
	Atrial septal defect			

Sheila Balakrishnan p 288 says —

- **Cardiac defects are the commonest (transposition of great vessels and VSD).**
- **Neural tube defects like anencephaly and spina bifida.**
- Caudal regression syndrome or sacral agenesis, which is very rare, is the congenital defect which is specific to diabetes.

"The most common single-organ system anomalies were cardiac (38%), musculoskeletal (15%) and central nervous system (10%)."   —*Williams Obs. 21/e, p 1369*

 Remember:

- Most common system involved = Cardiovascular system.
- IInd most common system involved = Nervous system
- Most common anomalies = VSD, ASD, TGA, Anencephaly, spina bifida
- In cardiac anomalies M/C is VSD but most specific is TGA.
- Anomaly most specific for gestational diabetes - Caudal regression syndrome/sacral agenesis.
- Congenital anomalies are seen in overt diabetes and not gestational diabetes
- Investigation of choice to predict the risk of congenital anomalies in diabetic patients-HbA1C
- Investigation of choice to detect the risk of congenital anomalies in diabetic patients-USG

---

14. **Ans. is a, i.e. Cardiac defect**
    Ref. Williams Obs. 24/e, p 1128; Fernando Arias 2/e, p 289; COGDT 10/e, p 312; Sheila Balakrishnan, p 288,

Cardiac anomalies are the most common single organ anomalies in case of diabetes.   —*Williams 21/e, p 1369*
This is supported by 24/e Williams which specifically mention, that cardiovascular anomalies are much common that CNS anomalies in babies of diabetic mothers   *(p 1128).*

Most common cardiac anomalies seen are:
- Ventricular septal defect[Q] (MC)
- Atrial septal defect[Q]
- Transposition of the great vessels[Q]
- Aortic coarctation[Q]

15. **Ans. is a, i.e. Ventricular septal defect**   *Ref: Nelson 20/e p898*
Most common congenital abnormality in a baby of diabetic women is ventricular septal defect.

16. **Ans. is d, i.e. Transposition of great arteries**   *Ref. Fernando Arias 3/e, p 454*
As VSD is not given in the options, transposition of great vessels is the single best answer.

17. **Ans. is d, i.e. Polycythemia**   *Ref. Dutta Obs. 7/e, p 285*

18. **Ans. is c, d and e, i.e. First trimester abortion, Unexplained fetal death and Caudal regression**
    Ref. Dutta Obs. 7/e, p 285; Sheila Balakrishnan, p 288, 291; Fernando Arias 3/e, p 445
Effect of diabetes on:

In Q17---
As far as hyperkalemia is concerned - It is not given directly whether there is hyperkalemia or hypokalemia in neonate of diabetic mother, but we all know that in neonate of diabetic mother hyperinsulinemia is seen.

"Insulin causes potassium to shift in to the cells by Na+ H+ antiporter and Na+ K+ ATPase pump thereby lowers plasma potassium concentration."   —*Harrison 16/e, p 262*
So, there is hypokalemia in infants of diabetic mother and not hyperkalemia.

In Q18---
Option a, i.e. brain enlargement as a part of macrosomia- is not true because be it IUGR, be it macrosomia—brain is the last organ to be affected
Most common organ affected = Abdomen
Most common USG parameter affected = Abdominal circumference   —*Ref. Fernando Arias 3/e, p 495*

19. **Ans. is a, i.e. Diabetes**   *Ref. Fernando Arias 3/e, p 454; COGDT 10/e, p 312*

"The lesion classically associated with diabetic embryopathy, the 'caudal regression syndrome', is rare, with an incidence of 1.3 per 1000 diabetic pregnancies".   —*Fernando Arias 3/e, p 454*

20. **Ans. is a, i.e. Transient tachypnea of the newborn**
    Ref. Ghai 6/e, p 166, 168; COGDT 10/e, p 316; Williams Obs. 22/e, p 1178, 23/e, p 1116

Friends don't get shocked by the answer, even I was perplexed *when I went through the texts given in all the standard reference books.*

Let's see what they have said.

Respiratory distress syndrome (RDS) or hyaline membrane disease (HMD)   *—Ghai 6/e, p 166*
- **RDS almost always occurs in preterm babies often less than 34 weeks of gestation.**
- It is the commonest cause of respiratory distress in a preterm neonate.

According to *Ghai* – RDS is seen in preterm babies and not the term babies (as is given in our question).

Now let's see what Ghai says about transient tachypnea of newborn:

Transient tachypnea of newborn (TTN)   *—Ghai 6/e, p 168*
- Transient tachypnea of the newborn is a benign self-limiting disease occurring usually in **term neonates** and is due to delayed clearance of lung fluid.
- These babies have tachypnea with minimal or no respiratory distress.
- Chest X-ray may show prominent vascular marking and prominent interlobar fissure.
- Oxygen treatment is often adequate and ventilatory support is necessary and prognosis is good.

But *Ghai* didn't mention any correlation between TTN and Diabetes. So, I had to search other books for more information.

COGDT 10/e, p 316 says:

Neonatal complications: *RDS and transient tachypnea are more common in infants of women with poorly controlled diabetics.*

In this way we can derive some correlation between diabetes and TTN.

Our answer is *further strengthened by Williams Obs. 22/e, p 1178, 23/e, p 1116 which says -*

Respiratory distress:

"Conventional obstetrical teaching through the late 1980s generally held that fetal lung maturation was delayed in diabetic pregnancies. Thus, these infants were at increased risk for respiratory distress (Gluck and Kulovich, 1973). Subsequent observations have challenged this concept, and gestational age rather than overt diabetes is likely the most significant factor associated with neonatal respiratory distress (Berkowitz and colleagues, 1996; Kjos and colleagues, 1990b)".

So, it is the gestational age and not diabetes which is the main factor causing neonatal respiratory distress.

In our question the baby is delivered at 40 weeks gestation (Full term) so, the answer cannot be Hyaline membrane disease rather it is transient tachypnea of newborn (*i.e. option 'a' is correct).*

21. **Ans. is a, i.e. B cell hyperplasia**   *Ref. Williams Obs. 22/e, p 1173, 23/e, p 1109; Sheila Balakrishnan p 288, 289*

It is seen that all fetal and neonatal complications are more in poorly controlled diabetes and are mainly due to the fetal hyperinsulinaemia.

This can be explained by the ***Penderson hypothesis*** which says - *Maternal hyperglycemia leads to fetal hyperglycemia which in turn stimulates the fetal pancreatic beta cells to produce more insulin. The fetal hyperinsulinemia is responsible for most of the perinatal problems.*

Maternal hyperglycemia
↓
Fetal hyperglycemia
↓
Fetal pancreatic beta-cell hyperplasia
↓
Hyperinsulinaemia
↓
Neonatal complications

22. **Ans. is b and d, i.e. High incidence of congenital heart anomalies is common; and Beta agonist drugs are contraindicated during delivery**
    Ref. Fernando Arias 3/e, p 454; Williams Obs. 22/e; p 1173, 1178, 23/e, p 1109, 1115, 1116

Maternal hyperglycaemia
↓
Fetal hyperglycaemia
↓
Fetal pancreatic beta-cell hyperplasia
↓
HYPERINSULINAEMIA

↓   ↓

Hypoglycemia in infant   Increase in growth factors IGF-I & II
(Blood glucose ≤ 40 mg/dl)   ↓

Macrosomia (Birth Weight ≥ 4 kg.^{Q})
With excessive fat deposition on
shoulders and trunk

So, option 'a' i.e. hyperglycemia occurs in all infants of diabetic mother and 'c' i.e. small baby are incorrect.
Coming on to *option 'b'* Fernando Arias 3/e, p 454 Says
"The most frequent abnormalities involve the heart and the central nervous system."
Thus option 'b' is correct

As far as option 'd' i.e. "Beta agonist drugs are contraindicated during delivery" is concerned.

"The use of intravenous beta adrenergic drugs to stop preterm labour in pregnant diabetic patients is to be discouraged. These agents increase glycogenolysis and lipolysis and, consequently, also increase the tendency toward metabolic acidosis. Most diabetic patients require continuous intravenous insulin to antagonize the diabetogenic effect of the labour-inhibiting medication. The potential morbidity from the intravenous administration of beta-adrenergic agents to diabetic pregnant patients contraindicates their use."
—*Fernando Arias 3/e, p 454*

There fore option 'd' is also correct.

23. **Ans. is a, b and c, i.e. Macrosomia, IUGR; and Congenital anomalies**   Ref. Dutta Obs. 7/e, p 284, 285

"Growth restriction is less commonly observed and is associated with maternal vasculopathy."
—*Dutta Obs. 6/e, p 287*

"Fetal growth restriction in women with diabetes may be seen and may be related to substrate deprivation from advanced maternal vascular disease or to congenital malformations".   —*Williams Obs. 24/e, p 1129*
Rest all details about Fetal and Neonatal complications of Maternal diabetes have been discussed earlier.

24. **Ans. is b, d and e, i.e. Hydramnios; Increased Congenital defect; and PPH**   Ref. Dutta Obs. 7/e, p 284, 285
- *As explained in the previous question maternal hyperglycaemia leads to fetal hyperglycaemia, which in turn causes polyuria and thus causes polyhydramnios.*
  - Polyhydramnios leads to preterm delivery and not post datism.
  - Excessive uterine enlargement because of polyhydramnios and macrosomia causes increased incidence of atonic PPH.
- Diabetes leads to increased incidence of congenital defects in fetus.
- Maternal hyperglycemia → to **fetal hyperglycemia** → hyperinsulinemia → to **neonatal hypoglycemia** at birth.

Remember:
  In Diabetes: There is: • Maternal and fetal   – hyperglycemia
                    •   Neonatal   – hypoglycemia.

25. **Ans. is c, i.e. Hyperglycemia in newborn**   Ref. Dutta Obs. 7/e p 285
Already explained

26. **Ans. is b and d, i.e. Chromosomal anomaly and Abruptio placenta**

Ref. Dutta Obs. 7/e, p 284, Williams 23/e, p 1114

All the options given in the question – stillbirth, NTD and fetal anomalies are know fetal complications of diabetes.

Chromosomal anomalies are not seen associated with diabetes.

The only data which I could get on it was from internet

"Chromosomal Abnormalities: Studies addressing the risk of aneuploidy with diabetes suggest that chromosomal abnormalities occurring with preexisting diabetes are likely associated with the risks of increasing maternal age. However, the paucity of data that include second trimester pregnancy terminations for chromosomal abnormalities may bias these finding"

27. **Ans. is b, i.e. 6–10% cases are associated with major congenital abnormality**

Ref: Dutta Obs. 7/e, p 218 for option c 284 for option a, Williams Obs. 24/e, p 1128

Lets see each option separately

Congenital disease in diabetes mellitus

Option a i.e. Results due to free radical injury - True

Congenital malformation in a case of diabetes can be due to variety of reasons like,   *Dutta Obs. 6/e, p 287*

• Genetic susceptibility
• Hyperglycemia - It is seen that good glycemic control indicated by HbAIC levels < %.9 can significantly lower the risk of fetal malformation.
• Arachidonic acid deficiency
• Ketone body formation
• Free Radical injury
• Somatomedin inhibition.

Option b–6 to 10% cases are associated with major congenital abnormality

Here we will have to read the option very carefully - the option is talking about Major congenital anomalies and not all anomalies.

Dutta Obs 6/e, p- 287 says overall incidence of congenital Malformations is 6-10%.

Williams 24/e p 1128. "The incidence of major malformations in women with type I diabetes is ~ 5%"

Hence **option b is incorrect**

Option c - 1 - 2% of newborns are associated with single umbilical artery

This option can be taken in + /– status because no where the incidence of single umbilical artery in a case of diabetes has been mentioned separately.

Whatever little information we have is from Dutta Obs. 6/e, p 220

Single umbilical artery:

• It is present in 1-2% cases (overall)
• May be due to failure of development of artery or due to its atrophy in later months
• It is seen in case of
    i. Twins
    ii. Babies born to diabetic mothers
    iii. In polyhydramines
• Single umbilical artery has been associated with congenital malformations of the fetus in 10-20% cases viz- Renal & Genital anomalies and fetal Trisomy
• There is increased incidence of abortions, prematurity, IUGR and increased perinatal mortality.

Option d- insulin can be given

There is no doubt as far as this option is concerned as insulin is the TOC for controlling hyperglycemia in case of diabetes in pregnancy.

So from above discussion it is clear that option 'b' is absolutely incorrect, so we are opting it out.

28. **Ans. is d, i.e. Phosphatidyl glycerol**

29. **Ans. is b, i.e. Phosphatidyl glycerol** *Ref. Fernando Arias 3/e, p 204; COGDT 10/e, p 256*

The best test to detect fetal lung maturity in diabetic mothers is presence of phophatidyl glycerol (PG) in amniotic fluid. If PG is present in amniotic fluid fetal lungs are considered mature and vice versa.

30. **Ans. is b, i.e. 92, 180, 153** *Ref. High Risk Pregnancy; Fernando Areas 4/e, p 213*

The cutoffs for diagnosis of Gestational diabetes mellitus following a 75 g Oral Glucose tolerance test are given below. Any one of the values above threshold level is diagnostic.

Threshold values for diagnosis of gestational diabetes:

	Threshold	
Plasma glucose	mmol/L	mg/dL
Fasting	5.1	92
1-hr PP	10.0	180
2-hr PP	8.5	153

31. **Ans. is a, b, c and d**

All are complications of shoulder dystocia.

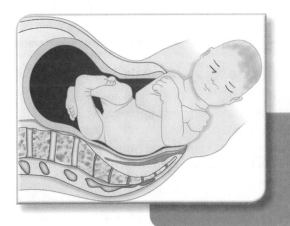

Chapter 24

Hypertensive Disorders in Pregnancy

Chapter at a Glance

- PIH
- Eclampsia
- Predictors of Pre-eclampsia

- Drugs to Prevent Pre-eclampsia
- Management Principles
- HELLP Syndrome

PIH

Definition

Hypertension in pregnancy is defined as systolic **BP ≥ 140 mm of Hg or diastolic BP ≥ 90 mm of Hg** on two occasions atleast 4 hours apart.

Diastolic BP is determined by the disappearance of sound (Korotkoff ph V). Korotkoff V is chosen as opposed to Korotkoff IV (muffing) as it is more reproducible and shows better correlation with the diastolic BP in pregnancy. For accuracy, mercury sphygmomanometer is preferred over automated ones.

Pregnancy induced hypertension	Chronic hypertension in pregnancy
(Means–a **normotensive patient has conceived and due to some placental pathology, her B/P increases)**	**Means a hypertensive female has conceived**
<ul><li>No past H/O hypertension</li><li>Increase in BP is seen after 20 weeks of pregnancy</li><li>BP comes back to normal before 12 weeks of pregnancy.</li></ul>	<ul><li>Past H/O hypertension present</li><li>Rise in B/P will be seen before 20 weeks</li><li>No proteinuria</li><li>B/P does not come back to normal within 12 weeks of delivery.</li></ul>

Types of PIH

Pre-eclampsia	Gestational Hypertension
<ul><li>In both these conditions, increase in BP is seen after 20 weeks and BP comes back to normal within 12 weeks of delivery</li><li>Proteinuria is seen or signs of end-organ damage are present.</li></ul>	<ul><li>Proteinuria and signs of end organ damage are absent.</li></ul>

Note: Earlier without proteinuria, pre-eclampsia was not diagnosed. Proteinuria was essential for its diagnosis. But now according to the new guidelines—if signs of end organ damage are present diagnosis of pre-eclampsia can be made irrespective of the presence or absence of proteinuria.

Proteinuria

- It is excretion of proteins more than 300 mg in 24 hours urine sample or more than 30 mg/dL of urine or urine protein: creatinine ratio ≥ 0.3 or Dipstick 1 + persistent.
- Proteinuria of pre-eclampsia is non-selective.

Signs of End Organ Damage

- Platelet count < 1 lacs
- Raised serum creatinine > 1.1 mg/dL
- Elevated liver enzymes to than 2 times their normal value
- Evidence of Pulmonary edema
- New onset of visual/cerebral symptoms.

Grades of Pre-eclampsia

Mild Pre-eclampsia	Severe Pre-eclampsia
• BP is more than 140/90 but less than 160/110	• BP is more than or equal to 160/110
• Signs of End organ damage are absent	• Signs of End organ damage are present

Note: Earlier grading of proteinuria was used to differentiate between mild and severe pre-eclampsia, but ACOG 2013 has removed that criteria. This is because, it is seen that there is no difference in maternal and perinatal outcome with different grades of proteinuria.

Criteria which have been removed to differentiate between mild and severe pre-eclampsia
- Proteinuria
- Oliguria
- IUGR

Also Know:
- **There is one more category and that is:**
  - **Chronic hypertension with superimposed pre-eclampsia.** The condition is diagnosed in a chronic hypertension pregnant female if:
- BP suddenly becomes incontrollable after 20 weeks.

  or
- New onset proteinuria after 20 weeks

  or
- Signs of end organ damage are seen after 20 weeks.

Risk Factors for Pre-eclampsia

- Previous H/O Pre-eclampsia (Recurrence rate: Mild pre-eclampsia = 15% Severe eclampsia = 25%)
- **Primigravida**
- **Obesity:** BMI > 35 kg/m² (*Note:* Normally obesity is > 30 kg/m² but here risk increased when BMI is > 35 kg/m²)
- Diabetes
- Chronic renal disease
- Extremes of maternal age (< 18 years or > 40 years).
- Molar pregnancy
- Twin pregnancy
- Rh negative pregnancy
- Metabolic X syndrome
- Anti phospholipid antibody syndrome

Protective Factor: Smoking.

ETIOPATHOGENESIS

Any satisfactory theory concerning the origins of preeclampsia must account for the observation that gestational hypertensive disorders are more likely to develop in women with the following characteristics:

- Are exposed to chorionic villi for the first time
- Are exposed to a superabundance of chorionic villi, as with twins or hydatidiform mole
- Have preexisting conditions associated with endothelial cell activation or inflammation, such as diabetes, obesity, cardiovascular or renal disease, immunological disorders, or hereditary influences
- Are genetically predisposed to hypertension developing during pregnancy.

A fetus is not a requisite for preeclampsia to develop. And, although chorionic villi are essential, they need not be intrauterine. For example, preeclampsia can develop with an abdominal pregnancy. *Regardless of precipitating etiology, the cascade of events leading to the preeclampsia syndrome is characterized by abnormalities that result in systemic vascular endothelial damage with resultant vasospasm, transudation of plasma, and ischemic and thrombotic sequelae.*

What Causes PIH

PIH is a placental pathology.

Normal: Placenta has villi and Intervillous spaces. The villi are lined by trophoblast and into the villi open fetal blood capillaries.

In the intervillous space, spiral arterioles carrying maternal blood open.

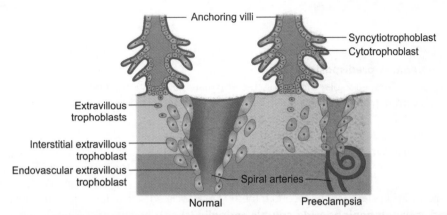

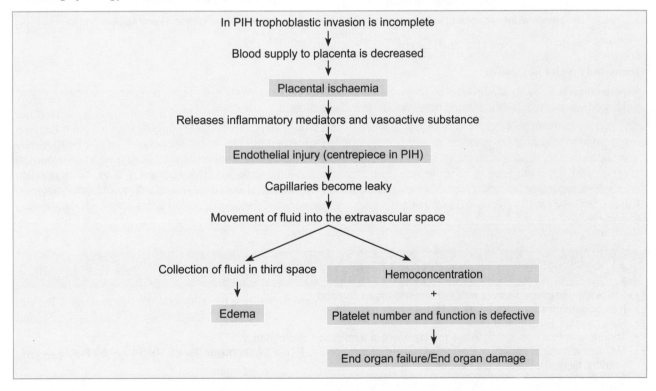

Fig. 24.1: Schematic representation of normal placental implantation shows proliferation of extravillous trophoblasts from an anchoring villus. These trophoblasts invade the decidua and extend into the walls of the spiral arteriole to replace the endothelium and muscular wall to create a dilated low-resistance vessel. With preeclampsia, defective implantation is characterized by incomplete invasion of the spiral arteriolar wall by extravillous trophoblasts. This results in a small-caliber vessel with high resistance to flow.

The endovascular trophoblast replaces the lining of these maternal spiral arteries, making them low resistance, low pressure and high flow vessels.

This is called as **Trophoblastic Invasion** which occurs in 2 steps (Fig. 24.1):

i. **1st step:** Time 16–18 weeks—invading uptil decidual segments of the artery.

ii. **2nd step:** Time 16–18 weeks—invading uptil myometrial segment of the artery.

In PIH: This trophoblastic invasion is incomplete, so maternal blood vessels have high resistance and high pressure causing PIH.

Pathophysiology of PIH.

In PIH trophoblastic invasion is incomplete
↓
Blood supply to placenta is decreased
↓
Placental ischaemia
↓
Releases inflammatory mediators and vasoactive substance
↓
Endothelial injury (centrepiece in PIH)
↓
Capillaries become leaky
↓
Movement of fluid into the extravascular space
↓
Collection of fluid in third space → Hemoconcentration
↓ +
Edema → Platelet number and function is defective
↓
End organ failure/End organ damage

Also Know:

- Apart from the explanations I have given just now to explain why PIH occurs—Remember:
    1. PIH also has **hereditary predisposition**
    2. **Immunological factors**—also play a role as discussed in maternal adaption in pregnancy: There are angiogenic factors like **VEGF & placental growth factors** which help in placental angiogenesis, so diameter of spinal arteries supplying the intervillous space increases & hence pressure decreases.

    In case of PIH: antiangiogenic factors increase like:
    (i) **Soluble fms-like tyrosine kinase 1 (sFlt–1)** is a receptor for VEGF. As depicted in Fig. 24.2, elevated maternal sFlt-1 levels inactivate and reduce circulating free placental growth factor (PIGF) and VEGF concentrations, leading to endothelial dysfunction. Importantly, sFlt-1 levels begin to rise in maternal serum months before preeclampsia is evident. These high levels in the second trimester are associated with a doubling of the risk for preeclampsia
    (ii) **A second antiangiogenic peptide, soluble endoglin (sEng),** inhibits various transforming growth factor beta (TGF-β) isoforms from binding to endothelial receptors. Endoglin is one of these receptors. Decreased binding to endoglin diminishes endothelial nitric oxide-dependent vasodilatation.

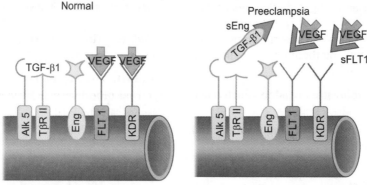

Fig. 24.2: Schematic of the receptor blocking action of sFlt-1 (soluble fms-like tyrosine kinase 1) and soluble endoglin (sEng).

    3. In PIH there is increased pressor response:

Increased Pressor Responses

In pregnant women normally develop refractoriness to infused vasopressors. Women with early preeclampsia, however, have enhanced vascular reactivity to infused norepinephrine and angiotensin II.

Several prostaglandins are thought to be central to preeclampsia syndrome pathophysiology. Specifically, the blunted pressor response seen in normal pregnancy is at least partially due to diminished vascular responsiveness mediated by endothelial prostaglandin synthesis. For example, compared with normal pregnancy, endothelial prostacyclin (PGI$_2$) production is lower in preeclampsia. This action appears to be mediated by phospholipase. At the same time, thromboxane A$_2$ secretion by platelets is increased, and the prostacyclin:thromboxane A$_2$ ratio declines. The net result favors greater sensitivity to infused angiotensin II and, ultimately, vasoconstriction. These changes are apparent as early as 22 weeks' gestation in gravidas who later develop preeclampsia.

 Key Concept

- PIH is a multisystem disorder with signs of end organ damage
- **Hemoconcentration—Hallmark of PIH**
- Main culprit in PIH—Placenta
- Therefore in PIH—always definitive management is termination of pregnancy
- M/C hematological finding in PIH is Decreased platelet count. PT/APTT/fibrinogen levels should not be tested in PIH patients, till platelet counts are normal.

Pathology

Kidney Changes

- RBF and GFR decrease in pre-eclampsia as total blood volume decreases in PIH.
- Since GFR is decreased, so levels of S. creatinine, Suric acid increase.
- Hallmark renal lesion is **Glomerular endotheliosis**.
- Acute renal failure is a rare complication of pre-eclampsia but pre-eclampsia is the M/C cause of obstetric ARF. ARF in pre-eclampsia is due to Acute Tubular necrosis.

Remember:
- M/C visual symptom in pre-eclampsia is: scotoma.
- Blindness mostly is due to vasospasm. Blindness can be due to pathology in occipital cortex or retina.
  - a. Occipital blindness is called **Amaurosis** and occurs due to occipital cortex edema.
  - b. Blindness secondary to retinal ischaemia or infraction is called **Purtscher's retinopathy**.
  - c. Blindness can occur secondary to retinal detachment. It is U/L and partial.
- Mostly blindness is reversible and corrects automatically after delivery.
- M/C ophthalmoscopic finding in a patient with severe pre-eclampsia is an increase in veinto-artery ratio and segmental vasospasm.
- No electrolyte imbalance in pre-eclampsia.
- Levels of Renin, angiotensin II and aldosterone area increased in normal pregnancy but in Pre-eclampsia, they are reduced but sensitivity of vessels is increased towards them.

ECLAMPSIA

- Eclampsia is **severe pre-eclampsia with generalised tonic-clonic convulsion or coma which cannot be attributed to any other cause**.
- In other words, eclampsia is an advanced stage of Severe pre-eclampsia.
- Maternal mortality is 4–6% and perinatal mortality is 45% in India due to Eclampsia.
- Incidence of Eclampsia
  - Globally—1 in 1500 or 1 in 2000 deliveries.
  - India—1 to 5%

Key Concept

Since eclampsia is an advanced stage of severe pre-eclampsia, there are certain signs and symptoms in a patient of severe pre-eclampsia which predict that patient is about to throw convulsions.

Signs/symptoms of impending eclampsia:
1. Epigastric pain (due to stretching of Glisson capsule of liver), nausea, vomiting
2. Headache and dizziness (due to cerebral hypoxia)
3. Visual symptoms like blurring/diplopia/scotomas/blindness
4. Oliguria

Why do convulsions occur in Eclampsia

In case of Severe pre-eclampsia—BP is very high

$\downarrow$

$$\text{Pressure } \alpha \; \frac{1}{\text{Volume}}$$

$\downarrow$

Hence volume of blood going to brain decreases

$\downarrow$

Cerebral hypoxia

$\downarrow$

Convulsions

Convulsions in eclampsia can first occur:

i. **In antepartum period:** This is called as **Antepartum eclampsia**

ii. **During delivery:** This is called as **Intrapartum eclampsia**

iii. **After delivery** (within 48 hours): This is called as **Postpartum eclampsia**.

Important One Liners

- M/C type of eclampsia: Antepartum eclampsia
- Eclampsia with worst prognosis: Antepartum eclampsia
- Factor determining prognosis/outcome of a patient with eclampsia: Duration of eclampsia, the longer a patient stays in this form, worse is the prognosis
- M/C MRI finding in eclampsia: Subcortical white matter edema
- M/C cause of death in eclampsia and pre-eclampsia: Intracranial bleeding.

(Fernando arias, High risk pregnancy 4/e, p223)

PREDICTORS OF PRE-ECLAMPSIA

Uterine Artery Doppler

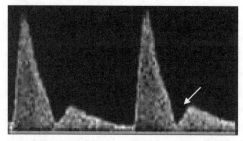

Fig. 24.3: Uterine artery Doppler showing diastolic notch

- Doppler of uterine artery shows a **diastolic notch** (**Fig. 24.3**).
- In normal pregnant female this notch disappears by **24 weeks**.
- **If the diastolic notch persists in uterine artery beyond 24 weeks, it predicts PIH.**

Giants rollover test:

The basis of Giants rollover test was Supine hypotension syndrome. As discussed earlier, if in late third trimester a normal pregnant female lies supine, her BP decreases. But if the female is about to develop PIH, instead of decreasing, her BP increases by 20 mm of Hg.

Giants rollover test is done between 28–32 weeks.

New Predictors for PIH

1. VEGF = decreased levels
2. Placental growth factor = decreased levels
3. sFlt-1: soluble fms-like tyrokinase kinase-1 = increased levels
4. Thromboxane A2- increased
5. Prostacyclin – decreases.

 Remember: **The following are findings and not predictors of PIH**
- Hemoconcentration
- Oedema
- Increased uric acid

DRUGS TO PREVENT PRE-ECLAMPSIA

1. **Aspirin ± Heparin**

   Aspirin: 50–150 mg/day prevents PIH (NICE-recommends 75 mg/day) by inhibiting thromboxane A$_2$ producing. It is to be given after 1st trimester and continued throughout pregnancy and stopped 7 days before delivery.

2. **Calcium supplementation** to prevent pre-eclampsia should be given only to those females who are calcium deficient (1–5 g/day). Otherwise in females with normal calcium levels, its role to prevent pre-eclampsia is not supported.

3. **Exercise:** Studies have shown regular exercise during pregnancy decreases the chances of PIH.

Measures proven to have no role in preventing Pre-eclampsia
• Salt restriction
• Supplementation of antioxidants
• Supplementation of Fish oil
• Supplementation of Vitamin C, D and E
• Progesterone
• Low dose Heparin alone

MANAGEMENT PRINCIPLES

- Always remember Pregnancy induced hypertension (Pre-eclampsia/Gestational hypertension) are raised BP conditions due to placental pathology (incomplete trophoblastic invasion) and always their definitive treatment would be Termination of pregnancy (throw out the defective placenta from the body).
- Antihypertensive of choice for Chronic hypertension in pregnancy—earlier Methyldopa, now being replaced by Labetalol.
- Antihypertensive of choice for pregnancy-induced hypertension (Pre-eclampsia/Gestational hypertension) is Labetalol > Alpha-methyldopa
- Antihypertensive of choice for Hypertensive crisis is— Labetalol > Hydralazine.

Antihypertensives in Pregnancy

Safe	Contraindicated
• Labetalol	• ACE inhibitors - like enalapril, captopril
• Calcium channel blockers - nifedipine	• Diuretics
• Hydralazine	• Losartan
• Alpha-methyldopa • Nitroglycerine	• Diazoxide
• Sodium nitroprusside (last resort)	

Key Concept

- As per ACOG guidelines antihypertensives should be used only if BP≥160/110 mm of Hg. As per NICE guidelines antihypertensives should be used only if BP≥150/100 mm of Hg. Thus role of antihypertensives in the management of mild PIH is not mandatory.
- Target BP in Pre-eclampsia—
  Systolic = 130–140 mm of Hg.
- Diastolic = 80–90 mm of Hg
- Target BP in Chronic hypertension during pregnancy:
  Systolic = 140–150 mm of Hg
  Diastolic = 90–100 mm of Hg
- Labetalol = oral dose = 100 mg BD or TDS
- Labetalol = I/v dose (used in acute hypertension)
  Max. total dose 220 mg
  Initially give: 20 mg I/v bolus
      ↓ Not effective within 10 minutes
  40 mg I/v
      ↓ within 10 minutes
  80 mg I/v
      ↓ within 10 minutes
  80 mg I/v
- Hydralazine = I/v dose = Initial dose 5 mg followed by 5–10 mg every 15–20 minutes
  Maximum dose = 30 mg

Management of Mild Pre-eclampsia

- Role of antihypertensives is +/–
- **Definitive management:** Termination of pregnancy at 37 weeks
- Mode of delivery: Vaginal delivery.

Management of Severe Pre-eclampsia

- Prevention of convulsions by giving $MgSO_4$ along with management of hypertension using antihypertensives.
- If lungs of baby are not mature: Give corticosteroids
- Definitive management: Termination of pregnancy at 34 weeks
- Mode of delivery: Vaginal delivery.

Indications for termination of pregnancy irrespective of the weeks of gestation in case of pre-eclampsia are:
  - Impending eclampsia
  - Eclampsia (give $MgSO_4$ first, followed by induction of labor)
  - HELLP syndrome.
  - Abruption of placenta
  - Previable fetus
  - Fetal compromise
  - Uncontrollable BP or rising S. creatinine levels.
  - Reversal of end diastolic flow in umbilical artery doppler

Management of Eclampsia

- **First line management in eclampsia is** always airway management.
- Drug of choice to control convulsions $MgSO_4$.
- Antihypertensive should be given to control B/P. DOC in hypertensive crisis is I/v Labetalol.
- **Definitive management:** Termination of pregnancy irrespective of gestational age.

Mode of delivery: Try vaginal delivery. In most of the cases spontaneous labor begins. If it does not occur within 24 hours of the last convulsion, do cesarean section.

Indications for cesarean in Eclampsia

- Prolonged fetal bradycardia
- Unripe cervix
- Gestational age < 32 weeks
- Poor progress in labor.
- IUGR
- Uncontrollable BP.

Prevention and Treatment of Convulsions with $MgSO_4$

- $MgSO_4$ is the drug of choice for prevention and management of convulsions in eclampsia.[Q]

Mechanism of action:

- It blocks NMDA receptors in brain
- It causes cerebral vasodilatation
- Blocks the calcium channel and decreases intracranial edema.

Regimens for $MgSO_4^-$

A. **Pritchard Regimen**
  - **Loading dose** = 4 gms of 20% $MgSO_4$ slow I/v
    - Followed by 10 gms of 50% $MgSO_4$ – 5 gms in each buttock
    - Total dose = 14 gms.
  - Maintenance dose – Given after every 4 hours
    - Dose= 5 gms of 50% $MgSO_4$, I/m in alternate buttock.

B. **Sibai Regimen**
  Currently ACOG recommends I/v $MgSO_4$ as it does not carry any risk of gluteal abscess.
  - **Loading Dose:** 6 gm I/v $MgSO_4$ (30 mL of 20% $MgSO_4$ in 100. Normal saline over 15–20 minutes)
  - Maintenance dose = 2 gm I/v infusion
  - If convulsion recurs—2 gm I/v bolus $MgSO_4$ is given. If seizure still occurs – Phenobarbitone is given.

For status epilepticus – If patient continues to have seizure in spite of $MgSO_4$= Thiopentone sodium 0.5 g dissolved in 20 mL of Dextrose (5%) is given under anesthetic supervision.

Note: Treatment with MgSO$_4$ is continued for 24 hours after delivery in order to avoid postpartum eclampsia.

Therapeutic range of MgSO$_4$ – 4 to 7 mEq/L

- There is a narrow range at which therapeutic effect and toxic effects of Magnesium occurs, therefore monitoring for magnesium toxicity is very essential.

Monitoring for magnesium toxicity is done before giving each maintenance dose:

i. Urine output should be at least 30 mL/hr^Q

ii. Deep tendon reflexes (Patellar reflex) should be present^Q

iii. Respiration rate should be more than 14/min.^{Q}

iv. Pulse oximetry should be ≥ 96%

 Remember: Repeat injection are given only if all (i to iv) of the above are present.
- If any of these are absent, maintenance dose is omitted

Absolute contraindication of MgSO$_4$

- Myasthenia gravis.^{Q}
- Deranged renal function.^{Q}

 Important One Liners

- Disappearance of patellar reflex is the first sign of impending toxicity of MgSO$_4$.^{Q}
- Patellar reflex is lost when Mg^{++} concentration reaches 10 mEq/L.
- Respiratory depression occurs with Mg concentration > 12 mEq/L and arrest at Mg concentration is ≥ 15 mEq/L.
- Cardiac arrest occurs when ≥ 30 mEq/L.
- Best marker of magnesium toxicity is pulse oximetry as oxygen saturation begins to drop before there is evidence of respiratory depression.
- The neuromuscular blocking action of MgSO$_4$ may be potentiated by calcium channel blockers. So, MgSO$_4$ should be used cautiously with nifedipine.
- It should be used with caution with general anaesthetics.

Antidote for MgSO$_4$ toxicity is 10 mL Injection of 10% calcium gluconate (Alternative-Calcium Chloride)

Uses of MgSO$_4$
1. Used prophylactically in severe pre-eclampsia
2. Used prophylactically in severe HELLP syndrome
3. Used prophylactically in severe Impending eclampsia
4. Used therapeutically in eclampsia
5. Short term tocolytic
6. Neuroprotective action, hence given in all protein labor patients to prevent cerebral palsy in neonate.

HELLP SYNDROME

 It was 1st described by Weinstein in 1985.

- It is the most severe hematological complication of severe pre-eclampsia.
- In 15% cases, BP of the patient is normal (so remember: Not in all patients of HELLP syndrome BP is high)
- M/C in 3rd trimester
- Maternal mortality rate—1%
- Recurrence rate—25%
- The acronym HELLP stands for:
  H = Evidence of hemolysis manifested by
  i. LDH ≥ 600 IU/L
  ii. Elevated bilirubin ≥ 1.3 mg/dL
  iii. Low serum haptoglobin **(most specific marker)**
  iv. Abnormal peripheral blood smear—showing schistocytes, Burr cells and helmet cells.

EL = **E**levated **l**iver enzymes, i.e. AST and ALT ≥ 70 IU/L

LP = **L**ow **p**latelet count (≤ 1 lac/mm³)

Criteria for Diagnosis of HELLP— Tennessee Criteria

- LDH ≥ 600 IU/L
- ASTH ≥ 70 IU/L
- Platelet count < 100,000/mm³

 Note: HELLP syndrome is not a variant of DIC, as all coagulation parameters (PT, PTT, fibrogen) are normal in HELLP syndrome unlike DIC.

Mississippi Classification of HELLP Syndrome

- **Class I** (severe): Platelet count < 50,000/mm³
- **Class II** (moderate): Platelet count is between 50 and 100,000/mm³
- **Class III** (mild): Platelet count is between 100,000 and 150,000/mm³ but AST and LDH are increased.

Management

- If pregnancy is ≥ 34 weeks = give prophylactic MgSO$_4$ and immediately deliver.
- If pregnancy is between 24 and 34 weeks, give MgSO$_4$ and corticosteroids (Betamethasone 12 mg I/m 2 doses, 24 hours apart) and deliver.

Mode of delivery: Vaginal delivery only if Cervix is ripe, gestational > 32 weeks and FHR is reactive, otherwise cesarean section.

New Pattern Questions

N1. Which type of eclampsia has the worst prognosis?
a. Antepartum
b. Postpartum
c. Intrapartum
d. Imminent

N2. Cause of convulsion in eclampsia:
a. Cerebral anoxia due to arterial spasm
b. Hypovolemia
c. Hypocalcemia
d. Shock

N3. A pregnant woman in 3rd trimester has normal blood pressure when standing and sitting. When supine, BP drops to 90/50. What is the diagnosis?
a. Compression of uterine artery
b. Compression of aorta
c. Compression of IVC (inferior vena cava)
d. Compression of internal iliac vessels

N4. The following are related to pre-eclampsia:
a. It is a totally preventable disease
b. Systolic rise of blood pressure is more important than the diastolic
c. Eclampsia is invariably preceded by acute fulminating pre-eclampsia
d. Endothelial dysfunction is the basic pathology

N5. In a pregnant female with BP 150/100 mm Hg, a protein/creatinine ratio of _____ suggests development of pre-eclampsia
a. > 0.20
b. > 0.30
c. < 0.20
d. < 0.30

N6. High-risk factor for gestational hypertension include all *except*:
a. BP ≥ 150/100 mm of Hg
b. Gestation age < 30 weeks
c. IUGR
d. Polyhydramnios

N7. A G2P1, female presenting at 37 weeks with increased reflexes, pedal edema and hypertension. All of the following can be seen *except*:
a. Increased uric acid levels
b. Increased creatinine levels
c. Increased SGOT/SGPT
d. Increased platelet counts

N8. Recurrence rate of HELLP syndrome:
a. 5%
b. 10%
c. 15%
d. 25%

N9. The most important reason to give antihypertensive drug in PIH is to decrease the:
a. Incidence of IUGR
b. Incidence of fetal death
c. Incidence of maternal complication like stroke
d. Incidence of placental abruption

N10. Pre-eclampsia M/C presents in:
a. 1st trimester
b. 2nd trimester
c. 3rd trimester
d. Postpartum

N11. A primigravida 32-year-old female is admitted to the antenatal ward at 35 weeks is found to BP of 160/110. Her urine does not contain albumin. Which of the following drugs should not be used in her management?
a. Frusemide
b. Hydralazine
c. Labetalol
d. Methyldopa
e. Nifedipine

N12. Remodelling of placental vasculature contains how many phases?
a. 2 phases
b. 3 phases
c. 4 phases
d. 5 phases

N13. All of the following increase in PIH *except*:
a. Uric acid
b. Thromboxane A2
c. sFlt-1
d. VEGF

N14. All of the following play a role in preventing PIH *except*:
a. Aspirin
b. Aspirin + Heparin
c. Heparin
d. Regular exercise

N15. Best predictive test for PIH:
a. PSV of MCA Doppler
b. Uterine artery Doppler
c. Umbilical artery Doppler
d. Giant roll over test

Previous Year Questions

1. **Risk factors for pre-eclampsia:** [PGI 06]
   a. Chronic hypertenstion
   b. Obesity
   c. Placental ischaemia
   d. Multigravida
   e. Antiphospholipid syndrome

2. **Risk factor for pre-eclampsia:** [PGI 07]
   a. Chronic hypertension
   b. Smoking   c. Obesity
   d. Multiparity   e. Placenta previa

3. **Risk factor for pre-eclampsia includes:**
   a. Age >35 years   [PGI May 2010]
   b. Obesity
   c. Previous h/o pre-eclampsia
   d. Multigravida
   e. Antiphospholipid syndrome

4. **Which of the following seen in pre-eclampsia?**
                                              [PGI 01]
   a. Hypertension   b. Proteinuria
   c. Convulsions   d. Pedal edema

5. **Indicator of severe pre-eclampsia:** [PGI Dec 09]
   a. IUGR
   b. Diastolic BP > 110 mm of Hg
   c. Pulmonary edema
   d. Systolic BP > 160 mm of Hg
   e. Oliguria

6. **All are prognostic indicators of pregnancy induced hypertension, except:** [AIIMS May 01]
   a. Low platelets
   b. Serum Na
   c. Elevated liver enzymes
   d. Serum uric acid

7. **All of the following indicate superimposed pre-eclampsia in a pregnant female of chronic hypertension except:** [AIIMS May 14]
   a. New onset proteinuria
   b. Platelet count < 75,000
   c. Increase in systolic BP by 30 mm Hg and diastolic by 15 mm Hg
   d. Fresh retinal hypertensive changes

8. **In PIH an impending sign of eclampsia is:**
   a. Visual symptoms   [PGI Dec 98]
   b. Weight gain of 2 lb per week
   c. Severe proteinuria of 10 g
   d. Pedal edema.

9. **All of the following may be used in pregnancy associated hypertension except:** [AI 04]
   a. Nifedipine   b. Captopril
   c. Methyldopa   d. Hydralazine

10. **Which of the following antihypertensives is not safe in pregnancy?** [AIIMS Nov. 05; May 05]
    a. Clonidine   b. ACE inhibitors/Enalapril
    c. α-Methyldopa   d. Amlodipine

11. **Which of the following antihypertensives is not given in pregnancy?** [AIIMS May 14,15]
    a. Enalapril   b. α-methyldopa
    c. Labetalol   d. Nifedipine

12. **All of the following can be administrated in acute hypertension during labour except:** [AIIMS May 14]
    a. IV labetalol   b. IV nitroprusside
    c. IV dihydralazine d. IV diazoxide

13. **Which is the drug of choice for severe pre-eclampsia?**
                                              [AI 08]
    a. Labetalol   b. Metaprolol
    c. α-methyldopa   d. Nifidipine

14. **DOC for PIH is:** [AIIMS Nov 2015]
    a. Atenolol
    b. Nitroprusside
    c. Enalapril
    d. Alpha methyldopa

15. **A 27 year primigravida presents with pregnancy induced hypertension with blood pressure of 150/100 mm of Hg at 32 weeks of gestation with no other complications. Subsequently, her blood pressure is controlled on treatment. If there are no complications, the pregnancy should be terminated at:** [AIIMS May 06]
    a. 40 completed weeks
    b. 37 completed weeks
    c. 35 completed weeks
    d. 34 completed weeks

16. **Which of the following is/are criteria for the expectant management in pre-eclampsia except:** [PGI Nov 2014]
    a. Platelet count <100000
    b. BP > 140/90
    c. Urine output < 400 mL/day
    d. Persistent headache
    e. Visual disturbances

17. **A 30-year-old primi with 36 weeks of pregnancy with blood pressure 160/110 and urinary albumin is 3+ and platelet count 80000/mm³. What will be the management?** [PGI June 09]

a. Betamethasone   b. $MgSO_4$
c. Labetalol   d. Urgent LSCS
e. Labour induction

18. **A gravida 2 patient with previous LSCS comes at 37 weeks, has BP = 150/100 mm of Hg. And on pervaginal examination, cervix is 50% effaced station-3, os is closed and pelvis is adequate. Proteinuria is +1, Most appropriate step at the moment would be:**
    a. Antihypertensive regime and wait for spontaneous labor   **[AIIMS Nov 2010]**
    b. Wait and watch
    c. Induced labor
    d. Caesarean section

19. **A female of 36 weeks gestation presents with hypertension, blurring of vision and headache. Her blood pressure reading was 180/120 mm Hg and 174/110 mm Hg after 20 minutes. How will you manage the patient?** **[AIIMS Nov 12]**
    a. Admit the patient and observe
    b. Admit the patient, start antihypertensives and continue pregnancy till term
    c. Admit the patient, start antihypertensives, $MgSO_4$ and terminate the pregnancy
    d. Admit oral antihypertensives and follow-up in out-patient department

20. **A 28-year-old eclamptic woman develop convulsions. The first measure to be done is:** **[AIIMS June 99]**
    a. Give $MgSO_4$
    b. Sedation of patient
    c. Immediate delivery
    d. Care of airway

21. **Which is not a feature of HELLP syndrome?**
    [AIIMS Feb 97]
    a. Thrombocytopenia
    b. Eosinophilia
    c. Raised liver enzyme
    d. Hemolytic anemia

22. **Which of the following is not a part of HELLP syndrome?** **[AIIMS May 2014]**
    a. Hemolysis
    b. Elevated liver enzymes
    c. Thrombocytopenia
    d. Retroplacental hemorrhage

23. **Concentration of $MgSO_4$ in the treatment of eclampsia in mEq/L:** **[PGI 99]**
    a. 7–10   b. 10–15
    c. 2–4   d. 4–7

24. **Side effects of magnesium sulfate includes:**
    a. Hypotension   **[PGI Dec 08]**
    b. Anuria
    c. Coma
    d. Pulmonary edema

25. **Earliest sign of Mg toxicity:** **[AI 2011]**
    a. Depression of deep tendon reflexes
    b. Respiratory depression
    c. Cardiac arrest
    d. Anuria

26. **Best drug for management of eclampsia:**
    [AIIMS Nov 2010]
    a. $MgSO_4$ b. Lytic cocktail regime
    c. Phenytoin   d. Diazepam

27. **$MgSO_4$ is/are indicated in:** **[PGI Nov 2012]**
    a. Severe pre-eclampsia
    b. Eclampsia
    c. Pre-term labour
    d. Prevention of cerebral palsy

28. **All statements(s) is/are about use of magnesium sulphate except:** **[PGI May 2013]**
    a. Therapeutic level is 4–7 mEq/L
    b. Used in spinal anesthesia
    c. Used in seizure prophylaxis
    d. Decrease neuromuscular blockage
    e. Used in pre-emptive analgesia

29. **True about $MgSO_4$ role in pre-eclampsia and eclampsia:** **[PGI May 2017]**
    a. Used for controlling hypertension in pre-eclampsia and eclampsia
    b. Therapeutic level for seizure control is 4-7mEQ/L
    c. Toxicity should be monitored
    d. Can be given as IV infusion
    e. Also can be given by intramuscular route

30. **Pregnancy aggravates which of the following condition(s)?** **[PGI May 2017]**
    a. Hypertension
    b. Anaemia
    c. Rheumatoid arthritis
    d. Acne

31. **Feature(s) of HELLP syndrome:** **[PGI May 2017]**
    a. Low platelets
    b. Increased AST and ALT
    c. Decreased lactate dehydrogenase
    d. Increased conjugated bilirubin
    e. Hemolysis

Answers with Explanations to New Pattern Questions

N1. **Ans. is a, i.e. Antepartum**   *Ref. Dutta Obs. 7/e, p233*

Eclampsia if associated with the following features has bad prognosis:

- Long interval between onset of fit and commencement of treatment
- *Antepartum eclampsia especially with long delivery interval*
- Number of fits > 10
- Coma in between fits
- Temperature > 102°F with pulse rate > 120/min
- BP > 200 mm of Hg systolic
- Oliguria (< 400 mL/24 hr) with proteinuria > 5 gm/24 hr
- Non response to treatment
- Jaundice.

N2. **Ans. is a, i.e. Cerebral anoxia due to arterial spasm**   *Ref. Dutta Obs. 7/e, p231*

Cause of convulsion is a case of eclampsia is cerebral irritation. This irritation may be provoked by:

Anoxia

↓

spasm of cerebral vessels due to HTN

↓

increased cerebral vascular resistance

↓

decrease in cerebral oxygen consumption

↓

Anoxia:
- Cerebral edema
- Cerebral dysrhythmia

N3. **Ans. is c, i.e. Compression of IVC (inferior vena cava)**   *Ref. Dutta Obs. 7/e, p 53, 54*

Supine hypotension syndrome:

- During **late pregnancy**[Q] the gravid uterus produces a compression effect on the inferior vena cava, when the patient is the supine position.
- This, generally results in opening up of collateral ciculation by means of paravertebral and azygous veins.
- In some cases (10%) when the collateral circulation fails to open, the venous return of the heart may be seriously curtailed which results in production of hypotension, tachycardia and syncope. Normal blood pressure is quickly restored by turning the patient to lateral position.

N4. **Ans. is d, i.e. Endothelial dysfunction is the basic pathology**   *Ref. Dutta Obs. 7/e, p 221*

Lets see each option separately:

Option a: It is a totally preventable disease incorrect as quoted by Dutta 7/e, on p 227.

"Pre-eclampsia is not a totally preventable disease" Dutta obs 7/e, p 22.

Option b: Systolic rise of BP is more important than diastolic—incorrect.

The rise in diastolic BP is more significant and first to occur.

Option c: Eclampsia is invariably preceded by acute fulminant pre-eclampsia—incorrect as in majority –80%. This is true but not in all.

Option d: Endothelial dysfunction is the basic pathology—true as explained in the text.

N5. **Ans. is b, i.e. > 0.30**   *Ref. Fernando Arias 4/e, p 189*

In patients with gestational hypertension, there are high chances (15-25%) of progressing to pre-eclampsia. Pre-eclampsia is heralded by the development of proteinuria.

Proteinuria ≥ + 2 in a random urine sample is diagnostic of pre-eclampsia in these patients. When proteinuria is + 1 or traces, it is necessary to send random sample to lab for determination of protein/ creatinine ratio and calcium/ creatinine ratio.

Protein/creatinine ratio = > 0.30 → indicates pre-eclampsia

Calcium/creatinine ratio = < 0.06 → indicates pre-eclampsia

Although the gold standard would be measuring protein in 24 hours urine sample, but it is cumbersome.

N6. Ans. is d, i.e. Polyhydramnios   *Ref. Fernando Arias 4/e*

Friends, first let's solve this MCQ by using common sense, even though we have not studied any risk factors for gestational hypertension.

As you know, in any kind of hypertension =

Matenal BP ↑

⇓

Now pressure and volume are inversely related

Therefore, volume of blood flowing to fetus decreases

⇓

Fetal blood flow ↓

⇓

Fetal renal blood flow ↓

⇓

GFR ↓

⇓

∴   Urine output of fetus ↓

⇓

Oligohydramnios (as fetal urine is the major contributor of amniotic fluid).

Therefore, in no case can polyhydramnios be seen in gestational HT. Hence it cannot be a high-risk factor.

Now coming to References:

Fernando Arias 4/e, page 188.

Criteria to Identify High Risk Women with Gastational Hypertension

- Blood pressure ≥ 150/100
- Gestational age < 30 weeks
- Evidence of end organ damage (Raised: S. Creatinine, liver enzymes, LDH; decreased platelet count)
- Oligohydramnios
- Fetal growth restriction
- Abnormal uterine/umbilical artery Doppler

N7. Ans. is d, i.e. Increased platelet count

In a PIH - platelet count is decreased and not increased.

N8. Ans. is d, i.e. 25%   *Ref. Fernando arias, high risk pregnancy 4/e p224*

Recurrence rate of HELLP syndrome is 25%

N9. Ans. is c, i.e. Incidence of maternal complication like stroke

Ref. Fernando arias, high risk pregnancy 4/e p 213)

"The objective of antihypertensive treatment in severe pre-eclampsia is to prevent intracranial bleeding and left ventricular failure".   *Ref. Fernando arias, 4/e pg 213*

N10. Ans. is c, i.e. 3rd trimester

N11. Ans. is a, i.e. Frusemide

In a PIH patient, furosemide is contraindicated as an anti-hypertensive because in PIH, the intravascular volume is low, giving a diuretic would further decrease it, which reduce placental perfusion.

 Remember: Diuretics are not contraindicated in pregnancy.
In a pregnant female with CHF, diuretics are used, then it is not contraindicated. Also diuretics can be used if there is pulmonary edema.

N12. **Ans. is a, i.e. 2 phases**

Trophoblastic invasion occurs in 2 phases.

N13. **Ans. is d, i.e. VEGF** *(Williams Obs 25/e p 716)*

See the text for explanation.

N14. **Ans. is c, i.e. Heparin** *(Williams Obs 25/e p 727, 728)*

Regular exercise during pregnancy is linked to a lower risk of developing preeclampsia. Also, in one systematic review, a trend toward risk reduction with exercise was noted (Kasawara, 2012). Only a few studies have been randomized, and thus, more research is needed. *(Williams Obs 25/e p 727)*

Antithrombotic Agents

As noted earlier preeclampsia is characterized by vasospasm, endothelial cell dysfunction, and inflammation, as well as activation of platelets and the coagulation-hemostasis system.

Low-molecular-weight heparin for prophylaxis has been studied in several randomized trials. Rodger and colleagues (2016) performed a metaanalysis using individual patient data from 963 women. The risk for recurrent preeclampsia, abruption, or fetal-growth restriction was similar in women receiving heparin or placebo.

Aspirin, in low oral doses of 50 to 150 mg daily, effectively inhibits platelet thromboxane A2 biosynthesis but has minimal effects on vascular prostacyclin production. Still, several clinical trials have shown benefits in preeclampsia prevention.

In recent dueling metaanalyses, Roberge and colleagues (2017) found that aspirin prophylaxis initiated before 16 weeks' gestation was associated with a significant risk reduction—about 60 percent for preeclampsia and fetal-growth restriction.

Meanwhile, the U.S. Preventive Services Task Force recommends low-dose aspirin prophylaxis from women at high risk for preeclampsia (Henderson, 2014). Because of this, the American College of Obstetricians and Gynecologists (2016b) issued a Practice Advisory that recommends low-dose aspirin be given between 12 and 28 weeks' gestation to help prevent preeclampsia in high-risk women. This includes those with a history of preeclampsia and those with twins, chronic hypertension, overt diabetes, renal disease, and autoimmune disorders. These results have also raised the question as to whether all pregnant women should be given aspirin (Mone, 2017). At this time, our answer is "no".

Low-dose aspirin coupled with heparin mitigates thrombotic sequelae in women with lupus anticoagulant. Because of a similarly high prevalence of placental thrombotic lesions found with severe preeclampsia, trials have assessed the possible merits of such treatments for women with prior preeclampsia. In two randomized trials, women with a history of early-onset preeclampsia were given an aspirin therapy or an enoxaparin plus aspirin regimen. Outcomes were similar. From their reviews, Sergis and associates (2006) reported better pregnancy outcomes in women with prior severe preeclampsia given low-molecular-weight heparin plus low-dose aspirin compared with those given low-dose aspirin alone. Similar findings were reported by de Vries and coworkers (2012). *(Williams Obs 25/e p 727, 728)*

Hence aspirin alone/Hepain + aspirin is useful in presenting preeclampsia but not Hepain alone.

N15. **Ans. is b, i.e. Uterine artery Doppler**

See the text for details

Answers with Explanations to Previous Year Questions

1. **Ans. is a, b, c and e, i.e. Chronic hypertension; Obesity; Placental ischaemia; and Antiphospholipid syndrome**

2. **Ans. is a and c, i.e. Chronic hypertension; and Obesity**

3. **Ans. is b, c and e, i.e. Obesity; Previous h/o pre-eclampsia; and Antiphospholipid syndrome**
   Risk factors for Pre-eclampsia:
   All the risk factors for PIH have been discussed in the preceding text
   Some which need explanation are: Placental ischaemia risk factor as per Dutta Obs 8/e, p256
   Age > 40 years is a risk factor, not > 35 years (JB Sharma p424)
   As far as smoking is concerned.

   "Although smoking during pregnancy causes a variety of adverse pregnancy outcomes, ironically, smoking has consistently been associated with a reduced risk of hypertension during pregnancy. Placenta previa has also been reported to reduce the risk of hypertensive disorders in pregnancy."   *Ref. Williams 23/e, p709*
   - Smoking is also protective for fibroids and endometriosis.

4. **Ans. is a and b, i.e. Hypertension; and Proteinuria**   *Ref. Fernando Arias 3/e, p 415; COGDT 10/e, p 320*
   Hypertension: It is defined as systolic BP $\geq$ 140 mm of Hg or diastolic BP $\geq$ 90 mm of Hg on 2 occasions atleast 6 hours apart seen in previously normotensive female after 20 weeks of gestation or mean arterial pressure $\geq$ 105 mm of Hg.
   Note: A systolic rise of 30 mm Hg or a diastolic rise of 15 mm Hg is no longer a diagnostic criterion.
   Proteinuria: Irreversible excretion of 300 mg of protein in 24 hours urine collection or atleast 30 mg/dL or 1+ dipstick in atleast 2 random urine samples is significant proteinuria.
   Note: Earlier presence of proteinuria was essential for the diagnosis of pre-eclampsia, but now pre-clampsia can be diagnosed in absence of proteins if signs of end organ damage are present.
   Oedema (which was included in diagnostic criteria of PIH is no longer a diagnostic criterion according to) *COGDT 10/e, p 320, Table 19-2* **and according to** *Fernando Arias 3/e, p 415 and all other books.*

   "Excessive weight gain and edema are no longer considered signs of pre-eclampsia. Large increases in body weight as well as edema of hands, face or both are common in normal pregnancy and the incidence of pre-eclampsia is similar in patients with or without generalised edema."

5. **Ans. is b, c and d, i.e. Diastolic BP > 110 mm of Hg; Pulmonary edema; and Systolic BP > 160 mm of Hg**
        Ref. Dutta Obs. 7/e, p 224

   Friends, now this question should be answered in light of the new guidelines of ACOG (2013) differentiating mild and severe pre-eclampsia.

Mild pre-eclampsia	Severe pre-eclampsia

• BP $\geq$ 140/90 but < 160/110 mm of Hg
• Signs of End organ damage absent
	• BP $\geq$ 160/110 mm of Hg
	• Signs of End organ damage present
	  – Platelet count < 1 lac
	  – S. creatinine > 1.1 mg/dL
	  – Elevated liver enzymes to more than 2 times their normal value
	  – Evidence of Pulmonary edema
	  – New onset visual/cerebral symptoms

6. **Ans. is b, i.e. Serum Na**
   - The question was before the new guidelines set by ACOG. Since electrolytes remain normal in all cases of Pre-eclampsia, be it mild and severe it was taken as the answer.

   - Criteria no longer used to differentiate mild and severe pre eclampsia are:
     – Oliguria
     – IUGR
     – Proteinuria

7. **Ans is c, i.e. Increase in systolic BP by 30 mm Hg and diastolic by 15 mm Hg**   *Ref. Fernando Arias 4/e, p 187*
Williams 24/e, p 730, 1007

As discussed in the text, **chronic hypertension with superimposed pre-eclampsia** is diagnosed in a pregnant female if:

i. Suddenly after 20 weeks her BP becomes uncontrollable
ii. After 20 weeks, there is new onset proteinuria
iii. After 20 weeks, signs of end organ damage are present.

So, option 'a' and 'd' are correct.

As far as option b, platelet count < 75,000 is correct—Criteria says platelet count should be < 1 lac so it is also taken as true.

Option 'c' increase in systolic BP more than 30 mm Hg and diastolic by 15 mm of Hg is not taken as any criteria now.

Remember:
- The incidence of superimposed pre-eclampsia for women with chronic HT is 20–30%
- As compared to pure pre-eclampsia, superimposed pre-eclampsia occurs earlier in gestation.
- It is associated with fetal growth restriction.
- ACOG recommends the use of $MgSO_4$ for patients with this condition to prevent seizures.

8. **Ans. is a, i.e. Visual symptoms**

Ref. Dutta Obs. 6/e, p 226; Sheila Balakrishnan 305; Williams Obs. 22/e, p 781, 23/e, p 729

As you know, severe pre-eclampsia progresses to eclampsia if not treated promptly, hence symptoms of severe pre-eclampsia can also be called as indicators of Impending eclampsia.

Signs of Impending or Imminent eclampsia/ Symptoms of severe pre-eclampsia/ Symptoms associated with poor prognosis	• Headache (severe) • *Blurring of vision/flashing lights* • Epigastric pain • Brisk deep tendon reflexes and ankle clonus • *Diminished urinary output (< 400 mL/24 hours).*

9. **Ans. is b, i.e. Captopril**   *Ref. Dutta Obs. 7/e, p 228; Williams Obs. 22/e, p 782, 23/e, p 731-732; KDT 5/e, p 517*

ACE inhibitors *(Captopril/Enalapril/Ramipril/Lisinopril/Perindopril)* are contraindicated in pregnancy as they can impair renal function causing fetal Oliguria and oligohydramnios. They also cause congenital defects in fetus viz.

- Bony malformation
- Persistent patent ductus arteriosus
- Respiratory distress syndrome
- Limb contracture
- Pulmonary hypoplasia
- Prolonged neonatal hypotension   *Ref. Williams Obs. 22/e, p 782*
- Neonatal death

10. **Ans. is b, i.e. ACE inhibitors/Enalapril**

11. **Ans. is a, i.e. Enalapril**   *Ref. Williams Obs. 23/e, p 731, 732, High Risk Pregnancy, Fernando Arias 4/e, p 196*
See the text for explanation

12. **Ans. is d, i.e. IV diazoxide**
Ref. http://www.drugs.com/pregnancy/diazoxie.html; http://www.rxlist.com/nitropress-drug/warnigs-precaution.htm

Although both sodium nitroprusside and diazoxide are not safe, still as a last resort sodium nitroprusside can be used but diazoxide is contraindicated.

13. **Ans. is a, i.e. Labetalol**   *Ref. Fernando Arias 4/e, p 213*

"Labetalol is the medication of choice for the treatment of acute severe hypertension in pregnancy and for maintenance treatment of hypertensive disorders in pregnancy. The reasons for being the first choice drug are its effectiveness, low incidence of side effects and the availability of oral and parenteral preparations."

... Fernando Arias 4/e, p 213

So this leaves no doubt that:
- *Antihypertensive of choice for severe pre-eclampsia is* - labetalol.

Hydralazine Versus Labetalol   *Ref. Williams 24/e, p 762*

Comparative studies of these two antihyperrensive agents show equlivalerar results (Umans, 2014). Labetalol lowered blood pressure more rapidly, and associated tachycardia was minimal. However, hydralazine lowered mean arterial pressures to safe levels more effectively. Maternal and neonatal outcomes were similar. Hydralazine caused significantly more maternal caused maternal hypotension and bradycardia. Both drugs have been associated with a reduced frequency of fetal heart rate accelerations (Cahill, 2013).

> *Also Know:*
>
> The objective of antihypertensive use in seizure pre-eclampsia is to prevent intracranial bleed and left ventricular failure.

14. Ans. is d, i.e. Alpha methyldopa

The answer to the question should have been labetalol.

But since it is not given in options we will go with alpha methyldopa. Methyldopa is used for chronic hypertension in pregnancy and mild pre-eclampsia but is not used in severe pre-eclampsia because of delayed onset of action.

15. Ans. is b, i.e. 37 completed weeks

Ref. Dutta Obs. 7/e, p229; Fernando Arias 3/e, p418-419,Bedside Obs. and Gynae-Richa Saxena 1/e, p217

The patient in the question has BP = 150/100 mm of Hg, i.e. mild hypertension (severe hypertension is when systolic BP is $\geq$ 160 mm or diastolic BP $\geq$ 110 mm of Hg) and has no other complications. Her BP is controlled on treatment, i.e. she is being managed expectantly.

In such patients pregnancy should be terminated at 37 weeks.

"If Pregnancy is beyond 37 completed weeks termination is to be considered without delay."

... Dutta Obs. 7/e, p229

16. Ans. is b, i.e. BP > 140/90

Ref. Fernando Arias 4/e, p 215, 216

Expectant Mgt of pre-eclampsia would be done in mild pre-eclampsia and severe pre-eclampsia before 34 weeks.

The main aspects of expectant management are:

Guidelines for the expectant management of severe pre-eclampsia less than 34 weeks:
• Hospitalization • Daily weight • Daily input and output • Antihypertensive treatment (Aldomet, labetalol, nifedipine) • Betamethasone (two 12 mg doses 24 hours apart) • Laboratory every other day or more frequently, if needed AST, ALT, LDH, platelet count, creatinine, bilirubin, 24-hour urinary protein • Daily fetal movement count • Weekly to as frequently as daily NST depending upon fetal growth status and liquor • Umbilical and middle cerebral Doppler twice every week • Amniotic fluid volume twice every week • Ultrasound for fetal growth every two weeks.

Patients with severe pre-eclampsia need meticulous attention. The criteria to interrupt expectant management and move to delivery are:

Criteria to interrupt expectant management and move to delivery— **Maternal:**
• Persistent severe headache or visual changes eclampsia • Shortness of breath, chest tightness with rales and/or SpO_2 < 94% at room air; pulmonary edema • Uncontrolled severe hypertension despite treatment • Oliguria < 500 mL in 24 hours or serum creatinine >1.5 mg/dL • Persistent platelet count < 100,000/mm³ • Suspected abruption, progressive labour and/or ruptured membranes
Fetal: • Severe growth restriction < 5th centile for gestational age • Reversed or end diastolic flow in umbilical artery Doppler • Persistent severe oligohydramnios • Biophysical profile < 4 dose • Fetal death

17. Ans. is b, c, and e, i.e. MgSO$_4$; Labetalol; and Labour induction

Ref. Fernando Arias 3/e, p 420-424, Flowchart 16-4 on p 424

In the Question patient has:
Blood pressure = 160/110 mm Hg
Platelet count = 80,000/mm^3 } indicating severe Pre-eclampsia
The gestational age is 36 weeks

Management of severe pre-eclampsia in Gestational age ≥ 34 weeks

Ref. Dutta Obs. 6/e, p 231; Fernando Arias 3/e, p 418, 419

"If Gestational age is ≥ 34 weeks, the best approach is to treat with magnesium sulphate for the prevention of seizures, give antihypertensive to control the blood pressure and delivery after stabilization."

—Fernando Arias 4/e, p 210

So this leaves us with no doubt that

- Magnesium sulphate
- Labetalol (the antihypertensive of choice in pre-eclampsia)
- Labor induction are all correct options as per Fernando Arias.
- As far as mode of delivery is concerned, vaginal delivery is preferred. If cervix is not ripe–prostaglandins are used to refer cause. If it fails then cesarean is done.

Betamethasone to hasten lung maturity is not required at 36 weeks as lungs are already mature by this time.

18. Ans. is c, i.e. Induced labor *Ref. Fernando Arias 3/e, p 420-424, Flowchart 16-4 on p 424, Williams Obs 23/e, p 729.*

This patient has

- BP: 150/100 mm Hg

Therefore, it is classified as mild pre-eclampsia.

In mild pre-eclampsia – if gestational age is > 37 weeks then labor should be induced

Remember, PIH is not a contraindication for VBAC (Vaginal birth after cesarean) and further more the pelvis of this patient is adequate – so there is no harm in inducing labour, rather it is advantageous, because it will help in developing lower uterine segment. At any point of time; if there is scar tenderness or if patients BP rises uncontrollably, immediate cesarean section can be performed.

19. Ans. is c, i.e. Admit the patient, start antihypertensives, MgSO$_4$ and terminate the pregnancy

Ref. Fernando Arias 'Practical Guide to High Risk Pregnancy and Delivery 3/e, p 417, 420, 424'

In the question, patient is presenting with:

- Headache
- Blurring of vision
- B/P = 180/120 mm of Hg (later 174/110 mm of Hg)

i.e. she is a case of severe pregnancy induced hypertension.

In severe pre-eclampsia there are 2 risks:

1. **Intracranial bleeding:** Give antihypertensive
2. **Convulsions:** Give MgSO$_4$

Definitive management is Termination of pregnancy at ≥ 34 weeks. Since this patient is 36 weeks pregnant, so option C is the best one.

First step in the management of this case would be to prevent seizures, i.e. give MgSO$_4$.

20. Ans. is d, i.e. Care of airway *Ref. Dutta Obs 6/e, p 235, COGDT 10/e, p 326*

Pre-eclampsia when complicated with convulsion and / or coma is called *eclampsia.*

Fits occurring in eclampsia are *Generalised tonic clonic seizure.*

In most cases seizures are self limited, lasting for 1 to 2 minutes.

Management:

"The first priorities are to ensure that the airway is clear and to prevent injury and aspiration of gastric content".

—COGDT 10/e, p 326

21. Ans. is b, i.e. Eosinophilia *Ref. Dutta Obs. 7/e, p 222; Fernando Arias 3/e, p 427, 428*

22. Ans. is d, i.e. Retroplacental hemorrhage

Discussed in detail in the text.

23. **Ans. is d, i.e. 4–7 mEq/L**

24. **Ans. is d, i.e. Pulmonary edema**

25. **Ans. is a, i.e. Depression of deep tendon reflexes**

26. **Ans. is a, i.e. MgSO$_4$**

No question needs explanation here.

Only in Q 24 I would like to point out that anuria/oliguria is not a side effect of MgSO$_4$. It is a sign of toxicity.

27. **Ans. is All** *Ref. Dutta Obs. 7/e, p 508, 509; Willams 23/e, p 737-739*

MgSO$_4$ is used in eclampsia and severe preclampsia both for prophyllaxis and treatment of convulsions. It is a tocoloytic agent also. As far as its role in preventing cerebral palsy is concerned the data which I could get from ncb through internet is:

"Cerebral palsy is a nonprogressive disorder of movement and posture and a leading cause of childhood disability. Preterm birth is a major risk factor for the development of cerebral palsy; gestational age at delivery has an inverse relationship to the risk of cerebral palsy. Observational studies over the past 15 years have suggested a possible protective role for MgSO$_4$. In some studies, children born preterm who were exposed prenatally to MgSO$_4$ for obstetric indications such as seizure prophylaxis or tocolysis had decreased rates of cerebral palsy as compared with children born preterm to women who were not exposed to MgSO$_4$. Randomized trials have been conducted to test the hypothesis that maternal MgSO$_4$ exposure had neonatal neuroprotective effects. These studies included women thought to be at risk of preterm delivery within 24 hours."

Thus option d is correct.

28. **Ans. is d, i.e. Decrease neuromuscular blockage**
Ref. Dutta Obs. 7/e, p 234, 235 and Intenet search Lee's Anaesthesia 13/e, p 674

We have read a lot about MgSO$_4$ so I will explain only the difficult options. You know option a and c are correct.
"The use of magnesium sulfate can induce prolong neuromuscular block" – *Lee 13/e, p 674 i.e. option d is incorrect*
"Preemptive analgesia is an antinociceptive treatment that prevents establishment of altered processing of afferent input, which amplifies postoerative pain" – *http://journals.lww.com/anesthesiology*
"Preemptive use of epidural magnesium sulfate to reduce narcotic requirements in orthopedic surgery" – *http://www.egyptja.org/articles/S1110 i.e option e is correct*
"The addition of intrathecal (IT) magnesium to spinal fentanyl prolongs the duration of spinal analgesia for vaginal delivery" i.e. option b is correct.

29. **Ans. is b, c, d and e, i.e. Therapeutic level for seizure control is 4–7 mEQ/L; Toxicity should be monitored; Can be given as IV infusion; Also can be given by intramuscular route**
(Ref: Dutta Obs 8th/273, 583; J B Sharma 1st/437-39)

Magnesium Sulphate
- Magnesium sulphate is drug of choice as anticonvulsant in Eclampsia and severe preeclampsia . It is not an antihypertensive, hence option a is incorrect.
- The therapeutic level of serum magnesium is 4-7 mEQ/L/ 4.8 to 8.4 mg/dL or 2 to 3.5 mmol/L
- Various regimens: Pritchard (IV+IM), Sibai (IV), Zuspan (IV) and Dhaka regimen (IV+IM).
- In India, most hospital use Pritchard regime but ACOG recommends IV regime due to chances of gluteal abscess with intramuscular regime
- Serum magnesium level may be monitored in selected cases (renal insufficiency, absent deep tendon reflex)
- Magnesium toxicity and serum magnesium level is seen in (a) loss of deep tendon reflex @ 10 mEq/L (b) respiratory depression more than 12 mEq , respiratory arrest @ 15mEq/l and (c) cardiac arrest @30 mEq/L

30. **Ans. is a and b, i.e. Hypertension and Anaemia**
(Ref: Dutta Obs 8th/255,303; J B Sharma 1st/541; William Obs 24th /1156)
"Acne usually improves in pregnancy"—J B Sharma 1st ed, pg 543
"There are no obvious adverse effects of rheumatoid arthritis on pregnancy outcome. The disease improves in majority (90%) of women during pregnancy" —*J B Sharma 1st ed pg 541*
"Up to 90 percent of women with rheumatoid arthritis will experience improvement during pregnancy" —*William Obs 24th ed, pg 1178*
"Hypertension is one of the common medical complications of pregnancy" —*Dutta Obs 8th ed pg 255*
"Anemia is the commonest haematological disorder that may occur in pregnancy, the others being rhesus isoimmunisation and blood coagulation disorders" —*Dutta Obs 8th ed pg 303.*

Note: T helper cells 2 increase and its cytokines i.e Interleukin 4 and 6 also increase in pregnancy hence SLE flares during pregnancy whereas T Helper cells 1 and its cytokines i.e IL 2 and interferon gamma decrease during pregnancy so Rheumatoid arthritis improves in pregnancy.

31. **Ans. is a, b, d and e, i.e. Low platelets; Increased AST and ALT; Increased conjugated bilirubin and Hemolysis**
    HELLP syndrome:
    It was first described by Weinstein

    > **H –stands for Hemolysis:**
    > Represented by LDH >/= 600 IU/L
    > Levels of bilirubin >1.2 mg/dl
    > Less haptoglobin levels
    > Peripheral blood smear shows Burr cells, schistocytes, helmet cells
    > **EL- Elevated liver enzymes**
    > **i.e AST and ALT ./=70IU/L**
    > **LP- Low platelet count (<1 lac)**

    Missisipi classification of HELLP Syndrome
    Class I = Severe = Plat count < 50,000
    Class II = Moderate = Plat count 50,000–1 lac
    Class III = Mild = Plat count ≥ 1 lac but AST and ALT > 70
    Management: Immediate Termination of pregnancy + MgSO$_4$.

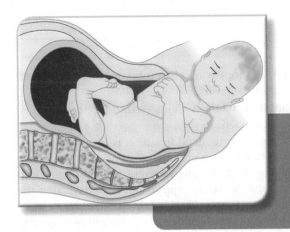

Chapter at a Glance

FETAL AND NEWBORN IMMUNOLOGY

- The active immunological capacity of the fetus and neonate is compromised compared with that of older children and adults.
- Fetal cell-mediated and humoral immunity begin to develop by 9 to 15 weeks' gestation.
- The primary fetal response to infection is immunoglobulin M (IgM). Passive immunity is provided by IgG transferred across the placenta.

- By 16 weeks, this transfer begins to increase rapidly, and by 26 weeks, fetal concentrations are equivalent to those of the mother.
- After birth, breastfeeding is protective against some infections, although this protection begins to decline at 2 months of age. Current World Health Organization (2013) recommendations are to exclusively breastfeed for the first 6 months of life with partial breastfeeding until 2 years of age.
- Vertical transmission refers to passage from the mother to her fetus of an infectious agent through the placenta, during labor or delivery, or by breastfeeding.

Table 25.1: Specific causes of some fetal and neonatal infections

Intrauterine	Intrapartum	Neonatal

• **Transplacental**
  – Viruses: Varicella zoster, coxsackie, human parvovirus B19, rubella, cytomegalovirus, HIV
  – Bacteria: Listeria, syphilis, borrelia Protozoa: Toxoplasmosis, malaria
• **Ascending infection**
  – Bacteria: Group B *streptococcus*, coliforms
  – Viruses: HSV
	• **Maternal exposure**
	  – Bacteria: Gonorrhea, chlamydia, group B *streptococcus*, tuberculosis, mycoplasmas
	  – Viruses: HSV, HPV, HIV, hepatitis B, hepatitis C
	• **External contamination**
	  – Bacteria: *Staphylococcus*, coliforms
	  – Viruses: HSV, varicella zoster
		Human transmission: *Staphylococcus*, HSV
		Respirators and catheters: *Staphylococcus*, coliforms

(HIV: Human immunodeficiency virus; HPV: Human papillomavirus; HSV: Herpes simplex virus.)

CHICKENPOX (VARICELLA ZOSTER)

- Chickenpox is caused by varicella zoster virus.
- Varicella virus is usually transmitted by the respiratory route.
- It can also be transmitted from pregnant women to their fetuses by the hematogenous transplacental route.
- Incubation period is 11 days
- Most common cause of maternal mortality in chickenpox is pneumonia.
- One of the risk factors for VZV pneumonia is smoking.
- Maternal varicella infection is usually diagnosed clinically. NAAT is also very sensitive.
- DOC for the treatment of pregnant female with chickenpox is Acyclovir. It should be used with caution before 20 weeks
- Acyclovir is initiated within 24 hours at the onset of rash, if the period of amenorrhea is more than 20 weeks gestation.
- There is no increased risk of abortion if chickenpox occurs in first trimester.
- Pregnant females who are exposed to patients of chickenpox should be given varicella immunoglobulin within 96 hours of exposure as prophylaxis but can be given up till 10 days after contact.

> **Remember:** VZ vaccine is not recommended for pregnant women as it is a live attenuated vaccine and should not be given to women who may become pregnant during the month following each vaccine dose. If VZ vaccine is given postpartum, breastfeeding is not contraindicated.

Varicella Infection in Pregnancy

- If varicella infection occurs in a pregnant female during first half of pregnancy (m/c time of transmission—13 to 20 weeks), it can result in **congenital varicella syndrome** in the fetus. A detailed USG is done at 5 weeks after infection or at 18-20 weeks.
- Amniocentesis is not routinely used in the diagnosis as risk of congenital varicella syndrome is low even if amniotic fluid is positive for VZV DNA (Amniocentesis has a strong negative predictive value but a poor positive predictive value).
- Congenital varicella syndrome is characterized by chorioretinitis, micro-ophthalmia, cerebral cortical atrophy, IUGR, hydronephrosis and skin or bone defects.
- Congenital varicella syndrome is an indication for doing MTP.
- Congenital defect rarely occurs if varicella infection occurs after 20 weeks.

- The terminology 'varicella embryopathy' is not used these days.
- **Neonatal varicella** is characterized by pneumonitis, hepatitis and DIC.
- The severity of neonatal infection is inversely related to the concentration of maternal antibodies present in the newborn circulation. Mother starts producing and transferring antibodies approximately 5 days after the onset of her disease. Thus babies born 5 days or more from the beginning of maternal disease will be protected.

—Fernando Arias 3/e, p 156

- Hence if there is no fetal or maternal risk in concerning the pregnancy delivery should be delayed for at least 7 days after the onset of rash, to allow time for maternal seroconversion and passive transfer of antibodies to fetus.
- Perinatal varicella exposure just before or during delivery poses a serious threat to newborns and so Varicella Ig should be given to all neonates of born to mothers who have clinical evidence of varicella 5 days before and upto 2 days after delivery.
- The use of VZIG decreases the chances of neonatal varicella and also modifies the clinical course but it does not always prevent severe or fatal varicella. Expectant treatment with close observation, followed by prompt initiation of antiviral therapy on suspicion of neonatal varicella is recommended.
- Antiviral treatment (acyclovir) is given to neonates only if they develop neonatal varicella syndrome.
- Vaccine is not secreted in breast milk. So, postpartum vaccination should not be delayed because of breastfeeding.
- Females with chickenpox can breastfeed their babies.

INFLUENZA

- Influenza viruses (RNA) are enveloped.
- Hemagglutinin (H) and neuraminidase (N) are present on the surface. Influenza strains are named according to their genus, species and H and N subtypes.
- The course of pregnancy remains unaffected unless the infection is severe.
- **Effects on pregnancy due to H1-N1 infection:** miscarriage, preterm labor, PROM, pneumonia, ARDS, renal failure, DIC and death. Severity of illness is high in pregnancy.
- There is no evidence of its teratogenic effect even if it is contracted in the first trimester. However, outbreak of Asian influenza showed increased incidence of congenital malformation (anencephaly) when the infection occurred in the first trimester.

- **Influenza (inactivated) vaccine is safe in pregnancy and also with breastfeeding.**
- **Diagnosis:** Rapid influenza diagnostic tests (RIDTs) are immunoassays, used for detection of viral RNA by RT-PCR.
- **Management:** Treatment is supportive care.
- During influenza season, all pregnant women should be given the inactivated vaccine (IM).

MEASLES

- The virus (RNA) is not teratogenic.
- However, high fever may lead to miscarriage, IUGR, microcephaly, oligohydramnios, stillbirth or premature delivery.
- Non-immunized women coming in contact with measles may be protected by intramuscular injection of immune serum globulin (5 mL) within 6 days of exposure.
- Mortality is high when complications like pneumonia and encephalitis develop.
- Diagnosis is made by assay of IgM and detection of viral RNA (RT-PCR).
- **Management** is supportive care. Antibiotics are given to prevent secondary bacterial infections.
- Ribavirin may be given for viral pneumonia.
- **Active vaccination (live attenuated) should not be given in pregnancy.**

RUBELLA (GERMAN MEASLES)

- Rubella is caused by an RNA virus.
- Transmission is by droplet infection.
- It is the most severe congenital infection.[Q]
- Maternal rubella infection is manifested by rash, malaise, fever, lymphadenopathy and polyarthritis
- If a pregnant woman is infected with rubella, there is a high risk of fetal affection due to transplacental transmission.
- Fetal transmission of Rubella can occur upto 20 weeks.
- Congenital Rubella syndrome:

Gestational age	Risk of transmission
1-12 weeks	80–85%
12-16 weeks	50%
16-20 weeks	25%

- The risk of fetal transmission of rubella is negligible infection occurs after the second trimester.
- With late second trimester and third trimester infection, malformations are uncommon, but mental retardation and hearing loss and IUGR can occur.[Q]

Congenital Rubella Syndrome

- It affects all the organs.
- Most common manifestation is mental retardation. Other manifestations are:
  - Sensorineural deafness
  - Eye effects: Cataract, Glaucoma
  - Congenital heart disease: PDA (Patent Ductus Arteriosus) and pulmonary artery stenosis
  - CNS defects like microcephaly, developmental delay and mental retardation
  - Thrombocytopenia
  - Hepatosplenomegaly

Extended Rubella Syndrome

It is delayed disease comprising of progressive panencephalitis, hearing loss and type 1 diabetes developing in the second or third decade of life in the neonate with rubella.

- Infants with congenital rubella syndrome may shed the virus for months and remain infective to other infants and adults and, hence, may require isolation.

  Perinatal Effects: Miscarriage, intrauterine or neonatal death. Stillbirth and congenital rubella syndrome.

Diagnosis

Maternal Diagnosis

- If there is suspicion of exposure to rubella, both maternal IgG and maternal IgM are done within seven to ten days of exposure and repeated after 3 weeks.
- If IgM is negative and IgG levels do not rise in both samples: No acute infection.
- If IgM is negative & IgG levels rise: It means infection may have occurred but there is a reduced risk of congenital rubella.
- If IgM is positive in any of the samples, it indicates acute rubella infection and is indication to do MTP.
- **Avidity test** is done to know whether infection is of recent ov late onset. Low avidity indicates recent infection lasts 2 months & high avidity indicates past infection.

Fetal Diagnosis

- Test for confirming fetal infection is PCR.
  - Prenatal diagnosis of rubella virus infection using PCR can be done from chorionic villi, fetal blood and amniotic samples.

Management

If a pregnant woman gets primary infection in the first and early second trimester, MTP is the best management.

Prevention

- Vaccines available to prevent rubella—MMR vaccine and Rubella vaccine.
- The rubella vaccine should be offered to all women of childbearing age.
- It can also be given at adolescence.
- Vaccination should not be given to pregnant women and pregnancy is best avoided for one month after the vaccination.

 Note: The American Academy of pediatrics has changed its recommendation from three months to one month now.
- If inadvertently the vaccine was given to a pregnant woman, then no need to terminate pregnancy as congenital rubella syndrome has never been described after vaccination.
  ... Williams Obs. 23/e, p 1215, Fernando Arias 4/e pg60

CYTOMEGALOVIRUS (CMV)

- It is the commonest cause of fetal and perinatal infection,[Q] but is asymptomatic in 90% of affected newborns.
- Material Infection is usually asymptomatic, the mother is generally unaware of being infected with CMV. A small portion of patients may experience mononucleosis-like symptoms like malaise, fever, generalized lymphadenopathy and hepatosplenomegaly.
- Routine screening for CMV during pregnancy is not recommended.
  - Being a herpes virus, latent infection and reactivation can occur especially in pregnancy.
  - Fetal infection can occur when mother is affected primarily or if reactivation of infection occurs in pregnancy and so previous infection does not prevent congenital infection. CMV infection 3 months before conception carries a risk of 9% transmission.
  - Neonate infection can occur at the time of delivery or during breastfeeding.
  - Pregnancy does not increase the risk or severity of maternal CMV infection.
  - Primary maternal CMV infection is trasmitted to fetus in 40% cases whereas recurrent or reactivated maternal infection infects fetus in 0.5-1% cases.

Manifestation of congenital CMV infection: CMV is the M/C infective cause of congenital brain abnormalities.

- Stillbirth   – IUGR
- Microcephaly   – Hepatosplenomegaly
- Choroidoretinitis   – Icterus
- Deafness   – Mental retardation
- Hemolytic anemia
- Intracranial calcifications (Distributed around periventricular zone, to be distinguished from toxoplasma in which calcification is scattered throughout the brain)
- Thrombocytopenia with petechiae and purpura
- Pneumonitis

  Note: CMV never leads to heart defects in the fetus.

  Late onset sequelae: Hearing loss, neurological deficit, chorioretinitis, psychomotor retardation and/or learning disabilities.

 Note: CMV is the main cause of SNHL during childhood.

Diagnosis

1. Maternal
- Routine screening of all the pregnant women for CMV is not cost-effective.
- Test: Detection of CMV–IgM antibody.
- **Best Test: Avidity test**—Avidity refers to the strength with which an antibody bends to antigen. In recent infection avidity is low and in past or chronic infection avidity is high.
- Women with positive anti CMV IgM antibodies and low avidity are ones how are at increased risk of transmitting infection to fetus.

2. Fetal
- CMV PCR of amniotic fluid is considered **as the gold standard for diagnosis** of fetal infections. Sensitivity of this test is highest when it is performed at least 6 weeks after maternal infection or after 20 weeks gestation.

Management

- The management of pregnant women with primary or recurrent CMV is symptomatic treatment.
- Passive to immunization with CMV-specific hyperimmune globulin lowers the risk of congenital CMV infection when given to pregnant women with primary disease.
- Till date there is no vaccine available for CMV.
- If fetus is found to be affected the pregnant female has two options—either she can continue her pregnancy because most of the infected fetuses (90%) develop normally or she can go for MTP.

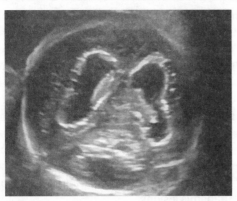

Fig. 25.1: Coronal view of cranial sonogram from a neonate with congenital cytomegalovirus infection showing multiple periventricular calcifications.

HERPES INFECTION

Herpes Simplex Virus in Pregnancy (Table 25.2)

Maternal HSV

- Maternal HSV infection can lead to varied outcomes, depending on whether the infection is a primary episode or it is a recurrent case. Therefore, first test done when a female comes with hSV is electron microscopy or PCR to identify the organism and type specific hSV antibody.
- If the infection is a recurrent one, the woman will have antibodies of the same type as the values isolated from genital swabs. If antibodies are absent, the infection is a primary one.

Table 25.2: Herpes infection

Type	Description	Manifestation in mother	Implication on pregnancy	Management
Primary infection	When an individual encounters either HSV 1 or 2 for first time and has no prior exposure, i.e. no antibodies present	U/L or B/L vesicular lesion with erythematous base located on sacral dermatomes These often become pustules and then ulcers (painful, multiple, shallow)	• Risk for neonatal infection is greatest when primary infection occurs in third trimester • If infection is acquired in first trimester. HSV does not lead to abortion • It can lead to prematurity, LBW and stillbirth.	Treatment with acyclovir (200 mg 5 times a day, for 5 days) and to restart daily from 36 weeks uptil delivery **Mode of delivery:** If a female acquires primary infection in last 6 weeks pregnancy, caesarean section. Is done in all cases before the rupture of membranes. (As risk of neonatal transmission is very high–41%)
Recurrent herpes infection			Antibodies IgG are present in mother. The maternal IgG antibodies are transferred to fetus, transplacental. Hence it is uncommon for fetus to develop infection in recurrent cases. However, if genital HSV lesion is present at the time of vaginal birth, risk of neonatal infection is less than 5%.	No treatment with acyclovir needed prior to 36 weeks, unless infection is severe Acyclovir–400 mg TDS to be taken from 36 weeks till delivery Cesarean is recommended only if genital ulcers are present or prodromal symptoms are present at the time of delivery. However, since the risk of neonatal infection is <5% with vaginal delivery also. Therefore, vaginal delivery can also be done. The choice depends on the patient.

TOXOPLASMOSIS

- Caused by *T. gondii* which is an obligate intracellular protozoan parasite.
- Cat is the definitive host.[Q]
- Maternal infection is acquired by eating undercooked meat.
- Primary infection causes immunity which is life-long and usually prevents reinfection, i.e. if a female has toxoplasma IgG antibody before pregnancy, there is no risk for a congenitally infected fetus.

Congenital Transmission

- The risk of transmission increases with the period of gestation, i.e. maximum chances of infection are during 3rd trimester.
- Severity of infection decreases with gestational age, i.e. most severe infection occurs when toxoplasma is transmitted in the first trimester.
- In acute maternal toxoplasma infection, patients are usually asymptomatic (in 80–90% cases).

- Some patients may present with posterior cervical lymphadenopathy (lymph nodes are nontender, discrete and firm), fever, fatigue, lassitude and maculopapular rash.
- DOC for Toxoplasma during pregnancy is spiramycin (1 g every 8 hours) i.e. 3 g/day.
- Spiramycin reduces the risk of congenital infection during pregnancy and should be continued (25 mg), till delivery.
- If fetal infection is confirmed, 3 weeks of spiramycin are alternated with, 3 weeks of pyrimethamine combination, and continued till delivery. This is because spiramycin can prevent fetal infection but cannot treat the infection if it is present. Pyrimethamine is not given in 1st trimester.
- Triad of congenital toxoplasmosis

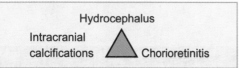

- Routine maternal screening for Toxoplasma is not done.
- If maternal infection is confirmed, by serology and avidity testing, then to confirm fetal infection, following tests are done:
  a. Gold standard: Isolation of toxoplasma in the amniotic fluid by PCR.
  b. Ultrasonography to detect fetal anomalies. If the fetus is infected and hydrocephalus is present, counselling for termination is to be done.
- Presence of IgM antibody in the neonate indicates congenital infection.
- Treatment with pyrimethamine should be continued in these babies till 1 year of age.

Note: A nonpregnant woman diagnosed with acute toxoplasma should avoid pregnancy for six months.

VARICELLA-ZOSTER VIRUS (CHICKEN POX IN PREGNANCY)

Maternal Infection

- Varicella-zoster virus (VZV) is a double-stranded DNA herpesvirus acquired predominately during childhood, and 90 percent of adults have serological evidence of immunity.
- Primary infection—*varicella or chickenpox*—is transmitted by direct contact with an infected individual, although respiratory transmission has been reported. The incubation period is 10 to 21 days, and a nonimmune woman has a 60- to 95–percent risk of becoming infected after exposure.

- Primary varicella presents with a 1- to 2-day flulike prodrome, which is followed by pruritic vesicular lesions that crust after 3 to 7 days. Infection tends to be more severe in adults. Affected patients are then contagious from 1 day before the onset of the rash until the lesions become crusted.
- Mortality is predominately due to VZV pneumonia, which is thought to be more severe during adulthood and particularly in pregnancy. Only 2 to 5 percent of infected pregnant women develop pneumonitis. Risk factors for VZV pneumonia include smoking and having more than 100 cutaneous lesions.

If primary varicella is reactivated years later, it causes *herpes zoster* or *shingles*. This presents as a unilateral dermatomal vesicular eruption associated with severe pain. Zoster does not appear to be more frequent or severe in pregnant women. Congenital varicella syndrome rarely develops in cases of maternal herpes zoster. Zoster is contagious if blisters are broken, although less so than with primary varicella.

Fetal and Neonatal Infection

- In women with varicella during the first half of pregnancy, the fetus may develop *congenital varicella syndrome*. Some features include chorioretinitis, microphthalmia, cerebral cortical atrophy, growth restriction, hydronephrosis, limb hypoplasia, and cicatricial skin lesions. When maternal infection developed before 13 weeks, only two of 472 pregnancies—0.4 percent —had neonates with congenital varicella syndrome. The highest risk was between 13 and 20 weeks. After 20 weeks gestation, the researchers found no clinical evidence of congenital infection.
- If the fetus or neonate is exposed to active infection just before or during delivery, and therefore before maternal antibody has been formed, the newborn faces a serious threat. Attack rates range from 25 to 50 percent, and mortality rates approach 30 percent. In some instances, neonates develop disseminated visceral and CNS disease, which is commonly fatal. For this reason, *Varicella-zoster immune globulin* (VZIG) should be administered to neonates born to mothers who have clinical evidence of varicella 5 days before and up to 2 days after delivery.

Diagnosis

Maternal varicella is usually diagnosed clinically. Infection may be confirmed by NAAT of vesicular fluid, which is very sensitive.

Management

Maternal Viral Exposure:

- Exposed gravidas with a negative history for chickenpox should undrgo VZY serological testing. At least 70 percent of these women will be seropositive, and thus immune. Exposed pregnant women who are susceptible (seronegative) should be given varicella-zoster immune globulin (VariZIG). Although best given within 96 hours of exposure, its use is approved for up to 10 day to prevent or attenuate varicella infection (Centers for Disease Control and Prevention, 2012, 2013d). In women with known history of varicella, VariZIG is not indicated.

Maternal Infection: *Any patient diagnosed with primary varicella infection or herpes zoster should be isolated from pregnant women.*

- Most women require only supportive care, but those who require intravenous (IV) fluids and especially those with pneumonia are hospitalized. IV acyclovir therapy is given to women requiring hospitalization—500 mg/m² or 10 to 15 mg/kg every 8 hours.

Vaccination: An attenuated live-virus vaccine is recommended for nonpregnant adolescents and adults with no history of varicella. Two doses of *Varivax* are given 4 to 8 weeks apart, and the seroconversion rate is 98 percent.

- *The vaccine is not recommended for pregnant women or for those who may become pregnant within a month following each vaccine dose.*
- The attenuated vaccine virus is not secreted in breast milk. thus, postpartum vaccination should not be delayed because of breastfeeding (American College of Obstetricians and Gynecologists, 2016c).

 Key Concept

Infections in Pregnancy
- Most common—CMV
- Most teratogenic—Rubella
- M/C time for rubella transmission to fetus—1st trimester (maxmimum—1 to 4 weeks), absent transmission—beyond 20 weeks.
- In Rubella—M/C single defect which occurs is—Sensorineural hearing loss.
- Heart defects seen in Rubella—Patent ductus arteriosus and Pulmonary artery stenosis.
- After rubella vaccine, pregnancy is contraindicated for 1 month.
- CMV—Transmission can occur in any trimester.
- Most severe infection occurs if transmission occurs in 2nd trimester.
- CMV transmission can occur during vaginal delivery and breastfeeding also.
- Primary infection—leads to 40% transmission.
- Recurrent infection—leads to 0.2%-2% transmission.
- **CMV Never Leads to Heart Defects in Fetus.**
- M/C time for toxoplasma infection—3rd trimester
- Fetus is affected maximum/most severely if fetal infection occurs in 1st trimester.
- Triad of toxoplasma infection—intracerebral calcification, chorioretinitis and hydrocephalus.
- Treatment—Spiramycin (prevents fetal transmission but it cannot treat fetal infection if it is present).
- Spiramycin + pyrimethamine and sulfonamide combination is given to treat fetal infection and prevent further transmission.

Drugs of Choice

Infection	DOC in Pregnancy
Bacterial vaginosis	Metronidazole to patient only 1st trimester—clindamycin
Pneumocystis carinii	Sulphamethozole-trimethoprim
Typhoid	Third gen cephalosporins/azithromycin
Syphilis <1 year >1 year	Benzathine penicillin 2.4 million UIM sigle dose Benzathine penicillin 2.4 million UIM weekly x 3 doses
Gonorrhea	Inj. Ceftriaxone 125 mg IM single dose or Tab cefixime 400 mg single dose or Inj. Spectinomycin 2 g i.m. single dose
Chlamydia	Azithromycin single dose or Amoxicillin 500 mg TDS × 7 days, 2nd choice—Erythromycin
Group B streptococci	Penicillin, 2nd best—Ampicillin. In patients who are penicillin-resistant—Cefazolin is the
Malaria—Prophylaxis	Chloroquine
Treatment	Chloroquine. For radical cure premaquine is advised after delivery
	In resistant cases (mostly d/t *P. falciparum*)—Quinine + clindamycin or mefloquine
Appendicitis	Immediate appendicectomy
Red degeneration	Conservative management (no termination of pregnancy and no myomectomy)

New Pattern Questions

N1. A woman develops chickenpox at a period of gestation of 8 weeks.

What is the best method to exclude foetal varicella syndrome?

a. Perform amniocentesis at 15 weeks and test for VZV DNA in the amniotic fluid

b. Perform an ultrasound scan at 20 weeks

c. Perform an ultrasound scan immediately

d. Perform chorionic villous sampling and test for VZV DNA

N2. A woman is exposed to chickenpox at a period of amenorrhea of 14 weeks. She does not give a history of having had the disease previously.

What is the next step in the management?

a. Administer the varicella vaccine as soon as possible after exposure

b. Administer varicella zoster immunoglobulin and varicella vaccine as soon as possible after exposure

c. Administer varicella zoster immunoglobulin as soon as possible after exposure

d. Test the maternal blood for antibodies against varicella zoster virus

N3. A woman is exposed to chickenpox at 12 weeks pregnancy weeks. She does not give a history of having had the disease previously.

What is the best management option if she does not have antibodies against varicella zoster virus?

a. Give varicella zoster vaccine as soon as possible after exposure

b. Administer varicella zoster immunoglobulin as soon as possible after exposure

c. Termination of pregnancy

d. Treatment with oral acyclovir if infection occurs

N4. A woman develops chickenpox at 39 weeks. She has a single fetus in the cephalic presentation. She has no other pregnancy complications.

What is the best method to prevent neonatal infection?

a. Continue the pregnancy for at least one week.

b. Give varicella zoster vaccine to the neonate soon after birth

c. Give VZIG to the neonate soon after birth

d. Induce labor immediately

N5. A woman who has developed chickenpox 2 days ago is admitted in labor.

What is the best method to prevent infection in the neonate?

a. Administer varicella zoster immunoglobulin (VZIG) to the neonate soon after birth

b. Administer varicella zoster vaccine to the neonate

c. Perform a cesarean section immediately

d. Prevent breastfeeding

N6. A 26-year-old woman is 38 weeks pregnant and presents to the labour room in active labour. She had fever for the past 2 days. Last night, she broke out in an itchy rash that has spread over her arms and torso. She is a teacher by profession and 2 weeks earlier, one of the children in her class was diagnosed with chickenpox. She didn't have chickenpox as a child.

The patient is worried: Which of the following is the best advice to give her?

a. Nothing needs to be done, chickenpox in children is mild and self-limiting

b. The chance of transmitting the virus of the baby is low and so we treat if symptoms develop

c. Baby must be treated immediately after birth as chickenpox is serious in newborns

d. Varicella virus is teratogenic and baby might have mild birth defects

N7. A 34-year-old primigravida at 11 weeks gestation presents to her obstetrics clinic with chief complaint of exposure to a rash. Her husband is HIV+ve and has broken out on a rash in his left buttock which consists of a grouped vesicles on a maculopapular base 4 days back. She has got her HIV testing done which is negative. Her P/R is 86/min, B/P = 100/60 mm of Hg, resp rate 10/min and temp = 98.7F. FHS is heard via Doppler.

What is the next step in the management?

a. Administer high-dose acyclovir to the infant at birth

b. Administer high-dose acyclovir to the patient now

c. Administer varicella immunoglobulin to the infant at birth

d. Administer varicella immunoglobulin to the patient

N8. A 37-year-old G2P1 woman at 38 weeks' gestation presents to the obstetrics clinic for a prenatal visit. The patient had difficulty becoming pregnant but was successful after using in vitro fertilization. She has a history of recurrent herpes outbreaks, and her first pregnancy was complicated by failure to progress, which resulted in a cesarean birth. Routine rectovaginal culture at 36 weeks was positive for Group B streptococci.

Which of the following would be an absolute indication for delivering the child by LSCS?

a. Current symptoms of genital pain and tingling

b. H/O previous cesarean section

c. IVF

d. Maternal colonization with group B streptococci

N9. A 25-year-old G1P0 female at 25 weeks of gestation comes to you for antenatal check-up. She has had an uncomplicated pregnancy but has 5 years of history of Genital Herpes infection. She is usually asymptomatic and has had 3 flares in the past 5 years. She is concerned about exposing her unborn child to infection. What is the most appropriate counsel to offer to this patient?
   a. Administer one dose of acyclovir if she has active genital herpes at the time of delivery
   b. Administer prophylaxis with acyclovir from now and uptil delivery whether she has active herpes or not
   c. Perform elective LSCS even if mother is asymptomatic at the time of delivery
   d. Perform elective LSCS only if mother has active herpes at the time of delivery

N10. A woman complains of discharge and soreness in the vulval region at 36 weeks of pregnancy. Examination reveals small discreet, tender ulcers in the labia majora, minora and perineum. She has not had a similar episode previously.
   a. Commence broad spectrum antibiotics and analgesics
   b. Commence oral acyclovir
   c. Identify the infecting organism by viral culture and test for type-specific antibodies
   d. Perform a cesarean section

N11. A woman complains of discharge and soreness in the vulval region at a POA of 36 weeks. Examination reveals small discreet, tender ulcers in the labia majora, minora and perineum. She has not had a similar episode previously. On viral culture and serological testing she did not have antibodies against the infecting strain.

   What is the best treatment option?
   a. Perform a cesarean section immediately
   b. Treat with oral acyclovir and induced labour as soon as the ulcers heal
   c. Treat with oral acyclovir and await spontaneous onset of labour
   d. Treat with oral acyclovir and perform an elective cesarean section at 38 weeks

GROUP B STREPTOCOCCAL INFECTION

N12. A 32-year-old G2P1 woman at 34 weeks' gestation presents to the labor and delivery floor with the chief complaint of regular contractions, bloody show, and a gush of fluids. A 2.3 kg (5 lb 1 oz) boy is delivered by spontaneous vaginal delivery without further complication 1 hour after presentation. Twenty-four hours later, the infant has developed irritability, fever, and respiratory distress. He is diagnosed with sepsis secondary to pneumonia. The mother has no complaints other than anxiety regarding the condition of her child. She denies rigors, chills, sweats, nausea, or vomiting. The mother's pulse is 60/min, blood pressure is 125/80 mm Hg, and temperature is 37°C (98.6°F). Physical examination reveals lungs that are clear to auscultation bilaterally, and no murmurs, rubs, or gallops are present on cardiac examination. The suprapubic region is not tender to palpation. Vaginal and cervical examination reveals no significant tears or bleeds.

   Which prenatal test would have provided the most useful information in preventing this condition:
   a. Cervical chlamydia culture
   b. Cervical gonorrhea culture
   c. ELISA for HIV
   d. Rectovaginal group B streptococcal culture

N13. A 19-year-old G2P1 woman at 9 weeks' gestation presents to the obstetrics and gynecology clinic for her second prenatal visit. She reports no complaints other than occasional nausea. She had her first child by spontaneous vaginal delivery without complications. She is taking no medications and denies ethanol, tobacco, or current drug use. While she does admit to a history of intravenous drug abuse, she denies using them since the birth of her first child. Over the past several months, she has had multiple sexual partners and does not use contraception. On physical examination, she is in no acute distress. Lungs are clear to auscultation bilaterally. Her heart has a regular rate and rhythm, with no murmurs, rubs, or gallops. She is informed that she will need the routine prenatal tests, including an HIV test. The physician informs her of the risks and benefits of the HIV test:

   What else should the physician inform the patient before performing the test?
   a. Despite the potential for fetal infection, she may opt out from the test
   b. Early retroviral therapy will absolutely decrease the chances of transmitting infection to the baby.
   c. CDC recommends screening only for patients with high risk factors
   d. Risk of the test includes potential for fetal loss

N14. Least rate of HIV transmission is seen in:
   a. Forceps delivery
   b. ARM
   c. Vacuum delivery
   d. Cesarean section

N15. A woman is exposed to rubella infection at a period of amenorrhea of 10 weeks.

   She has been vaccinated against rubella at the age of 15 years and had IgG antibodies against rubella on routine testing at 6 weeks.

   What is the most appropriate management?
   a. Administer acyclovir if the mother develops rubella
   b. Administer immunoglobulin to the mother
   c. Advice termination of pregnancy if she contacts rubella
   d. Reassure that she is unlikely to develop rubella

N16. A woman attends the antenatal clinic with a history of exposure to rubella infection at a period of amenorrhea of 10 weeks. Her immune status is not known.

What is the next step in the management?
a. Administer acyclovir if the mother develops symptoms of rubella
b. Administer immunoglobulin to the mother
c. Advice termination of pregnancy if she contacts rubella
d. Test maternal serum for rubella-specific IgG and IgM antibodies immediately and after 3 weeks

N17. Infections transmitted to the baby at delivery are all except:
a. Toxoplasmosis
b. Gonococcus
c. Herpes simplex type II
d. Hepatitis B

N18. Large placenta is seen in all of the following except:
a. IUGR
b. Syphilis
c. CMV
d. Rubella

N19. Cesarean section is preferred in:
a. Toxoplasmosis
b. Herpes
c. CMV
d. Varicella zoster virus

N20. DOC for intermittent preventive therapy during pregnancy in malaria is:
a. Proguanil
b. Pyrimethamine-dapsone
c. Sulfadoxine-pyrimethamine
d. Quinine

N21. DOC for pregnant females travelling to areas endemic to chloroquine resistant P-falciparum:
a. Primaquine
b. Doxycycline
c. Amodiaquine
d. Mefloquine

N22. Which of the following is a known effect of dengue to fetuses, if mother is affected:
a. Abortion
b. Teratogenicity
c. IUGR
d. None of the above

N23. DOC for symptomatic amebiasis during pregnancy:
a. No treatment
b. Metronidazole
c. Diloxanide furoate
d. Di-iodohydroxyquin

Previous Year Questions

TORCH INFECTIONS

1. Congenital infection in fetus with minimal teratogenic risk is: [AI 08]
   a. HIV
   b. Rubella
   c. Varicella
   d. CMV

2. Most common cause of intrauterine infection:
   a. Rubella
   b. Toxoplasma [AI 03]
   c. Hepatitis
   d. Cytomegalovirus

3. Congenital anomalies are most severe in: [AI 99]
   a. Rubella infection
   b. Mumps
   c. CMV
   d. Toxoplasma

4. Not implicated in congenital transmission is:
   a. Hepatitis A [UP 96]
   b. Toxoplasmosis
   c. Herpes
   d. Syphilis

5. Which of the following perinatal infections has the highest risk of fetal infection in the first trimester?
   a. Hepatitis B virus [AI 04]
   b. Syphilis
   c. Toxoplasmosis
   d. Rubella

6. Highest rate of transmission of toxoplasmosis during pregnancy is seen in: [AI 99]
   a. 1st trimester
   b. 2nd trimester
   c. 3rd trimester
   d. Puerperium

7. A pregnant lady had no complaints but mild cervical lymphadenopathy in first trimester. She was prescribed spiramycin but she was non-compliant. Baby was born with hydrocephalus and intracerebral calcification. Which of these is the likely cause? [AIIMS May 2010]
   a. Toxoplasmosis
   b. CMV
   c. Cryptococcus
   d. Rubella

8. Pregnant woman in 1st trimester is given spiramycin that she does not stick to. Baby born with hydro-cephalus infection was by: [AI 09]
   a. HSV
   b. Treponema pallidum
   c. Toxoplasma
   d. CMV

9. A lady G2P1 with 10 wks pregnancy with one live child has ocular toxoplasmosis. The risk of present baby to get infected is: [AIIMS Nov 99]
   a. 50%
   b. 25%
   c. 100%
   d. Nil

10. During pregnancy, baby can be affected in utero in all *except*: [AIIMS Nov 99]
    a. Candida
    b. Syphilis
    c. Toxoplasmosis
    d. Polio

11. Which of the following abnormalities is commonly seen in a fetus with congenital CMV infection: [AIIMS June 99]
    a. Colitis
    b. Myocarditis
    c. Blood dyscrasias
    d. Pulmonary cyst

12. Risk of transmittig LMV to fetus will be maximum in case mother has:
    a. Positive IgM antibodies; Low avidity
    b. Positive IgM antibodies; High avidity
    c. Positive IgG antibodies; Low avidity
    d. Positive IgM antibodies; High avidity

13. The drug of choice in treatment of typhoid fever in pregnancy is: [AIIMS Nov 05]
    a. Ampicillin
    b. Chloramphenicol
    c. Ciprofloxacin
    d. Ceftriaxone

14. A female presents with leaking and meconium-stained liquior at 32 weeks. She is infected with: [AI 10]
    a. CMV
    b. Listeria
    c. True toxoplasma
    d. Herpes

15. Regarding listerosis in pregnancy: [AI 12]
    a. Mode of transmission of infection is sexual
    b. Is associated with meningoencephalitis of the newborn
    c. May present with skin rash at birth
    d. In labour, liquor is meconium-stained

CHICKENPOX

16. A pregnant lady develops chickenpox. During which part of her pregnancy will it lead to highest chance of neonatal infection: [AIIMS May 02]
    a. Last 5 days
    b. 12-16 weeks
    c. 8-12 weeks
    d. 16-20 weeks

17. A pregnant lady acquires chickenpox 3 days prior to delivery. She delivers by normal vaginal route. Which of the following statements is true? [AIIMS Nov 08, AIIMS May 2011]
    a. Both mother and baby are safe
    b. Give antiviral treatment to mother before delivery
    c. Give antiviral treatment to baby
    d. Baby will develop neonatal varicella syndrome

HERPES SIMPLEX VIRUS

18. Transmission of herpes is maximum in: [AIIMS Nov 99]
    a. 2nd trimester
    b. 3rd trimester
    c. During parturition
    d. 1st trimester

SYPHILIS

19. Premature baby of 34 weeks was delivered. Baby had bullous lesion on the body. X-ray shows periostitis. What is the next investigation:
    a. VDRL for mother and baby [AIIMS]
    b. ELISA for HIV
    c. PCR for TB
    d. Hepatitis surface antigen for mother

20. DOC for syphilis in pregnancy: [AIPG 2012]
    a. Erythromycin
    b. Azithromycin
    c. Penicillin
    d. Cephalosporin/ceftriaxone

HIV IN PREGNANCY

21. During pregnancy, HIV transmission occurs mostly during: [AIIMS Nov 06]
    a. 1st trimester
    b. 2nd trimester
    c. 3rd trimester
    d. During labour

22. Most common cause of HIV infection in infant is: [PGI June 97]
    a. Perinatal transmission
    b. Breast milk
    c. Transplacement
    d. Umbilical cord sepsis

23. Risk of vertical transmission of HIV without intervention and without breastfeeding is: [AIIMS Nov 2013]
    a. 15 to 30%
    b. 5 to 10%
    c. 10 to 15%
    d. 2 to 5%

24. Which drug is given to prevent HIV transmission from mother to child: [AIIMS Nov 06, Nov 2011]
    a. Nevirapine
    b. Lamivudine
    c. Stavudine
    d. Abacavir

25. Drugs supplied by NACO for prevention of mother-to-child transmission: [PGI Dec 08]
    a. Nevirapine
    b. Zidovudine
    c. Nevirapine + Zidovudine
    d. Nevirapine + Zidovudine + 3TC

26. For an HIV +ve pregnant woman, true is: [PGI Dec 09]
    a. CS elective will decrease transmission to baby
    b. If she hasn't received prophylaxis, leave her alone for vaginal delivery
    c. Vaginal delivery will decrease risk for baby
    d. Start ART and continue throughout pregnancy, ART is safe for gestation
    e. Baby doesn't need drugs

27. **Transmission of HIV from mother to child is prevented by all the following except:** [AIIMS Nov 08, May 2013]
    a. Oral zidovudine to mother at 3rd trimester along with oral zidovudine to infant for 6 weeks
    b. Vitamin A prophylaxis to mother
    c. Vaginal delivery
    d. Stopping breastfeed

28. **HIV positive primi near term, advice given is:**
    [PGI Dec 08]
    a. Treatment should be started before labour
    b. Avoid mixing of blood intrapartam
    c. Vaginal delivery preferred
    d. Ceserean section would be to decrease transmission of HIV to baby

29. **All can be used to lower mother-to-child HIV spread except:** [AI 10]
    a. Elective CS
    b. Omitting ergometrine
    c. ART
    d. Intrapartum nevirapine

30. **Regarding transmission of HIV to infant from infected HIV mother, which statement(s) is/are true:**
    [PGI May 2010]
    a. Start zidovudine during labour.
    b. 25% chance of vertical transmission
    c. Avoid breastfeeding
    d. Vaccinate infant with OPV and MMR
    e. Cesarean section causes less transmission

Answers with Explanations to New Pattern Questions

N1. Ans. is b, i.e. Perform an ultrasound scan at 20 weeks.

A detailed ultrasound examination carried out 5 weeks after infection, or at 16-20 weeks is the best method to exclude fetal varicella syndrome.

Amniocentesis is not routinely advised because the risk of congenital varicella syndrome is low, even when amniotic fluid is positive for VZV DNA because amniocentesis has a strong negative productive value than a positive predictive valve.

N2. Ans. is d, i.e. Test the maternal blood for antibodies against varicella zoster virus

If a pregnant woman is exposed to chickenpox, the first step is to test the maternal blood for IgG antibodies against VZ virus. If antibodies are present, the mother is immune. So, she will not develop the disease and does not need any further treatment.

N3. Ans. is b, i.e. Administer varicella zoster immunoglobulin as soon as possible after exposure.

The best management option is to prevent her from infection. Therefore, if the mother is found to be non-immune after testing for antibodies, varicella zoster immunology should be given as soon as possible after exposure. The vaccine cannot be given in pregnancy as it is a live attenuated vaccine. Termination of the pregnancy is not indicated because fetal varicella syndrome is not common. Acyclovir is used for treating infection.

N4. Ans. is a, i.e. Continue the pregnancy for at least one week

If delivery can be postponed for at least 7 days, the mother will develop antibodies and there will be transplacental transfer of antibodies to the neonate. The neonate will have passive immunity and will not develop the infection. Therefore, the best method to prevent neonatal infection is to continue the pregnancy for at least one week after the mother develops the rash. If delivery occurs within one week, the baby should be given VZIG soon after birth.

N5. Ans. is a, i.e. Administer varicella zoster immunoglobulin (VZIG) to the neonate soon after birth

Since the mother developed the infection two days before the delivery, there is no time for the mother to develop antibodies. Therefore, the neonate will be non-immune and is at risk of developing chickenpox. Neonatal infection is prevented by giving VZIG to the neonate soon after birth.

N6. Ans. is c, i.e. Baby must be treated immediately after birth as chickenpox is serious in newborns.

In the question, patient is 38 weeks pregnant, is in labour and has chickenpox for past 2 days. As discussed in previous question, chances of transmitting infection to fetus is maximum just before or after delivery.

Thus, option 'c' is correct and options 'a' and 'b' are incorrect.

Perinatal varicella exposure just before or during delivery poses a serious threat to newborns and so Varicella-Zoster Immunoglobulin (VZIG) should be given to neonates born to mothers who have clinical evidence of varicella 5 days before and upto 2 days after delivery.

Coming to option 'd' – Birth defects are seen with varicella only if it occurs before 20 weeks of pregnancy. This female has acquired the infection at 38 weeks, hence no chances of birth defect in the fetus.

N7. **Ans. is d, i.e. Administer varicella immunoglobulin to the patient.**
- DOC for treatment of pregnant mothers infected with chickenpox is intravenous or oral acyclovir
- The pregnant woman is exposed to chickenpox rash, she does not have chickenpox. So, obviously we will not treat her or her baby with acyclovir. Now since the female herself does not have chickenpox, so why to give VZIG to the infant, rather this female should be given prophylactic VZIG so that she does not acquire chickenpox.

Varicella prophylaxis: Exposed pregnant women who are susceptible should be given Varicella IG within 96 hours of exposure to prevent or attenuate varicella infection.

N8. **Ans. is a, i.e. Current symptoms of genital pain and tingling**

N9. **Ans. is d, i.e. Perform elective LSCS only if mother has active herpes at the time of delivery.**
- As discussed in the text: Recurrent Herpes infection management
- Acyclovir from 36 weeks of pregnancy to decrease viral load at the time of delivery
- Vaginal deliveries are preferred
- Elective LSCS is done only if prodromal symptoms are present or active genital herpes infection is present (Ans. N8)

- If no active breast lesions are present, patient can breastfeed.
- Now let's have a look at the options given in N9.
- **Option a:** Administer one dose of acyclovir if she has active genital herpes at the time of delivery—incorrect as acyclovir should be given from 36 weeks onwards.
- **Option b:** Administer prophylaxis with acyclovir from now and uptil delivery, whether she has active herpes or not—again incorrect because, as such, recurrent herpes does not need Acyclovir treatment. It should be given after 36 weeks uptil delivery to decrease usual load.
- **Option c:** Perform elective LSCS even if mother is asymptomatic at the time of delivery – again incorrect
- **Option d:** Perform elective LSCS only if mother has active herpes at the time of delivery – correct

N10. **Ans. is c, i.e. Identify the infecting organism by viral culture and test for type-specific antibodies**

Patient is having shallow is mall multiple tender ulcers. Hence most probably it is herpes

The next step in the management is to determine whether the infection is primary or secondary, as the fetal effects and hence the obstetric management differ in both. The infecting organism and the strain (there are at least 2 infecting strains is identified by electron microscopy and viral culture from swabs obtained from the lesions. The maternal serum is tested for antibodies against the infecting strain. If antibodies are absent, it is a primary infection.

N11. **Ans. is d, i.e. Treat with oral acyclovir and perform an elective cesarean section at 38 weeks**

This is a case of primary herpes because she does not have type-specific antibodies. The best management option is to deliver by cesarean section at 38 weeks, if primary herpes occurs in the third trimester, especially during the last 6 weeks, as there is no time for the mother to develop antibodies. It is not necessary to perform a cesarean section immediately as transplacental transmission does not occur. Treatment with acyclovir is indicated in primary herpes as it reduces the severity and the duration of the maternal disease.

N12. **Ans. is d, i.e. Rectovaginal group B streptococcal culture**

Neonatal sepsis

- Group B streptococci, Streptococcus agalactiae is a major cause of neonatal mortality and morbidity.
- Neonates present with respiratory distress, apnea, hypotension, i.e. the neonate in the question is having neonatal sepsis due to Group B Streptococci.
- **ACOG recommends universal culture screening for rectovaginal Group B streptococci at 35–37 weeks in all pregnant females.**
- Samples are taken from lower third of vagina and rectum as colonization of the birth canal occurs secondary to colonization of anorectal region.

In the question, patient had delivered at 34 weeks and so her screening for group B streptococci by rectovaginal culture was not done. In all such cases, where patient presents with preterm labour or term labour with unknown GBS status, a shot of penicillin should be given prophylactically to protect her against GBS infection.

Prophylaxis Against GBS

Intrapartum prophylaxis is indicated	Intrapartum prophylaxis is not indicated
• **Previous infant with invasive GBS disease**	• Previous pregnancy with positive GBS screening
• **GBS bacteriuria during present pregnancy**	• Planned cesarean delivery performed in absence of labor or membrane rupture (regardless of maternal GBS culture status)

• Positive GBS screening or culture during present pregnancy unless LSCS is planned
• Unknown GBS status with any of the following:
  – Delivery at <37 weeks
  – Amniotic membrane rupture >18 hrs
  – Intrapartum temperature >100.4°F
	• Negative GBS vaginal and rectal screening culture

Drugs Used in GBS Prophylaxis

Best drug	Penicillin
Second best drug	Ampicillin
Penicillin-allergic patients	At low risk for anaphylaxis—cefazolin
	At high risk—idamycin/erythromycin/vancomycin

Note: Mode of delivery – In pregnant patients with GBS infection
- If treatment is given – vaginal delivery
- If treatment has not been given – cesarean section

N13. **Ans. is a, i.e. Despite the potential for fetal infection, she may opt out from the test.**

Ref. Williams Obs. 23/e p 1248

- The CDC and ACOG (2008) has recommended prenatal screening for HIV using an "opt-out approach". This means that the woman is notified that HIV testing is included in a comprehensive set of antenatal tests, but that testing may be declined.
- Women are given information regarding HIV but are not required to sign a specific consent.
- Screening is performed using an ELISA test which has a sensitivity of > 99.5%.
- A positive test is confirmed with either a western blot or immunofluorescence assay (IIFA), both of which have high specificity.
- According to CDC, antibody can be detected in most patients within 1 month of infection and thus antibody serotesting may not exclude early infection.

N14. **Ans. is d, i.e. Cesarean section**

Vertical HIV transmission was shown to be reduced by about half when cesarean was compared with vaginal delivery.

Ref. Williams 24/e p1282

N15. Ans. is d, i.e. Reassure that she is unlikely to develop rubella

This patient can be reassured that she is unlikely to develop rubella infection because she has been previously immunized against rubella and has rubella-specific IgG antibodies.

N16. Ans. is d, i.e. Test maternal serum for rubella specific IgG and IgM antibodies immediately and after 3 weeks.

Patient's immune status is not known. The first step in the management is to test maternal serum for rubella-specific IgG and IgM antibodies immediately to determine the immune status and after 3 weeks to detect the occurrence of infection. Presence of rubella-specific IgG antibodies in the initial serum sample indicates immunity. Presence of IgM antibodies in the first or second samples indicates acute infection with a high risk of congenital rubella.

N17. Ans. is a, i.e. Toxoplasmosis *Ref. Fernando Arias 2/e, p 375, Dutta Obs. 7/e, p 297*

Option 'a'	**Toxoplasma – Congenital transmission.** *"Most fetal transmission appears to be transplacental and usually occurs before labour as evidenced by cord antibody titre."* —Fernando Arias 2/e, p 375
Option 'b'	**Gonococcus** *"The baby may be affected during labour while passing through the birth canal, resulting in ophthalmia neonatorum."* —Dutta Obs. 7/e, p 294
Option 'c'	**HSV II** *"The fetus becomes affected by virus shed from the cervix or lower genital tract during vaginal delivery".* —Dutta Obs. 7/e, p 300
Option 'd'	**Hepatitis B** *"Neonatal transmission mainly occurs at or around the time of the birth through mixing of maternal blood and genital secretion."* —Dutta Obs. 7/e, p 292

N18. Ans. is a, i.e. IUGR *Ref. Dutta Obs. 7/e, p 497; Williams Obs 23/e, p 627; Fernando Arias 3/e, p 95-96 for causes of NIHF*

Large placenta is seen in case of Hydrops fetalis:

Hydrops fetalis

• There are two varieties of hydrops

Immune hydrops	Nonimmune hydrops fetalis (NIHF)
• It is due to Rh isoimmunization	• It is due to conditions other than Rh isoimmunization
• It accounts for 1/3rd cases of hydrops fetalis	• It accounts for 2/3 cases of hydrops fetalis

Nonimmune hydrops:

• It can be caused by a number of conditions (Discussed in detail in chapter 18).

Infections causing NIHF:

• Of all the PRATSCHEC agents (parvovirus, rubella, AIDS, toxoplasma, syphilis, cytomegalovirus, herpes, echovirus, and coxsackievirus), only AIDS has not been reported in association with Non-Immune Hydrops Fetalis. Parvovirus B-19 is the most common viral infection associated with NIFH.

 Note: In IUGR: Placenta is small and not big.

Note: In IUGR: Placenta is small and not big.

N19. Ans. is b, i.e. Herpes *Ref. Dutta Obs. 7/e, p 301*

Genital hepes is due to HSV 2

Effects of herpes on pregnancy:

• If there is primary infection in last trimester there are chances of premature labor or IUGR.
• Transplacental infection is not usual.
• The fetus becomes affected by virus shed from the cerivx or lower genital tract during vaginal delivery
• The baby may be infected in utero from the contaminated liquor following rupture of membranes.
• Risk of fetal infection is high in primary genital HSV at term due to high virus shedding compared to a recurrent infection.

- Cesarean delivery is indicated in an active primary genital HSV infection where the membranes are intact or recently ruptured and in females with prodromal symptoms of herpes.
- Drug of choice for genital herpes is acyclovir[Q] (when virus culture is positive).
- Breastfeeding is allowed[Q] provided mother avoids contact between her lesions, her hands and the baby.

Whether there is increased risk of abortion it is still not proved.

N20. Ans. is c, i.e Sulfadoxine – pyrimethamine

Ref. Williams 24/e, pg1257, high risk pregnancy fernando arias 4/e, pg 313

- **Intermittent Preventive Therapy** is a newer modification of prophylaxis. In chemo prophylaxis, the drugs have to be given daily or weekly, wherein in IPT the pregnant females are treated for malaria presumptively at fixed times (either twice or thrice) during pregnancy using drugs with long half life.
- The WHO allows for use of IPT during pregnancy. This consists of at least **two treatment doses of sulfadoxine-pyrimethamine in** second and third trimesters.
- DOC for chemoprophylaxis during pregnancy is chloroquine or hydroxyl chloroquine.

N21. Ans. is d, i.e Mefloquine

Ref. Williams 24/e, pg1257

Malaria	DOC
- Chloroquine sensitive malasias treatment - Chloroquine resistant *P. Falciparum* treatment - Intermittent Preventive therapy - Chloroquine sensitive malaria – prophylaxis - Chloroquin resistant *P. falciparum* – prophylaxis - Antimalarials contraindicated during pregnancy - Insufficient data for use in pregnancy	- Chloroquine followed by primaquine postpartum for radical cure. - Quinine sulphate + Clindamycin or Mefloquine - Sulfadoxine- pyrimethamine - Chloroquine/hydroxy chloroquine - Mefloquine - Primaquine - Doxycycline - Proguanil - Amodiaquine

N22. Ans. is, d i.e. None of the above

Ref. Fernando arias 4/e, pg313-314

Dengue Fever in Pregnancy

Material risks:
a. Associated with high maternal mortality
b. Deranged liver functions may mimic HELLP syndrome.

Fetal risks:
- No evidence of teratogenicity, abortion or IUGR following dengue infection during pregnancy.
- Vertical transmission is present.
- Newborn presents with fever, hepatomegaly and thrombocytopenia. In grave infection, newborn may show coagulopathy.

N23. Ans. is c, i.e. Diloxanide furoate

Ref. High risk pregnancy—F. arias 4/e, p 315

Infections	DOC
- Asymptomatic amebiasis - Symptomatic amebiasis - Severe infection - Giardiasis - Hookworm infection/Ascaris	No treatment Diloxanide furoate (500 mg B/D x 10 days) Diloxanide + metronidazole. Tinidazole 500 mg B/D for 3-5 days - Avoid any treatment in first trimester - Pyrantel pyruvate/Mebendazole/Albendazole can be used after 1st trimester

Answers with Explanations to Previous Year Questions

1. **Ans. is a, i.e. HIV** *Ref. Dutta Obs. 7/e, p 300*

   Teratogenic effects have not been documented with HIV infection

   Rubella, varicella and CMV infections have all been linked to a variety of congenital malformation in the fetus

Effects of maternal HIV infection in pregnancy	
On mother	**On fetus**
The course of HIV in mother remains unaltered as a result of pregnancy	No teratogenic effects have been reported. Preterm labor, IUGR
Maternal mortality or morbidity are not increased by HIV	
Main problems a/w HIV infection during pregnancy are related to preterm birth and IUGR.	

No teratogenic effects
• HIV
• Measles
• Influenza
• Mumps

Infections causing congenital malformation (teratogenic effect)	
• Rubella	• CMV
• Varicella	• Parvovirus
• Toxoplasmosis	
• Mumps	

2. **Ans. is d, i.e. Cytomegalovirus** *Ref. Williams Obs. 23/e, p 1216, 1217; Harrison 17/e, p 48*

   Most common cause of intrauterine infection is cytomegalovirus.

3. **Ans. is a, i.e. Rubella infection** *Ref. Williams Obs. 23/e, p 1214*

   "Rubella is one of the most teratogenic agents known." *Ref. Williams Obs. 23/e, p 1214*

   Rubella causes a number of serious defects in fetus. These defects may occur singly or in combination called *Congenital rubella syndrome.*

4. **Ans. is a, Hepatitis A** *Ref. Dutta Obs. 7/e, p 289*

   Hepatitis A is transmitted by feco-oral route. Vertical transmission is not seen.

5. **Ans. is d, i.e. Rubella**

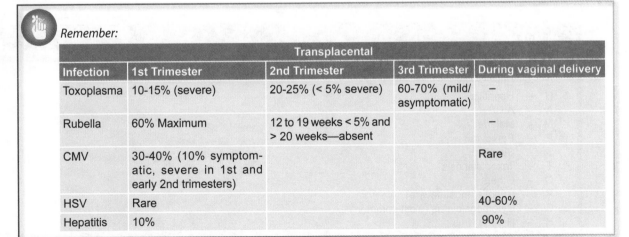

Remember:

Infection	Transplacental			
	1st Trimester	**2nd Trimester**	**3rd Trimester**	**During vaginal delivery**
Toxoplasma	10-15% (severe)	20-25% (< 5% severe)	60-70% (mild/ asymptomatic)	–
Rubella	60% Maximum	12 to 19 weeks < 5% and > 20 weeks—absent		–
CMV	30-40% (10% symptomatic, severe in 1st and early 2nd trimesters)			Rare
HSV	Rare			40-60%
Hepatitis	10%			90%

6. Ans. is c, i.e. 3rd Trimester   *Ref: Fernando Arias 3/e, p 161; Williams Obs. 23/e, p 1226*

"The incidence and severity of congenital infection depend on fetal age at the time of maternal infection. The risks for fetal infection increase with duration of pregnancy from 6% at 13 weeks to 72% at 36 weeks. Conversely, the severity of fetal infection is much greater in early pregnancy and fetuses are much more likely to develop clinical findings of infection."

Ref: Williams Obs. 24/e, p 1255

7. Ans. is a, i.e. Toxoplasmosis

8. Ans. is c, i.e. Toxoplasma

Ref: Williams Obs. 23/e, p 1226, Management of high risk pregnancy, Manju Puri, SS Trivedi p 462

In the question, patient had mild cervical lymphadenopathy for which she was prescribed spiramycin. But the patient was noncompliant and the baby was born with hydrocephalous and intracranial calcification, which are manifestations of congenital toxoplasmosis.

9. Ans. is d, i.e. Nil   *Ref. Harrison 17/e, p 1306*

The woman, who has already given birth to a child with congenital toxoplasmosis, now has no risk of transmitting it to the present baby because *"women who are seropositive before pregnancy usually are protected against acute infection and do not give birth to congenitally infected neonates".*

 Remember:

Timing of Maternal Infection	Risk of Transmission
• In previous pregnancy	• No risk in future pregnancy
• > 6 months before conception	• No risk in pregnancy
• < 6 months before conception	• Risk increases as the interval between infection and conception decreases
• In first trimester	• Risk is less (15%), but disease is severe
• In third trimester	• Risk is maximum (60%), but disease is mild

10. Ans. is d, i.e. Polio   *Ref. Nelson 16/e, p 933*

- In case of polio, only feco-oral transmission is known, no placental transmission has been reported yet
- All other diseases mentioned may be transmitted to fetus by mother
- I am in doubt about candida, because although congenital candidiasis can occur, the mode of transmission is not transplacental but ascending infection from external genitals of mother or during parturition.
- But as far as the answer is concerned it is undoubtedly "POLIO".

 Also Know:

We all know the Acronym TORCH for infection affecting the fetus or newborn. With certain additions, so that all infections can be included, it can be changed to: *—Shiela Balakrishnan, p 347*

 Mnemonic

CHAMP'S TORCH

C	–	Chickenpox
H	–	Hepatitis
A	–	AIDS
M	–	Malaria
P	–	Parvovirus
S	–	Syphilis
T	–	Toxoplasmosis
O	–	Others
R	–	Rubella (most severe)
C	–	Cytomegalovirus (most common)
H	–	Herpes virus

11. **Ans. is c, i.e. Blood dyscrasias**   *Ref. Dutta Obs. 7/e, p 300; Williams Obs. 23/e, p 1218*

- **Manifestation of congenital CMV infection:**
  - Stillbirth
  - Microcephaly
  - Choroidoretinitis
  - Deafness
  - Hemolytic anemia (Blood dyscrasias simply stands for any hematological disorder)
  - Pneumonitis
  - Thrombocytopenia with petechiae and purpura
  - IUGR
  - Hepatosplenomegaly
  - Icterus
  - Mental retardation
  - Have intracranial calcifications

 Note: CMV never leads to heart defects in the fetus.

12. **Ans. is a, i.e Positive IgM antibodies; Low avidity**   *Ref. Fernando Arias 4/e, p 54*
- If IgM antibodies are present—It means recent infection.
- Presence of IgG antibodies indicates chronic infection.
- Avidity refers to the ability of the antibody to bend to antigen. As time increases, avidity increases.

Hence:
- Low avidity indicates—Recent infection
- High avidity indicates—Past infection.

So, fetal transmission is maximum when IgM antibodies are positive and avidity is low.

13. **Ans. is d, i.e. Ceftriaxone**   *Ref. Harrison 17/e, p 958, 959*

Antibiotic therapy for Typhoid fever in Nonpregnant patients

Empirical:

- Ciprofloxacin
- Ceftriaxone/cefotaxime/cefixime

Alternative Drugs:

- Amoxicillin (second line)
- Azithromycin (in MDR patients)

Quinolones are contraindicated in pregnancy, therefore Ceftriaxone is the drug of choice for Typhoid in pregnancy.

14. **Ans. is b, i.e. Listeria**   *Ref: Williams Obs. 23/e, p 1224*

"Discolored brownish or meconium-stained amniotic fluid is common with fetal infection, even with preterm gestation."

Hence, the correct answer is Listeria, rest of the infections do not lead to preterm labour with meconium-stained liquor.

Listeriosis

- Causative organism—listeria monocytogenes (facultative intracellular gram positive bacillus)
- Mode of infection—Food-borne infection caused by eating food like raw vegetables, coleslaw, apple cider, melons, milk, fresh Mexican style cheese, smoked fish, processed foods.

Contd…

Contd…

- **Clinical features**
  - Can be asymptomatic
  - Can cause febrile illness.
- Maternal complications which can occur due to listeria infection are:
  - Preterm labor,
  - Chorioamnionitis,
  - Meconium-stained liquor,
  - Abortions,
  - Placental macroabscesses
- Maternal infection can lead to fetal infection characterized by:
  - Disseminated granulomatous lesions with microabscess in skin
  - Stillbirth
  - Overall perinatal mortality—50%.
- **Management**
  - Drug of choice is combination of Ampicillin + gentamicin or in case of pencillin allergy – Trimethoprim sulfamethoxazole
  - Maternal treatment may be effective for fetal infection
  - There is no vaccine for listeriosis.

15. **Ans. is a, i.e. Mode of transmission of infection is sexual**　　　　　*Ref. Williams 23/e, p 1224, 1225*
For explanation, see previous answer.

16. **Ans. is a, i.e. Last 5 days**

17. **Ans. is d, i.e. Baby will develop neonatal varicella syndrome**
　　　　　Ref. Fernando Arias 3/e, p 156; Williams Obs. 23/e, p 1211, 1212, CMDT 07, p 799, 800
This patient has developed chickenpox 3 days prior to delivery. So, antibodies are not formed in mother (which take at least 5 days' time to develop). Hence, fetus is not protected
Delivery during the viremic period can cause serious complications to mother and neonatal varicella syndrome
In this case, varicella immunoglobulin should be given to neonate.

18. **Ans. is c, i.e. During parturition**　　　　　*Ref. Dutta Obs. 7/e, p 301*
- In case of herpes infection, transplacental infection is not common. Instead the fetus becomes affected by virus shed from the cervix or lower genital tract during vaginal delivery.
- Baby may sometimes be affected in utero from contaminated liquor following rupture of membranes.

Remember: (Very Important)	
• Maximum risk of transmission in first trimester	Rubella
• Maximum risk if infection occurs before 20 weeks	Varicella zoster
• Maximum risk if infection occurs after 18–20 weeks	Syphilis
• Rate of transmission increases as pregnancy advances (i.e. maximum risk in third trimester)	Toxoplasmosis and Hepatitis
• No relation to gestational age	CMV
• Least risk of transmission during delivery	Toxoplasmosis
• Maximum risk of transmission during delivery	HIV and Herpes
• Cesarean section is indicated in	Active Herpes infection and HIV
• Most common congenital infection	CMV
• Most severe congenital infection	Rubella
• Congenital infection with minimal teratogenic risk	HIV

19. **Ans. is a,. i.e. VDRL for mother and baby**

20. Ans. is c, i.e Penicillin *Ref. Williams 23/e, p 1238*

Syphilis in Pregnancy

Congenital syphilis:

- Transmission of T pallidum across the placenta from a syphilitic woman to her fetus may occur at any gestational age.
- Untreated infection leads to fetal loss in 40% cases, IUD, stillbirth and abortions. (stillbirths being more common than abortions)

Early Congenital Syphilis	Late Congenital Syphilis	Residual Stigmata
• Appears within first 2 years of life, M/C time is 2-10 weeks age	• Appears after 2 years of life • Subclinical in most of the cases	• Hutchinson's teeth (Centrally notched widely spaced peg-shaped upper central incisor)
• Earliest manifestation—rhinitis/ snuffles	• Features—interstitial keratitis • Eighth nerve deafness	• Mulberry molars
• M/C bone changes— osteochondritis	• Recurrent arthropathy	
• Periostitis	• B/L knee effusion k/a Clutton's joint	
• Mucocutaneous lesion	• Asymptomatic neurosyphilis	
• Hepatosplenomegaly	• Gummatous periostitis	
• Lymphadenopathy		

Diagnosis of congenital syphilis innonates:

- Presence of antetrioponemal IgM antibodies in neonates is diagnostic of congenital syphilis (IgG antibodies are not specific for neonatal infection and may be the result of transplacental transmission from a mother who has been adequately treated).
- VDRL and RPR tests are used for rapid screening. A VDRL titre in neonates 4 times greater than the maternal titre is consistent with congenital syphillis.

In asymptomatic infants:

- If mother has been treated with penicillin in 1st/2nd trimester—No treatment for infant
- If mother has not been treated/received treatment with penicillin in third trimester – Treat infant with penicillin

SYPHILIS TREATMENT during pregnancy *Ref. Williams 23/e, p 1238*

- Syphilis therapy during pregnancy is given to eradicate maternal infection and to prevent congenital syphilis.
- Parenteral penicillin G remains the preferred treatment for all stages of syphilis during pregnancy.
- There are no proven alternative therapies for syphilis during pregnancy. Erythromycin may be curative for mother, but because of limited transplacental passage, it does not prevent all congenital diseases.

Women with H/O penicillin allergy, first penicillin desensitization should be done and then followed by penicillin injection.

In Question 19

- Bullous leisons on the body of the infant and presence of periostitis suggest the diagnosis of congenital syphilis. The only option related to syphilis is VDRL. Therefore, it is the answer.

21. Ans. is d, i.e. During labour

22. Ans. is a, Perinatal transmission *Ref. COGDT 10/e, p 692, 693; Dutta Obs. 7/e, p 301, 302; Harrison 17/e, p 1145; Williams Obs. 23/e, p 1248 onwards, Dutta Obs. 7/e, p 301-302*

Maternal transmission of HIV to child i.e. vertical transmission can occur:

- Antepartum (Transplacental)
- Peripartum (exposure to maternal blood and body fluids at delivery)—Maximum risk period
- Postpartum (breastfeeding).

Maximum risk of transmission is in peripartum period followed by labour

"In the absence of any intervention, an estimated 15–30% of mothers with HIV infection will transmit the infection during pregnancy and delivery, and 10–20% will transmit the infection, through breastfeeding. Vertical transmission of HIV-1 occurs mostly during the intrapartum period (50–70%)."   *—COGDT 10/e, p 692*

Note: If the choice is between intrapartum and peripartum period–better option is peripartum as the risk of transmission due to breastfeeding is also included in peripartum period.   *—Park 19/e, p 289, 290*

- Vertical transmission rate to neonates is ≈ 14 %-25%

Factors increasing vertical transmission:

- **Disease factors**
  - Maternal viral load i.e. maternal plasma HIV RNA burden (most important risk factor)
  - Seroconversion in pregnancy or early disease
  - Advanced maternal disease
  - Low CD4 count (i.e. risk of vertical transmission is inversely related to maternal immune status)
  - Vitamin A deficiency
  - Chorioamnionitis
- **Obstetric factors**
  - Vaginal delivery
  - Prolonged rupture of membranes (> 4 hrs)
  - Preterm delivery
  - Chorioamnionitis
  - Coexistent STD (specially HSV) and syphilitic
  - Low birth weight infection of placenta
  - Antepartum invasive procedures (amniocentesis, CVS, etc.)
  - Intrapartum invasive procedures (instrumental delivery, episiotomy, scalp electrodes, etc.)

---

23. **Ans. is a, i.e. 15 to 30%**   *Ref. Selected Topics in Obstetrics and Gynaecology-4: For Postgraduate by Daftary & Desai p29*

Timing	Transmission rate
During pregnancy	5 to 10%
During labour and delivery	10 to 15%
During breastfeeding	5 to 20%
Overall without breastfeeding	15 to 25%
Overall with breastfeeding upto 6 months	20 to 35%
Overall with breastfeeding from 18 to 24 months	30 to 45%

24. **Ans. is a, i.e. Nevirapine**   *Ref. Dutta Obs. 7/e, p 301, 302, Current concept in contraception and women health. p 186, 188; Shiela balakrishnan/text book of Obs p 360; Williams Obs. 23/e, p 1252; Harrison 17/e, p 1145*

- Traditionally the therapy being given to prevent fetomaternal transmission of HIV has been zidovudine.
- But the cost of the therapy makes it out of reach of many patients in the developing countries.
- One important study in Uganda demonstrated that a single dose of nevirapine given to the mother at the onset of labour followed by a single dose to the new born within 72 hours of birth decreased transmission by 50% compared with a regimen of zidovudine to the mother.

The cost of this regimen is much cheaper than that of zidovudine and thus is being used increasingly in developing countries for prevention of mother to child transmission.

According to *Harrison 17/e, p 1145*

Zidovudine treatment of HIV infected pregnant women from the begining of 2nd trimester through delivery and of infant for 6 weeks following birth dramatically decreased the rate of intrapartum and perinatal transmission of HIV infection from 22.6% in the untreated group to 5%.

It further says *"Short course prophylactic antiretroviral (ARV) regimens, such as single dose of nevirapine given to the mother at the onset of labour and a single dose of nevirapine to the infant within 72 hrs of birth are of particular relevance to low-to-mid income nations because of the low cost and the fact that in these regions, perinatal care is often not available and pregnant women are often seen by a health care provider for the first time at or near the time of delivery."*

> **Note:**
> - These days when a pregnant female presents with HIV in pregnancy-HAART, i.e combination of three or four drugs from atleast two different classes, is given to all pregnant female with HIV, irrespective of CD4 count or viral load
> - If a woman on HAART gets pregnant, her HAART is continued during pregnancy
> - HAART reduces the chances of vertical transmission by less than 2%
> - Zidovudine is given IV during labor and delivery to woman with HIV RNA viral load more than 400 copies per mL or who have unknown viral load near delivery

25. **Ans. is a, i.e. Nevirapine** *Ref. Parks PSM 20/e, p 373*

NACO is National AIDS Control Organization which was launched in India in the year 1987.The Ministry of Health and Family Welfare had setup NACO as a separate wing to implement and closely monitor the various components of the National Aids Control Programme.

NACO has established many integrated counselling and testing centres (ICTCs), where pregnant women are provided counselling and testing facilities.

"Women who are found to be HIV positive are given single dose of prophylactic Nevirapine at the time of labour and new born infant is also given a single dose of Nevirapine within 72 hrs of birth". —*Park 20/e, p 373*

26. **Ans is a and d, i.e. CS elective will decrease transmission to baby and Start ART and continue throughout pregnancy, ART is safe for gestation**

27. **Ans. is c, i.e. Vaginal delivery**

28. **Ans. is a, b and d, i.e. Treatment should be started before labour; Avoid mixing of blood intrapartum and Cesarean section would be to decrease transmission of HIV to baby**

29. **Ans. is b, i.e. Omitting ergometrine**
Ref. Harrison 17/e, p 1145; Dutta Obs. 7/e, p 302, 303; Williams 22/e, p 1316, 23/e, p 1252, 1253

> **For prevention of mother-to-child transmission, the following steps are advocated intrapartum.**
> 1. Nevirapine/zidovudine during labor
> 2. If viral copies are >1000/ml, then elective cesarean should be done, otherwise vaginal delivery can be attempted.
> 3. Women with HIV infection should be scheduled for induction of labour or cesarean delivery at 38 weeks of gestation. The reason for this timing of delivery is to avoid rupture of membranes before labour.
> 4. Avoid breastfeeding.
> 5. If vaginal delivery is being done, ARM during labour is avoided.
> 6. The newborn of HIV-infected mother is treated with oral zidovudine, 2 mg/kg every 6 hrs for the first 6 weeks of life.
> 7. There is no role of vitamin A supplementation in preventing transmission, but it is seen that vitamin A deficiency has been noted in pregnant females with HIV. So, vitamin A supplementation is done.

30. **Ans. is a, b, c and e, i.e. Start zidovudine during labour, 25% chance of vertical transmission. Avoid breastfeeding, Cesarean section cause less transmission.** *Ref: Dutta Obs. 7/e, p 301, Nelson 18/e, p 1430, 1431, 1441, Harrison 17/e, p 1146, Williams Obs. 23/e, p 1252, 1253*

According to the latest edition of Williams Obs 23/e, p 1252

> **An HIV-infected woman on no antiretroviral medication who presents in labour management** includes: Start zidovudine IV
> *OR*
> Start zidovudine plus a single dose of nevirapine. If nevirapine is initiated, consider adding lamivudine for 7 days postpartum to decrease nevirapine resistance. *Ref: Williams Obs 23/e, p 1251, Table 59-8, p 1252*

So, option a is correct
- Elective cesarean is the best mode of delivery as chances of transmission of HIV are less (i.e. option e is correct)
- Breastfeeding should be avoided except in those cases where mother cannot afford formula feeds (i.e. option c is correct).
- Vertical transmission to the neonates is about 14-25%[Q] (i.e. option b is correct). Transmission of HIV-2 is less frequent (1-4%) than for HIV-1 (15-40%).

> **Vaccination of HIV Infected Infant** (Nelson)
> - Live oral polio vaccine (OPV) and BCG vaccine should not be given (i.e. option d is incorrect).
> - Varicella and MMR are recommended for children in immune categories. 1 and 2, but neither varicella nor MMR vaccines should be given to severely immunocompromised children (immune category 3).

Other Problems in Pregnancy

LIVER DISEASES IN PREGNANCY

CHOLESTASIS IN PREGNANCY/UTERUS GRAVIDARUM

- Idiopathic cholestasis of pregnancy is the 2nd most common cause of jaundice in pregnancy (first one being viral hepatitis).
- It is characterized by accumulation of bile acids in the liver with subsequent accumulation in the plasma causing pruritus and jaundice due to estrogen excess.

Clinical Features

- Manifestations appear in the last trimester (beyond 30 weeks) and only occasionally in the late 2nd trimester.
- **The cardinal clinical finding/1st symptom to appear is severe generalized pruritis with a predilection for the palms and soles[Q].**
- Pruritis precedes laboratory findings by a mean of 3 weeks and sometimes by months[Q]. Jaundice is slight[Q] **(Bilirubin levels rarely exceed 5 mg)** and seen in 10% patients.
- Cholestasis tends to recur in subsequent pregnancies[Q] (recurrence rate = 50%), or with estrogen containing contraceptives, therefore **OCPs are contraindicated in females with h/o cholestasis during pregnancy.**

Investigation

- **Rise in S. bile acids is the earliest/the most consistent change/Best marker for cholestasis.** There is a 10–100 fold increase in s. cholic acid followed by s. chenodeoxycholic acid.
- Serum bilirubin levels are increased (rarely more than 5 mg%)[Q] and increase is always in direct bilirubin.
- Serum alkaline phosphatase is raised.[Q]
- SGOT/SGPT levels are normal to moderately elevated (seldom exceed 250 U/L).[Q]
- Liver biopsy, which is rarely done shows no necrosis, no inflammation but shows feature of intrahepatic cholestasis.
- Dyslipidemia is present.

Prognosis

- There is no increased incidence of maternal mortality.
- Symptoms disappear within two weeks postpartum. Jaundice usually disappears within weeks following delivery. Pruritis as a rule persists longer than jaundice.
- Increase chances of PPH and cesarean section.
- There is increased incidence of prematurity, low birth weight babies, sudden IUD and meconium aspiration in fetus.

Management of Intrahepatic Cholestasis—Medical Management

The most troublesome feature of intrahepatic cholestasis is pruritis (and pruritis is due to bile acid in blood):

- Pruritis can be managed temporarily with antihistaminics and topical emollients
- Ursodeoxycholic acid (10-15 mg/kg/d in 2 divided doses) relieves pruritis decreasing the concentration of bile acid in blood and it also improves biochemical abnormalities.

  "ACOG (2006) has concluded that ursodeoxycholic acid both alleviates pruritis and improves fetal outcomes, although evidence for the latter is not compelling."
  —Williams Obs 24/e, p 1085

As far as cholestyramine is concerned.

"Cholestyramine is no longer routinely used because of poor compliance" —COGDT 10/e, p 382

"Cholestyramine may be effective in 50-70% of women. This compound also causes further decreased absorption of fat soluble vitamins, which may lead to vitamin K deficiency, fetal coagulopathy may develop and there are reports of intracranial hemorrhage and still births."
—Williams Obs 24/e, p 1085

Corticosteroids:

"Cholestyramine is no longer routinely used because of poor compliance" —COGDT 10/e, p 382

"Dexamethasone in a dose of 12 mg/d for 1 week, improves biochemical abnormalities but does not improve pruritis however, it is less effective as compared to USCA."

—Management of High Risk Pregnancy, S S Trivedi Manju Puri, 1/e, p 357

Corticosteroids:

Antihistaminics relieve pruritis and have no effect on biochemical abnormally temporarily, (hence they are not DOC (only provide symptomatic relief).

Obstetric management: *(Management of High Risk Pregnancy—S S Trivedi Manju Puri, p358)*

In patients of intrahepatic cholestasis of pregnancy – there is increased perinatal mortality. Hence fetal surveillance is done with biweekly NST. Conventional antepartum testing, does not predict fetal mortality as there is sudden death in cholestasis due to acute hypoxia, hence delivery is recommended at 37–38 weeks. In those patients with jaundice (S bilirubin >1.8 mg%) termination of pregnancy should be done at 36 weeks.

ACUTE FATTY LIVER OF PREGNANCY/ACUTE YELLOW ATROPHY OF LIVER

- It is a rare condition occurring in third trimester (mean gestational age of 37.5 weeks)[Q]
- It is the M/C cause of acute liver failure during pregnancy.

Aetiology

- It is associated with disorders of fatty acid transport and oxidation-deficiency of LCHAD enzyme, i.e. long chair hydroxyl acyl coenz A dehydrogenase
- Risk is increased in case of:
  - First pregnancy, male fetuses, preeclampsia, maternal obesity and multiple pregnancy.

Histology: Pathology

- Liver is yellow, soft and greasy:
  - Swollen hepatocytes with central nuclei and cytoplasm filled with microvesicular fat[Q] Collectively called as
  - Periportal sparing Acute yellow atrophy
  - Minimal hepatocellular

  } Collectively called as Acute yellow atrophy

Clinical Features

- Patients present in the third trimester (generally at 37 weeks) with nonspecific symptoms like nausea, vomiting, anorexia, vague abdominal discomfort and malaise.
- In many women, persistent vomiting is the main symptom.
- AFP should also be suspected in any woman who presents with new onset nausea and malaise in third trimester.
- This is followed by jaundice (progressive in nature) after about one week.
- In 50% cases—features of preeclampsia viz-hypertension, proteinuria and edema are present.
- In almost all severe cases, there is profound endothelial cell activation with capillary leakage causing hemoconcentration, hepatorenal syndrome, ascites, and sometimes pulmonary edema. Fetal death is more common in cases with severe hemoconcentration. Stillbirth possibly follows diminished uteroplacental perfusion, but is also related to more severe disease and acidosis. There is maternal leukocytosis and thrombocytopenia.
- The syndrome typically continues to worsen after diagnosis. Hypoglycemia is common, and obvious hepatic encephalopathy, severe coagulopathy, and some

degree of renal failure develop in approximately half of women.

Investigations

- Liver function tests are abnormal:
  - Rise in serum bilirubin but less than 10 mg/dL
  - Increase in SGOT and SGPT (< 1000 IU/L)
  - Increase in alkaline phosphatase (moderately)
  - Prothrombin time may be increased
  - Clotting time prolonged.
- In severe cases, there may be disseminated coagulation failure.

Renal function test:
- ↑ S. creatinine (present in all patients)
- ↑ S. uric acid
- ↑ S. ammonia levels

Others:
- ↓ level of glucose (hypoglycemia)
- ↓ platelet count
- ↓ fibrinogen levels (< 100 mg)

Management

- Rapid delivery is essential
- Mode of delivery – Induction of labor followed by vaginal delivery
- Since the patient has coagulopathy, hence cesarean section is avoided, but still in practice cesarean is very common.

Complication

- Maternal mortality 10–75%
- Hepatic dysfunction resolves automatically in the postpartum period.

There are two associated complications which can develop during this period:

1. Transient diabetes insipidus
2. Acute pancreatitis

Fetal Prognosis

- Fetal prognosis is poor.
- If the fetuses survive, they may later on develop a Reye like syndrome of hepatic encephalopathy and severe hypoglycemia due to the defect in beta fatty acid oxidation.

VIRAL HEPATITIS IN PREGNANCY

Viral hepatitis is the commonest cause of jaundice in pregnancy in the tropics.

Hepatitis A (HAV)

- Infection is spread by fecal-oral route.
- Diagnosis is confirmed by detection of IgM antibody to hepatitis A (anti HAV Igm).
- Disease is usually self limited and fulminant hepatitis is rare.
- Perinatal transmission is rare, chronic carrier state does not exist.
- The virus is not teratogenic.
- Pregnant woman *exposed to HAV infection* should receive immunoglobulin 0.02 mL/kg within 2 weeks of exposure. She should also have hepatitis A vaccine single dose 0.06 mL IM. It is safe in pregnancy.

Hepatitis B virus (HBV)

- The virus is *transmitted by parenteral route, sexual contact, vertical transmission and also through breast milk.*
- The risk of transmission to fetus ranges from 10% in first trimester to as high as 90% in third trimester and it is specially high (90%) from those mothers who are *seropositive to hepatitis B surface antigen (HBsAg) and 'e'-antigen (HBeAg).*
- *Neonatal transmission* mainly occurs at or around the time of birth through mixing of maternal blood and genital secretions. Approximately 25% of the carrier neonate will die from cirrhosis or hepatic carcinoma, between late childhood to early adulthood.
- HBV is not teratogenic.

Maternal Infection

The acute infection is manifested by flu like illness as malaise, anorexia, nausea and vomiting. In majority, it remains asymptomatic. Jaundice is rare and fever is uncommon.

Clinical Course (HBV)

Nearly 90–95% of patients clear the infection and have full recovery.

1% develop fulminant hepatitis resulting massive hepatic necrosis.

10-15% become chronic and 10% of these chronic cases suffer from chronic active hepatitis, cirrhosis and hepatocellular carcinoma.

Diagnosis is confirmed by serological detection of HBsAg, HBeAg (denote high infectivity) and antibody to hepatitis B core antigen (HBcAg) and HBV DNA titer (10^7–10^{11}).

Screening

All pregnant women should be screened for HBV infection at first antenatal visit and it should be repeated during the third trimester for 'high risk' groups (intravenous drug abusers, sexual promiscuity, hemophiliacs, patients on hemodialysis or having multiple sex partners).

The best way to prevent infection in a child born to HBsAg positive mother is to give both active and passive immunization.

Infants born to HBsAg positive mothers should be given hepatitis immunoglobulin (0.5 mL IM) within 12 hours after birth. Along with this the first dose of hepatitis B recombinant vaccine is given.

This is followed by hepatitis B vaccine at 1 and 6 months.

Hepatitis B is not a contraindication for breastfeeding.

Hepatitis C (HCV)

It is recognized as the major cause of non-A, non-B hepatitis worldwide and is the leading cause of transfusion associated hepatitis. Transmission is mainly blood borne and to a lesser extent by fecal-oral route.

It is responsible for chronic active hepatitis and hepatic failure.

Perinatal transmission (10–40%) is high when coinfected with HIV and HBV.

Detection is by antibody to HCV by EIA, which develops usually late in the infection.

Confirmation is done by recombinant immunoblot assay (RIBA-3).

Chronic carrier state is present. Breastfeeding is not contraindicated.

Hepatitis D (HDV)

It is seen in patients infected with HBV either as a co-infection or super infection. Perinatal transmission is known.

Hepatitis E (HEV): Hepatitis E is the most important cause of non-A, non-B hepatitis in developing countries like India. Chronic carrier state is present.

Perinatal transmission is uncommon.

Maternal mortality is very high (15–20%).

Remember: Fulminant hepatitis is more common in hepatitis E, less common in hepatitis C and rare in hepatitis A. Maternal mortality is very high in fulminant type.

Medical termination of pregnancy does not alter the prognosis of the patient.

😀 Important One Liners

- Maximum risk of maternal mortality is with hepatitis E.
- Maximum risk of hepatic encephalopathy is with hepatitis E.
- Maximum risk of perinatal transmission is with hepatitis B.
- All pregnant females should be screened for HBV infection in their first antenatal visit and repeated in the last trimester.
- Screening of HBV is done by determination of HBsAg.
- Maximum transmission of HBB infection occurs at the time of deliveryQ. Hence MTP is not recommended in case of first trimester. There is no evidence that cesarean section lowers the risk of vertical transmission.
- Breastfeeding is not contraindicated in case of hepatitis.

KIDNEY DISEASE IN PREGNANCY

URINARY TRACT INFECTIONS IN PREGNANCY

Urinary tract infections in pregnancy:

These are the commonest bacterial infections seen in pregnancy.

Risk factors of UTI in pregnant as well as nonpregnant state:

• Urinary tract obstructions as in:
   – Tumors
   – Calculi
 • Neurogenic bladder dysfunction as seen in case of:
   – Diabetes
   – Spinal cord injury
	• Vesicoureteric reflux as in:
	   – Incompetence of vesicoureteral valve
	   – Congenital absence of intravesical part of ureter
	   – Intrarenal reflux
	   – Sickle cell disease and analgesics—which cause papillary necrosis predisposing to UTI

Best urine sample – Midstream clean catch sample

- Most common cause of clinical pyelonephritis – ascending infection
- MC organism causing UTI and pyelonephritis – *E. coli* 90% cases.

Principles for Management of UTI During Pregnancy

- Single dose therapy is preferred
- The antimicrobial agent should be appropriate to the mother and fetus, any one of the following drugs could be prescribed:
  - Ampicillin
  - Nitrofurantoin – DOC for prophylaxis of recurrent UTI in pregnancy
  - Cephalexin Cephalosporin
  - Amoxicillin clavulanic acid combination.

- Sulfonamides should not be given in the third trimester because they may interfere with bilirubin binding and thus impose a risk of neonatal hyperbilirubinemia and kernicterus.
- Fluoroquinolones are also contraindicated because of their potential teratogenic effects on fetal cartilage and bone.
- Tetracyclines, cotrimoxazole and ciprofloxacin are: contraindicated during pregnancy.

 Note: Before starting any antibiotic a midstream clean catch urine sample should be collected for culture.

Cranberry fruit juice is known to prevent recurrences of UTI. It prevents the adhesions of the pilins of E. coli to uroepithelium.

ASYMPTOMATIC BACTERIURIA IN PREGNANCY

- This refers to persistent, actively multiplying bacteria within the urinary tract in an asymptomatic woman.
- It is diagnosed when bacterial count of the same species is over 10^5/ml in mid stream clean catch specimen of urine on 2 occasions without symptoms of urinary infection
- Counts < 10^4/ml indicate contamination of urine from the urethra or external genitalia
- M/C offending organism = *E. coli* (90% cases)
- Incidence is similar in both non-pregnant and pregnant women, i.e. 1 to 10%

Risk Factors

- Low social economic status
- Multiparity
- ↑Age
- Faulty sexual practices
- Maternal diabetes
- Sickle cell trait[Q]

 Remember:

- Asymptomatic bacteriuria is twice as common in pregnant women with sickle cell trait and 3 times as common in pregnant women with diabetes or with renal transplant as in normal pregnant women.
- ACOG recommends screening for bacteria at the first prenatal visit.
- Screening can be done by dip slide technique (Leukocyte esterase- nitrate dipstick) in places where prevalence is <2% and where prevalence is high (5-8%)—urine culture should be done for screening.

Prognosis

- Asymptomatic bacteriuria can lead to

• UTI in 40% cases	• Fetal loss
• If untreated – acute pyelonephritis in 25% patients	• IUGR
• In treated cases incidence of pyelonephritis is 10%	• Prematurity
• Premature labor	
• Preeclampsia	
• Anemia	
• Risk of developing chronic renal lesions in later life (cystitis and pyelonephritis).	

 Note: Recurrent asymptomatic bacteriuria is associated with high incidence of urinary tract abnormality of the patient which may be congenital or acquired.

Management

Drugs used for its treatment are:

- Amoxicillin
- Ampicillin
- Cephalosporin
- Nitrofurantoin
- Trimethoprim-sulphamethoxazole combination
- In resistant cases, nitrofurantoin is the drug of choice
- Regardless of the treatment recurrence rate is 30%.

PYELONEPHRITIS IN PREGNANCY

Etiology

- Incidence in pregnancy is 1-3%
- More common in primigravida and young females
- Usually occurs in the second trimester after 16 weeks (>50%) but may occur in 1st and 3rd as well
- Generally bilateral, if unilateral it is more common on right side (in more than half of the cases)
- Most common organism responsible *E. coli* (70%), *Klebsiella* (10%).

Complications

Maternal	Fetal
• Renal dysfunction	• Preterm delivery/PROM
• Septicemia/Septic shock	• IUGR
• DIC	• IUD
• ARDS	
• Endotoxin induced hemolysis and anemia	

Note: Bacteremia is seen in 15-20% cases.

Management

Aggressive treatment with IV fluids and IV ampicillin/ cefazolin. Other drugs which can be used are gentamicin alone or along with amoxicillin or piperacillin tazobactam, combination, IV antibiotics are given for 10 days followed by oral drug for 7-10 days.

Antimicrobial suppression therapy is continued till the end of pregnancy to prevent recurrence (30-40%). Nitrofurantoin 100 mg daily at bed time is effective.

GYNECOLOGICAL DISORDERS IN PREGNANCY

OVARIAN TUMOR IN PREGNANCY

Most common ovarian tumor in pregnancy is benign cystic teratoma (dermoid cyst)[Q]

M/C complication of ovarian tumors in pregnancy is torsion (M/C time of torsion-8-10 weeks or early puerperium)

M/C ovarian tumor to undergo torsion in pregnancy **dermoid cyst**.

Remember:

- In case of complication — remove the tumor irrespective of gestational age.
- During labor, if it leads to obstruction—do cesarean section and simultaneously remove the tumor.
- During puerperium—Remove the tumor as early as possible.

M/C malignancies of ovary seen in pregnancy

Germ cell tumors > sex cord stromal tumors > low malignant potential tumors > epithelial tumors.

Management of ovarian cyst during pregnancy (*See flowchart*)

RETROVERTED GRAVID UTERUS

The incidence of retroverted uterus is about 10% during first trimester of pregnancy.

Course

- **In majority, of cases, retroverted gravid uterus rectifies spontaneously.** As the uterus grows, the fundus rises spontaneously from the pelvis beyond 12 weeks. Thereafter, the pregnancy continues uneventfully.
- In minority, spontaneous rectification fails to occur between 12 weeks and 16 weeks. The developing uterus gradually fills up the pelvic cavity and **becomes incarcerated**.
  - **In such cases the cervix is pointed upwards and forwards** the uterus continues to grow at the expense of the anterior wall called **anterior sacculation. There is retention of urine**.

Effects on Pregnancy

- Retroverted gravid uterus can lead to Miscarriage;
- If pregnancy continues with anterior sacculation, there is increased chance of
  (a) Malpresentation
  (b) Nonengagement of the head
  (c) Preterm delivery and prematurity, and
  (d) Rupture of the uterus during labor.

Treatment

Before incarceration: (1) Periodic checkup up to 12 weeks until the uterus becomes an abdominal organ.

After incarceration: (1) Continuous bladder drainage slowly with a Foley's catheter; (2) To put the patient in bed and advise her to lie on her face or in Sims' position; (3) Urine is sent for culture and sensitivity test and urinary antiseptics—ampicillin 500 mg is given 8 hourly daily. With this treatment, the uterus is expected to be corrected spontaneously within 48 hours.

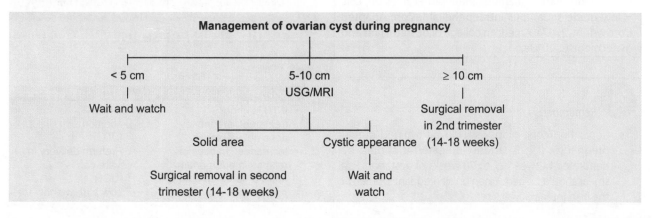

Management of ovarian cyst during pregnancy

If spontaneous correction fails:

- **Manual correction is done followed by insertion of a Hodge-Smith pessary (to be kept up to 18–20th week).**
- **In diagnosed cases of anterior sacculation** of the uterus, delivery by cesarean section is the method of choice.

CARCINOMA CERVIX IN PREGNANCY

- Cancer cervix is the M/C malignancy encountered during pregnancy (Incidence of invasive cancer cervix is 1 in 2500 pregnancies).
- Pap smear should be performed on all pregnant women at the first antenatal visit.
- Pregnancy does not accelerate cervical lesions
- Postpartum regressions is common

- Abnormal cytological result: In case of abnormal pap smear report during pregnancy the following guidelines are followed.

American Society for Colposcopy and Cervical Pathology (ASCCP) guidelines for initial management of epithelial cell abnormalities in pregnancy	
• Abnormality	Adults
• ASC-US	Repeat cytology or do colposcopy 6 weeks postpartum
• LSIL	Colposcopy during pregnancy (preferred) But may defer until 6 weeks postpartum
• HSIL	Colposcopy during pregnancy and repeated at 6 weeks postpartum if CIN2 or 3 are not seen or repeated after every 12 weeks if lesion worsens or cytology suggests invasion.

Note: Endocervical curettage and endometrial sampling are contraindicated in pregnancy. ASCUS = atypical squamous cells of unknown significance, HSIL = high-grade squamous intraepithelial lesion; LSIL = low-grade squamous intraepithelial lesion; Adapted from wright, 2007a; American college of obstetricians and gynecologists, 2013a.

Remember:

- Conization/cone biopsy should be avoided during pregnancy. If it is strictly indicated it should be performed between 12 to 20 weeks of gestation. Pap smear should be performed on all pregnant women at the first antenatal visit.

Management of CIN During Pregnancy

- CIN 1, 2, 3 are managed after delivery. Patient is allowed to deliver vaginally.
  Major risk during delivery is hemorrhage. Following vaginal delivery, these women should be reevaluated and treated at 6 weeks postpartum.
- Regression of CIN is common during pregnancy and postpartum.
- Adenocarcinoma in situ (AIS) is also managed like CIN i.e. after 6 weeks postpartum.

Management of Invasive Cervical Cancer During Pregnancy

- 70 % cases of cervical cancer diagnosed during pregnancy belong to stage I.
- **Stage 1A1:** Vaginal delivery and then simple extrafascial hysterectomy or therapeutic conization after 6 weeks postpartum. If cesarean is being done it can be followed by hysterectomy directly.
- **Stage 1A2:** Vaginal delivery and then Wertheim's hysterectomy and pelvic lymph node dissection after 6 weeks or immediately after cesarean section.
- **Stage 1B, IIA:** If detected in first trimester = immediate Wertheim's hysterectomy on pregnant uterus.
- **If detected in late second or third trimester:** Wait (treatment can be delayed up to 4-6 weeks) for fetal lung maturity and then classical cesarean section followed immediately by Wertheim's hysterectomy.
- **Stage IIB-IV:** If detected in first trimester: Immediate radiotherapy (patient will spontaneously abort before 4000 cGY are delivered
  If detected in late second or third trimester wait for fetal maturity, classical cesarean section and then radiotherapy begun postoperatively.

Mode of Delivery

The mode of delivery in cervical cancer is controversial. Vaginal delivery is not contraindicated but there may be significant haemorrhage and recurrence of cervical cancer in episiotomy scar. Hence, classical cesarean is the preferred route of delivery.

OTHER PROBLEMS IN PREGNANCY

TUBERCULOSIS IN PREGNANCY

Effect of pregnancy on TB	Effect of TB on pregnancy
• If TB is under treatment, pregnancy does not worsen it • Increased chances of relapse in puerperium and TB flares up during puerperium	– ↓ fertility – ↑ abortion – ↑ IUD – ↑ Preterm delivery in severe cases – ↑ IUGR – ↑ Low birth weight

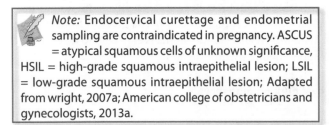

| Mode of infection for fetus:
 • Hematogenous route (through umbilical vein)
 • Ingestion of infected amniotic fluid during delivery
 • Postpartum infection. | |

 Remember: TB is not an indication for termination of pregnancy.

- TB during pregnancy, requires prompt treatment
- ATT can be given at any period in pregnancy, including the first trimester:
- **First line drug used are:**
  - INH, Rifampicin, ethambutol and pyrazinamide
  - Streptomycin is contraindicated during pregnancy[Q]
  - The 2 drugs which should be used throughout are – INH and Rifampicin
  - If a third drug is to be used it is usually ethambutol
  - Pyridoxine 50 mg is given along with chemotherapy.

Drug Regimen
Initial 3 drugs for 3 months followed by 2 drugs for 6 months
OR
Initial 4 drugs for 2 months followed by 2 drugs for 4 months

- Breastfeeding is not contraindication if the woman is on treatment[Q] but contraindicated if active lesions are present
- Baby should be given INH prophylaxis for 3 months. If montoux test is negative after 3 months, prophylaxis is stopped and BCG vaccination given.

 Important Concept

Antituberculosis drugs contraindicated in pregnancy:
K = Kanamycin
F = Fluoroquinolones
C = Capreomycin
A = Amikacin
S = Streptomycin
Mnemonic = KFC Always surprising

EPILEPSY IN PREGNANCY

- Epilepsy is the most common neurological disorder encountered in pregnancy.

- The most common cause for epilepsy in pregnant women is idiopathic.
- Seizure frequencies is unchanged in 50% increased in 30% and decreased in 20% of pregnant females
- Risk of congenital anomalies is about 4% and there is 5–10% risk of epilepsy in the child if parents are affected.
- All anticonvulsant drugs are associated with congenital anomalies as an interfere with folic acid metabolism
- **The malformations include:** Cleft lip and/or palate, mental retardation, cardiac abnormalities, limb defects and hypoplasia of the terminal phalanges. Sodium valproate is associated with neural tube defects. There is chance of neonatal hemorrhage and is related to anticonvulsant induced vitamin K dependent coagulopathy.

Antepartum Management

- In epilepsy during pregnancy:
  - Mono drug therapy is preferred
  - Lowest possible dose of the chosen drug is given
  - Therapeutic drug monitoring is done.
- All women on anticonvulsants should take folic acid: 4 mg/day for 12 weeks in the preconception period and throughout pregnancy.
- Prenatal screening: Maternal Serum Alphafetoprotein (MSAFP) at 16 weeks + level II USG (To detect neural tube defects)
- Vitamin K 10 mg/day orally from 36 weeks onward to prevent hemorrhagic disease of newborn.

Postpartum Management

- The newborn is given vitamin K (1 mg IM)
- Breastfeeding is not contraindicated as the dose excreted in breast milk is very small.
- There is no contraindication to Breastfeeding.

—Dutta Obs 7/e, p 291

- Antiepileptic medications are excerted into breast milk to a variable degree. Given the overall benefits of breastfeeding and the lack of evidence of long-term harm to the infant, by being exposed to antiepileptic drugs, mothers with antiepileptic drugs can be encouraged to breastfeed. *—Harrison 16/e p2372*

Contraception

ACOG has recommended oral contraceptives containing 50 mg of estrogen in women with epilepsy and taking anticonvulsants. *—Williams Obs. 23/e, p 1167*

DRUGS IN PREGNANCY

Food and Drug Administration (FDA) charted out categories for drugs, taking into account the possible fetal adverse effects:

Category A	Drugs which have no fetal risks as demonstrated by well-controlled studies in humans, e.g. *penicillin, ampicillin.*
Category B	Drugs which have shown no risk in animal studies but human studies do not exist, or also if any adverse effects have been seen in animal studies with no such effect in well-controlled human trials, e.g., paracetamol, ranitidine.
Category C	Drugs for which there are no studies either animal or human, or drugs in which there are adverse fetal effects in animal studies but no such data exists in human trials, e.g. chloroquine, *acyclovir, zidovudine.*
Category D	Drugs which have proven risks but their use is essential and the benefits outweigh the risks, e.g. *phenytoin, warfarin, propylthiouracil.*
Category X	Drugs which are clearly teratogenic and the risks outweigh the benefits and hence should be avoided.

SOME DRUGS AND THEIR TERATOGENIC EFFECTS

Friends, *Remember* CNS anomaly (NTD) + CVS anomaly + facial defects are seen with the use of isotretinoin.

Drug	Teratogenicity
Alcohol	**Fetal alcohol syndrome (dose related)** Pre and postnatal growth restriction. Facial abnormalities like shortened palpebral fissure, low set ears, smooth philtrum, thinned upper lip and midfacial hypoplasia. CNS defects like microcephaly, mental retardation and behavioral disorders.
Warfarin	**Fetal warfarin syndrome**[Q] Chondrodysplasia punctata[Q], epiphyseal stippling, nasal hypoplasia, optic atrophy and microcephaly.
Phenytoin	**Fetal hydantoin syndrome**[Q] Hypertelorism, broad nasal bridge, low set ears, hypoplastic nails and digits.
Sodium valproate	**Fetal valproate syndrome**[Q] Brachycephaly with a high forehead, hypertelorism, small nose and mouth, shallow orbits, overlapping long fingers and toes and hyperconvex nails.
Diethyl stilboestrol	**Neural tube defects**[Q] Vaginal and cervical adenosis, clear cell adenocarcinoma, uterine anomalies, cryptorchidism and testicular hypoplasia.
Isotretinoin	Cleft palate, neural tube defect, microcephaly, deafness, blindness, cardiac defects like atrial septal defect and great vessel defects.[Q]
ACE inhibitors	Renal tubular dysgenesis, anuria and oligohydramnios.
Androgens and danazol	Masculinisation of a female fetus.
Antineoplastic agents	IUGR, craniosynostosis, micrognathia, severe limb abnormalities.
Tetracyclines	Discoloration of deciduous teeth.
Cocaine	Microcephaly, limb reduction defects and genitourinary malformations due to cerebral infarction.

HIGH RISK PREGNANCY

High risk pregnancy is defined as one which is complicated by factor or factors that adversely affects the pregnancy outcome – maternal/perinatal or both.

THE HIGH RISK CASES

During Pregnancy

- Elderly primi (> 30 years) or age < 16 years
- Short stature primi < 140 cm
- Elderly grand multipara
- Pregnancies after prolonged infertility
- Threatened abortion and APH
- Malpresentation
- Preeclampsia and eclampsia (i.e. PIH)
- Anemia
- Previous stillbirth, IUD, manual removal of placenta, PPH
- Twins and hydramnios

- H/O of previous cesarean section and instrumental delivery
- Prolonged pregnancy
- Pregnancy associated with medical diseases.
- Rh negative pregnancy

During Labor

- PROM
- Prolonged labour
- Hand, feet or cord prolapse
- Placenta retained more than half an hour
- PPH
- Puerperal fever and sepsis.

 Note: Short stature worldwide is Ht < 150 cm and in Indian context it is Ht < 145 cm

New Pattern Questions

N1. A 25-year-old primigravida with 20 weeks of pregnancy has a first episode of a symptomatic bacteriuria. The risk of having pyelonephritis is:
a. No risk with first episode
b. 5%
c. 15%
d. 25%

N2. Regarding antibiotic of choice for urinary tract infection (UTI) during pregnancy at third trimester:
a. Cephalosporin   b. Quinolones
c. Aminoglycosides   d. Tetracyclines

N3. Regarding asymptomatic bacteriuria during pregnancy all are correct *except*:
a. Bacterial count is over 10^5/ml
b. Overall incidence is 5-10%
c. It should be treated with appropriate antimicrobial agent
d. Risk of progression to nephritis, if left untreated is rare

N4. Following is the emergency management of bleeding vulvar varices during pregnancy:
a. Pressure   b. Cautery
c. Simple vulvectomy d. Observation only

N5. Which of the following is not a complication of fibroid in pregnancy?
a. Preterm labor
b. Postpartum hemorrhage
c. Abortion
d. None of the above

N6. Procedure of choice in a woman with 12 weeks pregnancy and atypical pap smear is:
a. Cone biopsy   b. MTP with cone biopsy
c. Hysterectomy   d. Colposcopy

N7. Which female genital malignancy is most common in pregnancy?
a. Ovarian cancer
b. Vaginal vulvar cancer
c. Endometrial cancer
d. Cervical cancer

N8. A 23-year-old G1P0 woman at 10 weeks' gestation presents to the obstetrics clinic for her initial evaluation. She says she has been hospitalized several times for asthma exacerbations but has never required intubation or admission to an intensive care unit. She is controlled on daily inhaled corticosteroids and albuterol with adequate relief of her symptoms. She is concerned about taking these medications now that she is pregnant. Which of the following is true regarding asthma medications in pregnancy?
a. β_2 agonist are contraindicated during pregnancy
b. Both β_2 agonist and inhaled corticosteroids are both contraindicated in pregnancy

c. Both β_2 agonist and inhaled corticosteroids are safe in pregnancy
d. β_2 agonist and inhaled corticosteroids are both safe in pregnancy but during 2nd and 3rd trimester only
e. Inhaled corticosteroids are contraindicated in pregnancy

N9. Changes in the respiratory system in pregnancy:
a. Vital capacity is increased
b. Subcostal angle remains unchanged
c. Tidal volume remains unaltered
d. Residual volume is decreased

N10. For fetal lung maturation, all the corticosteroids can be used *except*:
a. Betamethasone   b. Dexamethasone
c. Hydrocortisone   d. Methylprednisolone

N11. True statements regarding epilepsy in pregnancy is:
a. Seizure frequency decreases in majority
b. Monotherapy is preferred to polydrug therapy
c. No increase in incidence of epilepsy in offspring
d. Breastfeeding is contraindicated

N12. A syndrome of multiple congenital anomalies including microcephaly, cardiac anomalies and growth retardation has been described in children of women who are heavy users of:
a. Amphetamines   b. Barbiturates
c. Heroin   d. Methadone
e. Ethylalcohol

N13. Smoking in pregnancy causes:
a. IUGR   b. PIH
c. Malpresentation   d. PPH

N14. High risk pregnancy includes all *except*:
a. Twins   b. 2–5 years old primi
c. Hydramnios   d. Previous LSCS

N15. Obesity in pregnancy causes all of the following complication *except*:
a. Abnormal uterine action
b. Fetal neural tube defect
c. Precipitate labor
d. Venous thrombosis

N16. All of the following are direct causes of maternal mortality *except*:
a. APH   b. PPH
c. Heart disease   d. Eclampsia

N17. Maternal near miss refers to:
a. Teenager becoming pregnant
b. Contraceptive failure in a teenager
c. A woman presenting with life threatening condition but has survived
d. A woman presenting with life threatening condition who has died

N18. Basic emergency obstetric services includes all, *except*:
 a. Parenteral oxytocics
 b. Antibiotics and anticonvulsants
 c. Manual extractions of the placenta
 d. Blood transfusions

N19. Fundal height is more than period of gestation in all *except*:
 a. Hydramnios   b. IUD
 c. Twin pregnancy   d. Hydatidiform mole
 e. Uterine myoma

N20. Large for date baby may be due to:
 a. Beckwith syndrome
 b. Diabetic mother
 c. Genetic predisposition
 d. All of the above

N21. Following are more common in multipara woman than primipara *except*:   [DNB 01]
 a. Anemia   b. Placenta previa
 c. PIH
 d. None of the above

Previous Year Questions

1. A pregnant woman developed idiopathic cholestatic jaundice. The following condition is not associated:
 a. Intense itching   [AI 02]
 b. SGOT, SGPT less than 60 IU
 c. Serum bilirubin > 5 mg/dL
 d. Markedly increased levels of alkaline phosphatise

2. Best diagnostic test for cholestasis of pregnancy:
 a. Serum bilirubin   [AI 11]
 b. Bile acid
 c. Serum alkaline phosphatase
 d. Serum transaminase

3. Regarding idiopathic cholestasis of pregnancy correct is: [PGI June 02]
 a. Deep jaundice is present
 b. Pruritus is the first symptom
 c. Maximum incidence during III trimester
 d. Increased liver transaminase
 e. Hepatic necrosis present

4. Cholestasis of pregnancy is characterized by: [PGI June 03]
 a. Commonly occur in 1st trimester of pregnancy
 b. Increased maternal mortality
 c. Increased perinatal mortality
 d. Recurrence in subsequent pregnancy
 e. Generalized pruritis

5. True statement regarding cholestasis in pregnancy: [PGI May 10]
 a. Recurs in subsequent pregnancy
 b. Ursodeoxycholic acid relieves pruritus
 c. Mild jaundice occurs in majority of patients
 d. Pruritus may precede laboratory findings
 e. Serum alkaline phosphatase is most sensitive indicaton

6. Suganti Devi is 30 weeks pregnant with idiopathic cholestasis, is likely to present with following features *except*:   [AIIMS Nov 00]

 a. Serum bilirubin of 2 mg/dL
 b. Serum alkaline phosphatase of 30 KAV
 c. SGPT of 200 units
 d. Prolongation of prothrombin time

7. Intrahepatic cholestasis treatment in pregnancy is: [AI 10]
 a. Cholestyramine   b. Ursodiol
 c. Steroids   d. Antihistamines

8. At what gestational age should be pregnancy with cholestasis of pregnancy be terminated?   [AIIMS May 10]
 a. 39 weeks   b. 36 weeks
 c. 38 weeks   d. 40 weeks

9. True about fatty liver of pregnancy: [PGI June 01]
 a. Common in third trimester
 b. Microvesicular fatty changes
 c. Lysosomal injury is the cause
 d. Alcohol is the main cause
 e. Recurrence is very common

10. A 36-year-old G1P0 at 35 weeks gestations presents with several days H/O generalized malaise, anorexia, nausea emesis and abd. discomfort. She has loss of apetite and loss of several pounds weight in 1 week. Fetal movements are good. There is no headache, visual changes, no vaginal bleeding, no regular uterine contractions or rupture of membranes. She is on prenatal vitamins. No other medical problem. On exaggeration she is mild jaundiced and little confused. Her temp is 100 degree F, PR-70, BP-100/62, no significant edema, appears dehydrated. FHR is 160 and is nonreactive but with good variability. Her WBC- 25000, Hct- 42.0, platelets- 51000, SGOT/SGPT- 287/350, GLUCOSE-43, Creatinine- 2.0, fibrinogen-135, PT/PTT- 16/50, S. Ammonia level- 90 μ mol/L. Urine is 3+ proteins with large amount of ketones. What is the recommended treatment for this patient?

a. Immediate delivery
b. Cholecystectomy
c. Intravenous diphenhydramine
d. MgSO$_4$ therapy
e. Bed rest and supportive measures since this condition is self limiting

11. **A 9-month-old pregnant lady presents with jaundice and distension, pedal edema after delivering normal baby. Her clinical condition deteriorates with increasing abdominal distension and severe ascites. Her bilirubin is 5 mg/dL, S. alkaline phosphatase was 450 u/L and ALT (345 Iu). There is tender hepatomegaly 6 cm below costal margin and ascetic fluid show protein less than 2 mg% diagnosis is:**
   a. Acute fatty liver of pregnancy
   b. HELLP syndrome
   c. Acute fulminant, liver failure
   d. Budd-Chiari syndrome

12. **Highest transmission of hepatitis B from mother to fetus occurs, if the mother is infected during:**
   [AI 07]
   a. Ist trimester   b. IInd trimester
   c. IIIrd trimester   d. At the time of implantation

13. **A mother is HBsAg positive and anti HBeAg positive. Risk of transmission of hepatitis B in child is:**
   [AIIMS June 99]
   a. 20%   b. 50%
   c. 0   d. 90%

14. **A pregnant lady is diagnosed to be HBsAg positive. Which of the following is the best way to prevent infection to the child?**   **[AIIMS May 01]**
   a. Hepatitis vaccine to the child
   b. Full course of hepatitis B vaccine and immunoglobulin to the child
   c. Hepatitis B immunoglobulin to the mother
   d. Hepatitis B immunization to mother

15. **Which of the following statements concerning hepatitis infection in pregnancy is true?**
   [AIIMS Nov 01]
   a. Hepatitis B core antigen status is the most sensitive indicator of positive vertical transmission of disease
   b. Hepatitis B is the most common form of hepatitis after blood transfusion
   c. The proper treatment of infants born to infected mothers includes the administration of hepatitis B Ig as well as vaccine which should be given within 12 hours of delivery
   d. Patients who develop chronic active hepatitis should undergo MTP

16. **Which of the following types of viral hepatitis infection in pregnancy, the maternal mortality is the highest?**   **[AIIMS May 06]**
   a. Hepatitis A   b. Hepatitis B
   c. Hepatitis C   d. Hepatitis E

17. **Differential diagnosis of Hyperemesis gravidarum:**
   a. Gastritis   **[PGI Dec 03]**
   b. UTI
   c. Toxemia of pregnancy
   d. Reflux oesophagitis

18. **When pregnancy is terminated in hyperemesis Gravidarum?**   **[TN 87]**
   a. Increased acetone in urine
   b. Decrease in renal output
   c. Vomiting is more than 3 months
   d. All of the above

19. **A 26-year-old woman in the first trimester of pregnancy has been admitted with retching and repeated vomiting with large hematemesis. Her pulse rate is 126/minute and blood pressure is 80 mm Hg systolic. The most likely diagnosis is:**   **[UPSC 95]**
   a. Mallory-Weiss syndrome
   b. Bleeding from esophageal varices
   c. Peptic ulcer
   d. Hiatus hernia

20. **In a female with appendicitis in pregnancy treatment of choice is:**   **[PGI Dec 06]**
   a. Surgery at earliest
   b. Abortion with appendectomy
   c. Surgery after delivery
   d. Continue pregnancy with medical Rx

21. **True statement regarding ulcerative colitis in pregnancy is:**   **[AIIMS Dec 97]**
   a. Severity increases in 3rd trimester
   b. Severity increases in 2nd trimester
   c. Disease become quiescent
   d. Disease remains as such

22. **A woman presents with amenorrhea of 6 weeks duration and lump in the right iliac fossa. Investigation of choice is:**   **[AI 01]**
   a. USG abdomen   b. Laparoscopy
   c. CT scan   d. Shielded X-ray

23. **Which of the following is normally present in urine of a pregnant woman in 3rd trimester:**
   [AIIMS Nov 10]
   a. Glucose   b. Fructose
   c. Galactose   d. Lactose

24. **Effect of PIH on GFR is:**
   a. GFR Increase
   b. GFR Decreases
   c. GFR remains the same
   d. GFR can increase or decrease

25. **All of the following conditions are risk factor for urinary tract infections in pregnancy except:** **[AI 04]**
   a. Diabetes   b. Hypertension
   c. Sickle cell anemia   d. Vesicoureteral reflux

26. **Following antibiotics are safe to treat UTI in pregnancy:** [PGI Dec 08]
    a. Aminoglycosides   b. Penicillin
    c. Cotrimoxazole   d. Ciprofloxacin
    e. Cephalosporins

27. **Asymptomatic UTI in pregnancy, true is:**
    [PGI Dec 08]
    a. Most are usually asymptomatic in pregnancy
    b. If untreated, progresses to pyelonephritis
    c. Early and prompt treatment prevents abnormalities in fetus
    d. Increase chance of premature infant
    e. Increase risk of chronic renal lesion

28. **With regards to acute pyelonephritis in pregnancy all of the following are true *except*:** [Manipal 06]
    a. Left kidney is involved in 50% of patients
    b. Most common isolate is *E. coli*
    c. More common in later half of pregnancy
    d. Responds to aminoglycosides

29. **Retention of urine in a pregnant woman with retroverted uterus is most commonly seen at:**
    [AI 99]
    a. 8-10 weeks   b. 12-16 weeks
    c. 20-24 weeks   d. 28-32 weeks

30. **A lady with 10-12 weeks pregnancy develops acute retention of urine. The likely cause is:**
    [AIIMS Nov 99]
    a. Retroverted uterus b. Urinary tract infection
    c. Prolapse uterus   d. Fibroid

31. **A 30-year-old lady develops retention of urine in the 2nd trimester. The most probable cause is:**
    a. Fibroid uterus   [AIIMS June 99]
    b. Bladder neck obstruction due to ovarian cyst
    c. Obstruction of uterus
    d. Retroverted uterus

32. **Following renal disorder is associated with worst pregnancy outcome:** [AIIMS May 03]
    a. Systemic lupus erythromatosus
    b. IgA nephropathy
    c. Autosomal dominant polycystic kidney disease
    d. Scleroderma

33. **In pregnancy, the most common cause of transient-diabetes insipidus is:** [AIIMS May 01]
    a. Severe preeclampsia
    b. Hydramnios
    c. Multiple pregnancy
    d. IUGR

34. **Ovarian cyst in postpartum patient, treatment is:**
    a. Immediate removal   [AI 07]
    b. Removal after 2 weeks
    c. Removal after 6 weeks
    d. Removal after 3 months

35. **A female having 6 weeks amenorrhea presents with ovarian cyst. The proper management is:** [AI 00]
    a. Immediate ovariotomy
    b. Ovariotomy at IInd trimester
    c. Ovariotomy 24 hours after delivery
    d. Ovariotomy with cesarean

36. **A 20-year-young female presented for antenatal checkup. She was in Ist trimester and was diagnosed to have ovarian cyst. Treatment of choice:**
    [AI 01; AIIMS June 99]
    a. Surgical removal in IInd trimester
    b. Removal after delivery
    c. Termination of pregnancy and cyst removal
    d. Observation

37. **Which of the following ovarian tumor is most prone to undergo torsion during pregnancy?** [AI 06]
    a. Serous cystadenoma
    b. Mucinous cystadenoma
    c. Dermoid cyst
    d. Theca lutein cyst

38. **Which of the following tumors is not commonly known to increase size during pregnancy?** [AI 06]
    a. Glioma   b. Pituitary adenoma
    c. Meningioma   d. Neurofibroma

39. **A pregnant woman with fibroid uterus develops acute pain in abdomen with low grade fever and mild leucocytosis at 28 weeks. The most likely diagnosis is:** [AIIMS Nov 03]
    a. Preterm labor
    b. Torsion of fibroid
    c. Red degeneration of fibroid
    d. Infection of fibroid

40. **A pregnant woman presents with red degeneration of fibroid; Management is:** [AI 01]
    a. Myomectomy   b. Conservative
    c. Hysterectomy   d. Termination of pregnancy

41. **Treatment of red degeneration of fibroid in pregnancy:** [PGI 03]
    a. Analgesics
    b. Laparotomy
    c. Termination of pregnancy
    d. Removal at cesarean section

42. **Which one of the following is the best drug of choice for treatment of bacterial vaginosis during pregnancy:** [AIIMS May 04]
    a. Clindamycin   b. Metronidazole
    c. Erythromycin   d. Rivamycin

43. **D/D of acute abdomen in pregnancy are all *except*:**
    a. Cystitis   [PGI Nov 2010]
    b. Threatened abortion c. Cervical incompetence
    d. Appendicitis   e. Ruptured ectopic

44. At what period does the tuberculosis flare up most commonly in a pregnant patient? [AI 06]
    a. First trimester   b. Second trimester
    c. Third trimester   d. Puerperium

45 A 6 week pregnant lady is diagnosed with sputum positive TB. Best management is: [AIIMS May 09/AI 11]
    a. Wait for 2nd trimester to start ATT
    b. Start category I ATT in first trimester
    c. Start category II ATT in first trimester
    d. Start category III ATT in second trimester

46. Antitubercular drug contraindicated in pregnancy: [PGI June 05, Dec 01; AI 03]
    a. Streptomycin   b. Refampicin
    c. INH   d. Ethambutol
    e. Pyrazinamide

47. Which of the following statements is incorrect in relation to pregnant women with epilepsy? [AI 05]
    a. The rate of congenital malformation is increased in the offspring of women with epilepsy
    b. Seizure frequency increases in approximately 70% of women
    c. Breastfeeding is safe with most anticonvulsants
    d. Folic acid supplementation may reduce the risk of neural tube defect

48 Which vitamin deficiency is most commonly seen in a pregnant mother who is on phenytoin therapy for epilepsy? [AI 06]
    a. Vitamin B_6 b. Vitamin B_{12}
    c. Vitamin A   d. Folic acid

49. True statement regarding use of antiepileptic drugs in pregnancy: [PGI Nov 10]
    a. Valproate is associated with NTD
    b. Multiple drug should be given
    c. Carbamazepine is used as monotherapy
    d. Phenytoin can produce foetal hydantoin syndrome

50. A 26-year-old primigravida with juvenile myoclonic epilepsy comes to you at 4 months with concern regarding continuing sodium-valproate treatment. Your advice is: [AIIMS Nov 11]
    a. Add lamotrigine to sodium valproate
    b. Taper sodium valproate and add lamotrigine
    c. Switch on to carbamazepine
    d. Continue sodium valproate with regular monitoring of serum levels

51. Antimalarial(s) to be avoided in pregnancy: [PGI June 01]
    a. Chloroquine   b. Quinine
    c. Primaquine   d. Antifolates
    e. Tetracyclines

52. Consequence of maternal use of cocaine is: [AI 01]
    a. Hydrops   b. Sacral agenesis
    c. Cerebral infarction d. Hypertrichosis

53. A pregnant mother is treated with oral anticoagulant. The likely congenital malformation that may result in the fetus is: [AI 98]
    a. Long bones limb defect
    b. Cranial malformation
    c. Cardiovascular malformation
    d. Chondrodysplasia punctata

54. Which does not cross placenta? [AIIMS Feb 97]
    a. Heparin   b. Morphine
    c. Naloxone   d. Warfarin

55. When heparin is given in pregnancy, which of the following is to be added? [AI 08]
    a. Iron folic acid   b. Copper
    c. Calcium   d. Zinc

56. A child born with multiple congenital defect including cleft palate, neural tube defect, atrial septal defect and microcephaly. Which of the following drug is used by mother during pregnancy? [AIIMS June 00]
    a. Erythromycin   b. Isotretinoin
    c. Ibuprofen   d. Metronidazole

57. Vasopressor of choice in pregnancy is: [AIIMS Nov 08]
    a. Ephedrine   b. Phenylephrine
    c. Methoxamine   d. Mephentermine

58. The following drug can be given safe in pregnancy: [AI 09]
    a. Propylthiouracil   b. MTX
    c. Warfarin   d. Tetracycline

59. Which of the following drug is category B (adequate studies in pregnant woman have failed to demonstrate a fetal risk)? [AIIMS Nov 14]
    a. Brimonidine   b. Pilocarpine
    c. Latanoprost   d. Dorzolamide

60. The use of the following drug during pregnancy can lead to Mobius syndrome: [AI 12]
    a. Warfarin   b. Phenytoin
    c. Mifepristone   d. Misoprostol

61. Which can be used in pregnancy?
    a. ACE inhibitors
    b. Aldosterone
    c. AT receptor antagonist
    d. Propylthiouracil

62. Comprehensive emergency obstetric care does not include: [AIIMS May 07]
    a. Manual removal of placenta
    b. Hysterectomy
    c. Blood transfusion
    d. Cesarean section

63. MMR is expressed in: [PGI June 05]
    a. Per 1000 live birth
    b. Per 10000 live birth
    c. Per 1 lac live birth
    d. Per 10 lac live birth

Answers with Explanations to New Pattern Questions

N1. **Ans. is d, i.e. 25%** *Ref. Dutta Obs. 7/e, p 299*

Twenty-five percent of these women are likely to develop acute pyelonephritis, usually in third trimester, if left untreated.

N2. **Ans. is a, i.e. Cephalosporin** *Ref. Williams Obs. 23/e, p 1033, 1036*

- UTI is the most common bacterial infections during pregnancy. Although asymptomatic bacteruria is the most common presentation, symptomatic infection includes cystitis, or pyelonephritis.
- Organisms that cause urinary infections are those from the normal perineal flora.

Drugs use for management of UTI

- As single dose or 3 days course:
  - Amoxicillin
  - Ampicillin
  - Cephalosporin
  - Nitrofurantoin
  - Trimethoprim-sulfamethoxazole.
- In treatment failure:
  - Nitrofurantoin 100 mg four times daily for 21 days.
- For suppression for bacterial persistence or recurrence:
  - Nitrofurantoin 100 mg at bedtime for remainder of pregnancy.

N3. **Ans. is d, i.e. Risk of progression to nephritis, if left untreated is rare** *Ref. Dutta Obs. 7/e, p 299*
As discussed earlier:

- Asymptomatic bacteriuria is when bacterial count of same species is over 10^5/ml (i.e. option a is correct).
- Overall incidence during pregnancy ranges between 2-10% (i.e. option b is correct).
- If left untreated, 25% of the women with asymptomatic bacteriuria develop acute pyelonephritis, hence it should be promptly treated (so option c is correct and option d is incorrect).

N4. **Ans. is d, i.e. Observation only** *Ref. Dutta Obs. 6/e, p 103; Williams Obs. 23/e, p 210–211*

Varicosities (lower leg, vulva, rectum) may appear for the first time or aggravate during pregnancy usually in later months.

- It is due to obstruction in the venous return by the pregnant uterus
- Specific treatment is better to be avoided
- Varicosities usually disappear following delivery
- Valvular varicosities may be aided by application of a foam rubber pad suspended across the vulva by a belt used with a perineal pad
- Rarely large varicosities may rupture leading to profuse hemorrhage.

N5. **Ans. is d, i.e. None of the above** *Ref. Dutta Obs. 6/e, p 309; Jeffcoates 7/e, p 493, 494*
Effects of Fibroid on Pregnancy
Infertility: It is either the cause or the effect of the fibroid:

- Leiomyomas are a sole cause of infertility in less than 3% of cases.[Q]
- It causes infertility by:
  a. Hindering the ascent of the spermatozoa by distorting the uterus and tubes
  b. By disturbances in ovulation and
  c. By interfering with implantation of the fertilized ovum
- Pregnancy rate following myomectomy is 40%.[Q]

During Pregnancy:

- ***Abortion[Q], Placental abruption[Q] and Premature labour[Q]*** Occurs when fibroid interferes with enlargement of uterus, initiates abnormal uterine contractions or prevents efficient placentation.
- ***Malposition[Q] and Malpresentation[Q] of Fetus:*** *Occur* as fibroid can prevent engagement of head.
- ***Obstructed labour:*** It can be caused by cervical[Q] and broad ligament tumours[Q] which are fixed in the pelvis and by pedunculated subserous leiomyomas which become trapped in the pouch of Douglas.

During Labour:
- If fibroid is situated above the presenting part: uneventful vaginal delivery.
- If fibroid is situated below the presenting part: trial for vaginal delivery should be given. Thus chances of cesarean section are increased.[Q]
- ***Postpartum Hemorrhage[Q]/Delayed Involution[Q]*** can occur if placenta is implanted[Q] over the leiomyoma.

 Also Know:

Effects of Pregnancy on Tumour:
- Red degeneration[Q]
- Increased growth of tumour[Q]
- Torsion of pedunculated subserous fibroid[Q]
- Infection during the puerperium.[Q]

N6. Ans. is d, i.e. Colposcopy *Ref. Dutta Obs. 6/e, p 307; Novak 14/e, p 1437–1438; Management of High Risk Pregnancy, SS trivedi, Manju Puri 1/e, p 504–505*

As discussed in the preceding text, all abnormal pap smears during pregnancy, should be followed by colposcopy

N7. Ans. is d, i.e. Cervical cancer *Ref. Williams Obs. 24/e, p 1221*
- *Combined together, genital tract cancers are the most common malignancies encountered during pregnancy.*
- *Most common genital malignancy during pregnancy is cervical cancer.*
  Proportion of malignancies during pregnancy is shown in Figure 24.1. —*Williams Obs. 24/e*

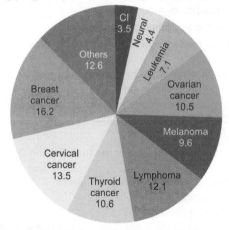

Fig. 24.1: Proportion of malignancies during pregnancy

N8. Ans. is c, i.e Both β_2 agonist and inhaled corticosteroids are safe in pregnancy

Asthma in Pregnancy – Important Points:
- Asthma is the most common chronic condition in pregnancy and affects 3–12% of gestations.
- **Effects of pregnancy on asthma:** The course of the disease is very much unpredictable. In about 20%, the condition improves, in 30%, it deteriorates and in 50%, it remains unchanged.
- It is more likely to deteriorate in women with severe asthma.
- Exacerbations are most frequent between 24 to 36 weeks gestation and are most commonly precipitated by viral respiratory infections and non compliance with inhaled corticosteroid regimens.
- Because asthma exacerbation can be severe, they should be treated aggressively in pregnancy.
- **Effects of asthma on pregnancy:** Preterm labor PROM, preeclampsia, LBW baby and slight increase in abruptio placenta.
- Severity of asthma correlates with FEV1 and PEFR (peak expiratory flow rate) FEV1 ideally is > 80% of the predicted value and PEFR FEV1 less than 1L or less than 20% of predicted value, correlates with severe disease.

Contd...

Contd...

Management of Asthma in Pregnancy:
- Mild asthma: Inhaled beta agonist (albuterol preferred because of more human data on safety in pregnancy).
- Mild persistent: Low dose inhaled corticosteroids (Budesonide preferred).
- Moderate: Low dose inhaled corticosteroids and long acting b agonist (Salmetrol preferred).
- Severe: High dose inhaled corticosteroid and long acting beta agonist and oral steroids if needed.

 Important Points
- PGF-2 alpha is absolutely C/I in patients of Asthma
- So, if in an asthmatic patient PPH occurs drug of choice is PGE1
- In asthmatic patients DOC for cervical ripening-PGE2 (PGE2 is not contraindicated in asthmatics).

N9. Ans. is d, i.e. Residual volume is decreased   *Ref. Dutta Obs. 7/e, p 55*

Changes in respiratory system during pregnancy:
- With the enlargement of the uterus, specially in the later months, there is elevation of the diaphragm by 4 cm.
- Total lung capacity is reduced by 5% due to this elevation.
- Breathing becomes diaphragmatic. Total pulmonary resistance is reduced due to progesterone effect.
- The subcostal angle increases from 68° to 103°, the transverse diameter of the chest expands by 2 cm and the chest circumference increases by 5–7 cm.
- A state of hyperventilation occurs during pregnancy leading to increase in tidal volume and therefore respiratory minute volume by 40%.

Increase	Decrease	Unchanged
Tidal volume	Residual volume	Respiratory
Minute ventilation	Total lung capacity	Vital capacity
Airway	Functional residual capacity	Maximum breathing capacity
conductance	Expiratory reserve volume	Inspiratory capacity
		Inspiratory reserve volume

N10. Ans. is d, i.e. Methylprednisolone

DOC for fetal lung maturation is betamethasone. Methylprednisolone is not effective because of poor placental transfer.

N11. Ans. is b, i.e. Monotherapy is preferred to polydrug therapy   *—Dutta Obs 7/e, p 291*

As discussed earlier, seizure frequency remains unchanged in majority during pregnancy.
"Frequency of convulsions is unchanged in majority (50%) and is increased in some."   *—Dutta 7/e, p 291*
"The risk of developing epilepsy to the offspring of an epileptic mother is 10%."   *—Dutta 7/e, p 291*
So, option c is incorrect.
"There is no contraindication for breastfeeding."   *—Dutta 7/e, p 291*
so option d is incorrect.
We have read time and again that monotherapy is preferred in pregnant epileptic patient.

N12. Ans. is e, i.e. Ethylalcohol   *Ref. Williams Obs. 23/e*

Maternal abuse-and abnormalities associated with it.
Smoking leads most commonly to IUGR:
- There are increased chances of preterm delivery, placenta previa, abruptio and Abortion.
- It leads to congenital heart defects, gastroschisis and small intestine atresia, cleft lip and palate in the fetus along with IUGR and low birth weight baby.

Maternal alcohol abuse-leads to   *Ref. Williams Obs. 23/e, p 317*
Fetal Alcohol Syndrome diagnostic criteria—all required
i. Dysmorphic facial features:
   a. Small palpebral fissures
   b. Thin vermilion border
   c. Smooth philtrum
ii. Prenatal/and or postnatal growth impairment
iii. CNS abnormalities:
   a. Structural: Head size < 10 percentile, significant brain abnormality on imaging
   b. Neurological
   c. Functional global cognitive or intellectual deficits, functional deficits in atleast three domains.

Alcohol Related Birth Defects:
i. **Cardiac:** atrial or ventricular septal defect, aberrant great vessels, conotruncal heart defects.
ii. **Skeletal:** radioulnar synostosis, vertebral segmentation defects, joint contractures, scoliosis.
iii. **Renal:** aplastic or hypoplastic kidneys, dysplastic kidneys, horse shoe shaped kidney, ureteral dilatation.
iv. **Eyes:** Striabismus, ptosis, retinal vascular abnormalities, optic nerve hypoplasia.
Ears: Conductive or neurosensory hearing loss.
Minor: Hypoplastic nails, clinodactyly, pectus carinatum or excavatum, camptodactyly, **hockey stick** palmar crease, **railroad track** ears.
Maternal opiate abuse: After birth children generally appear normal or have small head size, have tremors, irritability, sneezing, and vomiting:
• Symptoms lasts for <10 days
• Abnormal respiratory function during sleep can lead to sudden death.

N13. **Ans. is a i.e. IUGR;** *Ref. Dutta Obs. 7/e, p 100, 255; Williams Obs. 23/e, p 180, 181*

Smoking increase the risk of:
• Preterm labour
• Fetal growth restriction
• Low birth weight
• Attention deficit/Hyperkinetic disorder typically identified by school age
• Behavioural learning problems
• Besides the above fetal problems it increase the risk of pregnancy complications related to vascular damage, such as placental insufficiency and placental abruption.

Note:

• Carbon monoxide and nicotine are responsible for the adverse fetal effects.
• Both active and passive smoking are associated with these risks.
• Cessation of smoking increases birth weight of fetus.

• Smoking does not affect maternal weight during pregnancy
• Smoking is protective against PIH.

N14. **Ans. is b, i.e. 2-5-year-old primi** *Ref. Dutta Obs. 7/e, p 632*

High risk pregnancy is defined as one which is complicated by factor or factors that adversely affects the pregnancy outcome – maternal/perinatal or both.

The high risk cases are:
During pregnancy:
• Elderly primi (> 30 years) or age < 16 years
• Elderly grand multipara
• Threatened abortion and APH
• Preeclampsia and eclampsia (i.e. PIH)
• Previous stillbirth, IUD, manual removal of placenta, PPH
• H/O of previous cesarean section and instrumental delivery
• Pregnancy associated with medical diseases.

• Short stature primi < 140 cm
• Pregnancies after prolonged infertility
• Malpresentation
• Anemia
• Twins and hydramnios
• Prolonged pregnancy
• Rh negative pregnancy

During labour
• PROM
• Hand, feet or cord prolapse
• PPH

• Prolonged labour
• Placenta retained more than half an hour
• Puerperal fever and sepsis.

Note: Short stature worldwide is Ht < 150 cm and in Indian context it is Ht < 145 cm

N15. Ans. is c, i.e. Precipitate labour   *Ref. Dutta Obs. 7/e, p 344; Williams Obs. 23/e, p 951, 952*

Obesity in Pregnancy
Body weight > 90 kg or BMI > 30 kg/m² is considered obese.
(BMI = 20-24 is normal) > 25 kg/m² Overweight
Obesity is associated with increased incidence of:
During pregnancy:
- Dyspnoea on exertion
- Hypertension (essential and PIH)
- Diabetes
- Anomalies is increased
- Difficulty in diagnosis of presentation and in hearing the FHS.
During labour:
- Abnormal uterine contractions
- Prolonged labour (and not precipitate labour)
- Shoulder dystocia
- Operative interference/anesthetic complications.
In puerperium:
- Venous thrombosis
- Lactation failure.
Note: Obese pregnant females should be considered under 'High Risk group'
Risk to the fetus in case of maternal obesity:
- ↑ incidence of first trimester abortions
- ↑ Incidence of fetal anomalies – especially neural tubal defects
- Macrosomia which in turn leads to ↑chances of shoulder dystocia, birth injury and ↑incidence of low apgar
- Scores and perinatal death (Ref High risk pregnancy Manju puri SS. Trivedi, p 493)
- ↑Still birth rate
- In adult life – such fetuses have increased chances of obesity and heart diseases.

N16. Ans. is c, i.e. Heart disease   *Ref. Dutta Obs. 7/e, p 602*

Maternal Death – Death of a woman while pregnant or within 42 days of termination of pregnancy irrespective of the duration and site of pregnancy, from any cause related to or aggravated by the pregnancy or its management but not from accident or incidental causes is called as maternal death.

Maternal Mortality Ratio (MMR)	Maternal Mortality Rate
No. of maternal deaths per 100,000 live births In India: MMR is 212 per 100,000 live births **Note:** The MMR is expressed in per lac live births[Q]	No. of maternal deaths divided by the number of women in reproductive age (15-49). It is expressed per 100,000 women of reproductive age per year. In India, it is 120 as compared to 0.5 in US

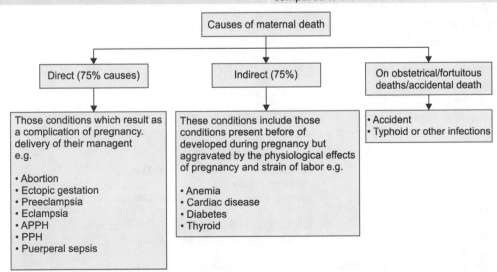

So, heart disease is an indirect cause of maternal death and not a direct cause.

N17. **Ans. is c, i.e. A woman presenting with life-threatening conditions but has survived.**

Ref. Master Pass in Obs/Gynae Konar, p 341

A woman presenting with any life-threatening condition and survived, is considered as a Maternal Near Miss case.

Maternal Near Miss is a retrospective event. From the definition point of view, woman can only be recognized as a maternal near miss, when she survives the server complications in pregnancy, labour or postpartum six weeks.

N18. **Ans. is d, i.e. Blood transfusions**

Ref. Internet search

Basic emergency obstetric services include	Comprehensive emergency obstetric services include
Parenteral oxytocics	Basic services
Antibiotics and anticonvulsants	Cesarean sections
Assisted deliveries	Blood transfusions
Manual extraction of the placenta	Neonatal resuscitation facility
Removal of retained products	

N19. **Ans. is b, i.e. IUD**

Ref. Dutta Obs. 7/e, p 78

Condition where the Height of Uterus is more than the Period of Amenorrhea:
- Mistaken dates
- Twins
- Polyhydramnios
- Big baby
- Pelvic tumours - Ovarian/fibroid
- H mole
- Concealed accidental hemorrhage.

Conditions where the Height of Uterus is less than the Period of Amenorrhea:
- Mistaken dates
- Scanty liquor
- Fetal growth restriction
- Intrauterine fetal death.

N20. **Ans. is d, i.e. All of the above**

Ref. Harrison 17/e, p 413 for option a; Wiliams 23/e, p 854

Beckwith syndrome: It is characterized by macrosomia, macroglossia and omphalocele. Cytogenetic location is 11q15 and is associated with Wilm's tumour of kidney.

—Harrison 17/e, p 413

Diabetic mother: Maternal diabetes is an important risk factor for development of fetal macrosomia.

Other risk factors which favour the risk likelihood of large fetus are:

—Williams 23/e, p 854

- Large size of parents specially the mother who is obese *(Option "c")*
- Multiparity
- Prolonged gestation
- Increased maternal age
- Male fetus
- Previous infant weighing more than 4 kg
- Race/ethnicity.

N21. **Ans. is c, i.e. PIH**

Ref. Dutta Obs. 7/e, p 262

Disorders most common in Multiparae during Pregnancy:
• Anemia	• Abortion	• H mole
• Twins (5th gravida onwards)	• Placenta previa	• Abruptio placentae
• Rh isoimmunization	• Prematurity	• Precipitate labour

During Labour:
• Cord prolapse	• Cephalopelvic disproportion	• Obstructed labour
• Rupture uterus	• Post partum hemorrhage	• Shock
• Operative interference		

Disorders most common in Nullipara:
• Hyperemesis gravidarum	• PIH	• Pyelonephritis in pregnancy

Answers with Explanations to Previous Year Questions

1. **Ans. is c, i.e. Serum bilirubin > 5 mg/dL**

2. **Ans. is b, i.e. Bile acid**

3. **Ans. is b, c and d, i.e. Pruritus is the first symptom, Maximum incidence during III trimester, Increased liver transaminase**

4. **Ans. is c, d and e, i.e. Increased perinatal mortality, Recurrence in subsequent pregnancy, Generalized pruritis**

5. **Ans. is a, b, c and d, i.e. Recures in subsequent pregnancy, Ursodeoxycholic acid relieves pruritus, Mild jaundice occurs in majority of patients, Pruritus may precede laboratory findings**

Ref. Dutta Obs. 6/e, p 291; Robbin's 7/e, p 921; Williams Obs. 23/e, p 1063, 1064; Mgt of High Risk Pregnancy –
SS Trivedi, Manju Puri, p 355, 356

Coming to the Question No. 1

A pregnant female with idiopathic cholestatic jaundice – is associated with

Option a – intense itching → True

Option b – SGDT, SGPT < 60 IU → True

Option c – S bilirubin >5 mg/dL → Incorrect

In Idiopathic cholestasis of pregnancy bilirubin levels are rarely more than 5 mg as supported by –

"Bilirubin levels rarely exceed 5 mg%" —*Williams 22/e, p 1126*

"Hyperbilirubinemia, results from retention of conjugated pigments; but total plasma concentration rarely exceeds 4-5 mg/dL".—*Williams 23/e, p 1064*

"Hyperbilirubinemia occurs in 20% of women and is almost exclusively direct reacting Bilirubin levels are usually between 2-5 mg/dL." —*Mgt of High Risk Pregnancy*—*S S Trivedi, Manju Puri Jaypee Publication p 356*

Option d – Markedly increased levels of alkaline phosphatase → Incorrect.

In cholestasis of pregnancy alkaline phosphatase may be mildly elevated and is not markedly elevated

Both option c and d are incorrect but, if I have to choose one option I would mark option 'c' as my answer – based on the fact that alkaline phosphatase as such does not carry much significance in the diagnosis of cholestasis (whether it is mildly/markedly elevated).

"Alkaline phosphatase increases above the normal elevation but is not much helpful in diagnosis."

Mgt of High Risk Pregnancy – S S Trivedi Manju Puri Jaypee Publication p 356

 Extra Edge

Pruritis of cholestasis during pregnancy and physiological pruritis gravidarum in pregnancy can be differentiated by – levels of serum – Glutathione S. transferase (GST) – It rises in cholestasis, at least 9 weeks before bile acid.

6. **Ans. is d, i.e. Prolongation of prothrombin time**

Ref. Dutta Obs. 6/e, p 291; Robbin's 7/e, p 921; Williams Obs. 23/e, p 1063, 1064

Let's see each option separately.

Option "a" Serum bilirubin of 2 mg/dL.

Bilirubin level rarely exceed 5 mg%.

Bilirubin levels are usually between 2-5 mg/dL i.e. Option "a" is correct.

Option "b" Serum alkaline phosphatase of 30 KAU.

"Alkaline phosphatase may be mildly elevated."—*Robbins 7/e, p 921*

i.e. alkaline phosphatase levels may be normal also. Hence, option b is correct.

Option "c" SGPT of 200 units.

"Serum transaminases levels are normal to moderately elevated but seldom exceed 250 IU/L."

—*Williams Obs. 23/e, p 1064*

i.e. Serum transaminases (SGPT) may be 200 units.

Option "d" Prolongation of prothrombin time

"Prothrombin time is usually normal unless there is malabsorption."

Mgt of High Risk pregnancy – SS Trivedi, Manju Puri, p 356

Prothrombin is coagulant factor II. Its formation in liver is dependent on fat soluble vitamin K. Absorption of vitamin K occurs with bile acid. In cholestasis absorption of bile acid (vitamin K) is not affected, rather there is accumulation of bile acids, so levels of vitamin K and clotting factors dependent on vitamin K are also normal. The prothrombin time therefore, remains normal in cholestasis.

Only when ursodeoxycholic acid or cholestyramine are being given to patients of cholestasis. Prothrombin time needs to be monitored because these drugs decrease the absorption of bile acids and can therefore cause prolongation of prothrombin time.

7. **Ans. is b, i.e. Ursodiol**

8. **Ans. is c, i.e. 38 weeks**

    Ref. COGDT 10/e, p 382; Williams Obs 24/e, p 1085, Mgt of High Risk pregnancy—S S Trivedi Manju Puri, p 357.

> **Management of Intrahepatic Cholestasis – Medical Management**
> The most troublesome feature of intrahepatic cholestasis is pruritis (and pruritis is due to bile acid in blood):
> *   Pruritis can be managed temporarily with antihistaminics and topical emollients
> *   Ursodeoxychotic acid (10-15 mg/kg/d in 2 divided doses) relieves pruritis decreasing the concentration of bile acid in blood and it also improves biochemical abnormalities.
> *"ACOG (2006) has concluded that ursodeoxycholic acid both alleviates pruritis and improves fetal outcomes, although evidence for the latter is not compelling."* —Williams Obs 24/e, p 1085
> As far as cholestyramine is concerned.
> *"Cholestyramine is no longer routinely used because of poor compliance"* —COGDT 10/e, p 382
> *"Cholestyramine may be effective in 50-70% of women. This compound also causes further decreased absorption of fat soluble vitamins, which may lead to vitamin K deficiency, fetal coagulopathy may develop and there are reports of intracranial hemorrhage and still births."* —Williams Obs 24/e, p 1085
> **Corticosteroids:**
> *"Cholestyramine is no longer routinely used because of poor compliance"* —COGDT 10/e, p 382
> *"Dexamethasone in a dose of 12 mg/d for 1 week, improves biochemical abnormalities but does not improve pruritis however it is less effective as compared to USCA."*
> —Management of High Risk Pregnancy, S S Trivedi Manju Puri, 1/e, p 357
> **Corticosteroids:**
> Antihistaminics relieve pruritis and have no effect on biochemical abnormally temporarily, (hence they are not DOC (only provide symptomatic relief).
> **Obstetric management**—*Mgt of High Risk Pregnancy—S S Trivedi Manju Puri, p 358*
> In patients of intrahepatic cholestasis of pregnancy – there is increased perinatal mortality. Hence fetal surveillance is done with biweekly NST. Conventional antepartum testing, does not predict fetal mortality as there is sudden death in cholestasis due to acute hypoxia, hence delivery is recommended at 37-38 weeks. In those patients with jaundice (S bilirubin >1.8 mg%) termination of pregnancy should be done at 36 weeks.

9. **Ans. is a and b, i.e. Common in third trimester and Microvesicular fatty changes**

    Ref. Williams Obs 23/e, p 1065, 1066; COGDT 10/e, p 382

    See the text for explanation

10. **Ans is a, i.e. Immediate delivery**
    Ref. Williams 23/e, p 1067

    A 35-year-old pregnant patient having:

• Nausea, vomiting • Jaundice • Hypoglycemia • ↑ ammonia levels • ↓ platelet levels • Raised SGOT, SGPT	leave no doubt that she is a case of acute fatty liver of pregnancy

    This is not HELLP syndrome as her B/P is normal and not raised.

    In AFP: Termination of pregnancy is the first step as spontaneous resolution usually follows delivery.

    Read the management of AFP as given by Williams 23/e, p 1067.

"The key to a good outcome is intensive supportive case and good obstetrical management. Spontaneous resolution usually follows delivery. In some cases, the fetus may be already dead when the diagnosis is made, and the route of delivery is less problematic. Many viable fetuses tolerate labor poorly. Because significant procrastination in effecting delivery may increase maternal and fetal risks, we prefer a trial of labor induction with close fetal surveillance. Although some recommend cesarean delivery to hasten hepatic healing, this increases maternal risk when there is a severe coagulopathy. Transfusions with whole blood or packed red cells, along with fresh-frozen plasma, cryoprecipitate, and platelets, are usually necessary if surgery is performed or if obstetrical lacerations complicate vaginal delivery."

11. Ans. is d, i.e. Budd-Chiari syndrome *Ref. Harrison 16/e, p 1862*

The most common causes of acute severe liver injury in a young pregnant women are:
- Viral hepatitis (HAV, HBV)
- Eclampsia, preeclampsia (HELLP syndrome)
- Acute fatty liver of pregnancy
- Budd-Chiari syndrome.

Let us discuss each option separately

Preeclampsia and eclampsia/HELLP syndrome:
- It is the most common cause of abnormal liver function test in women.
- Amniotransferases are modestly elevated.
- But in these cases delivery of the fetus is followed by rapid normalization of the hepatic abnormalities.
- Moreover the question does not mention any history of PIH, hemolysis and thrombocytopenia (HELLP syndrome).

Acute fatty liver of pregnancy:
- Acute fatty liver develops in the third trimester.
- Jaundice develops a few days after the onset. The serum bilirubin is rarely above 10 mg/dL.
- Alkaline phosphate is markedly elevated.
- Aminotransferases are moderately elevated.
- A markedly raised serum ammonia is the most diagnostic finding in establishing the diagnosis of acute fatty liver of pregnancy and symptoms rapidly abate with parturition in most patients.

Fulminant hepatic failure:
- The patient presents with features of severe acute hepatitis leading to the development of hepatic encephalopathy within 8 weeks of onset.
- The bilirubin increases to 20-30 mg/dL.
- The aminotransferase levels are very high (>1000)
- Alkaline phosphatase moderately elevated.
- Delivery is usually the best treatment.

Budd-Chiari syndrome:
- It is a disorder characterized by thrombotic occlusion of the hepatitis veins.
- It is a rare complication of pregnancy.
- Most of the cases presents within few weeks of delivery but in several cases onset occurs during pregnancy.
- Clinical triad of Budd-Chiari syndrome includes sudden onset of abdominal pain, hepatomegaly and ascites (ascites with high protein content is almost always present) near term or shortly after delivery.
- Tender hepatomegaly is one of the hallmark of Budd-Chiari syndrome.
- Aminotransferases are mildly elevated.
- Jaundice is seen in only half of the cases.

12. Ans. is c, i.e. IIIrd trimester

Hepatitis B virus (HBV):
- The virus is *transmitted by parenteral route, sexual contact, vertical transmission and also through breast milk.*
- The risk of transmission to fetus ranges from 10% in first trimester to as high as 90% in third trimester and it is specially high (90%) from those mothers who are *seropositive to hepatitis B surface antigen (HBsAg) and 'e'-antigen (HBeAg).*
- *Neonatal transmission* mainly occurs at or around the time of birth through mixing of maternal blood and genital secretions. Approximately 25% of the carrier neonate will die from cirrhosis or hepatic carcinoma, between late childhood to early adulthood.

13. **Ans. is a, i.e. 20%**   *Ref. Fernando Arias 3/e, p 158; Harrison 17/e, p 194, Dutta Obs. 7/e, p 292*

The risk of perinatal transmission of HBV depends upon the presence of HBeAg or Anti-HBe antibody.

"The likelihood of perinatal transmission of HBV correlates with the presence of HBeAg. 90% of HBeAg positive mother, but only 10-15% of anti-HBe positive mothers transmit HBV infection to their offspring."   *Harrison 17/e, p 1940*

According to Fernando Arias 3/e, p 158:

"The higher risk for vertical transmission of HBV is attributed to chronic carriers with positive HBeAg.

These patients are highly infective and as many as 90% of their newborns will be infected. Mothers with positive anti-HBe antibody have a 25% probability of transmitting the infection. If both HBeAg and anti-HBe are not present, there is a 10% probability of neonatal infection."

14. **Ans. is b, i.e. Full course of hepatitis B vaccine and immunoglobulin to the child**

         Ref. Dutta Obs. 7/e, p 292; Fernando Arias 3/e, p 158

The best way to prevent infection in a child born to HBsAg positive mother is to give both active and passive immunization.

Infants born to HBsAg positive mothers should be given hepatitis immunoglobulin (0.5 m–1m) within 12 hours after birth. Along with this, the first dose of hepatitis B recombinant vaccine is given.

This is followed by hepatitis B vaccine at 1 and 6 months.

Hepatitis B is not a contraindication for breastfeeding.

15. **Ans. is c, i.e. The proper treatment of infants born to infected mothers includes the administration of hepatitis B Ig as well as vaccine which should be given within 12 hours of delivery**

         Ref. Dutta Obs. 7/e, p 292; Fernando Arias 3/e, p 158

Persons at increased risk of hepatitis B infection include homosexuals, abusers of intravenous drugs, healthcare personnel, and people who have received blood or blood products.

However, because of intensive screening of blood for type B hepatitis, hepatitis C has become the major form of hepatitis after blood transfusion (i.e. option b is incorrect).

The most sensitive indicator of positive vertical transmission of disease is HBe antigen (i.e. option a is incorrect).

The proper treatment of infants born to infected mothers includes administration of hepatitis B immune globulin as well as vaccine.

Chronic acute hepatitis does not necessarily warrant therapeutic abortion (i.e. option d is incorrect). Fertility is decreased, but pregnancy may proceed on a normal course as long as steroid therapy is continued. Prematurity and fetal loss are increased, but there is no increase in malformations.

16. **Ans. is d, i.e. Hepatitis E**   *Ref. Dutta Obs. 7/e, p 292; Robbin's 6/e, p 862*

- Maximum risk of maternal mortality is with hepatitis E.
- Maximum risk of hepatic encephalopathy is with hepatitis E.
- Maximum risk of perinatal transmission is with hepatitis B.
- All pregnant females should be screened for HBV infection in their first antenatal visit and repeated in the last trimester.
- Screening of HBV is done by determination of HBsAg.
- Maximum transmission of HBB infection occurs at the time of delivery[Q]. Hence MTP is not recommended in case of first trimester. There is no evidence that cesarean section lowers the risk of vertical transmission.
- Breastfeeding is not contraindicated in case of hepatitis.

17. **Ans. is a, b and d, i.e. Gastritis; UTI; and Reflux of oesophagitis**

         Ref. Dutta Obs. 7/e, p 155, 157; Current Diagnosis and Treatment of Gastroenterology 2/e, p 180, 181

- Nausea and vomiting of pregnancy commonly termed *'morning sickness'* is a normal phenomenon in pregnancy, occurring in about 70% of all pregnancies.
- In most women, it is limited to the first trimester or till 16 weeks of pregnancy, but a few may continue to have symptoms throughout pregnancy.

Contd...

Contd…

- Hyperemesis gravidarum is the other end of the spectrum characterised by severe nausea and intractable vomiting sufficient to interfere with nutrition causing weight loss, dehydration, ketosis, alkalosis and hypocalcemia.
- **Risk Factors:**
  - Maternal age > 35 years
  - Nulliparity
  - Cigarette smoking
  - Fetal loss
  - Unplanned pregnancy
  - Hyperthyroidism
  - High body weight
  - H mole
  - Twin pregnancy
  - Positive family history
- **Clinical features are due to:**
  - Dehydration
  - Starvation
  - Ketoacidosis

Management: Mild to moderate nausea and vomiting of pregnancy – usually needs no treatment except reassurance and frequent small meals. Vitamin B_6 alone or with doxylamine is safe and can be considered.

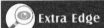 **Extra Edge**

- Vitamin deficiencies associated with hyperemesis gravidarum: *—Williams Obs. 23/e, p 1051*
  - Thiamine deficiency leading to Wernicke encephalopathy.
  - Vitamin K deficiency.
- Level of various minerals in hyperemesis gravidarum:
  - Plasma zinc levels increased.
  - Plasma copper levels decreased.
  - Plasma magnesium levels unchanged.

18. **Ans. is b, i.e. Decrease in renal output**
    Ref. Dutta Obs. 7/e, p 157; Current Diagnosis and Treatment of Gastroenterology 2/e, p 180, 181

    Indications for therapeutic termination in hyperemesis gravidarum:
    - Steady deterioration in spite of therapy
    - Rising pulse rate of 100/min or more
    - Temperature constantly above 38°C (100.4°F)
    - Gradually increasing oliguria and proteinuria[Q]
    - Appearance of jaundice[Q]
    - Appearance of neurological complications.

19. **Ans. is a, i.e. Mallory-Weiss syndrome**   *Ref. Williams 24/e, p 1074*

    Upper gastrointestinal bleeding:

    "Occasionally, persistent vomiting may be accompanied by worrisome upper gastrointestinal bleeding. The obvious concern is that there is a bleeding peptic ulceration. However, most of these women have minute linear mucosal tears near the gastroesophageal junction. Women with these so called Mallory-Weiss tears usually respond promptly to conservative measures."   *—Ref. Williams 23/e, p 1053*

    With persistent retching the less common but more serious oesophageal rupture– **'Boerhaave syndrome'** may develop.

20. **Ans. is a, i.e. Surgery at earliest**   *Ref. Williams Obs. 24/e, p 1074*

    Diagnosis of appendicitis during pregnancy is difficult as symptoms of appendicitis viz nausea, vomiting anorexia are normally present in pregnancy.

    But once the diagnosis is made immediate surgery should be done.

    "If appendicitis is suspected, treatment is prompt surgical exploration. Even though diagnostic errors sometimes leads to removal of a normal appendix, it is better to operate than to postpone intervention until generalized peritonitis has developed."

    Route:

    Before 20 weeks– Laparoscopy

    After 20 weeks–Laparotomy (Incision should be made at McBurney's point)

    Earlier it was believed CO_2 pneumoperitoneum created during laparoscopy can cause fetal acidosis and hypoperfusion, but now it is not so considered.

21. **Ans. is a or b, i.e. Severity increases in 3rd trimester; or Severity increases in 2nd trimester**

Ref. Williams Obs. 23/e, p 1056

Ulcerative colitis and pregnancy:

"In a meta-analysis of 755 pregnancies, Fonager and Colleagues (1998) reported that ulcerative colitis quiescent at conception worsened during pregnancy in about a third of cases. In woman with active disease at the time of conception, 45% worsened, 25% remained unchanged, and only 25% improved. These observations were similar to those previously described in an extensive review by Miller."

 Also Know:

Inflammatory bowel disease and pregnancy: Both forms of chronic inflammatory bowel disease are relatively common in woman of childbearing age. Donaldson concluded the following:
- Pregnancy does not increase the likelihood of an attack of inflammatory bowel disease. If the disease is quiescent in early pregnancy, then flares are uncommon, but if they develop, they may be severe (do not get confused, this statement is a generalised statement for IBD whereas the above statement is specific for ulcerative colitis).
- Active disease at conception increases the likelihood of poor pregnancy outcome.
- Diagnostic evaluations should not be postponed, if their results are likely to affect management.
- Many of the usual treatment regimens may be continued during pregnancy, and if indicated, surgery should be performed.

Effect of ulcerative colitis on pregnancy: In mild or quiescent UC and CD, fetal outcome is nearly normal Spontaneous abortions, stillbirths, and developmental defects are increased with increased disease activity, not medications.

—Harrison 16/e, p 1788

From the above text it is clear that severity of ulcerative colities increases during pregnancy. But sorry friends, no where it is mentioned, whether severity increases in second or third trimester. If anyone of you guys get to know the correct answer, do tell us.

22. **Ans. is a, i.e. USG abdomen**

The answer is quite obvious and I do not think you need any reference for this one.

X-ray and CT scan should be avoided during pregnancy due to risk of radiation exposure.

23. **Ans. is a, i.e. Glucose**

Ref. Williams 23/e, p 124, Dutta Obs. 7/e, p 281

- Glycosuria during pregnancy is normally seen in 5-50% cases
- Reason = Increase in GFR + impaired tubular reabsorptive capacity for filtered glucose
- Mostly seen in mid-pregnancy
- For detecting glycosuria **second fasting morning sample** is collected
- Fasting glycosuria, if present, is omnious
- If glycosuria is seen on one occasion before 20 weeks or on 2 or more occasions thereafter or if glycosuria is present in a pregnant female who has a positive family H/O diabetes or has previously given birth to a macrosomic baby
- Glucose tolerance test should be done.

Management – Glycosuria does not require any treatment and it disappears after delivery.

- **Also Remember**

Questions asked on urine sample collection:
Q1. For urine pregnancy test → Best sample is – first voided morning urine sample.
Q2. For detecting glycosuria – Best sample is second voided morning urine sample.
Q3. For detecting urine infection – Best samples is – midstream clear catch urine sample.
Q4. For detecting proteinuria in PIH. Best sample – do not use 1st voided urine as it may be concentrated and may give a false high reading.
    Hence after 1st urine, any urine sample can be used.
Q5. In a patient with urinary fistula – urine sample can be collected by Foley's catheterization.

24. **Ans. is b, i.e. GFR decreases**

Ref. Dutta Obs. 7/e, p 222, Williams Obs. 23/e, p 719

In normal pregnancy – changes which occur in renal system are:

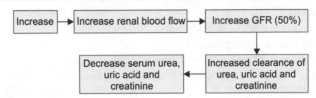

In case of PIH, as blood pressure increases, renal blood flow decreases (because pressure and volume are inversely related). So, GFR decreases in pregnancy and serum uric acid, urea and creatinine are increased in severe pre-eclampsia.

 Also Remember: Characteristic lesion in PIH is seen in the kidney, i.e. Glomeruloendotheliosis.
One of the earliest lab manifestations of pre-eclampsia is hyperuricemia.

25. **Ans. is b, i.e. Hypertension** *Ref. Sheila Balakrishnan 1/e, Paras Publication, p 320; Robbins 7/e, p 997*

Urinary tract infections in pregnancy:

These are the commonest bacterial infections seen in pregnancy.

Risk factors of UTI in pregnant as well as nonpregnant states:

• Urinary tract obstructions as in:
  – Tumors
  – Calculi
• Neurogenic bladder dysfunction as seen in case of:
  – **Diabetes**
  – Spinal cord injury
	• Vesicoureteric reflux as in:
	  – Incompetence of vesicoureteral valve
	  – Congenital absence of intravesical part of ureter
	  – Intrarenal reflux
	  – **Sickle cell disease and analgesics** – which cause papillary necrosis predisposing to UTI

26. **Ans. is b and e, i.e. Pencillin and cephalosporin** *Ref. Dutta 7/e, p 297; CMDT 07 p 800, 801; COGDT 10/e, p 375*

Principles for management of UTI during pregnancy:

• Single dose therapy is preferred
• The antimicrobial agent should be appropriate to the mother and fetus. Any one of the following drugs could be prescribed:
  – Ampicillin
  – Nitrofurantoin – DOC for prophylaxis of recurrent UTI in pregnancy
  – Cephalexin Cephalosporin
  – Amoxicillin-Clavulanic acid combination.
• Sulfonamides should not be given in the third trimester because they may interfere with bilirubin binding and thus impose a risk of neonatal hyperbilirubinemia and kernicterus.
• Fluoroquinolones are also contraindicated because of their potential teratogenic effects on fetal cartilage and bone.
• Tetracyclines, cotrimoxazole and ciprofloxacin are: contraindicated during pregnancy.

 Note: Before starting any antibiotic a midstream clean catch urine sample should be collected for culture.

Cranberry fruit juice is known to prevent recurrences of UTI. It prevents the adhesions of the pilins of E. coli to uroepithelium.

27. **Ans. is a, b, d and e, i.e. Most are usually asymptomatic in pregnancy, if untreated, progresses to pyelonephritis, Increase chance of premature infant and increase risk of chronic renal lesion.**

Ref. Williams Obs. 23/e, p 1035, 1036, COGD T, 10/e, p 374r

See the text for explanation.

28. **Ans. is a, i.e. Left kidney is involved in 50% of patients** *Ref. Fernando Arias 3/e, p 491; Dutta Obs. 7/e, 298*

Pyelonephritis in Pregnancy:

Etiology:

• Incidence in pregnancy is 1-3%
• More common in primigravida and young females
• Usually occurs in the second trimester after 16 weeks (>50%) but may occur in 1st and 3rd as well
• Generally bilateral, if unilateral it is more common on right side (in more than half of the cases)
• Most common organism responsible *E. coli* (70%), *Klebsiella* (10%).

29. Ans. is b, i.e. 12–16 weeks *Ref. Dutta Obs. 7/e, p 311; Jeffcoates 7/e, p 299*

Retroverted uterus is present in early weeks of pregnancy (in 15% cases).

Outcome of retroverted uterus in pregnancy:

Mostly spontaneous rectification occurs by 10–12 weeks.

In rare cases fundus fails to clear the promontory of sacrum and becomes impacted in pelvis at 12-14 weeks and blocks the opening of internal urethral sphincter leading to acute retention of urine (at 12-14 weeks) Management is immediate catheterization.

30. Ans. is a, i.e. Retroverted uterus *Ref. Dutta Obs. 7/e, p 311, 312, Jeffcotes Gynae Combination 7/e, p 493*

Well friends amongst the options given UTI and prolapse of uterus- cause increased frequency of urination and not retention. So we are left with 2 options – fibroid and irritability uterus.

Intrauterine fibroid commonly causes bladder irritability due to its weight leading to diurnal frequency.

Retroverted uterus: It is common during pregnancy and can lead to retention between 12 and 16 weeks. It is the best answer.

31. Ans. is d, i.e. Retroverted uterus *Ref. Dutta Obs. 7/e, p 311, 312*

In the question:

- Both fibroid and retroverted uterus can cause acute retention of urine during early pregnancy.
- But retroverted uterus will be the more correct option as:
  - It is common during pregnancy
  - Most common time of occurrence of urinary retention is second trimester – 12 to 16 weeks.

Also Know:

Other causes of retention of urine in pregnancy:

Early pregnancy   **During puerperium**

- Due to diminished bladder tone
- Retroverted uterus
- Impacted pelvic tumor

32. Ans. is d, i.e. Scleroderma *Ref. Williams Obs. 21/e, p 212; Fernando Arias 3/e, p 500, 501*

Prognostic indicators in renal disease and pregnancy:

- Most reliable prognostic indicator of the outcome of pregnancy is the presence of hypertension[Q]. The fetal prognosis for women with chronic renal disease is favorable as long as they do not develop superimposed preeclampsia.
- Second to hypertension, the most valuable prognostic index for patients with chronic renal disease during pregnancy is the degree of renal function impairment:
  - In patients with normal or only mildly impaired renal function, pregnancy does not accelerate renal damage
  - In patients with moderate renal insufficiency (serum creatinine of 1.4 mg/dL or greater before pregnancy or creatinine clearance <30 ml/min. there is a decline in renal function during pregnancy).
- Another important prognostic sign is the presence or absence of proteinuria. As a general rule, if the patient has 2+ or more protein in qualitative tests or 3 g or more in 24 hours urine collections at the beginning of pregnancy, the tendency will be toward increased protein losses and development of nephritic syndrome during pregnancy.
- The **histologic characteristics** of the renal lesion also have prognostic value.

Renal Disease	Effects
IgA nephropathy	Good prognosis
Systemic lupus erythematosus	Expect more problems than most glomerular diseases, but prognosis is most favourable, if disease is in remission for at least 6 months before conception.
Periarteritis nodosa and scleroderma	Associated with maternal deaths. Reactivation of quiescent scleroderma can occur during pregnancy and postpartum therapeutic abortion should be considered Fetal prognosis is poor.
Diffuse glomerulonephritis, membrano proliferative glomerulonephritis focal glomerulo sclerosis	Poor outcome

33. Ans. is a, i.e. Severe preeclampsia *Ref. COGDT 10/e, p 395; CMDT 07, p 1132*

Diabetes insipidus can be caused by:

Deficiency of antidiuretic hormone Resistance of ADH action
↓ ↓
Central diabetes insipidus Nephrogenic diabetes insipidus.

- A transient form of DI occurs during pregnancy due to:
  - Excessive placental production of vasopressinase
  - Decreased hepatic clearance due to abnormal liver function there in case of:
    a. Preeclampsia
    b. Fatty liver
    c. Hepatitis.
- Approximately 60% of women with previously known DI worsen, 20% improve and 20% do not change during pregnancy.
- Worsening is attributed to excessive placental vasopressinase production.
- Some females with DI who develop placental insufficiency show DI improvement, which is attributed to decreased vasopressinase production by the damaged placenta.

Symptoms: • Polyuria (4-15 liters/day)
 • Intense thirst particularly for ice cold fluids.

Diagnosis: is confirmed by water deprivation test.

Treatment: of choice intranasal L-deamino 8D arginine vasopressin (DDAVP) which is a synthetic analogue of ADH and is resistant to vasopressinase.

34. Ans. is a, i.e. Immediate removal *Ref. Dutta Obs. 7/e, p 310, Shiela Balakrishnan 1/e, p 265*

As discussed in the text, ovarian tumour in puerperium should be immediately removed.

35. Ans. is b, i.e. Ovariotomy at IInd trimester

36. Ans. is a, i.e. Surgical removal in IInd trimester *Ref. Dutta Obs. 7/e, p 310, Shiela Balakrishnan 1/e, p 265*

- Patient is presenting in the first trimester with ovarian cyst.
- The principle of treatment in case of ovarian tumour is to remove the tumour as soon as the diagnosis is made. But this principle should not be followed in the first trimester.
- Surgery in the first trimester is best avoided, as during surgery a corpus luteal cyst or ovary might be removed which will be detrimental to the pregnancy, which may end up in a miscarriage.
- Therefore, all such cases should be operated (ovariotomy/cystectomy) in the second trimester.
- *Therefore, the best time of elective operation for an ovarian tumor in pregnancy is between 14 to 18 weeks, as the chances of abortion are less and access to the pedicle is easy.*

37. Ans. is c, i.e. Dermoid cyst *Ref. Novak 14/e, p 510; Dutta Obs. 6/e, p 310*

"Incidence of dermoid cyst increases two times in pregnancy and it becomes the most commonly diagnosed ovarian tumour during pregnancy." —Dutta Obs. 7/e, p 310
"A benign cystic teratoma is the most common neoplasm to undergo torsion." —Novak 14/e, p 510

 Note: Benign cystic teratoma is another name for dermoid cyst.
From the above two lines it is clear that dermoid cyst is the most common ovarian tumour to undergo torsion during pregnancy.
For more details on dermoid cyst and other ovarian tumours kindly see *"Self Assessment and Review Gynaecology"* by the same author.

38. Ans. is a, i.e. Glioma

Ref. Williams Obs. 23/e, p 1140 for option b and d for option d, 1255; COGDT 10/e, p 398, for option c and d

Let us have a look at each option one by one
Pituitary adenoma (option b): Enlargement of both microadenomas and macroadenomas (≥ 10 mm) is seen during pregnancy, less in case of microadenoma and more in case of macroadenoma. —*Williams 23/e, p 1140*
"Neurofibromas and meningiomas although brain tumors are not specifically related to gestation, meningiomas, angiomas and neurofibromas are thought to grow more rapidly with pregnancy." —*COGDT 10/e, p 398*
"Lesions of neurofibromatosis may increase in size and in number as a result of pregnancy."
—*Williams 23/e, p 1191*

I did not get any text specifically mentioning the relationship between glioma and pregnancy but by exclusion the answer is Glioma.

 Remember: Tumours which increase in pregnancy:
- Meningioma   • Angioma
- Neurofibroma   • Pituitary microadenoma).

39. **Ans. is c, i.e. Red degeneration of fibroid** *Ref. Shaw 14/e, p 318, 326; Dutta Obs. 6/e, p 314, Fernando Arias 2/e, p 77*

Friends, the answer is quite obvious but let's see how other options can be ruled out.

Option "a" **Preterm labour.**

Points in favour	Points against
• Patient is pregnant • Pain in abdomen at 28 weeks (Preterm labour is where the labour starts before 37th completed weeks. The lower limit is 28 weeks in developing countries and 20 weeks in developed countries	• Preterm labour is diagnosed: – When there are regular uterine contractions (not acute pain), with or without pain at least once in every 10 minutes – Dilatation of cervix is ≥ 2 cm – Effacement of cervix = 80% – Length of cervix as measured by TVS ≤ 2.5 cm and funneling of the internal OS – Pelvic pressure, backache, vaginal discharge or vaginal bleeding. **None of the above criteria are being fulfilled** • Presence of leucocytosis and fever can also go against it as even if there is intraamniotic infection causing preterm labour: – Features like: *fever, leukocytosis, uterine tenderness* and *fetal tachycardia* are absent. Rather, if these features are present it means a final stage of uterine infection has reached. And here, our patient is having fever and leukocytosis without regular uterine contractions but with acute pain in abdomen so, *option "a"* is ruled out .

Option "b" **Torsion of fibroid**

Points in favour	Points against
• Patient has fibroid (though no mention has been made whether it is pedunculated or not, remember torsion is seen in subserous pedunculated myomas)[Q] • Patient is complaining of acute pain in abdomen.	• Orsion is not associated with fever and leucocytosis • It is rare.

Option "d" **Infection of fibroid**

Points in favour	Points against
Resence of fibroid (*Remember:* Infection is common in submucous fibroids)[Q] Fever Leucocytosis.	Acute pain in abdomen (infection of fibroid will not cause acute pain in abdomen) Infection of fibroid occurs following abortion or labour (here patient is pregnant but there is no history of abortion or labour) and m/c time for occurrence in pregnancy is puerperium Infection causes blood stained discharge (not seen in this patient).

So, from above discussion infection can be kept in +/– status. If we have no better option we can think about it.

Option "c" **Red degeneration of fibroid**

Red degeneration of fibroid: also called as *Carneous degeneration.*

- **It is seen mostly during mid pregnancy**[Q] (but can occur at other times, as well as in nonpregnant females also)[Q]
- It is an aseptic condition[Q]
- The myoma suddenly becomes acutely painful[Q], enlarged[Q] and tender[Q]

- *Patient presents with:*   – Acute abdominal pain[Q]   – Vomiting[Q]
  -    – Malaise[Q]   – Slight fever[Q]
- *Lab investigations:*   – Moderate leucocytosis[Q]   – Raised ESR[Q]

Pathological changes in the tumour:
- Fibroid becomes soft, necrotic or homogenous especially in its centre
- It is stained *Salmon pink*[Q], or red (due to diffusion of blood pigments from the thrombosed vessels)
- It has *fishy odour*[Q] (due to secondary infection with coliform organisms)
- *Histologically:* There is evidence of *thrombosis* in some vessels[Q]
- *Pathogenesis:* There is *subacute necrosis* of the myoma caused by an interference in blood supply *(aseptic infarction).*[Q]

Diagnosis is by ultrasound.

Differential diagnosis:
- Appendicitis[Q], Twisted ovarian cyst[Q], Pyelitis[Q] and Accidental hemorrhage[Q]
- So amongst above options — Red degeneration is the correct answer.

Management:
- *Conservative management*[Q]
- Patient is advised rest[Q]
- *Analgesics* are given to relieve the pain[Q]
- The acute symptoms subside in 3-10 days[Q] and pregnancy proceeds uneventfully.

40. Ans. is b, i.e. Conservative

41. Ans. is a, i.e. Analgesics   *Ref. Shaw 14/e, p 326; Dutta Obs. 6/e, p 309; Jeffcoate 7/e, p 502*

Management of Red degeneration of fibroid.
- Patient is managed conservatively[Q]
- Patient is put to bed rest and given analgesics[Q] (to relieve the pain), sedatives[Q] and, if required antibiotics[Q]
- If because of mistaken diagnosis laparotomy is done, abdomen is closed without doing anything
- Myomectomy should never be contemplated during caesarean section as vascularity of fibroid is increased during pregnancy (due to increased estrogen) leading to increased blood loss during cesarean section.[Q]

42. Ans. is b, i.e. Metronidazole   *Ref. Shaw 14/e, p 118; COGDT 10/e, p 601; Harrison 17/e, p 827*

Bacterial Vaginosis:
- It is an alteration in the normal vaginal flora (so, termed as vaginosis and not vaginitis)
- Polymicrobial in nature
- It is transmitted sexually[Q]
- Infection is favoured by decrease in the number of protective bacteria of vagina (*"Doderlein bacteria"* which release hydrogen peroxide and help in maintaining the acidic pH of vagina[Q])
- Symptoms:
  - 50% are asymptomatic
  - Rest complain of malodorous vaginal discharge with no irritation.[Q]

Diagnosis: By Amsel's criteria.
- Vaginal secretions are grey – white and thinly coat the vaginal walls[Q]
- pH > 4.5 (≈ 5 – 5.5) (i.e. increased vaginal pH)[Q]
- Whiff's test/Amine test is positive, i.e. addition of 10% KOH to vaginal secretions produces *Fishy odour*[Q]
- Presence of *'clue cells'* (> 20% of epithelial cells).[Q]

CLUE CELLS: are epithelial cells with granular cytoplasm.

Microscopic examination shows:
- Clue cells[Q]
- ↑ Number of gardnerella vaginalis[Q]
- ↓ Number of lactobacilli[Q]
- ↓ Leucocytes (conspicuously absent).[Q]

Treatment:
- DOC Metronidazole 500 mg twice daily for 7 days[Q]
- Treatment of male sexual partner does not improve therapeutic response and is not recommended.[Q]
- **In pregnancy:**
  - TOC is oral metronidazole after 1st trimester[Q]
  - Alternatively, clindamycin can be given
  - Topical application of metronidazole gel should be avoided during pregnancy.[Q]

43. Ans. is a, d and e, i.e. Cystitis, Appendicitis and Ruptured Ectopic

Ref. Dutta Obs. 7/e, p 305, Textbook of Obs. Sheila Balakrishnan, p 397

Causes of Acute Abdomen in Pregnancy:

Obstetrical		Non Obstetrical		
Early	Late	Medical	Surgical	Gynaecological
• Abortion • Ruptured ectopic pregnancy	• Abruptio placenta • Preterm labour • Polyhydramnios • Repture uterus • Severe pre-eclampsia and HELLP syndrome • Severe preeclampsia and liver rupture	• Pyelonephritis • Cystitis • Pancreatitis • Pyelitis	• Ac appendicitis • Ac cholecystitis • Intestinal or gastric perforation • Intestinal obstruction • Volvulus • Renal or ureteric • Calculi	• Torsion of ovarian cyst • Red degeneration of fiibroid • Retention of urine due to retro verted gravid uterus

From above table it is clear:

Cystitis (Option 'a'), appendicitis (Option d) and ruptured ectopic (Option e) can lead to acute abdomen in pregnancy. Although abortions can also cause acute abdomen, but then it is incomplete or inevitable abortions which are painful.

In case of threatened abortion

> **"The patient presents with amenorrhea followed by vaginal bleeding which is usually painless, but may be associated by mild abdominal pain backache."** —*Shiela Balakrishann 1/e, p 175*

Threatened Abortion

"Bleeding is usually painless but there may be mild backache or dull pain in lower abdomen." —*Dutta Obs 7/e, p 161*

This rules out threatened abortion.

Now coming to cervical incompetence – (option 'c')

In cervical incompetence patient typically presents with painless cervical dilatation and escape of liquor amnii followed by painless expulsion of products of conception.

Thus, it is also ruled out.

44. Ans. is d, i.e. Puerperium

Ref. Sheila Balakrishnan 1/e, p 386; Medical Disorders in Pregnancy and Update FOGSI, p 107

Tuberculosis in Pregnancy

Effect of pregnancy on TB

• If TB is under treatment, pregnancy does not worsen it
• Increased chances of relapse in puerperium and TB flares up during puerperium

 Remember: TB is not an indication for termination of pregnancy.

45. Ans. is b, i.e. Start category I ATT in first trimester

Ref. Textbook of Obs. Sheila Balakrishnan 1/e, p 387, Indian Journal of Tuberculosis

• TB during pregnancy, requires prompt treatment
• ATT can be given at any period in pregnancy, including the first trimester:
• **First line drug used are:**
    – INH, Rifampicin, ethambutol and pyrazinamide
    – Streptomycin is contraindicated during pregnancy[Q]
    – The 2 drugs which should be used throughout are – INH and Rifampicin
    – If a third drug is to be used it is usually ethambutol
    – Pyridoxine 50 mg is given along with chemotherapy.

Drug Regimen
Initial 3 drugs for 3 months followed by 2 drugs for 6 months
OR
Initial 4 drugs for 2 months followed by 2 drugs for 4 months

- Breastfeeding is not contraindication if the woman is on treatment[Q] but contraindicated if active lesions are present
- Baby should be given INH prophylaxis for 3 months. If montoux test is negative after 3 months, prophylaxis is stopped and BCG vaccination given.

46. Ans. is a, i.e. Streptomycin   *Ref. Harrison 17/e, p 1018; Williams Obs. 23/e, p 1005, 22/e, p 1065*

We all know streptomycin is contraindicated during pregnancy; earlier their were some doubts regarding the safety profile of pyrazinamide- but now it is absolutely clear that it can be given safely in pregnancy.

"The regimen of choice for pregnant women is 9 months of treatment with isoniazid and rifampicin, supplemented by ethambutol for the first 2 months. When required pyrazinamide may be given, although there are no data concerning its safety in pregnancy. Streptomycin is contraindicated because it is known to cause 8th cranial nerve damage in the fetus." —Harrison 16/e, p 962

"The 6 months regimen with pyrazinamide can probably be used safely during pregnancy and is recommended by the WHO and the international union against tuberculosis and lung disease." —Williams Obs. 22/e, p 1065

"Recommended initial treatment for pregnant patients is a three- drug regimen with isoniazid, rifampicin, and ethambutol. If the organism is susceptible the regimen is given for a total of 9 months. According to Bothamley (2001), all of these drugs are safe during pregnancy. Pyrazinamides added, if necessary. Indeed, the World Health Organization recommends initial therapy with the four-drug regimen for 6 months, as prescribed for nonpregnant adults."

So from above text it can be concluded that pyrazinamide is not contraindicated during pregnancy.

 Mnemonic

Antituberculosis drugs contraindicated in pregnancy:
K = Kanamycin
F = Fluoroquinolones
C = Capreomycin
A = Amikacin
S = Streptomycin
Mnemonic = KFC Always Surprising

47. Ans. is b, i.e. Seizure frequency increases in approximately 70% of women
Ref. Dutta Obs. 7/e, p 291; Harrison 17/e, p 2512; Sheila Balakrishnana 1/e, p 393, 394

Epilepsy in pregnancy:
- **Epilepsy is the most common neurological disorder encountered in pregnancy.**
- **The most common cause for epilepsy in pregnant women is idiopathic.**
- **Seizure frequencies is unchanged in 50% increased in 30% and decreased in 20% of pregnant females.**
- **Risk of congenital anomalies is about 4% and there is 5–10% risk of epilepsy in the child if parents are affected.**
- **All anticonvulsant drugs are associated with congenital anomalies as an interference with folic acid metabolism.**
- **All women on anticonvulsants should take folic acid: 4 mg/day for 12 weeks in the preconception period and throughout pregnancy.**

ACOG has recommended oral contraceptives containing 50 mg of estrogen in women with epilepsy and taking anticonvulsants.   —Williams Obs. 23/e, p 1167

48. Ans. is d, i.e. Folic acid   *Ref. KDT 7/e, p 414; Katzung g/e, p 383; Goodman Giliman 11/e, p 510*

- Hypotension and arrhythmias occur only on iv injection.
- Vitamin deficiencies associated with phenytoin: — Folic acid (most common)
    - Vitamin D
    - Vitamin K

These vitamin deficiencies occur in all patients an phenytoin therapy and have nothing do with pregnancy. Hence all patients on phenytoin are advised to take folic acid supplementation.

49. **Ans. is a, c and d, i.e. Valproate is associated with NTD, Carbamazepine is used as monotherapy and Phenytoin can produce foetal hydantoin syndrome** *Ref. Willams 24/e, p 1190*

Drug and associated abnormalities

Drug (Brand name)	Abnormalities Described
Valproate (Depakote)	Neural-tube defect, clefts, cardiac anomalies; associated developmental delay
Phenytoin (Dilantin)	Fetal hydantoin syndrome-craniofacial anomalies, fingernail hypoplasia, growth deficiency, developmental delay, cardiac anomalies, clefts
Carbamazepine; oxcarbazepine (Tegretol;Trileptal)	Fetal hydantoin syndrome, as above; spina bifida
phenobarbital	Clefts, cardiac anomalies, urinary tract malformations
Lamotrigine (Lamictal)	Increased risk for clefts (registry data)
Topiramate	Clefts
Levetiracetam (Keppra)	Theoretical— skeletal abnormalities; impaired growth in animals

50. **Ans. is d, i.e. Continue sodium valproate with regular monitoring of serum levels**
Ref. Williams Obs 23/e, p 1166, 1167, Textbook of Obs by Sheila Balakrishnan, p 394, Harrison 18/e, p 3266

As per ACOG and RCOG guidelines, there is no particular drug of choice for epilepsy in pregnancy

Valproate increases chances of birth defects much more than phenytoin, carbamazepine or phenobarbitone and hence if valproate is being used, it should be substituted by a lesser teratogenic drug.

Now in this question:

A 26-year-old primigravida with juvenile myoclonic epilepsy who has been using valproic acid comes to you at fourth month of pregnancy for advice.

Logically speaking if patient has myoclonic epilepsy in non pregnant states-DOC is valproic acid —Harrsion 18/e, p 3266 or lamotrigine, so her physician must have prescribed valproic acid to her. Ideally valproic acid should not be used during pregnancy as it is associated with a high risk of congenital malformations in the fetus. So if this patient would have come in the first trimester, I would have substituted it with some other antiepileptic drug like lamotrigine.

> *Note: "Carbamazepine, oxcarbazeine and phenytoin can worsen certain types of generalised seizures including myoclonic, tonic and atonic seizures."*
> —*Harrison 18/e, p 3266*
>
> • But since this patient is coming at 4th month, I will continue using valproic acid as the period of maximum teratogenicity is over. In addition I will do a lever II USG scan to rule out congenital anomalies and give folic acid supplementation 4 mg/day – therapeutic dose, to be continued throughout pregnancy.

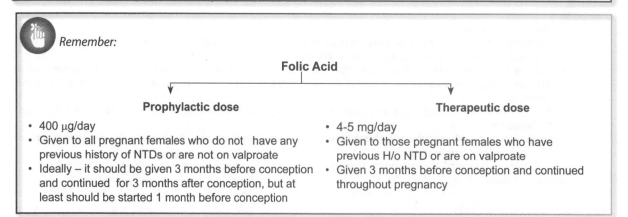

Remember:

Folic Acid

Prophylactic dose
- 400 µg/day
- Given to all pregnant females who do not have any previous history of NTDs or are not on valproate
- Ideally – it should be given 3 months before conception and continued for 3 months after conception, but at least should be started 1 month before conception

Therapeutic dose
- 4-5 mg/day
- Given to those pregnant females who have previous H/o NTD or are on valproate
- Given 3 months before conception and continued throughout pregnancy

- Dose of folic acid in tablets distributed free of cost by Government of India = 500 µg
- **Vitamin K 10 mg/day is given orally from 36 weeks onward to prevent hemorrhagic disease of new born.**

51. **Ans. is c and e, i.e. Primaquine and Tetracyclines** *Ref. Dutta Obs. 7/e, 296, 297; Harrison 17/e, p 1289, 1291, 1293*

- Malaria is life threatening in pregnancy, therefore benefits of treatment outweigh the potential risk of antimalarials.
- The commonly used antimalarials are not contraindicated in pregnancy.

- Chloroquine is the drug of choice for treatment and prophylaxis (even in pregnancy) of all varieties of malaria.

—Harrison 17/e, p 1293, Williams Obs. 24/e, p 1257

- According to Williams 24/e chloroquine should be used throughout pregnancy and primaquine should be used during postpartum period for malaria in pregnant moment.
- In chloroquine resistant P. vivax malaria-mefloquine is the DOC.
- In chloroquine resistant P. falciparum malaria-mefloquine or quinine is the drug of choice.

Chemoprophylaxis:

- Pregnant women in endemic areas are candidates for chemoprophylaxis.
- It is also recommended for travel to endemic areas.
- *Chloroquine is the drug of choice for prophylaxis* in pregnancy.
- Mefloquine is the only drug adviced for pregnant women who travel to areas with drug resistant malaria. This drug is generally considered safe in 2nd and 3rd trimester of pregnancy and the limited data on 1st trimester exposure are reassuring.

—Harrison 17/e, p 1293

- *"Proguanil is considered safe for antimalarial prophylaxis in pregnancy."*   *—Harrison 17/e, p 1293*

Antimalarials contraindicated in pregnancy:

- *"Tetracycline and doxycycline cannot be given to pregnant women".*

—Harrison 17/e, p 1291, 1289

- *"Primaquine should not be given to pregnant women and neonates.*   *—Harrison 17/e, p 1293*
- *"Primaquine and doxycycline are contraindicated in pregnancy".*   *—Williams 24/e, p 1257*

52. **Ans. is c, i.e. Cerebral infarction**   *Ref. Sheila Balakrishnan, p 696; Williams Obs. 22/e, p 364, 23/e, p 326, 327*

Cocaine addiction can cause – *miscarriage, intrauterine fetal death, PROM, preterm labour* **and** *IUGR.*

It can lead to the following Malformations in the fetus:

- Microcephaly, cutis aplasia, porencephaly, subependymal and periventricular cysts, ileal atresia, cardiac anomalies, visceral infarcts, limb reduction defects and genitourinary malformations.
- It produces cerebral infarction and periventricular leukomalacia in the fetus.
- The risk of malformations in the embryo/fetus is highest after the first trimester.

53. **Ans. is d, i.e. Chondrodysplasia punctata**   *Ref. Dutta Obs. 7/e, p 511*

Warfarin is an anticoagulant drug.

Action : Interferes with the synthesis of the vitamin K dependent factors like II, VII, IX and X.

Side effects:

- Hemorrhage
- *It leads to:* – Contradi's syndrome : skeletal and facial anomalies in the fetus
           – Chondrodysplasia punctata in the fetus.
- Miscarriage, IUGR and stillbirths accentuates neonatal hypothrombinemia.

54. **Ans. is a, i.e. Heparin**   *Ref. Dutta Obs. 7/e, p 511*

Heparin does not cross placenta and is safe during pregnancy.

It is the drug of choice for the management and prophylaxis of venous thromboembolism during pregnancy.

55. **Ans. is c, i.e. Calcium**   *Ref. KDT 6/e, p 598, 599; Harrison 17/e, p 2400*

Heparin can lead to osteoporosis. or hypocalcemia so, calcium supplementation is advisable with the use of heparin.

Also Know:

Durgs which may lead to hypocalcemia and hence calcium supplementation is necessary:

• Corticosteroids	• Cyclosporine
• Anticonvulsants	• Cytotoxic drugs
• Excessive alcohol	• Aromatase inhibitor
• Increase dose of thyroxine	• Aluminium
• GnRH	• Heparin
• Lithium	

56. Ans. is b, i.e. Isotretinoin *Ref. KDT 5/e, p 801; Sheila Balkrishnan, p 684*

Friends, *Remember* CNS anomaly (NTD) + CVS anomaly + facial defects are seen with the use of isotretinoin.

Drug	Teratogenicity
Alcohol	**Fetal alcohol syndrome (dose related)** Pre and postnatal growth restriction. Facial abnormalities like shortened palpebral fissure, low set ears, smooth philtrum, thinned upper lip and midfacial hypoplasia. CNS defects like microcephaly, mental retardation and behavioural disorders.
Warfarin	**Fetal warfarin syndrome[Q]** Chondrodysplasia punctata[Q], epiphyseal stippling, nasal hypoplasia, optic atrophy and microcephaly.
Phenytoin	**Fetal hydantoin syndrome[Q]** Hypertelorism, broad nasal bridge, low set ears, hypoplastic nails and digits.
Sodium valproate	**Fetal valproate syndrome[Q]** Brachycephaly with a high forehead, hypertelorism, small nose and mouth, shallow orbits, overlapping long fingers and toes and hyperconvex nails.
Diethyl stilboestrol	**Neural tube defects[Q]** Vaginal and cervical adenosis, clear cell adenocarcinoma, uterine anomalies, cryptorchidism and testicular hypoplasia.
Isotretinoin	Cleft palate, neural tube defect, microcephaly, deafness, blindness, cardiac defects like atrial septal defect and great vessel defects.[Q]
ACE inhibitors	Renal tubular dysgenesis, anuria and oligohydramnios.
Androgens and danazol	Masculinisation of a female fetus.
Antineoplastic agents	IUGR, craniosynostosis, micrognathia, severe limb abnormalities.
Tetracyclines	Discolouration of deciduous teeth.
Cocaine	Microcephaly, limb reduction defects and genitourinary malformations due to cerebral infarction.

Maximum sensitivity to teratogens is seen between 3-8 weeks.

57. Ans. is a, i.e. Ephedrine *Ref. COGDT 10/e, p 459*

Vasopressor of choice in pregnancy is ephedrine.

Vasopressors	
Which stimulate α adrenergic receptor. ↓ ↓ uterine tone and ↓ uteroplacental flow ↓ Fetal hypoxia so are not preferred. e.g.: Phenylephrine Methoxamine Mephentermine	**Which stimulate α + β adrenergic receptors** ↓ β₂ mediated vasodilation ↓ Less chances of fetal hypoxia ↓ Therefore they are the vasopressors of choice in pregnant females e.g.: Ephedrine

58. Ans. is a, i.e. Propylthiouracil *Ref. Dutta Obs. 7/e, p 288' KDT 6/e, p 250*

Propylthiouracil is used for medical management of hyperthyroidism during pregnancy. As far as other 3 options are concerned.

"Tetracycline and doxycycline cannot be given to pregnant women or to children <8 years of age."

—Harrison 17/e, p 1291

Tetracyclines should not be used in pregnant women and children <8 years because of the risk of dental discolouration/damage and inhibition of growth. *—Dutta Obs. 7/e, p 513, KDT 6/e, p 714*

"Anticancer drugs are contraindicated during pregnancy". —*Dutta Obs, 7/e, p 512*
(Methothexate)

"Warfarin can lead to contradis syndrome (skeletal and facial anomalies), optic atrophy, microcephaly and chondrodysplasia punctata." —*Dutta Obs, 7/e, p 510*

59. **Ans. is a, i.e. Brimonidine** *Ref. Internet search*

Drug	Category	Adverse effects
Beta-blockers	**Category C** (for oral beta-blockers) No specific categorization for topical beta-blockers	• Timolol can cross the placental barrier, thus resulting in fetal bradycardia and cardiac arrhythmia. • Furthermore, beta-blockers can be secreted into breast milk and may cause similar effects in newborn infants.
Alpha-2 Agonists	Category B	• Brimonidine poses substantial risk to the newborn, having been reported to cause central nervous system depression and apnea. • The drug penetrates the blood-brain barrier, and can cross the placenta and possibly excrete into breast milk, posing a real risk of apnea or hypotension in infants. • Thus, even if brimonidine is used during pregnancy, it should be discontinued before labor and during breastfeeding to prevent potential fetal apnea in the infant.
Prostaglandin analogues	Category C	• Associated with a high incidence of miscarriage in animal studies. • Oral or vaginal use of misoprostol in pregnancy is associated with an increased risk of Moebius syndrome and terminal transverse limb defects. • Prostaglandins can also stimulate uterine contractions producing premature labor.
Topical carbonic Anhydrase inhibitors Brinzolamide, Dorzolamide	Category C	• There were malformations of the vertebral bodies in rabbits exposed to dorzolamide during pregnancy, suggesting that brinzolamide may be a better alternative. • It is uncertain, if these medications are excreted in human milk.
Oral carbonic Anhydrase inhibitors Acetazolamide	Category C	• Systemic high dose carbonic anhydrase inhibitors in rats can result in forelimb anomalies. • Acetazolamide may also result in potential metabolic complications to the newborn or breast-feeding child.

Drugs for Glaucoma

Group	Drugs	Mechanism of Action	Adverse-effects
Miotics: • Direct acting • ACHE inhibitor	Pilocarpine Physostigmine	Trabecular outflow	• Blurred vision (induced myopia) • Headache, brow pain • Cataract formation • Iris cysts • Corneal hypoesthesia
Beta-blockers: • Nonselective (beta-1 and beta-2) • Selective (beta-2)	Timolol, Levobunolol Carteolol Betaxolol	Aqueous formation	• Allergic blepharoconjunctivitis • Transient stinging • Acquired nasolacrimal duct obstruction
Carbonic anhydrase inhibitors	Dorzolamide Brinzolamide	Aqueous formation	• Ocular allergy • Corneal edema • Bitter taste
Alpha-2 agonists	Apraclonidine Brimonidine	Aqueous formation	• Lid retraction • Dry mouth • Anterior uveitis • Drowsiness
Alpha-1 agonists	Dipivefrine Adrenaline	Trabecular and uveoscleral outflow	• Ocular allergy • Conjunctival hyperemia
Prostaglandin F2-alpha	Latanoprost Bimatoprost	Uveoscleral outflow	• Iris pigmentation • Growth of eyelashes • Macular edema

60. Ans. is d, i.e. Misoprostol   *Ref. Katzung Pharmacology 11/e, p 1029*

- **Möbius syndrome** is an extremely rare congenital neurological disorder which is characterized by facial paralysis and the inability to move the eyes from side to side.
- Most people with Möbius syndrome are born with complete facial paralysis and cannot close their eyes or form facial expression.
- They have normal intelligence.
- Möbius syndrome results from the underdevelopment of the VI and VII cranial nerves.
- Causes: The causes of Möbius syndrome are poorly understood. Möbius syndrome is thought to result from a vascular disruption (temporary loss of blood flow) in the brain during prenatal development. There could be many reasons for the vascular disruption leading to Möbius syndrome. The use of the drugs misoprostol or thalidomide or cocaine by women during pregnancy can lead to mobius syndrome.

61. Ans. is d, i.e. Propylthiouracil   *Ref. KDT 6/e, p 251,484,488,Dutta Obs 7/e, p 288*

Propylthiouracil is used for hyperthyroidism during pregnancy.

ACE inhibitors and Losartan should be avoided during pregnancy.

ACE inhibitors can cause fetal renal tubular dysplasia when used in second and third trimester leading to oligohydramnios, fetal limb contractures, craniofacial deformities and hypoplastic lung development.

62. Ans. is b, i.e. Hysterectomy (emergency obstetrics for doctors and midwives, course handbook, Milman School of Public Health)

Setting standards of emergency obstetrics and newborn care:

Basic emergency obstetric and newborn care provided in health centres, large or small include the facilities for:

- Administration of antibiotics, oxytocics and anticonvulsants.
- Manual removal of the placenta.
- Removal of retained products following miscarriage or abortion.
- Assisted vaginal delivery preferably with vacuum extractor.

Comprehensive emergency obstetrics and newborn care, typically delivered in district hospital, includes all basic functions above, plus cesarean section, safe blood transfusion and care to sick and low birth weight newborns including resuscitation.

It is recommended that for every 5,00,000 people there should be 4 facilities offering comprehensive essential obstetric care.

63. Ans. is c, i.e. Per 1 lac live birth   *Ref. Park 22/e, p 517*

The maternal mortality rate should be expressed as a rate per 1000 live births.

Maternal Mortality Rate:

$$\frac{\text{Total number of female deaths due to complications of pregnancy,}}{\text{children or within 42 days of delivery from "puerperal causes"}}{\text{in an area during a given year}} \times 100$$

In developed countries MMR has declined significantly so multiplying factor 100,000 instead of 1000 to avoid fractions in calculating MMR.

Also Know:

- Maternal mortality rate in India (2000 census) = 212 per 1 lac live birth.
- Most common cause of maternal mortality in India = Hemorrhage (38%) > sepsis (11%) > abortion (8%) > obstructed labour (5%) > hypertension (5%).
- Late maternal death is death of woman from direct or indirect obstetric causes more than 42 days but less than one year after termination of pregnancy.

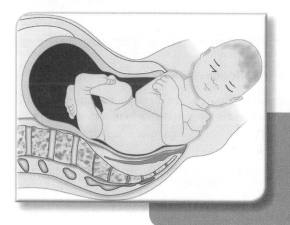

Chapter 27

Puerperium and its Abnormalities

Chapter at a Glance

➢ Definition
➢ Physiological Changes

➢ Menstruation and Ovulation

DEFINITION

Normal puerperium is the period 6 weeks after delivery during which the pelvic organs return to near prepregnant state and the physiological changes of pregnancy are reversed. *Involution is the process by which the genital organs revert to their prepregnant stage.*

Duration

Normal puerperium starts from expulsion of placenta and lasts up to 6 weeks. The period can be divided into the following three time periods:

1. **Immediate puerperium:** The first 24 hours after delivery.
2. **Early puerperium:** It is the period of the first week after delivery, beyond 24 hrs
3. **Remote puerperium:** Starts from the second week to six weeks postdelivery.

PUERPERIUM: PHYSIOLOGICAL CHANGES

Uterine Changes

Involution of the Uterus

- Just after delivery, the fundus of the contracted uterus is felt slightly below the umbilicus and is about 13 cm above the pubic symphysis. After 48 hours, the uterus begins to shrink at a rate of 1.25–1.5 cm (about 1/2 inch) per day and lies at level of pubic symphysis by 10th–12 day after delivery to become a pelvic organ in 2 weeks time and regains its non-pregnant position 4 weeks after delivery.

- Uterus weighs 1000 g at delivery, 500 g after one week, 300 g after two week and 100 g after end of 3 weeks 60 gm non-pregnant size at end of 6 weeks.

Contd...

Contd...

Clinical significance
- The ideal time to do tubectomy is within 1 week of delivery and called as **postpartum sterilization**
- Beyond 1 week, Tubectomy is done after 16 weeks of delivery called as **Interval sterilization.**
- **Postpartum sterilization** is done by Minilaparotomy. Laparoscopy cannot be done in postpartum period .

- Total number of muscle cells do not decrease but their size decreases significantly. This is due to increase in activity of uterine collagenase and release of proteolytic enzymes as a result of withdraw of estrogen and progesterone in puerperium.

 Note: Delayed involution is called subinvolution.

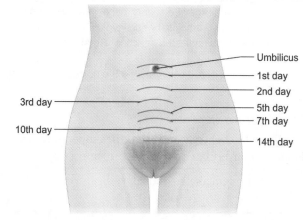

Umbilicus
1st day
2nd day
3rd day
5th day
7th day
10th day
14th day

Fig. 27.1: Involution of uterus during the first two weeks of puerperium.

Causes of Subinvolution

1. Infection like endometritis
2. Retained product of conception
3. Fibroid uterus
4. Uterus was overdestended

Investigations: to do: USG

Management: Gentle curettage and antibiotics

 Note: Postpartum curettage can lead to Asherman syndrome.

Endometrial Regeneration

- The superficial part of the decidua becomes necrotic, sloughs off and is shed in the form of lochia.
- The basal layer of the endometrium near the myometrium remains intact.
- Regeneration of the endometrium is very fast covering the epithelium within a week and is completed in exactly 16 days.
- Regeneration is slowest at placental site (approximately 6 weeks).

LOCHIA:
- It is the vaginal discharge for the first fortnight during puerperium
- The discharge originates from the uterine body, cervix and vagina.
- It has got a peculiar offensive fishy smell.
- Its reaction is alkaline tending to become acid towards the end.
- Depending upon the variation of the color of the discharge, it is named as:
  - Lochia rubra (red) 1-4 days. (RBC)
  - Lochia serosa (5-9 days) — (the color is yellowish or pink or pale brownish).
  - Lochia alba — (pale white) — 10-15 days

Composition:
- **Lochia rubra** consists of blood, shreds of fetal membranes and decidua, vernix caseosa, lanugo and meconium.
- **Lochia serosa** consists of less RBC but more leukocytes, wound exudate, mucus from the cervix and microorganisms (anaerobic streptococci and staphylococci).
- **Lochia alba** contains plenty of decidual cells, leukocytes, mucus, cholestrin crystals, fatty and granular epithelial cells and microorganisms.

 Note:

- The average amount of discharge for the first 5–6 days, is estimated to be 250 mL.
- The normal duration may extend up to 24–36 days (Williams 24/e, p 670). The red lochia may persist for longer duration especially in women who get up from the bed for the first time in later period.

Clinical importance:
- The discharge may be scanty, especially following premature labors or in case of infection or may be excessive in twin delivery or hydramnios, or subinvolution of uterus and retained bits of conception.
- If malodorous, indicates infection. Retained plug or cotton piece inside the vagina can also be a cause should be kept in mind.
- Persistence of red color beyond the normal limit signifies subinvolution or retained bits of conceptus.

Temperature

There may be slight reactionary rise in temperature of 0.5 °F following delivery but it comes down to normal by 12 hours.

 Note: Temperature should not be more than 37.2°C (99 °F) in first 24 hours.

Breast engorgement may cause slight rise in temperature on third day but it should not last for more than 24 hours.

Urinary Tract

The bladder in puerperium has increased capacity and is insensitive to the raised intravesical pressure due to trauma to the nerve plexus during delivery. Therefore, the bladder can be overdistended and incomplete emptying is common in the puerperium which can lead to UTI.

Gastrointestinal Tract

Constipation is common due to slight intestinal paresis.

Loss of Weight

There is an immediate loss of about 5 kg due to delivery of the fetus, placenta, amniotic fluid and blood loss. At the end of 6 weeks, most women lose the excess 4 kg weight accumulated during pregnancy through excretion of the fluids and electrolytes.

Fluid Loss

About 2 L of fluid is lost within the first week and 1.5 L in the next 5 weeks after delivery through loss of extracellular fluid.

Endometritis

- Infection of uterine endometrium
- M/C site: Site where placenta was attached
- M/C manifestation: Puerperal pyrexia, i.e. temperature ≥ 100.4°F.

Remember:

- M/C cause of puerperal pyrexia: Endometritis
- M/C organism responsible: Group A streptococci
- M/C organism for late onset endometritis—chlamydia.
- Apart from this in most cases: It is a mixed infection (aerobic + anaerobic)
- Highest risk of endometritis—is with cesarean section (cesarean has 13 times more chances of endometritis than vaginal delivery).

Other Risk Factors

- Iron deficiency anemia
- Prolonged labour
- PROM
- Bacterial vaginosis

M/C route of spread: Direct spread from cervix and vagina.

Signs of Endometritis: Fever and uterine tenderness are present. All Inflammatory markers are raised (ESR, WBC & CRP)

Management: Broad spectrum antibiotics, i.e. gentamicin + clindamycin or ampicillin

Changes in Cervix

- **External OS:** In a nulliparous female: The cervix is pinpoint or circular
- After delivery, the cervix is transverse slit like
- Transformation zone rebuilds in this time and is very susceptible to infection.

Vagina: Comes back to normal size and shape

- Its rugosities appear by 3 weeks
- But its elasticity is not properly regained, that contributes to occurrence of prolapse
- Not only this, birth trauma itself is a risk factor for prolapse[Q]

Hematocrit Changes

Hypercoagulable state is seen in early puerperium due to rise in platelets and coagulation factors making women more prone for thromboembolism.

Breast

- **Hormone responsible for milk secretion—Prolactin**
- **Hormone responsible for milk ejection—Oxytocin**

Prolactin

- Maximum levels of **prolactin seen during pregnancy (not lactation)[Q]**
- Increased Prolactin leads to amenorrhea due to its inhibitory effect on GnRH.[Q]
- This is the reason for lactational amenorrhea
- DOC for hyperprolactinemia: Cabergoline
- DOC for hyperprolactinemia in infertile female: Bromocriptine
- Drugs which are needed for increasing milk secretion (Galactogogue):
    - Metoclopramide
    - Nipple stimulation
    - Breast pump
- Drugs to suppress milk secretion (in case of IUD)
    - DOC—Cabergoline
    - Bromocriptine
    - Injection Mixogen (high dose estrogen)
- This is not used as it can a lead to venous thrombosis.

C/I for Breastfeeding

- Mother is alcoholic
- Mother is I/V drug abuser
- Mother has breast cancer or is on any anticancer drug
- Active herpes lesion on breast

- Active pulmonary TB
- Baby has lactose intolerance/Galactosemia

 Remember: HIV in mother is not a C/I for breast-feeding in developing countries.

Mastitis
- Infection of breast parenchyma.
- M/C organism Staphylococcus aureus

Psychological Problems

Mnemonic: <u>Bi</u><u>pa</u>rietal <u>di</u>ameter

	Seen in	Onset	Symptoms	Due to
Bi: Postpartum blues	50-60%	• Occurs within 10 days of delivery • Gradual onset	Mildest variety T/t: form reassurance and care needed	Progesterone withdrawal
Parietal: Postpartum psychosis	< 1%	• Sudden onset • Occurs in 10-14 days of delivery	Most dangerous variety T/t: antipsychotic drug	
Diameter: Postpartum depression	10-20%	• Gradual occurs in 4-6 months of delivery	Moderate form T/t: SSRI: Fluoxetine	Changes in HPO axis

Thrombophlebitis
- Endometritis of placental site can lead to thrombophlebitis
- Hence M/C site for thrombophlebitis: Placental site
- M/C vein involved: Right side ovarian vein.
- In patients of endometritis if cropite of antibiotics, patient has pain and spikes of fever or sometimes a tender mass can be palpated at the cornua of uterus.
- IOC: CT or MRI
- Management: High dose antibiotics + heparin.

MENSTRUATION AND OVULATION IN PUERPERAL FEMALE

- In non-lactating women, menstruation may resume in about 40% by the 6th week and 70–80% by the 12th week. In lactating women, menses may not appear so long as the infant is breast fed.
- Ovulation returns @ 7 weeks (between 5–11 weeks).
- *Lactating mothers usually do not menstruate or ovulate because of increased levels of prolactin which suppresses the release of LH and inhibits the ovarian response of FSH.*

CONTRACEPTIVE OF CHOICE IN LACTATING FEMALES

IUCD (Best answer)   Progesterone only pills
↓   (2nd best answer)
Copper IUCD.

- M/C source of infection—Infant's nose and mouth
- Symptoms: Seen in 3-4 weeks
- It is mostly unilateral. Patient complains of fever, breast tenderness

 Note: It is not a C/I for breastfeeding. In 10% cases it can lead to breast abscess. Its management is incision and drainage.

Management: Penicillin/Dicloxacillin and milk expression

Time of insertion of Cu IUCD

- **Post placental insertion:** It has higher expulsion rate but is highly effective. Government of India advocates post- placental insertion of CuT 380A.
- Insertion within 48 hours of delivery called as **postpartum insertion**
- Or it can be inserted after 6-8 of weeks of delivery.

Timings of Other Contraceptives

	Non breastfeeding	Breastfeeding
LNG-IUCD	Immediately	4 weeks
Progesterone only pills	Immediately	4-6 weeks
Combined oral pills	3 weeks	6 months
Barrier contraceptive	After female	After female
	Resumes coital activity	Resumes coital activity

 Note: Females should be adviced to resume, coital activity minimum after 6 weeks of delivery.

New Pattern Questions

N1. A 24-year-old P2+0 woman presents to the emergency department complaining of pain in her right breast. The patient is postpartum day 10 from an uncomplicated spontaneous vaginal delivery at 42 weeks. She reports no difficulty breast-feeding for the first several days postpartum, but states that for the past week her daughter has had difficulty latching on. Three days ago her right nipple became dry and cracked, and since yesterday it has become increasingly swollen and painful. Her temperature is 38.3°C (101°F). Her right nipple and areola are warm, swollen, red, and tender. There is no fluctuance or induration, and no pus can be expressed from the nipple.
   a. Continue breastfeeding from both the breasts
   b. Breastfeed from unaffected breast only
   c. Immediately start antibiotics and breastfeed only when antibiotics are discontinued.
   d. Pump and discard breastmilk till infection is over and then continue breatfedding
   e. Stop breastfeeding immediately.

N2. Sarita, a 30-year-old woman develops a deep vein thrombosis in her left calf on fourth postoperative day following cesarean section done for fetal distress. The patient is started on heparin and is scheduled to begin a 6 weeks course of warfarin therapy. The patient is a devoted mother who wants to breastfeed her baby. What is the advice which is given to the patient:
   a. Patient may continue breastfeeding at her own risk
   b. Patient should breastfeed her baby only if her INR is at <2.5
   c. Patient can breastfeed her baby after 6 weeks course of warfarin is over
   d. Warfarin is not a contraindication for lactation
   e. Warfarin is absolutely contraindicated during lactation

N3. You are called to a maternity ward to see a 23 year-old primi patient who had delivered a 2.7 kg baby boy 2 days back. She had a normal vaginal delivery and placenta delivered spontaneously. Now she complains of bloody vaginal discharge with no other signs. O/E you notice a sweetish odour bloody discharge on the vaginal walls and introitus. Sterile pelvic examination shows a soft nontender uterus. Her P/R-78/min, B/P-110/76 mm of hg, temp-37°C,R/R-16/min. Her WBC count =10,000 with predominant granulocytes. What is the most appropriate step?
   a. Currettage
   b. Oral antibiotics
   c. Reassurance
   d. Order urinalysis
   e. Vaginal culture

N4. Which of the following sets of condition is attributed to normal physiology of puerperium?
   a. Tachycardia and weight gain
   b. Retention of urine, constipation and weight gain
   c. Constipation, tachycardia and retention of urine
   d. Retention of urine and constipation

N5. The uterus becomes pelvic organ after delivery in:
   a. 10 to 12 days
   b. 12 to 14 days
   c. 14 to 16 days
   d. 16 to 18 days
   e. 18 to 20 days

N6. Without breastfeeding the first menstrual flow usually begins – weeks after delivery:
   a. 2-4 weeks
   b. 4-6 weeks
   c. 6-8 weeks
   d. 8-10 weeks
   e. More than 10 weeks

N7. Common route of spread of puerperal sepsis:
   a. Lymphatic
   b. Direct invasion
   c. Skip lesion
   d. Hematogenous

N8. The cause of 'postpartum blues' is:
   a. Decreased estrogen
   b. Decreased progesterone
   c. Increased prolactin
   d. Decreased estrogen and progesterone

N9. All are complication of formula fed baby over human milk fed baby *except*:
   a. Necrotizing enterocolitis
   b. Otitis media
   c. Hypocalcemia
   d. Vitamin K deficiency

N10. All of the following are true regarding after pains *except*:
   a. M/C in multiparous females
   b. Pain worsens when infant suckles
   c. Decreases in intensity by 5th day
   d. They become more pronounced as parity increases

N11. For first 2 hrs after delivery, temperature should be recorded:
   a. Every 5 mins
   b. Every 15 mins
   c. Every 30 mins
   d. Hourly

N12. M/C nerve injured during normal vaginal delivery is:
   a. Femoral N
   b. Lateral femoral cutaneous N
   c. Iliohypogastric N
   d. Ilio inguinal N

N13. Which of the following steps has proven benefit in decreasing puerperal infection following cesarean section:
   a. Non closure of peritoneum
   b. Single layer uterine closure
   c. Administration of single dose of ampicillin or 1st generation cephalosporin at the time of cesarean delivery
   d. Skin closure with staples than with suture

Previous Year Questions

1. **Postpartum decidual secretions present are referred to as:** [AI 97/ MAHE 05]
   a. Lochia
   b. Bleeding per vaginum
   c. Vasa-previa
   d. Decidua-capsularis

2. **Lochia in correct order: during puerperium:**
   a. Rubra, serosa, alba [AIIMS Nov 2013]
   b. Serosa, rubra, alba
   c. Alba, serosa, rubra
   d. Alba, mucosa, serosa

3. **Likely size of uterus at 8 weeks postpartum is:**
   a. 100 gm   b. 500 gm   [AI 97]
   c. 700 gm   d. 900 gm

4. **A pregnant female has past history of embolism in puerperium. What medical management she should take in next pregnancy to avoid this:** [AIIMS Nov 99]
   a. Cumpulsory prophylaxis with warfarin start at 10 weeks
   b. To take warfarin after delivery
   c. Chance of thromboembolism increases by 12% in next pregnancy
   d. Does not need anything

5. **Initiation of lactation is affected by:** [PGI Dec 01]
   a. Oxytocin   b. Prolactin
   c. HPL   d. Thyroid hormone
   e. Progesterone

6. **Decrease lactation seen in:** [PGI Dec 03]
   a. Maternal anxiety   b. Antibiotic therapy
   c. Cracked nipple   d. Breast abscess
   e. Bromocriptine therapy

7. **Contraindication to breast milk feeding:**
   a. Mother is sputum negative [PGI June 01]
   b. Bromocriptine therapy for mother
   c. Heavy breast engorgement
   d. Ca breast
   e. Mother on domperidone

8. **Contraindications for breastfeeding are all *except*:**
   a. Hepatitis-B infection of mother [PGI June 00]
   b. Lithium treatment of mother
   c. Acute bacterial mastitis
   d. Tetracycline treatment of mother

9. **About colostrum true statements are:** [PGI 03]
   a. Secreted after 10 days of childbirth
   b. Rich in immunoglobulin
   c. Contains more protein
   d. Contains less fat
   e. Daily secretion is about 10 ml/day

10. **In comparison to breast milk, colostrum has higher content of:**
    a. Carbohydrates   b. Fat
    c. Sodium   d. Potassium

11. **Which of the following is more correct about breast infection during lactation?** [AI 08]
    a. Due to bacteria from Infant's GIT
    b. Mastitis does not affect the child
    c. *E. coli* is the only organism
    d. Can lead to abscess and I and D may be required

12. **Contraceptive method of choice in lactating mothers is:** [AI 09]
    a. Barrier method
    b. Progesterone only pill
    c. Oral contraceptive pills
    d. Lactational amenorrhea

13. **Most common immunoglobulin secreted by mother in milk and colostrum is:** [PGI June 97]
    a. IgA   b. IgG
    c. IgE   d. IgD

Answers with Explanations to New Pattern Questions

N1. **Ans. is a, i.e. Continue breastfeeding from both the breasts**
Ref. Dutta Obs, 7/e, p 439; William Obs, 22/e, p 703, 23/e, p 653; COGDT 10/e, p 245

A postpartum lady coming with H/o pain in breast and fever and nipples being warm, red, swollen, with no induration, fluctuance and no pus extruding from them - leaves no doubt that the patient is having mastitis. As discussed in question 9, mastitis is not a contraindication for breastfeeding. She should continue feeding from both the breasts.

N2. **Ans. is d, i.e. Warfarin is not a contraindication for lactation**

 Remember:

- Warfarin is contraindicated in the first trimester of pregnancy as it can lead to contradi syndrome comprising of microcephaly, optic atrophy, nasal hypolplasia and chondrodysplasia punctate. It can also lead to IUGR, abortions and IUD.
- But warfarin is absolutely safe during lactation as an extremely minute quantity of it is excreted in breast milk.

N3. **Ans. is c, i.e. Reassurance**
Ref. Dutta Obs 7/e, p 146

This patient is a puerperal female who is complaining of bloody vaginal discharge with no other significant abnormal signs. On examination there is a sweetish odour bloody discharge on the vaginal walls and introitus. Her vitals are normal suggesting that this cannot be PPH (The most common cause of secondary PPH is retained bits of placenta for which curettage is done, but here it is not required).

Slight amount of bloody discharge called as lochia is absolutely normal for the first 15 days after delivery and does not require any treatment, so we will reassure the patient and do nothing.

Do not get confused with the finding of WBC count, 10,000 with predominant granulocytes as this is a normal finding in the puerperal period. Note- leucocytes can rise to as high as 25000 during puerperium probably as a response to the stress of labor). Since lochia has no foul smell it means no infection and so no need for culture or antibiotics.

N4. **Ans. is d, i.e. Retention of urine and constipation**
Ref. Dutta Obs. 7/e, p 146
General Physiological Changes in Puerperium

Pulse	• It increases for few hours after delivery and then settles down to normal.
Temperature	• In the first 24 hrs-temp should not be above 99°F • – On day 3, due to breast engorgement there may be slight rise of temperature. (**Note:** Rule out UTI if there is rise of temperature).
Weight	• Loss of 2 kg (5 lb) occurs due to diuresis.
Blood volume	• Decreases after delivery and returns to pre-pregnant levels by the second week.º
Cardiac output	• Rises after delivery to 60% above the pre-labour value, and returns to normal within one week.
Fibrinogen levels and ESR	• Remain high up to the second week of puerperium, ESR levels also remain high.
Urinary tract	• Retention of urine is common. • Patient should be encouraged to pass urine following delivery.
GIT tract	• Thirst increased • Constipation (due to intestinal paresis)

N5. **Ans. is a, i.e. 10 to 12 days**
Ref. Dutta Obs. 7/e, p 145; COGDT 10/e, p 222, 223, Fig 12-1
Now, this is a tricky one :
Till now we have studied that by the end of 2 weeks uterus becomes a pelvic organ i.e. involution is complete. But as far as number of days are concerned some of you may think, 12-14 days as the correct answer. *COGDT 10/e, p 222 says—*

"At the end of first postpartum weeks, it (uterus) will have decreased to the size of a 12 week gestation and is just palpable at pubic symphysis. At 7th day it is at the level of pubic symphysis and by 10th day it is an intrapelvic organ.

Suppose even if we did not have COGDT reference still-

Dutta says– Just after delivery uterus is 13.5 cm above pubic symphysis and thereafter its size decreases by 1.25 cm/ day which means by 10-12 days it will be an intrapelvic organ (i.e. below the level of pubic symphysis).

N6.   Ans. is c, i.e. 6–8 weeks   *Ref. Williams 24/e, p 678, p 147*

Women not breastfeeding have return of menses usually within 6 to 8 weeks.   *—Dutta Obs. 7/e, p 147*

Also Know: Ovulation occurs at a mean of 7 weeks, but ranges from 5–11 week.

The Rule of 3's:

- In the presence of FULL breastfeeding, a contraceptive method should begin in the ***3rd postpartum month***.
- With PARTIAL breastfeeding or no breastfeeding, a contraceptive method should begin during the ***3rd postpartum week.***

N7.   Ans. is b, i.e. Direct invasion   *Ref. Dutta Obs 7/e, p 433; Williams Obs. 22/e, p 714, 23/e, p 663*

- ***Puerperal pyrexia*** – is defined as a rise of temperature reaching 100.4° F (38° C) or more (measured orally) on 2 separate occasions at 24 hours apart (excluding first 24 hours) within first 10 days following delivery.
- Any infection of genital tract which occurs as a complication of delivery is called as ***Puerperal sepsis.***
- ***Most common site*** of Puerperal infection – Placental site. In vaginal delivery and uterine incision in cesarean section.
- ***Most common manifestation*** of Puerperal infection – Endometritis.
- ***Most common cause*** of Puerperal sepsis – Streptococcus.
- ***Most common route*** of infection – Direct spread.
- Single most significant risk factor for development of puerperal sepsis (uterine infection) = Route of delivery (It is M/C in cesarean delivery than vaginal delivery)
- ***Mgt:*** Clindamycin + Gentamicin ± Ampicillin

N8.   Ans. is d, i.e. Decreased estrogen and progesterone   *Ref. Dutta Obs 7/e, p 443; COGDT 10/e, p 1020*

Puerperal Blues/3 Days Blues/Baby Blues
- It is transient state of mental illness observed 4–5 days after delivery in nearly 50% of postpartum women.
- Postpartum blues occurs at the height of hormonal changes.   *—COGDT 10/e, p 1025*
- Patients present with *depression, anxiety, fearfulness, insomnia, helplessness and negative feelings towards infant.*
- It may last from a few days to 2–3 weeks.
- Generally self limited, 20% of women may develop depression in the first postpartum year.

Treatment: Reassurance and psychological support of family members.

Postpartum Depression
- It is observed in 10-20% of mothers.
- It is more gradual in onset over the first 4-6 months following delivery or abortion.
- Changes in hypothalamo-pituitary-adrenal axis may be a cause.
- Manifested by loss of energy and appetite, insomnia, social withdrawal, irritability and even suicidal attitude.
- **Risk of recurrence 50-100% in subsequent pregnancies.**

Treatment: Should be started early. Fluoxetine or paroxetine is effective and has fewer side effects.

According to Kaplan, the cause of postpartum blues is :

"The sudden decrease in estrogen and progesterone immediately after delivery may also contribute to the disorder, but treatment with these hormones are not effective."

N9.   Ans. is d, i.e. Vitamin K deficiency
            Ref. Net Search (www.uspharmacist.com) Infant Formula vs Breast Milk; Ghai 6/e, p 164, 177, 331

Formula feeds contain a host of vitamin and minerals, as well as trace elements (zinc, mangnese, copper, iodine) and electrolytes.

In formula feeds vitamin K is added in higher levels than in breast milk to reduce the risk of hemorrhagic diseases in new born. So, vitamin K deficiency can never be a complication of formula fed babies.

Now let's see what *Ghai 6/e, p 164, 331, 177* has to say on the rest of options.

Option *"a"*   i.e. **Necrotizing enterocolitis**

"Almost all patients of neonatal necrotizing enterocolitis (NEC) are artificially fed prior to the onset of illness. Breast milk is protective for NEC."   —Ghai 6/e, p 164

Option *"b"*   i.e. **Otitis media**

"Otitis media is one of the most common infections of early childhood. Anatomic features which make this age group particularly susceptible to ear infection include shorter, more horizontally placed and compliant eustachian tube, which permits reflux of nasopharyngeal secretions into the middle year. A high incidence of bacterial carriage in the adenoids may also contribute to the frequency of otitis media in children. Other risk factors include exposure to cigarette smoke, over crowding, bottle feeding, cleft palate, allergic rhinitis, Down's syndrome and disorders of mucocilliary transport."   —Ghai 6/e, p 331

Option *"c"*   i.e. **Hypocalcemia**

"In the neonatal period there is transient hypoparathyroidism. As a result, less phosphate is excreted in the urine. Human milk is low in phosphate, but cow's milk is rich in phosphate. Immature parathyroid in the neonates cannot easily cope with excess phosphate in cow's milk leading to hypocalcemia in top fed babies".   —Ghai 6/e, p 177

N10. **Ans. is c, i.e. Decreases in intensity by 5th day**   *Ref. Williams 24/e, p 670*

- **After pains** – In primiparous women, uterus tends to remain tonically contracted following delivery. In multiparas, however, it often contracts vigorously and gives rise to after pains.
- After pains are similar to uterine contractions but milder than them.
- More pronounced as parity increases.
- Worsen with suckling of breast by infant.
- Decrease in intensity and become mild by 3rd day following delivery.

N11. **Ans. is b, i.e. Every 15 minutes**   *Ref. Williams 24/e, p 675*

Hospital care after delivery:
- For 2 hours after delivery, BP and pulse should be taken every 15 minutes.
- Temperature assessed every 4 hours for the first 8 hours and then 8 hourly subsequently.
- Amount of vaginal bleeding should be monitored.
- Fundus of uterus palpated to ensure that it is well contracted (uterus should be closely monitored for at least 1 hour after delivery because of risk of PPH)

N12. **Ans. is b, i.e. Lateral femoral cutaneous N**   *Ref. Williams 24/e, p 677*

Obstetrical neuropathies:
- M/C nerve injured during vaginal delivery- **Lateral femoral cutaneous nerve** followed by femoral nerve
- Risk factors: Nulliparity, prolonged second stage of labor, pushing for a longer period in semifowler position
- M/C nerves injured during cesarean section- Iliohypogastric N and Ilioinguinal N.

N13. **Ans. is c, i.e. Administration of single dose of ampicillin or 1st generation cephalosporin at the time of cesarean delivery**   *Ref. William 24/e, p 685*

- The only proven way of decreasing uterine infection following cesarean section is administering a single dose of ampicillin or 1st generation cephalosporin at the time of cesarean delivery.
- Rest none of the steps like single layer closure of uterus, closure of peritoneum, use of stapler to close skin incision instead of surtures, etc. are not proven to have any benefits as far as incidence of infection is considered following surgery.

Answers with Explanations to Previous Year Questions

1. **Ans. is a, i.e. Lochia** Ref. Dutta Obs. 7/e, p 146

2. **Ans. is a, i.e. Rubra, serosa, alba** Ref. Dutta Obs. 7/e, p146

LOCHIA:
- It is the vaginal discharge for the first fortnight during puerperium
- The discharge originates from the uterine body, cervix and vagina.
- It has got a peculiar offensive fishy smell.
- Its reaction is alkaline tending to become acid towards the end.
- Depending upon the variation of the color of the discharge, it is named as:
  - Lochia rubra (red) 1-4 days.
  - Lochia serosa (5-9 days) — the color is yellowish or pink or pale brownish.
  - Lochia alba — (pale white) — 10-15 days.

Composition:
- **Lochia rubra** consists of blood, shreds of fetal membranes and decidua, vernix caseosa, lanugo and meconium.
- **Lochia serosa** consists of less RBC but more leukocytes, wound exudate, mucus from the cervix and microorganisms (anaerobic streptococci and staphylococci).
- **Lochia alba** contains plenty of decidual cells, leukocytes, mucus, cholestrin crystals, fatty and granular epithelial cells and microorganisms.

Note:
- The average amount of discharge for the first 5–6 days, is estimated to be 250 mL.
- The normal duration may extend up to 24–36 days (Williams 24/e, p 670). The red lochia may persist for longer duration especially in women who get up from the bed for the first time in later period.

Clinical importance:
- The discharge may be scanty, especially following premature labors or in case of infection or may be excessive in twin delivery or hydramnios, or subiinvolution of uterus and retained bits of conception.
- If malodorous, indicates infection. Retained plug or cotton piece inside the vagina can also be a cause should be kept in mind.
- Persistence of red color beyond the normal limit signifies subinvolution or retained bits of conceptus.

3. **Ans. is a, i.e. 100 gm** Ref. Dutta Obs. 7/e, p 145; Williams Obs. 24/e, p 669

Weight of uterus :

Immediately after delivery	–	1000 gm
At the end of 1 week	–	500 gm
At the end of 2 weeks	–	300 gm
At the end of 4 weeks it weighs	–	100 gm (Pre-pregnant state)
At the end of 6 weeks it weighs	–	60 gm

Also Know:
- Immediately following delivery, the fundus is just below the umbilicus (13.5 cm above the symphysis pubis/ 20 weeks gestational age size.).[Q]

Involution of the uterus
- After 24 hours of delivery, height of uterus decreases by 1.25 cm/day.[Q]
- Uterus is a pelvic to organ.[Q] by the end of 2 weeks.

- Uterus returns almost to its normal size (pre-pregnant size) by the end of 8 weeks.
- The process by which the postpartum uterus returns to its pre-pregnant state is called as *Involution.*
- Involution is achieved by decrease in the size of muscle fibres[Q] (and not in the number).[Q]
- **Placental site involution:** Immedietly after delivery placental site is palm size. By the end of 2 weeks it is 3–4 cm in diameter.

 Note: Doppler USG shows continuously increasing uterine artery vascular resistance during first five days postpartum.

4. **Ans. is b, i.e. To take warfarin after delivery**   *Ref. Williams 23/e, p 1028, 29, Table 47.6*

Friends venous thromboembolism in pregnancy, is one of those topics which we do not study in detail during undergraduation. So, I am giving in brief, all the important points you need to remember:

Venous thromboembolism in pregnancy
- Venous thromboembolism is the leading cause of maternal deaths in developed countries.
- Pregnancy increases the risk of thromboembolism 6 times as all components of *Virchow's triad* are increased.[Q]

A. Deep vein thrombosis:
- Left sided DVT is more common than right sided DVT.
- Homans sign-i.e. pain in calf muscles on dorsiflexion of foot is positive.

Investigations
- Recommended method during pregnancy: Doppler ultrasound
- Gold standard (in conditions other than pregnancy): Venography
- Though objective evidence is ideal, treatment should be started on clinical grounds, if confirmatory tests are not available.

Management

- **Drug of choice in pregnancy is** unfractionated heparin
- Low molecular weight heparins (enoxaparin, dalteparin) are safe during pregnancy and breastfeeding. But they should not be used in
  - i. Women with prosthetic valves
  - ii. Renal failure
  - iii. With regional analgesia

Warfarin is not safe during pregnancy as it crosses placenta and can cause fetal malformations (Conradi syndrome). The single undisputed use for warfarin in pregnancy is in women with prosthetic heart valves.

Monitoring is done by – APTT and Platelet count.

Protocol

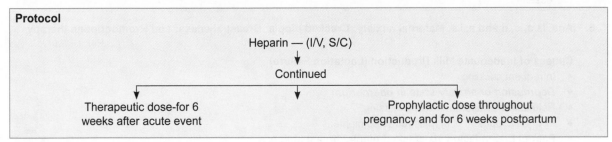

Heparin — (I/V, S/C)

↓

Continued

Therapeutic dose-for 6 weeks after acute event   Prophylactic dose throughout pregnancy and for 6 weeks postpartum

For postpartum venous thrombosis, treatment with IV heparin and warfarin are started simultaneously 6-8 hours after vaginal delivery and 24 hours after cesarean section and once INR is between 2 and 3, heparin is discontinued and warfarin is continued for 6 weeks.

 Note: Warfarin is absolutely safe in lactation.

Thromboprophylaxis

Women at risk of venous thromboembolism during pregnancy have been grouped into different categories depending on the presence of risk factors. Thromboprophylaxis to such a woman depends on the specific risk factor and the category.

(1) A low risk woman has no personal or family history of VTE and are heterozygous for factor V Leiden mutation. Such a

woman need no thromboprophylaxis, (2) A high risk woman is one who has previous VTE or VTE in present pregnancy, or antithrombin–III deficiency. Such a woman needs low molecular weight heparin prophylaxis throughout pregnancy and postpartum 6 weeks. Women with antithrombin-III deficiency can be treated with antithrombin-III concentrate prophylactically. Now lets have a look at the question: It says a female with previous history of embolism becomes pregnant, what medical management should be given to her.

Option 'a' i.e. Compulsory prophylaxis with warfarin at 10 weeks.

• It is absolutely wrong as warfarin is not given during pregnancy.

Option 'b' i.e. to take warfarin after delivery - As discussed above, in all high risk patients, post partum prophylaxis with warfarin has to be given as peuperium is the time of greatest risk for embolism/thromboembolism. Thus option b is correct.

During pregnancy: A women with previous H/O embolism becomes high risk patient. In such patients prophylaxis with heparin needs to be given. Hence option 'd' is incorrect.

5. **Ans. is a, b, c and e, i.e. Oxytocin; Prolactin; HPL; and Progesterone**

Ref. COGDT 10/e, p 238 239, Dutta 7/e, p 148-149, 239

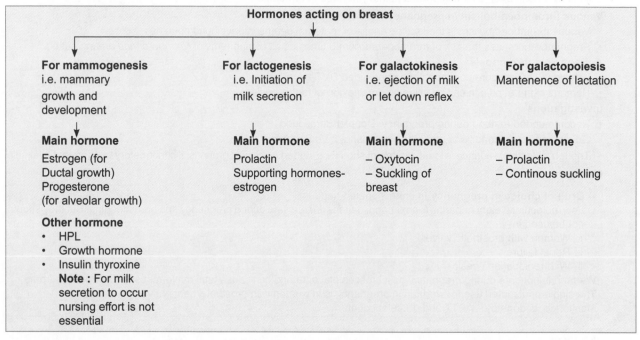

6. **Ans. is a, c, d and e, i.e. Maternal anxiety; Cracked nipple; Breast abscess; and Bromocriptine therapy**

Ref. Dutta Obs. 7/e, p 439

Causes of Inadequate Milk Production (Lactation Failure)

• Infrequent suckling.
• *Depression or anxiety state in puerperium*
• Reluctance or apprehension to nursing.
• Poor development of nipples/retracted nipple.
• **Painful breast lesion viz cracked nipple/ breast abscess.**
• Endogenous suppression of prolactin.
• Prolactin inhibition (ergot preparation, diuretics, pyridoxine, bromocriptine).

Note: Lactation suppressors and galactagogues

Lactation suppressors	Galactagogues/drugs milk secreting
1. Bromocriptine/cabergoline	1. Nipple stimulation
2. Testosterone	2. Breast pump
3. Ethinyl estradiol	3. Metoclopramide
4. Pyridoxine	4. Intranasal oxytocin
5. Sulpiride	

7. **Ans. is b and d, i.e. Bromocriptine therapy for mother; and Ca breast**   *Ref. COGDT 10/e, p 242, 702; 23/e, p 652*

CONTRAINDICATIONS TO BREASTFEEDING
- Mother on IV drug abuse/excess alcohol.
- In females undergoing treatment for breast cancer (ACOG 2000)
- Mother on anticancer drugs or other teratogenic drugs.
- Active Herpes simplex lesions of the breast.
- Active/untreated pulmonary tuberculosis in mother.
- Galactosemia and congenital lactose intolerance in infant.
- *HIV-positive mother if she can afford formula feeds.*

Hepatitis B/C infections are concerned they are not contraindications to breastfeeding.
Infants of seropositive hepatitis B mothers should be given Hepatitis B Immunoglobulin (IM) within 12 hours of birth.

 Also Know:

HIV in developing countries is not a contraindication for breastfeeding.

Medications contraindicated during lactation.   *—COGDT 10/e, p 242*

Medication	Reason
Bromocriptine	Suppresses lactation; may be hazardous to the mother
Cocaine	Cocaine intoxication
Cyclophosphamide	Possible immune suppression; unknown effect on growth or association with carcinogenesis;
Cyclosporine	neutropenia
Doxorubicin	Possible immune suppression; unknown effect on growth or association with carcinogenesis;
Ergotamine	Possible immune suppression; Unknown effect on growth or association with carcinogenesis;
Lithium	Vomiting, diarrhea, convulsions (at doses used in migraine medications)
Methotrexate	Possible immune suppression; unknown effect on growth or association with carcinogenesis;
Phencyclidine	Neutropenia
Phenindione	Potent hallucinogen
Radioactive iodine	–

8. **Ans. is a, c and d, i.e. Hepatitis B infection of the mother; Acute bacterial mastitis; and Tetracycline treatment of mother**   *Ref. COGDT 10/e, p 242; Williams Obs. 22/e, p 702, 704; 23/e, p 652-654*
Breastfeeding is not contraindicated in case of maternal hepatitis B infection as explained in previous question.
Option 'b' Lithium is contraindicated during pregnancy and lactation (*see* Answer 7)
Option 'c' i.e. Acute bacterial mastitis.
"In case of acute bacterial mastitis breastfeeding should be continued as it is helpful in avoiding abscess formation. If the infected breast is too tender to allow suckling, gentle pumping until nursing can be resumed is recommended."   *—Williams Obs. 22/e, p 704*
Option 'd' Tetracycline : according to KDT
"Tetracycline is secreted in breast milk and can cause teeth discoloration and impaired growth in infants and children therefore is contraindicated during lactation."   *—KDT 5/e, p 850*
But all other books and extensive internet search (*see* Drug.com/Rxlist.com) says that tetracycline is not contraindicated during lactation but should be used cautiously in nursing mothers.

9. **Ans. is b, c and d, i.e. Rich in immunoglobulin; Contains more protein; and Contains less fat**
    Ref. Dutta Obs. 7/e, p 148; Ghai 6/e, p 150; COGDT 10/e, p 240;

10. **Ans. is c, i.e. Sodium**   *Ref. Dutta Obs 7/e, p 148*
Colostrum is a deep yellow serous fluid secreted from breasts *starting from pregnancy and for 2-3 days after delivery.*
Composition
- It has higher specific gravity and *higher protein, Vitamin A, D, E, K, immunoglobulin, sodium and chloride content than mature breast milk.*

- It has lower *carbohydrate, fat and potassium* than mature milk.

Advantages

- Antibodies (IgA, IgG, IgM) and humoral factor (lactoferrin) provide immunological defence to the new born.
- Laxative action due to fat globules.
- It is an ideal natural starter food.

Extra Edge

	Protein	Fat	Carbohydrate	Water
Colostrum	8.6	2.3	3.2	86
Breast milk	1.2	3.2	7.5	87

11. Ans. is d, i.e. Can lead to abscess formation for which I and D may be required

Ref. Dutta Obs 7/e, p 439; William Obs 24/e, p 691; COGDT 10/e, p 245

Mastitis is parenchymatous infection of breast.

Most common organism causing breast infection: *Staphylococcus aureus*
Others: • Coagulase negative Staphylococci • Viridian Streptococci. • Symptoms appear in the 3rd or 4th week. • Infection is almost always unilateral

"The immediate source of organism that cause mastitis is almost always the infant's nose and throat."

—*William Obs. 24/e, p 691*

(Not GIT so *option "a"* is incorrect)

- Predisposing factors : fissures/abrasions or cracks in nipples.
- Mastitis is not a contraindication for breastfeeding.

Treatment

In patients not sensitive to penicillin	Patients allergic to penicillin
Dicloxacillin (DOC for emperical therapy)	Erythromycin

- Treatment to be given for 10-14 days.
- About 10% of women with mastitis develop an abscess due to variable destruction of breast tissue.

    If abscess is formed - surgical drainage is done under general anaesthesia (i.e. *option "d"* is correct).

12. Ans. is b, i.e. Progesterone only pill

Ref: Williams Obs, 23/e, p 694, Dutta Obs, 7/e, p 558

"According to the American college of obstetries and gynaecologist (2000), progestin only contraceptives are the preferred choice in most of the cases. In addition IUD's may be recommended for the lactating sexually active woman after uterine involution."

—*Williams, Obs 24/e, p 715*

Lactational amenorrhea

"For mothers who are nursing exclusively, ovulation occurring during the first 10 weeks after delivery is unlikely. But it is not a reliable method if mother is nursing only in day time. Waiting for first menses involves a risk of pregnancy because ovulation usually antedates menstruation."

—*Willams 24/e, p 715*

Safe period method – In this method the fertile period is calculated and the female should refrain from having sex during that period

The basic prerequisite of this method is that cycles should be regular which is usually not the case with lactating mothers – safe period method is not applicable in them.

IUCD's – According to Williams 23/e p 644 IUCD's can be used as an alternative to progesterone only pills by lactating mothers but only following complete uterine involution in woman who are sexually active.

Remember in Nutshell
1st contraceptive of choice in lactating mother – Progesterone only pill or progesterone implant or DMPA injection. IUCD can also be used.

13. **Ans. is a, i.e. IgA**   *Ref. Dutta Obs. 7/e, p 148; Ghai 6/e, p 97*

Composition of Breast Milk:
Carbohydrate – Lactose is present in high concentration in breast milk.
Protein content is low, as the baby cannot metabolise a high protein diet. The proteins are mainly lactalbumin and lactoglobulin, which are easily digestible. It is also rich in the aminoacids taurine and cysteine, which are necessary for neurotransmission and neuromodulation.
Fats - Breast milk is rich in polyunsaturated fatty acids (PUFA) needed for myelination.
Water and electrolytes - The water content is 86-87%.
Immunological superiority - Breast milk contains immunoglobulins, especially IgA and IgM, lysozyme, lactoferrin (which protects against enterobacteria), bifidus factor (to protect against E.coli), PABA (which protects from malaria).
"Breast milk has a high concentration of secretory IgA, IgM".   —*Ghai 6/e, p 97*
"Colostrum –Contains antibody (IgA) produce locally".   —*Dutta Obs. 6/e, p 149*

Therefore, IgA is the option of choice.

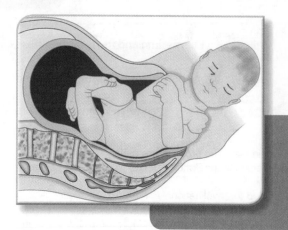

Chapter 28

Fetal Growth Disorders

Chapter at a Glance

➢ Fetal Growth
➢ IUGR
➢ Macrosomia

FETAL GROWTH

- Fetal growth is characterized by sequential patterns of tissue and organ growth, differentiation, and maturation.
- Fetal growth has been divided into three phases. The initial phase of hyperplasia occurs in the first 16 weeks and is characterized by a rapid increase in cell number. The second phase, which extends up to 32 weeks' gestation, includes both cellular hyperplasia and hypertrophy. After 32 weeks, fetal growth is by cellular hypertrophy, and it is during this phase that most fetal fat and glycogen are accumulated. The corresponding fetal-growth rates during these three phases are 5 g/day at 15 weeks' gestation, 15 to 20 g/day at 24 weeks, and 30 to 35 g/day at 34 weeks.
- Insulin and insulin-like growth factors, particularly insulin-like growth factor-I (IGF-1), have an important role in regulation of fetal growth and weight gain.
- Other hormones implicated in fetal growth are hormones derived from adipose tissue. These hormones are known broadly as adipokines and include leptin, the protein product of the *obesity gene*. Fetal leptin concentrations increase during gestation, and they correlate with birth weight.
- Fetal growth is also dependent on an adequate supply of nutrients. Both excessive and diminished maternal glucose availability affect fetal growth. Reducing maternal glucose levels may result in a lower birth weight. Excessive glycemia produces macrosomia.

Gestational Age and Birth Weight

Previously, the birth weight of ≤ 2500 g was taken as the index of prematurity without taking any consideration of the gestational period or any other factors. But infants born at term or post-term may weigh ≤ 2500 g and occasionally a baby of diabetic mother may weigh much more than 2500 g even before 37 weeks. Therefore, survival outcome of an infant depends both on the gestational age as well as on the birth weight. Gestational age and birth weight are related by the following terms:

a. **Small for gestational age (SGA):** Birth weight less than 10th percentile for gestational age.

b. **Appropriate for gestational age (AGA):** Birth weight lies between the 10th and 90th percentiles for gestational age.

c. **Large for gestational age (LGA):** Infant's birth weight above the 90th percentile for gestational age.

   – **Low birth weight (LBW) infant is defined as one whose birth weight is less than 2500 g irrespective of the gestational age.** *Very-low birth weight (VLBW)* infants weigh 1500 g or less and *extremely-low birth weight (ELBW)* infants weigh 1000 g or less (WHO).

   – **Preterm**—Preterm Birth (PTB) is defined as one when birth occurs before completion of 37 menstrual weeks of gestation regardless of birth weight. The growth potential may be normal and appropriate for the gestational period (10th to 90th percentile).

– **Small for gestational age (SGA)**—About 70% of infants with a birth weight below the 10th percentile are found normally grown. **They are constitutionally small and not at any increased risk for adverse outcome**. They present at the end of the normal spectrum for growth. The remaining 30% are truly growth restricted.

Types of SGA Fetus

Based on clinical evaluation and ultrasound examination:

Type I	• Fetuses that are small and healthy • They have normal ponderal index, normal subcutaneous fat and usually have uneventful neonatal course.
Type II	• Fetuses where growth is restricted by pathological process (true IUGR) • These are further divided into symmetrical IUGR (20%) and asymmetrical IUGR (80%).

IUGR

Intrauterine growth restriction (IUGR) is said to be present in those babies whose birth weight is below the tenth percentile of the average for the gestational age. Growth restriction can occur in preterm, term or post-term babies.

Depending upon the relative size of their head, abdomen and femur, the fetuses are subdivided into: (a) Symmetrical or Type I (b) Asymmetrical or Type II.

Symmetrical (20%): The fetus is affected from the noxious effect very early in the phase of cellular hyperplasia. The total cell number is less. This form of growth retardation is most often caused by structural or chromosomal abnormalities or congenital infection (TORCH). **The pathological process is intrinsic to the fetus and involves all the organs including the head**.

Asymmetrical (80%): The fetus is affected in later months during the phase of cellular hypertrophy. The total cell number remains the same but size is smaller than normal. The pathological processes that too often result in asymmetric growth retardation are maternal diseases extrinsic to the fetus. These diseases alter the fetal size by reducing uteroplacental blood flow or by restricting the oxygen and nutrient transfer or by reducing the placental size.

Comparison of Symmetric and Asymmetric IUGR

Symmetric IUGR (20%)	Asymmetric IUGR (80%)
• Symmetrically small	• Head is larger than abdomen
• Head/abdomen and femur/abdomen ratios normal	• Elevated head/abdomen and femur/abdomen ratios
• Normal ponderal index associated with genetic disease, infection	• Low ponderal index due to mainly placental vascular insufficiency
• Total number of cells—decreased	• Total number of cells—same
• Cells size—normal	• Cells size—decreased
• Poor prognosis	• Good prognosis

Causes of IUGR

Maternal	Fetal	Placental	Unknown (~ 40%)
• Constitutional[Q]: Small mothers	• Structural anomalies – Cardiovascular – Renal – Osteogenesis imperfecta	• Causes leading to poor uterine blood flow to the placental site for long time, i.e. placental insufficiency (MC) – Placenta praevia[Q] – Abruption[Q] – Infarction – Placental hemangiomas – Chronic villitis – Hemorrhagic endovasculitis	
• Poor maternal nutrition[Q]: During pregnancy	• Chromosomal abnormalities – Trisomy 13, 18, 21[Q] – Turner syndrome[Q]		

Contd...

Contd...

Maternal	Fetal	Placental	Unknown (~ 40%)

• Social deprivation[Q]	• Infections (fetal infection)
	  – Rubella, CMV, Herpes simplex virus, Varicella virus, and HIV
	  – Malaria		

• Maternal diseases
  – Chronic hypertension/PIH[Q]
  – Thrombophilia[Q], hemoglobinopathy
  – Heart disease[Q] Class III and IV
  – Chronic renal disease
  – Collagen vascular disease
  – Diabetes with vascular lesion
  – Sickle cell anemia
	• Multiple pregnancy		

• *Toxins*: Alcohol, Smoking[Q], Heroin, Morphine, Cocaine			
• *Drugs*: Chemotherapeutic agents, Warfarin and Phenytoin			

Diagnosis

Diagnosis of IUGR by Clinical Method

- **Maternal weight gain:** *Maternal weight gain is an insensitive index of fetal growth.* The association between poor maternal weight gain and small babies has been demonstrated in one study but most of the studies have found that this association has questionable clinical value and that the weight gain is normal in a significant number of mothers who deliver small babies.

- **Uterine fundal height:** Measurement of the uterine fundal height is the most common method used to clinically estimate fetal growth. Fundal height is measured in centimeters from the upper border of the pubic symphysis to the top of the fundus of the uterus.

- **Symphysiofundal height (SFH):** Measurement in centimeters closely correlates with gestational age after 24 weeks. A lag of 4 cm or more suggests growth restriction. It is a fairly sensitive parameter (30-80%). Serial measurement is important.

Biochemical markers have also been used to assist the diagnosis. Erythropoietin level in cord blood is high in IUGR fetuses.

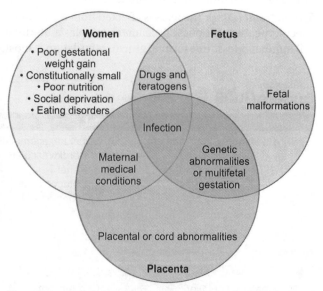

Fig. 28.1: Risk factors and causes of impaired fetal growth centering on the mother, her fetus and the placenta

Diagnosis of IUGR by Ultrasound Examination

Parameter	Feature
Biparietal diameter	Serial measurement of BPD can diagnose IUGR but has low sensitivity and low specificity as the head is one of the last organs affected by fetal malnutrition. Also, late in pregnancy, the fetal head begins to undergo a moulding process as it dips into the pelvis, making it difficult to obtain adequate measurements.
Abdominal circumference	Abdominal circumference (AC) is the single most sensitive parameter to detect IUGR. Serial measurements of AC and estimations of fetal weight are more diagnostic to fetal growth restriction. It has a negative predictive value of 99%, i.e. normal AC rules out the possibility that the baby is small.
Estimated fetal weight	Fetal weight estimates are usually within 5–10% of the true fetal weight. It is valuable in the diagnosis of small fetuses but does not differentiate between IUGR babies and babies who are small and healthy.
Head to abdomen ratio (HC/AC)	The ratio compares the most preserved organ in the malnourished fetus, i.e. the brain, with the most compromised organ, the liver. The AC should be measured at the level of the bifurcation of the hepatic vein in the center of the fetal liver.
	The fetal head circumference should be measured at the level of thalami. An advantage of using the head circumference instead of the BPD is that the effect of head moulding is minimised. Fetal malnutrition should be suspected when the HC/AC ratio is abnormally high. In asymmetric IUGR, HC is ↑, HC/AC >> 1. In symmetric IUGR, both HC and AC are decreased. So HC/AC remains normal.
Femur to abdomen ratio	Normally the femur to abdomen ratio remains constant after 20 weeks. Normal value 22 ± 2 High femur to abdomen ratio suggests fetal growth restriction.
Fetal ponderal index $PI = \dfrac{Estimated\ fetal\ wt.}{(FL)^3}$	The degree of fetal wasting is judged by fetal PI. PI is independent of gestational age and has constant value throughout the second part of pregnancy. Normal PI = 8.325 ± 2.5 Fetal PI ≤ 7 should be considered abnormal, which strongly suggests fetal malnutrition.
Oligohydramnios	It is a late manifestation of fetal malnutrition.
Doppler velocimetry Most Important	Abnormal umbilical artery Doppler velocimetry findings—characterized by absent or reversed end-diastolic flow—have been uniquely linked with fetal-growth restriction. It has also been correlated with hypoxia, acidosis and fetal death. Umbilical artery Doppler velocimetry is considered standard in the evaluation and management of the growth-restricted fetus. American College of Obstetricians and Gynecologists (2013a) notes that umbilical artery Doppler velocimetry has been shown to improve clinical outcomes.

Complications

Fetal: (a) Antenatal—Chronic fetal distress, fetal death

(b) Intranatal—Hypoxia and acidosis

(c) After birth.

Immediate: (1) Asphyxia, bronchopulmonary dysplasia and RDS. (2) Hypoglycemia due to shortage of glycogen reserve in the liver. (3) Meconium aspiration syndrome (4) Microcoagulation leading to DIC. (5) Hypothermia. (6) Pulmonary hemorrhage. (7) Polycythemia, anemia, thrombocytopenia. (8) Hyperviscosity-thrombosis. (9) Necrotizing enterocolitis due to reduced intestinal blood flow. (10) Intraventricular hemorrhage (IVH). (11) Electrolyte abnormalities: hypocalcemia, hyperphosphatemia, hypokalemia due to impaired renal function. (12) Multiorgan failure. (13) Increased perinatal morbidity and mortality.

Late: Asymmetrical IUGR babies tend to catch up growth in early infancy. The fetuses are likely to have: (1) retarded neurological and intellectual development in infancy. The worst prognosis is for IUGR caused by congenital infection, congenital abnormalities and chromosomal defects. **Other long-term complications** are: (2) Increased risk of metabolic syndrome in adult life: obesity, hypertension, diabetes and coronary heart disease (CHD). (3) LBW infants have an altered orexigenic mechanism that causes increased appetite and reduced satiety. (4) Reduced number of nephrons—causes renal vascular hypertension.

Management

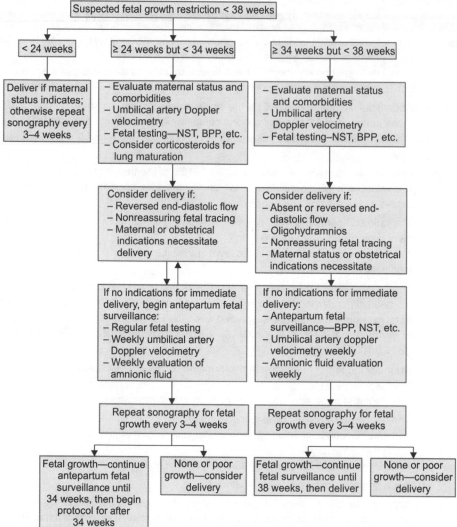

MACROSOMIA

The recommended definition is fetal (neonatal) weight exceeding two standard deviations or above 90th centile for the appropriate normal population.

According to ACOG, birth weight of ≥ 4500 g is called macrosomia.

In the Indian context, birth weight of ≥ 4000 g is called macrosomia.

Risk factors associated with macrosomia are:	
– Maternal diabetes	– Maternal obesity (If maternal BMI is > 30 kg/m², it is associated with increased risk)
– Multiparity	– Prolonged gestation
– Increased maternal age	– Male fetus
– Race and ethnicity (Hispanic ethnicity is a/w increased risk)	– Previous infant weight more than 4000 g

Grades of Macrosomia

Grade I	–	4000–4499 g
Grade II	–	4500–4999 g
Grade III	–	≥ 5000 g

- A major concern in the delivery of macrosomic infants is shoulder dystocia and permanent brachial plexus injury (seen in < 10% of all shoulder dystocia cases).

- There are increased chances of operative delivery with macrosomia.

- Some clinicians proposed labor induction when fetal macrosomia is diagnosed in nondiabetic women but it is not supported by ACOG.

- Planned LSCS may be done in diabetic women with an estimated fetal weight exceeding 4500 g and in nondiabetics, if expected fetal weight is > 5000.

—Williams Obs, 23/e

New Pattern Questions

N1. Which is not done in case of IUGR ?
a. Nonstress test
b. Oxytocin challenge test
c. Ultrasound abdomen
d. Amniocentesis

N2. The characteristics of caput succedaneum include all of the following *except*:
a. Crosses midline
b. Crosses the suture line
c. It does not disappear within 2-3 days
d. It is a diffuse edematous swelling of the soft tissues of the scalp

N3. Hematoma of the sternomastoid muscle detected in a 16 days old infant requires:
a. Immediate surgical evacuation
b. Surgical intervention within 2 weeks
c. Prophylactic antibiotic therapy
d. No immediate therapy

N4. Meconium is excreted by a newborn till...days:
a. 2   b. 3
c. 6   d. 4

N5. The number of fontanelles present in a newborn child is:
a. 1   b. 2
c. 4   d. 6

N6. Consider the following in a newborn:
1. Heart rate of 110
2. Slow and irregular respiratory effort
3. Flaccid muscle tone
4. No reflex irritability
5. Blue colour

What is the Apgar score in this case?
a. 1
b. 3
c. 5
d. 7

N7. A 25-year-old woman had premature rupture of membranes and delivered a male child became lethargic and apneic on the 1st day and went into shock. The mother had a previous history of abortion 1 year back. On culture, her vaginal swab growth of a hemolytic colonies on blood agar was found. On staining these were found to be gram positive cocci. Which of the following is the most likely etiological agent:
a. Streptococcus pyogenes
b. Streptococcus agalactiae
c. Peptostreptococci
d. Enterococcus faecalis

N8. The commonest cause of perinatal death in India:
a. Prematurity
b. Asphyxia
c. Intracranial haemorrhage
d. Congenital malformation

N9. Regarding IUGR
a. Abdominal circumference (AC) is the least sensitive parameter for detection of IUGR
b. In asymmetric IUGR head circumference/abdominal circumference (HC/AC) is reduced
c. Serial biparietal diameter (BPD) is the only important measurement in IUGR
d. AC indirectly reflects fetal liver size and glycogen storage

Previous Year Questions

1. IUGR is defined when: [AI 97]
a. Birth weight is below the tenth percentile of the average of gestational age
b. Birth weight is below the 20 percentile of the average of gestational age
c. Birth weight is below the 30 percentile of the average of gestational age
d. Weight of baby is less than 1000 gm

2. All are the causes of intrauterine growth retardation except: [AI 05]
a. Anemia
b. Pregnancy induced hypertension
c. Maternal heart disease
d. Gestational diabetes

3. IUGR is seen in: [PGI Dec 02]
a. Rubella   b. Syphilis
c. CMV   d. Chickenpox
e. HPV

4. **IUGR is characterized by all** *except*:
   a. Polycythemia   [PGI June 01]
   b. Meconium aspiration syndrome
   c. HMD
   d. Hypocalcemia

5. **True statement about symmetrical IUGR with respect to asymmetrical IUGR:**   [PGI May 2013]
   a. Worse prognosis
   b. Neurological defects
   c. Head larger than abdomen
   d. Less common
   e. Total number of cell is normal

6. **IUGR can be detected by USG:**   [PGI Dec 05]
   a. ↓ Fetal weight
   b. ↓ BPD
   c. ↑ HC/AC
   d. ↓ Head circumference
   e. ↑ Amniotic fluid volume

7. **Best parameter for ultrasound evaluation of IUGR is:**
   a. Placental membrane   [AIIMS June 97]
   b. Length of femur
   c. Abdominal circumference
   d. BPD

8. **A lady of 150 cm height with Hb of 11gm%, BP of 160/110 mm Hg and 12 kg gain during her pregnancy delivered an IUGR baby, the causes in this cases are:**
   a. Maternal infection   [PGI Dec 03]
   b. Short stature
   c. HTN
   d. ↑ Weight gain
   e. ↓ Hb%

9. **Birth weight of a baby can be increased by:**
   a. Cessation of smoking   [AIIMS May 07]
   b. Aspirin
   c. Ca++ and vitamin D supplement
   d. Bed rest

10. **Difference between prematurity and IUGR is that premature baby has:**   [PGI June 08]
    a. Sole creases all over feet
    b. Breast nodule 2 mm
    c. Ear cartilage well formed - good clastic recoil
    d. Skin glistening, thin
    e. Poor muscle tone

11. **A large baby is born with which complication in pregnancy:**   [AI 07]
    a. Gestational diabetes
    b. Gestational hypertension
    c. Cardiac disease
    d. Anaemia

12. **Caudal regression syndrome is seen in babies of mother having:**   [AI 07]
    a. Gestational diabetes
    b. PIH
    c. Cardiac disease
    d. Anaemia

13. **Hypoglycemia in newborn is seen in:**
    a. IUGR   [PGI Dec 01]
    b. Mother with hypothyroidism
    c. Rh incompatibility
    d. Macrosomia
    e. Hyperthyroidism

14. **Intrauterine fetal distress is indicated by:**
    a. Acceleration of 15/min   [PGI June 04]
    b. Deceleration of 30/min
    c. Variable deceleration 5-25/min
    d. Fetal HR<80/min
    e. Fetal HR 160-180/min

15. **A pregnant lady with persistent late, variable deceleration with cervical dilatation of 6 cm shifted to OT for surgery. Which of the following is not done in M/n:**   [AIIMS May 01]
    a. Supine position   b. O₂ inhalation
    c. IV fluid   d. Subcutaneous terbutaline

16. **Most common cause of post neonatal mortality is:**   [AIIMS Dec 98]
    a. Genetic cause
    b. Maternal health during pregnancy
    c. Environmental causes
    d. Conditions effecting in early neonatal period

17. **Cephalhematoma:**   [AI 02]
    a. Is caused by oedema of the subcutaneous layers of the scalp
    b. Should be treated by aspiration
    c. Most commonly lies over the occipital bone
    d. Does not vary in tension with crying

18. **All are the risk factors associated with macrosomia** *except*:   [AI 05]
    a. Maternal obesity
    b. Prolonged pregnancy
    c. Previous large infant
    d. Short stature

19. **Macrosomia is/are associated with:**   [PGI Nov 09]
    a. Gestational diabetes mellitus
    b. Maternal obesity
    c. Hypothyroidism
    d. Hyperbilirubinemia
    e. Fetal goitre

Answers with Explanations to New Pattern Questions

N1. Ans. is d, i.e. Amniocentesis　　　　*Ref. Fernando Arias 2/e, p 313, 314; COGDT 10/e, p 294*

Bedside Obs and gynae by Richa Saxena p 192

Antepartum Surveillance of IUGR Fetus

Majority of the fetal deaths in IUGR occur after 36 weeks. Therefore, correct diagnosis and timely intervention is vital.
There is no best method for monitoring a fetus with suspected IUGR.

Following investigation should be done in case of IUGR.

Test	Timing
Fetal movement count	Daily
Amniotic fluid volume	Weekly
Nonstress test	Twice weekly
Biophysical profile	Weekly if NST is abnormal
Oxytocin challenge test	Every fortnightly, if biophysical profile is less than 8
Umbilical artery Doppler	**Every 2-3 weeks**

Test	Significance
Amniocentesis	*"In selected cases, amniocentesis may be indicated for determination of fetal pulmonary maturity with an uncertain date of conception, for assessment of fetal karyotype, or for diagnosis of fetal infection."* —COGDT 10/e, p 294
Cordocentesis	*"Fetal blood sampling has a limited role in the evaluation of IUGR fetuses. Also, umbilical cord sampling is dangerous in the IUGR fetus, and these babies frequently develop prolonged, severe bradycardia during this procedure, requiring emergency cesarean delivery."* —Fernando Arias 2/e, p 314

So, from the above text it can be concluded that NST, CST and USG are done routinely in case of IUGR whereas amniocentesis is required in selected cases.

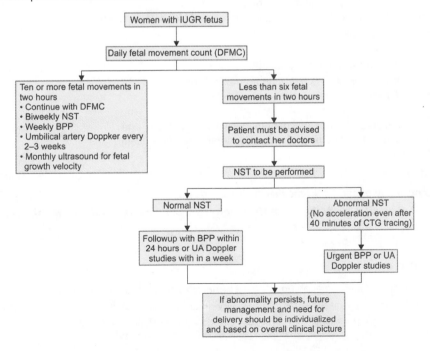

N2. **Ans. is c, i.e. It does not disappear within 2-3 days** *Ref. Dutta Obs. 7/e, p 86, 87*

Caput succedaneum
* This is a localised swelling of the scalp due to effusion of serum above the periosteum.

Pathology:
* There is obstruction of venous and lymphatic return due to pressure by the cervix.

  ↓
* Stagnation of fluid

  ↓

Edema over scalp
* **Site:** of the caput depends upon the position of the head.
* It is present at birth and disappears by about 24-36 hours.
* The size indicates the amount of pressure on the head.

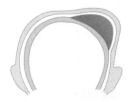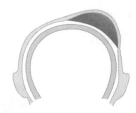

Cephalhematoma	Caput succedaneum
Sharply circumscribed	Diffuse
Soft but does not pit on pressure	Soft and pits on pressure
Under the periosteum	Above the periosteum
Does not cross suture lines	Lies over and crosses suture lines/midline
Fixed in one place	Movable over dependant part
May be associated with fracture	Not associated with fracture
Appears sometime after birth, grows larger and disappears only after weeks or months	Largest at birth, immediately starts to regress and disappears in a few hours

N3. **Ans. is d, i.e. No immediate therapy** *Ref. Dutta Obs. 7/e, p 486*

Sternomastoid tumour/Hematoma
* Presents at about 7-10 days after birth
* Situated at the junction of upper and middle third of the muscle
* **Etiology:** rupture of sternocleidomastoid muscle fibres and blood vessels, due to:
  - hematoma and cicatricial contracture
  - Difficult breech delivery
  - Attempted delivery after shoulder dystocia
  - Excessive lateral flexion of neck following normal delivery.
* Clinical features: Transient torticollis
* **Treatment:**
  - No treatment required, disappears spontaneously by 6 months of age
  - Gentle movements and stretching of muscle done after feeds is useful
  - Do not massage.

N4. **Ans. is b, i.e. 3 days** *Ref. Dutta Obs. 7/e, p 446; Williams Obs. 23/e, p 600*

"Meconium is normally passed 3-4 times a day for 2-3 days." —Dutta Obs. 6/e, p 448

"For the first 2-3 days after birth, the contents of colon are composed of soft, brownish green meconium." —Williams Obs. 22/e, p 643

 Also Know:

* A delay in initial passage of meconium for > 12 hours after birth requires observation.
* In breast-fed infants – stools are soft, golden yellow in colour, sour smelling and acid in reaction.
* In bottle fed infants – the stools are hard, pale, foul smelling and alkaline in reaction.

N5. **Ans. is d, i.e. 6** *Ref. Dutta Obs. 7/e, p 84*

6 fontanelles are present in fetal skull:
- Anterior fontanelle (bregma)   – 1
- Posterior fontanelle (lambda)   – 1
- Anterolateral fontanelle   – 1
- Posteriolateral fontanelle   – 1

N6. **Ans. is b, i.e. 3** *Ref. Dutta Obs. 7/e, p 470*

Signs	0	1	2
• Respiratory effort	Absent	Slow, irregular	Good, crying
• Heart rate	Absent	Slow (< 100)	> 100
• Muscle tone	Flaccid	Flexion of extremities	Active body movement
• Reflex irritability	No response	Grimace	Cry
• Colour	Blue, pale	Body pink, extremities blue	Complete pink

Total score   = 10
No depression   = 7-10
Mild depression   = 4-6
Severe depression   = 0-3
In this case :
Heart rate   = 110 means score of 2
Respiratory effort   = slow and irregular means a score of 1
Muscle flaccid   = score 0
Blue color   = score 0
Reflex irritability none   = 0
Total score in this case = 3

N7. **Ans. is b, i.e. Streptococcus agalactiae** *Ref. Nelson 17/e, p 627, Williams Obs, 23/e, p 1220*

Streptococcal (agalactiae) infection is characterised by:
- Asymptomatic bacteremia to septic shock (as is the case here).
- Early onset disease may present at birth, and generally within 6 hours of birth (patient is presenting here on the first day).
- In utero infection may result in fetal asphyxia, coma or shock.
- In 10% of infants with early onset disease, meningitis occurs.
- Diagnosis is made by isolation and identification of organism from sterile site.
- The demonstration of gram positive organism in pairs or chain in buffy coat or other sterile fluid indicates infection.
- Drug of Choice: Penicillin G/Ampicillin

If patient is allergic to penicillin → cefazolin is recommended.

N8. **Ans. is b, i.e. Asphyxia** *Ref. Park 22/e, p 522*

The WHO's definition, more appropriate in nations with well-established vital records of stillbirths is as follows:

$$PMR = \frac{\text{Late foetal deaths (28 weeks gestation and more) + early neonatal deaths (first week) is one year}}{\text{Live births + late foetal deaths (28 weeks gestation and more) in the same year}} \times 100$$

The WHO'S definition, more appropriate in nations with less well-established vital records, is:

$$\text{Perinatal mortality rate} = \frac{\text{Late foetal deaths (28 weeks of gestation) + postnatal deaths (first week) in a year}}{\text{Live births in a year}} \times 1000$$

Causes of perinatal mortality   *—Park 22/e, p 522*
About two-thirds of all perinatal deaths occur among infant with less than 2500 g birth weight. The causes involve one or more complications in the mother during pregnancy or about, in the placenta or in the foetus or neonate.

Main causes
The main causes of death are intrauterine and birth asphyxia, low birth weight, birth, and intrauterine or neonatal infection.
Important causes of perinatal mortality   *Ref. Dutta Obs 7/e, p 607*

Causes	Percent
Infections (Sepsis, Meningitis, Pneumonia, Neonatal tetanus, Congenital syphilis)	33
Birth asphyxia and trauma hypothermia	28
Preterm birth and/or low birth weight	24
Congenital malformations and others	15

N9. **Ans. is d, i.e. AC indirectly reflects fetal liver size and glycogen storage** *Ref. Dutta Obs 7/e, p 462, 463*

'AC is the single most sensitive parameter to detect IUGR' —*Dutta Obs 7/e, p 462*

'Serial measurements of AC (not BPD) and estimation of fetal weight are more diagnostic to fetal growth restriction'
—*Dutta Obs 7/e, p 462*

Head circumference (HC) and abdominal circumference (AC) ratios: In a normally growing fetus the HC/AC ratio exceeds 1.0 before 32 weeks. It is approximately 1.0 at 32 to 34 weeks. After 34 weeks, it falls below 1.0. If the fetus is affected by asymmetric IUGR, the HC remains larger. The HC/AC is then elevated. In symmetric IUGR, both the HC and AC are reduced. The HC/AC ratio remains normal. Using HC/AC ratio, 85% of IUGR fetuses are detected.

Pathophysiology: Basic pathology in small for gestational age is due to reduced *availability* of nutrients in the mother or its reduced transfer by the placenta to the fetus. It may also be due to reduced *utilization* by the fetus. Brain cell size (asymmetric–SGA) as well as cell numbers (symmetric-SGA) are reduced. Liver glycogen content is reduced. AC indirectly reflects the decreased fetal liver size and glycogen content.

Answers with Explanations to Previous Year Questions

1. **Ans. is a, i.e. Birth weight is below the tenth percentile of the average of gestational age** *Ref. Dutta Obs. 7/e, p 461*
   Intrauterine growth restriction is said to be present in those babies whose birth weight is below the tenth percentile of the average for the gestational age.

2. **Ans. is d, i.e. Gestational diabetes** *Ref. Dutta Obs. 7/e, p 287,463, 464; Fernando Arias 3/e, p 11 for a,115 for d,106 for b*

   As far as, Pregnancy induced hypertension and maternal heart disease are concerned, there is no doubt that both these conditions cause IUGR.

   For 'Anemia' *Dutta Obs. 6/e, p 463* says: **Anemia causes IUGR.**

   Williams Obs. 23/e, p 848 says: "**In most cases, maternal anemia does not causes fetal growth restriction, Exception include sickle cell disease.**"

   Fernando Arias 3/e, p111 says: "**Sickle cell anemia causes fetal growth retardation.**"

   "**Awathi et al (2001) reported an incidence of IUGR of 37% among Indian women suffering from moderately severe anemia.**"

   So sickle cell anemia and moderately severe anemia with Hb < 8 g/dL causes IUGR.

   As far as diabetes is considered: "**Growth restriction is less commonly observed and is associated with maternal vasculopathies**". —*Dutta Obs. 7/e, p 287*

   Fernando Arias 3/e, p 106 says: Diabetes with vascular disease is a cause of IUGR.

   It is further supported by following lines from Fernando Arias 3/e, p 115.

   "**Insulin dependant diabetes with microvascular disease are at high risk for having IUGR fetuses.**"

   "**Diabetic Vasculopathy and excessively tight control of diabetes mellitus in pregnancy has been linked to intrauterine growth restriction**"

   Mgt of High Risk Pregnancy, SS Trivedi and Manju Puri p 328, 329

   But here friends all texts refer to overt diabetes complicated with vasculopathies leading to IUGR, gestational diabetes is diabetes which is first recognised during pregnancy and it does not lead to vasculopathies so no IUGR. Rather gestational diabetes leads to macrosomia.

3. **Ans. is a, b, c and d, i.e. Rubella; Syphilis; CMV; and Chickenpox** *Ref. Dutta Obs. 7/e, p 462; COGDT 10/e, p 290, Mgt of High Risk Pregnancy, SS Trivedi and Manju Puri, p 178, Bedside Obs and Gynae Richa, Saxena, p 184*

One spermatogonia gives rise to 16 primary spermatocytes.
Congenital infections leading to IUGR:
    Viral: CMV, Rubella, Herpes, Varicella zoster, Influenza, Poliovirus, HIV
    Protozoan: Toxoplasma, Malaria, Trypanosoma
    Bacterial: Listeria monocytogenes, Tuberculosis and Syphilis

—*COGDT 10/e, p 289, 290*
—*Fernando Arias 3/e, p 110*

4. **Ans. is c, i.e. HMD** *Ref. COGDT 10/e, p 293; Dutta Obs. 7/e, p 464.*

Fetal complications of IUGR

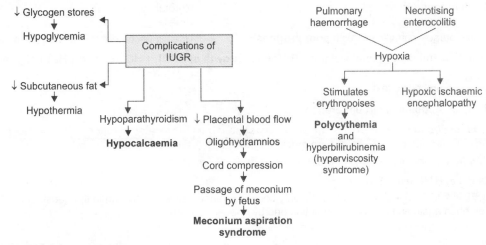

Long-term complications of IUGR:
- Low IQ, learning and behaviour problems
- Major neurologic handicaps (seizure disorders, cerebral palsy, mental retardation)
- Adult diseases—these children are supposed to be at increased risk of developing disorders like obesity, diabetes mellitus, cardiovascular disease.

Now let's see what *Ghai 6/e, p 166* says about Hyaline membrane disease (RDS).
In RDS the basic abnormality is surfactant deficiency.
***"RDS almost always occurs in preterm babies** often less than 34 weeks **of gestation. It is the commonest cause of respiratory distress in a preterm neonate"**.*

- The overall incidence is 10-15% but can be as high as 80% in neonates < 28 weeks.
OGDT 10/e, p 293 **says:** ***"Hypoxia in IUGR fetus is the result of increasing fetal requirement during pregnancy and not due to hyaline membrane disease (i.e. surfactant deficiency)."***

According to Fernando Arias, 3/e p 112.....RDS/HMD is seen in preterm fetal growth restricted infants. The RDS is not because of IUGR but due to prematurity, so I am ruling it out because **the question is not asking about Preterm IUGR**

5. **Ans. is a and d, i.e. Worse prognosis and Less common** *Ref. Dutta Obs. 7/e p 462*
Intrauterine growth restriction is said to be present in those babies whose birth weight is below the tenth percentile of the average for the gestational age. Growth restriction can occur in preterm, term or post-term babies.
Depending upon the relative size of their head, abdomen and femur, the fetuses are subdivided into:
- Symmetrical or Type I
- Asymmetrical or Type II

Symmetrical (20%):
The fetus is affected from the noxious effect very early in the phase of cellular hyperplasia. The total cell number is less. This form of growth retardation is most often caused by structural or chromosomal abnormalities or congenital infection (TORCH). The pathological process is intrinsic to the fetus and involves all the organs including the head.

Asymmetrical (80%):

The fetus is affected in later months during the phase of cellular hypertrophy. The total cell number remains the same but size is smaller than normal. The pathological processes that too often result in asymmetric growth retardation are maternal diseases extrinsic to the fetus. These diseases alter the fetal size by reducing uteroplacental blood flow or by restricting the oxygen and nutrient transfer or by reducing the placental size.

Features of symmetrical and asymmetrical IUGR fetuses	
Symmetrical (20%)	**Asymmetrical (80%)**
Uniformly small	**Head larger than abdomen**
Ponderal index (Birth weight/Crown-heel length³)—normal	Low
HC: AC and FL: AC ratios—normal	Elevated
Etiology: Genetic disease or infection—(Intrinsic to fetus)	Chronic placental insufficiency—(Extrinsic to fetus)
Total cell number—less Cell size—normal	Normal Smaller
Neonatal course—complicated with **poor prognosis**	Usually uncomplicated having good prognosis

6. **Ans. is a, b, c and d, i.e. ↓ fetal weight; ↓ BPD (less growth of BPD); ↑ HC/AC; and ↓ Head circumference**
   Ref. Dutta Obs. 7/e, p 463; Fernando Arias 2/e, p 307-309

   For detail see preceding text.

7. **Ans. is c, i.e. Abdominal circumference** *Ref. Dutta Obs. 7/e, p 463; Fernando Arias 3/e, p 308*

   "Abdominal circumference (AC) is the single most sensitive parameter to detect IUGR. Serial measurements of AC and estimations of fetal weight are more diagnostic to fetal growth restriction." —Dutta 7/e, p 463

   "The biometric parameters, AC is most affected by fetal growth" —Williams 24/e, p 199

8. **Ans. is c, i.e. HTN (hypertension)** *Ref. Dutta Obs. 7/e, p 97, p 260, 51*

   Friends, It is a tricky question which needs only common sense. Answer is hidden in the question itself. So, lets read the question once again and rule out each option one by one.

   The lady in our question is of 150 cm height (~ 5 feet).

   "While an arbitrary measurement of 5 ft. is considered as short stature in western countries, it is 4' 7" in India considered the low average height." —Dutta Obs. 6/e, p 98

   So, the lady is not constitutionally small. *i.e. options 'b' is ruled out.*

   Her Hb is 11 gm%.

   "According to the standards laid down by WHO, anemia in pregnancy is present when the haemoglobin concentration in the peripheral blood is 11gm% or less". —Dutta Obs. 6/e, p 262

   So, according to the WHO standard 11gm% is borderline for anemia.

   Also-as discussed in answer 2 anemia leads to IUGR when it is moderately severe i.e. Hb<8 gm% or if it is sickle cell anemia (Fernando arias, 3/e, p 41)

   So, *option 'e'* is ruled out.

   Her BP is 160/110 mm Hg

   Hypertension: is an absolute rise of BP of at least 140/90 mm Hg, if the previous BP is not known. So, there is no doubt that the patient is hypertensive.

   Prolonged hypertension leads to placental insufficiency which ultimately results in IUGR.

   So, option 'c' is correct.

   Her weight gain is 12 kg.

   "Ideally weight gain should depend on prepregnancy body mass index (BMI) level. Weight gain for a woman with normal BMI (20-26) is 11 to 16 kg" —Dutta Obs. 6/e, p 51

   So, the weight gain comes under normal range, *option 'd'* ruled out.

   Though maternal infection during pregnancy also causes IUGR, here in our question no such history has been mentioned. So, *option 'a'* is also ruled out. Hence the answer of this question is, **IUGR is due to hypertension.**

9. **Ans. is a, i.e. Cessation of smoking** *Ref. COGDT 10/e, p 293; Williams Obs. 22/e, p 354,23/e, p 329*

   "Smoking is the single most preventable cause of IUGR in infants born in the united states—women who quit smoking at 7 months gestation have newborns with higher mean birthweights than do women who smoke throughout the pregnancy. Women who quit smoking before 16 weeks of gestation are not at any increased risk for an IUGR infant." —COGDT 10/e, p 293

The answer is further supported by   *Williams 24/e, p 882*

"In prevention of fetal growth restriction – smoking cessation is critical"   —*Williams 24/e, p 882*

10. **Ans. is b, d and e, i.e. Breast nodule 2 mm; Skin glistening, thin; and Poor muscle tone**
        Ref. Dutta Obs. 7/e, p 457, 462, 447; Meharban Singh's Clinical Method 3/e, p 243

> **Prematurity**
> * Definition: Baby born before 37 completed week of gestation are preterm/premature baby.
> * Incidence: 20-25%

Difference between Prematurity and IUGR.

Prematurity	IUGR
• Definition: Baby born before 37 completed weeks of gestation	• Babies whose birth weight is below 10th percentile of the average for gestational age
• Incidence: 20-25%	• 2-8%
• Weight and height: 2500 gm or less & length is usually less than 44 cm and length is unaffected	• Weight deficit at birth is about 600 gm below the minimum in percentile standard
• Head and abdomen: are relatively large	• Scaphoid abdomen
• Head circumference (HC): disproportionately exceeds that of the chest • {Normally HC is greater than the circumference at birth, the difference is about 1.5 cm}	• Head circumference is relatively large than the body in asymmetric variety
• Pinnae of ears are soft and flat. Poor recoil	• Pinna of ear has cartilaginous ridges
• Eyes: kept closed	• Eyes are open
• Skin: thin, red shiny, covered by plentiful lanugo and vernix caseosa[Q].	• Dry and wrinkled, skin thin meconium stained vernix caseosa and thin umbilical cord
• Muscle tone is poor[Q]	• Reflexes are normal including Moro's reflex, baby alert active and normal cry
• Plantar creases are not visible before 34 weeks	• Plantar crease are well-defined
• Nails are not grown right upto the finger tips	• Nails grown
• Breast nodule < 5 mm and nipple small or absent	

11. **Ans. is a, i.e. Gestational diabetes**   *Ref. Dutta Obs. 7/e, p 284; Williams Obs. 23/e, p 854*

> *Large baby is called as **macrosomia** which is defined as fetal (neonatal) weight exceeding two standard deviations or above 90th centile for the appropriate normal population.*
> *According to ACOG: birth weight of ≥ 4500 gm is called as macrosomia.*
> In Indian context birth weight of ≥ 4000 gm is called as macrosomia.
> **Macrosomia is seen in:**
> * Maternal diabetes
> * Multiparity
> * Increased maternal age
> * Maternal obesity
> * Prolonged gestation

12. **Ans. is a, i.e. Gestational diabetes**   *Ref. Dutta Obs. 7/e, p 284; Fernando Arias 3/e, p 454*
     Gestational diabetes is associated with increased risk of congenital malformation in the newborn.
     The malformation most specific for gestational diabetes is caudal regression syndrome.

     "The lesion classically associated with diabetic embryopathy, the caudal regression syndrome, is rare, with an incidence of 1.3 per 1000 diabetic pregnancies." —*Fernando Arias 3/e, p 454*

13. **Ans. is a and d, i.e. IUGR and Macrosomia**
        Ref. Dutta Obs. 7/e, p 285; Williams Obs. 23/e, p 1131, 1132; Ghai 6/e, p 177, 487; KDT 5/e, p 227

Hypoglycemia is defined as blood glucose of less than 40 mg/dL, irrespective of the gestational age.

Causes of hypoglycemia

Let us see each option one by one.

Option 'a' **IUGR**

"Hypoglycemia is due to shortage of glycogen reserve in the liver as a result of chronic hypoxia" —Dutta Obs. 6/e, p 465

Option 'b' **Mother with hypothyroidism**

Maternal hypothyroidism can cause hypoglycemia if it leads to fetal hypothyroidism also but "Maternal TSH receptor blocking antibodies can cross the placenta and cause fetal thyroid dysfunction. They however have little or no effect on fetal thyroid function even though they too cross the placenta." —Williams 23/e, p 1131, 1132

So according to latest edition of Williams, maternal hypothyroidism does not lead to fetal hypothyroidism, thus it does not cause fetal hypoglycemia.

Option 'c' **Rh incompatibility**

There is no definite correlation between Rhincompatibility and hypoglycemia.

Option 'd' **Macrosomia**

Macrosomia usually is due to maternal diabetes which inturn results in fetal hyperinsulinemia due to beta cell hyperplasia, which further results in neonatal hypoglycemia. —Dutta Obs. 6/e, p 287

Option 'e' **Hyperthyroidism:** Hyperthyroidism is a diabetes like state with increased insulin resistance.

Increased thyroid hormone		
↑ Glycogenolysis	↑ Gluconeogenesis	↑ BMR
↓	↓	↓
Hyperglycemia	Hyperglycemia	Hypoglycemia

Though utilization of sugar by tissues is increased (mainly secondary to increased BMR), glycogenolysis and gluconeogenesis in liver more than compensates for it and result in hyperglycemia. —KDT 5/e, p 227

 Also Know:

Causes of hypoglycemia in neonates —Ghai 6/e, p 177

Common

- Inadequate substrates, especially, if feeding is delayed or is suboptimal: small for dates and preterm babies.
- Relative hyperinsulinism in infants of diabetic mothers.
- Secondary to polycythemia.
- Secondary to stressful conditions such as hypothermia, sepsis, asphyxia and respiratory distress.

Rare

- Hyperinsulin states: Beta cell hyperplasia (nesidioblastosis), adenoma of beta cells.
- Deficiency of hormones such as glucagon, GH, epinephrine, adrenal and ACTH.
- Metabolic disease such as glycogen storage disease, fructose intolerance, ketotic hypoglycemia, maple syrup urine disease, etc.

14. **Ans. is b, c, d and e, i.e. Deceleration of 30/min; Variable deceleration 5-25/min; Fetal HR < 80/min; and Fetal HR 160-180/min** *Ref. Williams Obs. 22/e, p 461; 23/e, p 429-431, Dutta Obs. 7/e, p 612*

Fetal distress is an ill-defined term, used to express intrauterine fetal jeopardy, as a result of intrauterine fetal hypoxia.

Indicators of Fetal Distress:

Clinical	Biochemical
• Prolonged tachycardia (> 160 bpm)	• Fetal scalp blood pH < 7.2
• Prolonged bradycardia (< 110 bpm for atleast 5 minutes)	
• Absence of acceleration	
• Reduced fetal heart rate variability	
• Severe variable and late deceleration	

Also Know:

Meconium in Amniotic fluid

Earlier meconium in amniotic fluid was considered as a potential warning of fetal asphyxia.

But now it is considered that the high incidence of meconium observed in the amniotic fluid during labour often represents fetal passage of gastrointestinal contents in conjunction with normal physiological process. Although normal, such meconium becomes an environmental hazard when fetal acidemia supervenes.

15. Ans. is a, i.e. Supine position   *Ref. Dutta Obs. 7/e, p 614*

"Deceleration is defined as a decrease in fetal heart rate below the base line of 15 beats per minute or more."
Variable deceleration is seen in case of cord-compression/prolapse.

In case of cord-compression/prolapse patient should not be allowed to rest in supine position as it will lead to more pressure on the cord. In cord prolapse the patient is allowed to rest in exaggerated elevated Sims position with a pillow under the hip.

Management of Non-reassuring fetal status (Fetal Distress)
- Lateral positioning avoids compression of vena cava and aorta by the gravid uterus. This increases cardiac output and uteroplacental perfusion.
- Oxygen is administered to the mother with mask to improve fetal SaO_2.
- Correction of dehydration by IV fluids (crystalloids) improves intravascular volume and uterine perfusion.
- Correction of maternal hypotension (following epidural analgesia) with immediate infusion of 1 litre of Crystalloid (Ringer's solution).
- Stoppage of oxytocin to improve fetal oxygenation. Fetal hypoxia may be due to strong and sustained uterine contractions. With reassuring FHR and in absence of fetal acidemia, oxytocin may be restarted.
- Tocolytic (Injection terbutaline 0.25 mg S.C.) is given when uterus is hypertonic and there is nonreassuring FHR.
- Amnioinfusion is the process to increase the intrauterine fluid volume with warm normal saline (500 ml). Indications are:
    - Oligohydramnios and cord compression
    - To dilute or to wash out meconium
    - To improve variable or prolonged decelerations.

Advantages: Reduces cord compression, meconium aspiration, and improves Apgar score.

16. Ans. is c, i.e. Environmental causes   *Ref. Park 19/e, p 452*

Deaths occurring from 28 days of life to under one year are called postneonatal death.

The postneonatal mortality rate $= \dfrac{\text{Number of deaths of children between 28 days and one year of age in a given year}}{\text{Total live births in the same year}} \times 1000$

Park 19/e, p 452 says:
"Whereas neonatal mortality is dominated by endogenous factors, postneonatal mortality is dominated by exogenous factors (e.g. environmental and social factors)."
- Main causes in developing countries:
    - Diarrhoea
    - Respiratory tract infection
    - Malnutrition.
- Main causes in developed countries:
    - Congenital anomalies.

> ### Extra Edge
>
> **Some important definitions:**
> - *Perinatal period* extends from the 28th week of gestation up to the 7th day of life.
> - *Extended perinatal period* is the period from the 22nd week up to the 7th day of life.
> - *Neonatal period* extends from birth up to 28 days of life. The early neonatal period refers to the first 7 days and the late neonatal period from 7 days to 28 days.
> - Stillbirth: A stillbirth is the birth of a newborn after 28th completed week (weighing 1000 gm or more) when the baby does not breathe or show any sign of life after delivery. Such deaths include antepartum deaths (macerated) and intrapartum deaths (fresh stillbirths). Stillbirths rate is the number of such deaths per 1000 total births (live and still births).
> - **Perinatal mortality rate (PNMR):** Perinatal mortality is defined as deaths among, fetuses weighing 1000 gm or more at birth (28 weeks gestation) who die before or during delivery or within the first 7 days of delivery. The perinatal mortality rate is expressed in terms of such deaths per 1000 total births. Perinatal deaths are thus the sum of stillbirths plus early neonatal deaths.

Causes: Infection > Birth asphyxia and trauma > Preterm birth and/or LBW > Congenital malformation.
- Neonatal mortality rate (NMR): It is the death of the baby within 28 days after birth. Neonatal mortality rate is the number of such deaths per 1000 live births. Majority of the deaths occur within 48 hours of birth.

Most common cause of Neonatal mortality is Prematurity.

17. **Ans. is d, i.e. Does not vary in tension with crying**   *Ref. Dutta Obs. 7/e, p 483*

Cephalhaematoma:
- Collection of blood in between the pericranium and the flat bone of the skull due to rupture of a small emissary vein from the skull. It may be associated with fracture of the skull bone.
- Usually unilateral.
- Lies over a parietal bone.
- Caused generally by forceps delivery but may also be met with following a normal labour.
- Ventouse application does not increase the incidence of cephalhaematoma.
- It is never present at birth but gradually develops after 12-24 hours of birth and disappears by 6-8 weeks[Q].
- It is circumscribed, soft, fluctuant, and incompressible.
- The swelling is limited by the suture lines of the skull[Q] as the pericranium is fixed to the margins of the bone.
- No active treatment is necessary.
- Prognosis is good.

Meningocele always lies over a suture line or fontanelle and there is impulse on crying.

18. **Ans. is d, i.e. Short stature**

19. **Ans. is a and b, i.e. Gestational diabetes mellitus and Maternal obesity**   *Ref. Williams Obs. 22/e, p 905, 23/e, p 854*
Macrosomia is the term used to describe a large fetus.

The recommended definition is fetal (neonatal) weight exceeding two standard deviations or above 90th centile for the appropriate normal population.
According to ACOG: birth weight of ≥ 4500 gm is called as macrosomia.

In Indian context birth weight of ≥ 4000 gm is called as macrosomia.

Risk factors associated with macrosomia are:	
• Maternal diabetes	• Maternal obesity (If maternal BMI is > 30 kg/m², it is a/w increased risk)
• Multiparity	• Prolonged gestation
• Increased maternal age	• Male fetus
• Race and ethinicity (hipanic ethnicity is a/w increased risk)	• Previous infant weight more than 4000 g

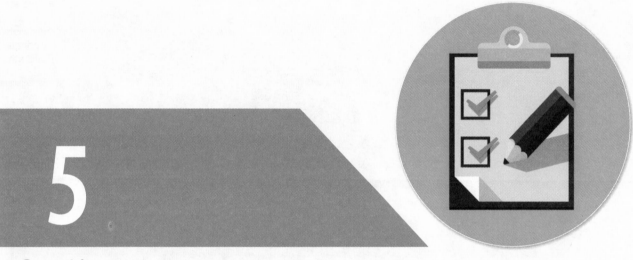

5
Section

Latest Papers

Latest Papers

AIIMS NOVEMBER 2018

1. **Which of the following is not in quadruple test for antenatal detection of Down syndrome?**
   a. AFP
   b. β- hCG
   c. Estradion
   d. Inhibin B

2. **Maternal mortality ratio expressed in:**
   a. Maternal death per 10,000 lives
   b. Maternal death per 100,000 lives
   c. Maternal death per 1,000,000 lives
   d. Maternal death per 100 lives

3. **Possible cause of choriocarcinoma after hydatidiform mole is all except:**
   a. Rising hCG
   b. More Theca lutein cysts
   c. Increase uterus size
   d. Sub urethral nodule

4. **What should be the time of termination of pregnancy of a female with insulin dependent diabetes?**
   a. 40 weeks
   b. 38 weeks
   c. 37 weeks
   d. 34 weeks

5. **Active management of third stage of labor includes except:**
   a. Ergometrine after anterior shoulder delivery
   b. Uterine massage
   c. Cord traction
   d. Oxytocin infusion

6. **Placenta grade 3, 35+3 weeks pregnancy, and absent end diastolic flow in Doppler; next management is:**
   a. Dexamethasone and terminate after 48 hours
   b. Terminate after 37 weeks
   c. Talk with pediatrician and termination
   d. Monitor and do nothing

Answers With Explanations

1. **Ans. is d, i.e. inhibin B**
   - **Quadruple test** is the second trimester measurement of maternal serum
   - Alpha fetoprotein (MSAFP)
   - Unconjugated estriol
   - hCG
   - Inhibin-A

   It is done between 15-20 weeks.

	MS-AFP	Estriol	Inhibin A	β-hCG
Trisomy 18	↓	↓	↓	↓
Trisomy 21	↓	↓	↑	↑

2. **Ans. is b, i.e. Maternal death per 100,000 lives**

   $$MMR = \frac{\text{No. of maternal deaths}}{\text{Total number of live births}} \times 100{,}000$$

3. **Ans. is b, i.e. More theca lutein cysts**

   Suburethral Nodule indicates metastases choriocarcinoma. All others are very well seen in the conversion of a complete hydatidiform mole into choriocarcinoma except more theca lutein cyst.
   - It is not the number of cyst but size of cyst ($\geq$ 6 cms) which indicate neoplastic conversion.
   - Suburethral nodule may be a manifestation of vaginal metastasis from choriocarcinoma.
   - Metastatic choriocarcinoma is however seen in only about 4% of patients after evacuation of a complete mole and vaginal metastasis that may present with suburethral nodule occur in only 30% of patients with such metastatic disease. Hence it is an unusual indicator.
   - Raised β-hCG level present in choriocarcinoma.

4. **Ans. is b, i.e. 38 weeks**

   Ideally the answer to this question should be $\geq$ 39 weeks to 39 weeks + 6 days.
   But since this option is not given and we don't want till 40 weeks in insulin controlled diabetes, so here the best anwser is 38 weeks.

Type of diabetes	Time of delivery
GDM controlled on diet	≥ 39 weeks to 40 weeks + 6 days
GDM controlled on insulin	≥ 39 weeks to 39 weeks + 6 days
Overt diabetes	37 weeks to 37 weeks + 6 days

5. **Ans. is b, i.e. Uterine massage**

   Uterine massage is not a core component of Active Management of Third Stage of Labor (AMTSL).
   AMTSL recommended by WHO is a triad including:
   - Immediate administration of prophylactic uterotonic (Oxytocin)
   - Controlled cord traction during placental delivery
   - Delayed cord clamping
   - Intermittent assessment of uterine tone

6. **Ans. is c, i.e. Talk with paediatrician and termination**   *Ref: Williams 25/e p 855*
   - Absent end diastolic flow: Fetal compromise (hence terminate pregnancy by caesarean section if > 34 weeks)
   - Reverse end diastolic flow: Impending doom of death (terminate pregnancy irrespective of gestational age).
   - Steroids are given if pregnancy < 34 weeks.

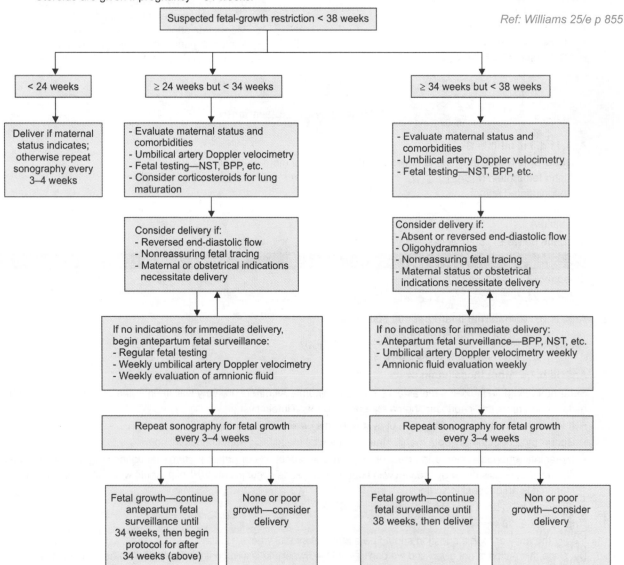

AIIMS May 2018

1. **A pregnant female with known cardiac disease presents to you in the first trimester with history of warfarin embryopathy, what should be advised now?·**
   a. Continue warfarin throughout the pregnancy
   b. Replace warfarin with heparin in First trimester
   c. Give isocoumarin
   d. Use LMW heparin

2. **A 28-week Pregnant female presents with the fetal distress on examination and the test performed (MCA Doppler study) is given below. What should be the next step in management?**

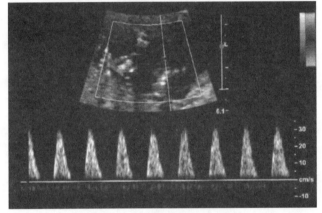

   a. Immediate termination of pregnancy
   b. Give steroid cover and monitor with doppler and BPP, and plan delivery
   c. Give steroid and take up for CS immediately
   d. Go for normal vaginal delivery as baby is very small

3. **Identify the instrument shown?**

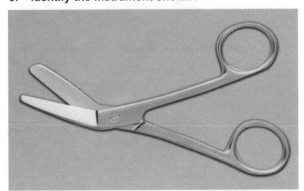

   a. Episiotomy scissor   b. Cutting scissors
   c. Babcock forceps   d. Ovum forceps

4. **A 32 weeks pregnant female presented with labor pains and minimal vaginal discharge, on analysis of the cervicovesical discharge showed fibronectin. What is the probable diagnosis?**
   a. Preterm labour
   b. IUGR
   c. IUD
   d. Cervical infection

5. **Identify the given procedure done in labor room:**

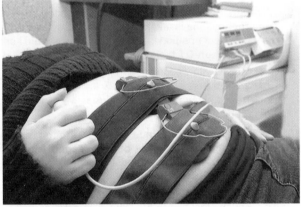

   a. NST
   b. Amniotic fluid index
   c. Amniocentesis
   d. MCA Doppler

6. **All of the following indicate Fetal lung maturity except?**
   a. Lecithin/Sphingomyelin ratio >2
   b. Positive shake test
   c. Increased phosphatidyl glycerol
   d. Blue cells in Nile Blue Test

7. **Identify the anomaly based on the image below**

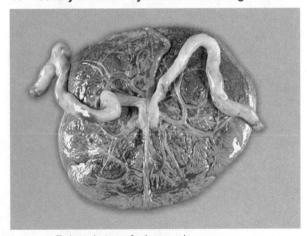

   a. Twin-twin transfusion syndrome
   b. Monochorionic diamniotic pregnancy
   c. Monochorionic monoamniotic pregnancy
   d. Dichorionic diamniotic pregnancy

8. **A pregnant woman with G3P2LO presented to you with a pregnancy at period of gestation of 9 weeks. She has a history of conization one year back currently on follow up with no recurrence on PAP smear. She also has the history of preterm births at 30 and 32. weeks during her last 2 pregnancy. What is your next step in the management of This patient?**
   a. USG to see cervical length
   b. Cervical cerclage
   c. Complete bed rest
   d. Abdominal cerclage

9. **A pregnant female presents with prolonged labor in emergency. She is taken for Cesarean Section. What is the correct position in which the nurse should keep the patient on OT table?**
   a. Supine with wedge under right hip
   b. Semi fowlers
   c. Trendelenburg with legs in stirrup
   d. Prone position

10. **A female come to gynae OPD for preconceptual counselling, with history of two second trimester abortions. What is the next investigation you will advice**
    a. TVS   b. Hysteroscopy
    c. Endometrial biopsy d. Chromosomal abnormalities

11. **A pregnant female delivered a baby with normal expulsion of an intact placenta. After half hour she started bleeding per vaginaly. On examination she was hypotensive and boggy mass is palpated per abdomen. USG showed. retained placental tissues. What is the likely diagnosis?**
    a. Placenta succenturiata
    b. Adenomyosis
    c. Placenta accreta
    d. Membranous placenta

12. **Following are the features of the color of normal amniotic fluid during delivery?**
    a. Milky to yellowish green with mucus flakes
    b. Amber colored
    c. Clear colorless to pale yellow
    d. Golden color

13. **A lady presented with 7 weeks amenorrhea presented with slight vaginal spotting. CRL was 5mm with well-formed gestational sac with calculated GA of 5.6 weeks on TVS. Next line of management?**
    a. Wait for another 1 week and repeat TVS
    b. Surgical or medical evacuation
    c. Wait for another 4 weeks
    d. Serum hCG levels

Answers With Explanations

1. **Ans. is b, i.e. Replace warfarin with heparin in first trimester**
   As discussed in Chapter 22, warfarin is replaced by heparin in 1st trimester

2. **Ans. is b, i.e. Give steroid cover and monitor with doppler and BPP, and plan delivery**
   The Doppler shows absent end diastolic flow. The period of pregnancy is 28 weeks. In all cases of absent End diastolic flow-pregnancy termination is done at 34 weeks.
   Till then patient is managed expectantly.

3. **Ans. is a, i.e. Episiotomy scissor**
   It is Braun episiotomy scissor. It is non-ratcheted, finger ring scissors, angled with smooth, blunt/blunt tips, and has a length of 5-1/2 inches.
   • Babcock's forceps:

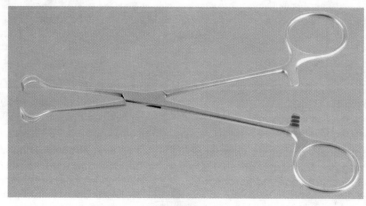

Finger ring ratcheted, non-perforating forceps used to grasp tubular and delicate structures.

- Ovum forceps

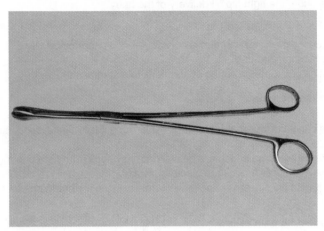

They don't have lock, used to remove retained products of conception.

4. **Ans. is a, i.e. Preterm labour** *Ref: Williams Obstetrics 25/e*
   - Fibronectin can be detected in cervicovaginal secretions before membrane rupture and is a marker for impending preterm labour.
   - It reflects stromal remodelling of the cervix before labour.
   - It is measured sing an enzyme-linked immunosorbent assay, and values exceeding 50 ng/mL are considered positive.

5. **Ans. is a, i.e. NST** *Ref: Williams's Obstetrics, 25/e*
   Answer should be CTG as the picture shown has toco probe but since that's not in the option then the next best answer will be NST since both measure the same parameters.

6. **Ans. is d, i.e. Blue cells in Nile Blue Test**
   All of the above are correct except that it is the presence of more than 50% orange coloured cells in Nile Blue test that suggests fetal pulmonary maturity.
   - Other tests for assessment of fetal pulmonary maturity are:
   - Foam Stability Index (FSI): It is calculated by utilising serial dilutions of amniotic fluid to quantitate the amount of surfactant present. FSI > 47 excludes the risk of RDS.
   - Saturated phosphatidyl choline > 500 ng indicates pulmonary maturity.
   - Fluorescence polarization: This utilises polarised light to quantitate surfactant in amniotic fluid. Presence of > 55 mg of surfactant per gram indicates fetal lung maturity.
   - Amniotic fluid optical density: at 650 mm greater than 0.15 indicates lung maturity.
   - Lamellar body – lamellar body count more than 30,000/ul indicates pulmonary maturity.

7. **Ans. is c, i.e. Monochorionic monoamniotic pregnancy**
   - Two umbilical cords are seen arising from the same placenta and there is no intervening amniotic membrane; it is monochorionic monoamniotic placenta.
   - Monochorionic diamniotic placenta: There will be one placenta and intervening 2 layers of amnion on gross examination as shown in the above picture.

8. **Ans. is a, i.e. USG to see cervical length** *Ref: NICE guidelines; ACOG guidelines; SOGC guidelines*
   The current review from ACOG recommends cervical cerclage for women with a current singleton pregnancy, prior spontaneous preterm birth at less than 34 weeks of gestation, and cervical length less than 25 mm.
   NICE guidelines recommend either prophylactic vaginal progesterone or prophylactic cervical cerclage to women:
   - With a history of spontaneous preterm birth or midtrimester loss between 16 and 34 weeks of pregnancy and in whom a transvaginal ultrasound scan has been carried out between 16 and 24 weeks of pregnancy that reveals a cervical length of less than 25 mm.
   The patient has history of 2 preterm births and conisation, next step would be to measure the cervical length as history of preterm labor and conisation increases the risk of preterm births but not necessarily cervical insufficiency.

9. **Ans. is a, i.e. Supine with wedge under right hip**   *Ref: DC Dutta's textbook of Obstetrics, 9th ed*

In caesarean section, patient is placed in supine position. In order to prevent venocaval compression, 15-degree tilt is given by placing a wedge under the right hip till delivery of the baby.

10 **Ans. is a, i.e. TVS**   *Ref: Williams Obstetrics 24th ed*

Most common cause of second trimester abortion is cervicouterine abnormalities. Next step would be to do an ultrasound and look for any structural uterine anomaly.

Chromosomal abnormalities are common cause of abortions in first trimester.

11. **Ans. is a, i.e. Placenta succenturiata**   *Ref: DC Dutta's textbook of Obstetrics, 9th ed*

Placenta succenturiata has one (usual) or more small lobes of placenta placed at a varying margin from the main placental margin. A leash of vessels connects the small lobe with the main lobe. Many times, succenturiate is retained and it presents as postpartum haemorrhage which may be primary or secondary.

Placenta membranacea is unduly large and thin. The placenta develops from both chorion frondosum and chorion leave. It increases chances of placenta previa, retained placenta, PPH.

In placenta accreta, all or part of the placenta attaches abnormally to the myometrium. So, either whole or a part of placenta comes out causing PPH.

12. **Ans. is c, i.e. Clear colorless to pale yellow**   *Ref: Dc Dutta's textbook of Obstetrics, 9th ed*
   - Green yellow with flakes (meconium stained)—Fetal distress
   - Golden color—Rh incompatibility
   - Greenish yellow (Saffron)—postmaturity
   - Dark colored—concealed accidental hemorrhage
   - Dark brown (tobacco juice)—intrauterine demise

13. **Ans. is a, i.e. Wait for another 1 week and repeat TVS**   *Ref: Williams obstetrics, 24th ed*
   - An intrauterine gestational sac is reliably visualized with transvaginal sonography by 5 weeks, and an embryo with cardiac activity by 6 weeks.
   - The embryo should be visible transvaginally once the mean sac diameter has reached 20 mm, otherwise the gestation is anembryonic.
   - Cardiac motion is usually visible with transvaginal imaging when the embryo length has reached 5 mm. If an embryo less than 7 mm is not identified to have cardiac activity, a subsequent examination is recommended in 1 week.

JIPMER MAY 2017

1. **AMSTL criteria include all except:**
   a. Controlled cord traction
   b. Uterine massage
   c. Oxytocin
   d. Methergine

2. **Longest fetal diameter:**
   a. Biparietal
   b. Suboccip tobregmatic
   c. Occipitofrontal
   d. Mentovertical

Answers With Explanations

1. **Ans is b, i.e. Uterine massage**

   Active management of third stage of labor earlier included uterine massage but now it has been replaced by intermittent assessment of uterine tone. Hence now uterine massage is not a part of AMTSL.

   As far as methergine is concerned, WHO recommends oxytocin as DOC for AMTSL but if it is not available then Methergine is given.

2. **Ans is d, i.e. Mentovertical**

   Fetal diameters–AP diameters are always longer than Transverse diameter of fetal head.

   Longest diameter is–Mentovertical diameter (14 cms) followed by submentovertical diameter.

JIPMER DECEMBER 2016

1. **Triple test includes:**
   a. Maternal AFP + HCG + Estradiol
   b. Maternal AFP + HCG + PAPPA
   c. Maternal AFP + PAPPA + Estradiol
   d. TSH + HCG + Estradiol

2. **Cordocentesis is done at what gestation age?**
   a. 14–18 weeks
   b. 10-12 weeks
   c. Anytime more than 8 weeks
   d. 18–20 weeks

3. **A postnatal mother presents with inability to void along with abdominal pain and pallor following normal vaginal delivery. She complains of severe pain in the perineal region. Digital exam shows no bleeding but full bladder is palpable. Her HR is 130 per minute and BP is 90/60 mm of Hg. What is the most probable diagnosis?**
   a. Urethral injury
   b. Para vaginal hematoma
   c. Retained placental bits
   d. Atonic bladder

4. **A 34 weeks pregnant with complaints of leaking vaginal discharge. What examination will confirm premature rupture of membranes in this patient?**
   a. Digital examination   b. USG exam
   c. Speculum exam   d. Urine exam

5. **A 22 weeks primigravida had her LMP on June 10 She had regular 32 days cycles prior to that Her EDD would be**
   a. March 17th   b. March 22nd
   c. March 13th   d. March 21th

6. **A 45 years old female, who has underwent sterilization 8 years back, now presents with an ectopic pregnancy. USG reveals gestational sac of 4 cm with beating fetal heart. Best management for this patient?**
   a. Methotrexate
   b. Laparoscopic salpingectomy
   c. Linear salpingostomy
   d. Excision of tubes and anastomosis

7. **Which of the following is diagnostic of GDM by 75 g GTT as per NICE 2015 criteria?**
   a. FBG > 5.1 mmol/L
   b. FBG > 7.0 mmol/L
   c. Fasting blood glucose 5.6 mmol/L
   d. 2 hr PP OGTT more than 5.8 mmol/L

8. **Labor is said to be prolonged when the first and second stage extend arbitrarily beyond:**
   a. 12 hours   b. 18 hours
   c. 24 hours   d. 6 hours

9. **Spigelberg criteria is used in:**
   a. Ovarian pregnancy
   b. Abdominal pregnancy
   c. Cervical pregnancy
   d. Tubal pregnancy

10. **All are true in pregnancy with epilepsy except:**
    a. Seizure risk is decreased by 30%
    b. Valproate causes adverse fetal outcomes
    c. AED causes malformations in 15% cases
    d. Monotherapy is better

11. **Growth restriction during intrauterine period is estimated by which sonographic parameter?**
    a. Femur length
    b. BPD
    c. Abdominal circumference
    d. Head circumference

12. **Drug of choice of PPH resistant to Oxytocin and Ergometrine:**
    a. Carboprost
    b. Dinoprostone
    c. Dinoprost
    d. Misoprostol

13. **A term G2P1L1 presents with active labor. Her cervix is 8 cm dilated; fetal head station +2, MSL+, Type 2 deceleration seen in NST. What is the next step in management?**
    a. Vacuum   b. Forceps
    c. LSCS   d. Wait for spontaneous

14. **In a pregnant mother with hypothyroidism, the dose of levothyroxine in 1st trimester of pregnancy should be:**
    a. Remain same
    b. Decreased by 50%
    c. Increased by 30%
    d. Stopped since levothyroxine is associated with congenital anomaly.

15. **Most common site of ectopic pregnancy is:**
    a. Ampullary portion of fallopian tube
    b. Isthmus
    c. Interstitium
    d. Abdomen

Answers With Explanations

1. **Ans. is a, i.e. Maternal AFP + hCG + Estradiol**

    This is a repeat question and doesn't need explanation- actually it is estriol levels and not estradiol levels which are checked but since in options only estradiol is mentioned so we go with it.

2. **Ans. is d, i.e. 18–20 weeks**   *Ref: see chapter 7of this book for answer and explanation*

3. **Ans. is b, i.e. Para vaginal hematoma**

    This patient is complaining of inability to void, abdominal pain, pallor, severe pain in perineal area and inability to pass urine after vaginal delivery, now all this indicates there is a hematoma.

    For more details see chapter 10 of this book for more details.

4. **Ans. is c, i.e. Speculum exam**   *Ref: Current obs and gynae 10/e, pg 257*

    In a case of PROM …digital examination is contraindicated as it may lead to infection viz chorioamnionitis. For differentiating between PROM and vaginal discharge best is sterile Per speculum examination.

    "A most important step in accurate diagnosis is examination with a sterile speculum. This examination is the key to differentiate PROM from hydrorrhea gravidarum, vaginitis, increased vaginal secretions and urinary incontinence. "

5. **Ans is d, i.e. 21 March**

    We know EDD is calculated using Naegles formula

    EDD= First day of the last menstrual period +9

    Months +7 days

    This formula is for cycle of 28 days.

    Now whatever EDD comes by this formula add or subtract the number of days cycle is above or below the 28 day cycle.

    For e.g., here for 28 day cycle EDD would be= 10 June + 9 months =10 March

    Now add 7 days= 17 March

    Now this females cycle is 32 days i.e. 4 days more than 28 days so add 4 days to the EDD = 21 st march

6. **Ans. is b, i.e. Laparoscopic salpingectomy**   *Ref: Williams' Textbook of Gynecology*

    In this patient gestational sac is 4 cm and cardiac activity is present – as discussed in the text in chapter 17 if cardiac activity is present sac size should be < 3.5 cm then only methotrexate can be given.

    Hence medical management cannot be done.

    This means we have to do surgical management. Now since her ectopic is unruptured we will go for laparoscopic surgery. And if this patient underwent sterilization it means her family is complete we will go for laparoscopic salpingectomy as the surgery of choice.

7. **Ans. is c, i.e. Fasting blood glucose 5.6 mmol/L**

    NICE 2015 guidelines for diagnosing Gestational diabetes

    Gestational Diabetes

    • Diagnose gestational diabetes if the woman has either:
        – A fasting plasma glucose level of 5.6 mmol/litre or above **or**
        – A 2-hour plasma glucose level of 7.8 mmol/litre or above.   *[New 2015]*

    Also know – Metabolic goals as per NICE 2015

    Advise pregnant women with any form of diabetes to maintain their capillary plasma glucose below the following target levels, if these are achievable without causing problematic hypoglycaemia:

    • Fasting: 5.3 mmol/litre **and**

    • 1 hour after meals: 7.8 mmol/litre **or**

    • 2 hours after meals: 6.4 mmol/litre.   *[New 2015]*

8. **Ans. is b, i.e. 18 hours**

    As per the criteria used earlier Labor was said to be prolonged if combined first and second stage extended beyond 18 hours.

9. **Ans. is a, i.e. Ovarian pregnancy**

Site of ectopic	Criteria for diagnosis
Ovarian ectopic	Spigelberg criteria
Abdominal ectopic	Studdiform ectopic
Cervical ectopic	Rubin criteria/ Palmann criteria

10. **Ans. is a, i.e. Seizure risk is decreased by 30%**

In pregnancy the seizure risk increases and doesnot decrease, hence our answer is but obvious.

Now here I want to tell you about antiepileptic drugs and malformations associated with them.

Anti epileptic drugs and malformations:

- In Women with epilepsy not exposed to Anti epileptic drugs (AEDs), the incidence of major congenital malformations is similar to the background risk for the general population. A prospective Finnish population-based study reported a 2.8% (26/939) rate of congenital malformations in the offspring of Women with epilepsy who were not taking AEDs in the first trimester.
- In Women with epilepsy who are taking AEDs, the risk of major congenital malformation to the fetus is dependent on the type, number and dose of AED. Among AEDs, lamotrigine, and carbamazepine monotherapy at lower doses have the least risk of major congenital malformation in the offspring.
- The most common major congenital malformations associated with AEDs are neural tube defects, congenital heart disorders, urinary tract and skeletal abnormalities and cleft palate. Risk of major malformations is 3-5%.
- A milder form of malformations may be present in 8-15% cases.
- Sodium valproate is associated with neural tube defects, facial cleft and hypospadias; phenobarbital and phenytoin with cardiac malformations; and phenytoin and carbamazepine with cleft palate in the fetus.
- A systematic review and meta-analysis of 59 studies provided estimates of incidence of congenital malformation in fetuses born to women taking various AEDs.
- The risk was highest for women taking sodium valproate (10.7 per 100, 95% CI 8.16–13.29) or AED polytherapy (16.8 per 100, 95% CI 0.51–33.05) compared with the 2.3 per 100 (95% CI 1.46–3.1) observed in mothers without epilepsy.
- Data from the EURAP study group13 suggest that the lowest rates of malformation were observed in women exposed to less than 300 mg per day of lamotrigine (2 per 100, 95% CI 1.19–3.24) and to less than 400 mg per day of carbamazepine (3.4 per 100, 95% CI 1.11–7.71).

11. **Ans. is c, i.e. Abdominal circumference**

As discussed in chapter 6 for growth of fetus there is only one ultrasound parameter which is useful and that is abdominal circumference.

Now whether it is Macrosomia/ IUGR – best remains Abdominal circumference.

12. **Ans. is a, i.e. Carboprost**   *Ref: High Risk pregnancy, Fernando Arias 4/e, pg 394*

13. **Ans. is c, i.e. LSCS**

Now in this patient who is in labor, Type 2 deceleration seen i.e. late Deceleration which indicates fetal distress. Now the cervix is 8 cm dilated and not fully dilated so forceps cannot be applied.

Vacium although can be used in 8 cm dilated cervix but in fetal distress vacium cannot be used. Hence the only option is cesarean section.

14. **Ans is c. i.e. Increased by 30%**   *Ref: Williams obs 24/e,pg 1153*

In pregnancy the dose of thyroxine is increased. Increased requirements begin as early as 5 weeks.

15. **Ans. is a, i.e. Ampullary portion of fallopian tube**

As discussed in chapter on ectopic pregnancy, most common site of ectopic pregnancy is ampulla.

JIPMER MAY 2016

1. **A primigravida presents in emergency room with painless bleeding at 12 weeks of gestation. Cervix is closed and normal. What is the diagnosis?**
   a. Threatened abortion
   b. Incomplete abortion
   c. Inevitable abortion
   d. Placenta previa

2. **A pregnant woman at 32 weeks gestation presents to OPD for routine antenatal checkup and an examination she has pedal edema and her BP on repeated recordings is 150/100 mm of Hg. Her urine protein is 2+. Which of the following will be the first line drug of choice in the patient?**
   a. Metoprolol
   b. Methyl dopa
   c. Losartan
   d. Nifedipine

3. **A RH negative patient delivers a RH positive fetus. Which of the following tests should be done before giving Anti D injection to the mother?**
   a. Indirect Coomb's test
   b. Direct Coomb's test
   c. Detection of fetal cells in maternal circulation
   d. Serum bilirubin in cord blood

4. **A primigravida is admitted at 38 weeks of gestation in labor. Admission NST is reactive. However, during active labor, the baseline FHR increased from 140 to 160 bpm with presence of variable decelerations during contractions. The patient was taken for emergency LSCS. The most important reason for the decision is:**
   a. Fetal acidemia
   b. Fetal distress
   c. Non reassuring FHR Pattern
   d. Fetal hypoxic encephalopathy

5. **A 25 years old woman attends the OPD with complaints of having missed her periods. Her urine Pregnancy test is positive and USG reveals a CRL of 12 weeks. She is concerned because she has received MMR vaccine 4 months back. The most appropriate step is:**
   a. Vaccine risk is nil, MTP is completely inappropriate
   b. Vaccine risk is normal, not a reason by itself for MTP
   c. Vaccine risk is high, MTP should be strongly considered
   d. Vaccine risk is high, MTP is mandatory

6. **A primigravida at 42 weeks of pregnancy, Group B Streptococcal (GBS) cultures positive (GBS) is admitted induction of labor. Her Bishop's score is 2. She is started on intravenous Ringer lactate and cervix is ripened with PGE2 gel inserted intracervically. After 1 hour, the FHR drops to 90 bpm as the uterus is contracting every minute with minimal relaxation in between contractions. The cause for uterine hyperstimulation is:**
   a. GBS infection
   b. PGE2 gel
   c. Post term pregnancy
   d. IV fluids

7. **Indications for USG at 32-36 weeks are all except:**
   a. If anomaly scan not done at 1st trimester
   b. In multiple pregnancy
   c. To diagnose IUGR
   d. To determine positioning of placenta

8. **A pregnant lady came for routine follow up at 12 weeks of pregnancy. USG done showed increased nuchal translucency. Which of the following is true regarding nuchal translucency?**
   a. Always due to venous congestion
   b. Increased NT sensitive for cardiac problems
   c. Specific for trisomy 21
   d. Increased in twin to twin transfusion syndrome in monozygotic twins

9. **A woman at term 39 weeks came with history of previous two C-sections out of which classical scar was given in the first one for non-reassuring heart rate, the second one was C section(uneventful). History of appendectomy 10 years back. Major contraindications for VBAC will be which one of the following?**
   a. Previous two C- sections
   b. Classical scar in the first one
   c. Scar of appendectomy 10 years back
   d. Indications was non reassuring heart rate

Answers With Explanations

1. **Ans. is a, i.e. Threatened abortion**

   In this patient bleeding is occurring at 12 weeks so placenta previa is ruled out...where bleeding occurs in third trimester.
   Now because os is closed so inevitable abortion and incomplete abortion are ruled out.
   Hence our answer is Threatened abortion.
   IN Threatened abortion internal os is closed and patient complains of painless bleeding.

2. **Ans. is d, i.e. Nifedipine**

   This patient came for antenatal checkup and was detected with high BP at 32 weeks which indicates that it is PIH. In PIH Metoprolol and Losartan is contraindicated. Now the choice is between Methyldopa and Nifedipine. Between the two, methyldopa is used for the management of chronic hypertension and Nifedipine is used for the management of PIH.

3. **Ans. is b, i.e. Direct Coomb's test**   *Ref: DC Dutta, TB of obstetrics, 8th edition, Pg330*

   In Rh Negative female when a baby is born, following tests are done:
   • Fetal blood group and Rh status
   • Direct Coomb's test
   If fetus is Rh positive and Direct coombs test is negative then Anti D is given

4. **Ans. is c, i.e. Non reassuring FHR Pattern**

   Variable deceleration indicates cord compression and such decelerations are common during labor and do not indicate fetal compromise.
   Variable Decelerations which are > 60 beats in depth or > 60 secs in duration or take a longer time to return to baseline rate are non reassuring and warrant immediate delivery.

5. **Ans. is b, i.e. Vaccine risk is normal, not a reason by itself for MTP**   *Ref: Williams obs 24/e, pg 1243*

   MMR vaccination should be avoided 1 month before or during pregnancy because it contains live attenuated virus. Although there is a small theoretical risk of up to 2.6%, there is no observed evidence that the vaccine induces malformations. MMR vaccination is not an indication for pregnancy termination.

6. **Ans. is b, i.e. PGE2 gel**

   PGE2 or dinoprostone can lead to hyperstimulation of uterus. This patient was inserted PGE2 and after 1hour has fetal distress and uterus is contracting every minute, which indicates hyperstimulation.

7. **Ans. is a, i.e. If anomaly scan not done at 1st trimester**

   For anomaly scan copy USG is done in 1st trimester and repeated at 16 to 20 weeks. There is no use getting a scan done in third trimester as MTP cannot be done beyond 20 weeks.

8. **Ans. is b, i.e. Increased NT sensitive for cardiac problems**

   Increased nuchal translucency is seen in aneuploidy- Downs syndrome, Turners syndrome, Congenital heart disease.

9. **Ans. is b, i.e. Classical scar in the first one**   *Ref: Williams 25/e, pg 594-595*

   Classic cesarean section and T shaped incision in prior pregnancy is an absolute contraindication for VBAC.
   Previous 2 cesarean sections and non reassuring fetal heart rate pattern although are contraindications but not major.

1. The smallest anteroposterior diameter of the pelvic inlet is called the:
   a. Interspinous diameter
   b. True conjugate
   c. Diagonal conjugate
   d. Obstetric conjugate

2. A 25 years of primigravida delivered at term by a normal vaginal delivery. The mother and the baby were during the post natal period. She is very concerned about her vaginal discharge at the time of the discharge. The most appropriate advice for her regarding the discharge is:
   a. Will be present for 2 weeks
   b. Level correlates with lactation
   c. Color changes from bright red to yellow to brown
   d. It is an abnormal phenomenon to have vaginal discharge

3. A pregnant 35-year-old patient is at highest risk for the concurrent development of which of the following malignancies?
   a. Cervix   b. Ovary
   c. Breast   d. Vagina

4. A 26 years old primigravida at 30 weeks of gestation on clinical examination, has blood pressure values of 142/100 mm Hg. 150/94 mmHg and 150/100 at 6 hours intervals. The next line of management is:
   a. Add captopril
   b. Add atenolol
   c. Add methyldopa
   d. No medical management is necessary at present

5. A 32 years old primigravida presents in labor and on examination, the cervix is 2 cm dilated. The fetal heart rate is 148/min and rises to twenty second, then again falls back to 146/min. This type of presentation is suggestive of:
   a. It's a normal pattern
   b. Fetal head compression
   c. Intrauterine fetal bleed
   d. Cord compression

6. A 22 years old female underwent suction evacuation for molar pregnancy. Beta HCG levels are persistently high following evacuation. The next line of management is:
   a. Follow up at 1 year
   b. Monitor until HCG becomes 0

   c. Hysterectomy
   d. Methotrexate

7. A 30 years old female G2P2L2 at 38 weeks gestation presents with labor pains. On examination, cervix is 5 cm dilated and the fetus was found to be in face presentation with left mento anterior position. The next step in management is:
   a. LSCS
   b. Forceps
   c. Expectant management
   d. Vacuum delivery

8. Monochorionic monoamniotic twins occur when splitting of zygote occurs:
   a. At bilaminar germ disc stage
   b. At 8 cell stage
   c. At 2 cell stage
   d. At early blastocyst stage

9. An abnormal attitude is illustrated by?
   a. Breech presentation
   b. Face presentation
   c. Transverse position
   d. Occiput posterior

10. Which of the following is the most accurate way of dating the pregnancy?
    a. Determination of uterine size on pelvic examination
    b. Quantitative serum HCG level
    c. Crown rump length on abdominal or vaginal ultrasound
    d. Determination of progesterone level along with serum HCG level

11. A 28 years old primi, with 28 weeks of gestation presents to the obstetrics department. On obstetrics scan, it is found that she is harboring a twin pregnancy and the first baby is in vertex presentation and the second one in breech presentation. She was very concerned about the course of her labor. The most appropriate advice for her would be:
    a. She has to be delivery by LSCS as the second baby is in breech presentation
    b. She can be allowed for vaginal delivery as the first baby is in vertex presentation
    c. Vaginal delivery and LSCS both can be expected
    d. Vaginal delivery of the first and caesarian delivery of the second twin may be required

Self Assessment & Review: Obstetrics

Answers With Explanations

1. **Ans. is d, i.e. Obstetric conjugate**

    As discussed in the chapter on maternal pelvis, the smallest AP diameter of pelvic inlet is obstetric conjugate.

2. **Ans. is a, i.e. Will be present for 2 weeks**

    Lochia – vaginal discharge after delivery is seen till 2 weeks after delivery. The sequence of discharge is Lochia Rubra, followed by Lochia Serosa and Lochia Alba. That is color changes from red to yellow to white (not brown).

    It is a normal physiological phenomenon to have discharge after delivery. Lochia has no relation to breastfeeding.

3. **Ans. is a, i.e. Cervix**

    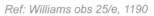
    Ref: Williams obs 25/e, 1190

    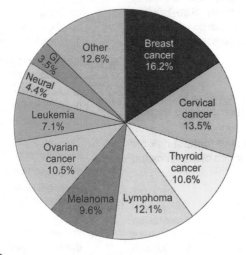

4. **Ans. is c, i.e. Add methyldopa**

    In this case although patient has mild elevated BP but her BP is continuously increasing which means she needs antihypertensive. The antihypertensive which can be used in pregnancy is Methyldopa.

5. **Ans. is a, i.e. It's a normal pattern**

    Fetal accelerations are normal and indicate a healthy fetus

6. **Ans. is d, i.e. Methotrexate**

    Persistently raised βhCG levels after H mole evacuation indicate the patient may develop GTN, and is an indication for Prophylactic methotrexate therapy.

7. **Ans. is c, i.e. Expectant management**

    Vaginal delivery is possible in Mento Anterior position and hence we should wait for fetus to deliver spontaneously.

    In mento posterior cesarean section is mandatory

8. **Ans. is d, i.e. At early blastocyst stage**

    Monochorionic: Monoamniotic twins are seen when division occurs at more than 8 days which means Blastocyst is formed s we all know Implantation occurs in stage of blastocyst and implantation begins by 6 to 7 days after fertilization and is completed by 10th day after fertilization. Hence between this time the stage is Blastocyst.

9. **Ans. is b, i.e. Face presentation**

    Face presentation means head of the fetus is extended. Normal attitude of fetus is that of flexion, hence in face there is abnormal attitude.

10. **Ans. is c, i.e. Crown rump length on abdominal or vaginal ultrasound**

    Best method for dating of pregnancy is ultrasound in first trimester. The best parameter is Crown Rump length.

11. **Ans. is c, i.e. Vaginal delivery and LSCS both can be expected**

    Since first baby is in vertex hence vaginal delivery is possible but because second baby is breech and also due to the risks involved in breech vaginal delivery, we should tell her beforehand that cesarean should be expected.

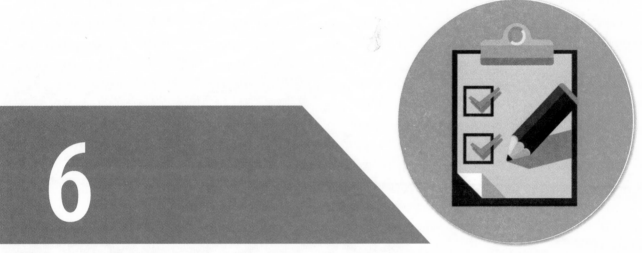

6

Section

Most Recent Papers

1. **In Atonic PPH, which of the following is done?**
   a. Uterine massage is first step in the management
   b. Suction of uterus
   c. IV methylergometrine is given to all patients
   d. B-Lynch suture is put if medical management fails
   1. If a, b, c are correct
   2. If a and c are correct
   3. If b and d are correct
   4. If all four (a, b, c, and d) are correct

2. **IV loading dose of MgSO$_4$ Prophylaxis in Pre-eclampsia is?**
   a. 8 mL MgSO$_4$ + 10 mL of 0.9% NS
   b. 10 mL MgSO$_4$ + 10 mL of 0.9% NS
   c. 8 mL MgSO$_4$ + 12 mL of 0.9% NS
   d. 12 mL MgSO$_4$ + 8 mL of 0.9% NS

3. **True/False regarding the management of a 36 weeks primigravida female diagnosed with transverse lie:**
   a. Repeat USG to confirm the position
   b. Prepared for CS at onset of labor
   c. First breech part is extracted during CS
   d. Most probable cause in this case is placenta previa
   e. Admit at 36 weeks

4. **In GTN, lung metastasis belongs to which stage?**
   a. Stage-1
   b. Stage-2
   c. Stage-3
   d. Stage-4

5. **Anti-D prophylaxis administered in all of the following cases except:**
   a. MTP at 63 days
   b. Manual removal of placenta
   c. Amniocentesis at 16 weeks
   d. Intrauterine blood transfusion at 28 weeks

6. **The given below instrument used in:**

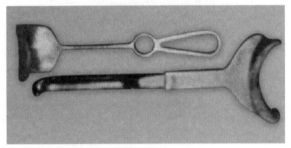

   a. Cesarean section
   b. Vaginal hysterectomy
   c. Fothergill surgery
   d. Suction evacuation

7. **Criteria for high risk infant:**
   a. Have not taken 100 days folic acid
   b. Working mothers
   c. Preeclampsia in pregnancy
   d. Malpresentation during birth

1. **Ans. is 3, i.e. b and d are correct**

   Now before discussing the correct answer, let us discuss each option separately.

   Option a: Uterine massage is the first step in management:

   In a patient of Atonic PPH, the recent guidelines say that initial management includes uterotonic drugs along with uterine massage. Uterine massage which was earlier a part of AMTSL has now been removed from there and included in management of PPH by WHO.

   So, option a is correct.

   Option b: Suction of uterus:

   See, while attempting questions on PPH you will have to be very careful with the language of question.

   If question says, "methods recommended by WHO to treat PPH then suction of uterus will not be included.

   But like this question is saying simply — In ATONIC PPH, which of the following are done.

   Then you will include suction in correct options.

   Principle behind using suction

   When suction of uterus is done, it results in aspiration of all the blood collected in uterine cavity. The quantity of blood sucked larges from 50–300 mL. This causes the inner surface of the uterine cavity to get strongly sucked and the bleeding stops.

   Option c: IV Methylergometrine is given to all patients

   IV ergometrine leads to severe hypertension that is why it should not be used in all patients i.e. option c as incorrect.

   Option d : B-lynch suture is put if medical management fails

   True: B-lynch suture is put if medical management fails

2. **Ans. is c, i.e. 8 mL of $MgSO_4$ + 12 mL of 0.9% NS**

   As per the PRITCHARD regime -
   The loading dose of $MgSO_4$ is:
   I/V = 4 gm (20% $MgSO_4$)
   I/M = 10 gm (50% $MgSO_4$)
   Followed by maintenance dose of 5 gm, $MgSO_4$ I/M in alternate buttock.
   • Now the vial available for $MgSO_4$ has 50% $MgSO_4$ i.e. a 10 mL vial has 5 gm of $MgSO_4$ (0.5 g/mL).
   So for I/M doses: this is appropriate as for loading dose = 10 gm I/M is given, i.e. 1 vial in each buttock.
   And for maintenance dose = 1 vial is given I/M in alternate buttock.
   For I/V: the concentration needed is 20%. The vail available in market has 50% concentration so we will have to make 20% solution, hence take *a 20 mL syringe and add 8 mL of $MgSO_4$ (50%)*.
   8 mL means 4 gm.
   Now add 12 mL of normal saline. So in total 20 mL there is 8 mL of $MgSO_4$ which makes it 20%.

   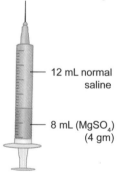

   12 mL normal saline

   8 mL ($MgSO_4$) (4 gm)

3. **Ans. Option (a) True**
   (b) True
   (c) True
   (d) True
   (e) False

We have already dealt with transverse lie in detail. Here we will look at each option separately and decide whether it is true or false.

Options a: Repeat USG to confirm the position

In case of transverse lie, most of the times diagnosis can be made by palpation (in 70%) cases. But for an obese female this is difficult. So USG is done to confirm lie, presentation and position of fetus and also to rule out placenta previa.

Read what operative Obstructive-Munro Kerr 11/e, p 133 has to say—

In transverse lie

"Diagnosis may be suspected by simply inspecting the abdomen, where the uterus is enlarged transversely and shortened vertically. With palpation the emptiness of the lower pole of the uterus is obvious and the head and breech can usually be felt at each side connected by the transverse or obliquely lying fetal back. Only in cases of considerable maternal obesity should it be necessary to resort to an ultrasound to confirm the diagnosis. However, ultrasound is usually advisable to rule out placenta previa or structurally fetal anomaly"

Option b: Prepared for CS at the onset of labor.

This is a true statement, as patient in transverse lie should be prepared for cesarean section. CS is the only management of choice.

Option c: First breech part is extracted during CS – True.

The important points which should be kept in mind for caesarean of Transverse lie:

"Cesarean section for transverse and oblique lie requires careful appraisal of the lower uterine segment once the abdomen has been entered. Unless the membranes are intact and a broad well developed lower uterine segment is present, which is not likely in these circumstances, a vertical incision should be made starting in lower uterine segment. This incision will usually have to be extended into the upper uterine segment to allow adequate room to manoeuvre the fetus into the position of delivery. If accessible it is usually better to deliver the feet first, unless the head is much lower. Munro Kerr 11/e, p 134

Option d: Most probable cause in this case is placenta previa---true

In case of transverse lie: Placenta previa should be considered in all cases. Munro kerr 11/e, p 132

But remember the M/C cause of transverse lie is prematurity.

Option e: Admit at 36 weeks – False.

There is no need to admit the patient at 36 weeks in case of transverse lie. Rather at ≥ 36 weeks, with membranes intact – external cephalic version is attempted which is on OPD procedure.

4. **Ans. is c, i.e. Stage-3**   *Ref. William Gyne, 3/e, p 788, Williams Obs 25/e, p 394*

FIGO staging of GTN

Stage   Involvement
Stage 1   Confined to uterus
Stage 2   Cancer spreads outside the uterus but is limited to structure of genital tract, e.g. vegina
Stage 3   Lung metastasis with or without uterine, pelvic or vaginal involvement
Stage 4   Distant metastasis, e.g. to brain, liver.

5. **Ans. is d, i.e. intrauterine blood transfusion at 28 weeks**   *Ref. Williams Obs 25/e, p 302 Table 15-2*

Causes of fetomaternal hemorrhage which need Anti D

Pregnancy loss	Procedures	Others
Ectopic pregnancy Spontaneous abortion Elective abortion Fetal death (any trimester)	• Chorionic villi sampling • Amniocentesis • Fetal blood sampling • Evacuation of molar pregnancy • Delivery • External cephalic version • Manual removal of placenta	• Abdominal trauma • Placental abruption • Unexplained vaginal bleeding in pregnancy

Note:
- Intrauterine blood transfusion (IUT) means that patient already has developed antibodies against Rh antigen which have crossed the placenta and can lead to hemolysis fetus because of which IUT is being done. Hence, now there is no use of giving Anti D.

Remember: In Rh negative pregnancy—if Rh isoimmunization is suspected, i.e. indirect Coombs test is positive. Peak systolic velocity of middle cerebral artery is determined and if PSV of MCA is >1.5 MOM for gestational age, we obtain fetal blood by cordocentesis for Hb determination.

Indications for giving IUT are:
1. If hemoglobin of fetus is more than two standard deviation below the mean value for that gestational age
2. If hematocrit is less than 30%.

6. **Ans. is a, i.e. Cesarean section**
   - The image given in the question is of Doyen retractor.
   - Doyen retractor is used for retracting the bladder during abdominal operations like LSCS, abdominal hysterectomy, and laparotomy.
   - The smooth edge and the curvature help to retract the bladder protects it during surgeries like cesarean section and hysterectomy.

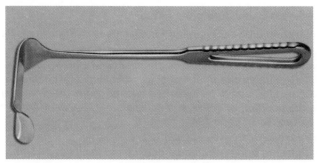

Morris Retractor

Morris retractor is used to retract strong structures like abdominal wall muscles and give space to work.

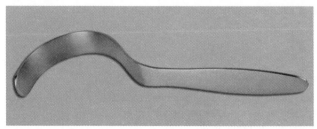

Deaver's Retractor

It helps to retract the soft intra-abdominal visceral organs in procedures like Hysterectomy.

7. **Ans. is c, i.e. Pre-eclampsia in pregnancy**

Infants can be classified as:

Well Infants	High risk Infants
• Born at term	• Infants born preterm on post-term
• Weight appropriate for gestational age	• All LBW infants
• H/O pregnancy, labor, post delivery paused normal	• Infants underweight or overweight for age
• Vital signs are normal in examination	• Wasted infant
	• Infants who have low 1 minute Apgar score
	• Infants born to mothers with complication in pregnancy (like preeclampsia diabetes)
	• Infants with one or more clinical problems since delivery
	• Infants who were sick but are now normal

1. A 30 years old G3P2 patient visits an antenatal clinic at 20 weeks. She reveals during history that her first baby weighed 4.6 kg, second baby weighed 4.8 kg and both were delivered by C-section. The gynecologist suspects gestational diabetes and orders a GTT. The blood sugar level after 50 gm of oral glucose are 206 mg% and the patient is thus confirmed as a case of gestational diabetes. All of the following are known complications of this condition *except*?
   a. Susceptibility for infection
   b. Fetal hyperglycemia
   c. Congenital malformation in fetus
   d. Neonatal hypoglycemia

2. A pregnant lady is suffering from SLE. Which of the following autoantibodies would be responsible if her child has congenital heart block?
   a. Anti-Sm
   b. Anti-dsDNA
   c. Antiphospholipid antibody
   d. Anti-Rho

3. Arrange the following antenatal investigations in sequential order:
   a. NTNB scan
   b. Triple marker test
   c. Anomaly scan
   d. Growth scan

4. Which of the following drugs has neuroprotective action on the fetus when used in preterm birth?
   a. $MgSO_4$
   b. Oxytocin
   c. Nicardipine
   d. Salbutamol

5. What is the best treatment for impending eclampsia at 35 weeks period of gestation?
   a. Steroids
   b. Emergency cesarean section
   c. Induce labor
   d. Magnesium sulfate

6. Multiple correct type. Uterotonic drugs amongst the following are:
   a. Oxytocin
   b. Misoprostol
   c. $PGF_{2\alpha}$
   d. Dinoprostone
   e. None

7. Which of the following types of trophoblast cells invade the spiral arterioles?
   a. Villous
   b. Endovascular
   c. Interstitial
   d. None of the above

Answers with Explanations

1. **Ans. is c, i.e. Congenital malformation in fetus**
    - As explained in the chapter on diabetes if mother's blood sugar levels are increased there is increased susceptibility for infection (hence option a is correct).
    - The fetus is dependent on the mother for glucose, so there is fetal hyperglycemia.
    - Congenital malformations are seen in case of overt diabetes but not in case of gestational diabetes as in gestational diabetes, blood sugar levels are increased from 24–28 weeks onwards, so free radicals are formed from 24–28 weeks onwards (hence option c is incorrect).
    - In neonates of diabetic mothers there is hypoglycemia as the source of increased sugar i.e. condition with mother is no longer there but neonate has increased insulin levels which being about hypoglycemia.

2. **Ans. is d, i.e. Anti-Rho**   *Ref. Williams Obs 25/e, p 1139-1140*

    Friends—SLE in pregnancy is one of the upcoming topics. Read everything about it from the notes I have given in appendix in front of the book.

    As far as congenital heart block is concerned in babies of mothers with SLE—Read what Williams 25/e, has to says—

    "Fetal and neonatal heart block results from diffuse myocarditis and fibrosis in the region between the atrioventricular node and bundle of His. Congenital heart block develops almost exclusively in fetuses of women with antibodies to the SS-A or SS-B antigens."   *Williams 25/e, p 1142*

    > *Note:*
    > - Anti SS-A antibodies are also called as Anti-Rho antibodies.   *Williams 25/e, p 1139*

3. **Ans. is a, b, c and d i.e. NTNB scan; Triple marker test; Anomaly scan; Growth scan**

    > *Note:*
    > - NT = Nuchal translucency   NB = Nasal bone measurement

    NTNB

    Scan is done in 1st trimester as a part of aneuploidy screening. Time 11 to 13 weeks

    Triple marker test is done in second trimester between 15–20 weeks. (Best time = 16–18 weeks)

    Anomaly scan is done in all pregnant females by end of second trimester (18–20 weeks)

    Growth scan is performed in the third trimester for assessing the growth parameters of fetus.

    Hence the sequential order for doing the test is: NTNB scan, triple marker test, anomaly scan, growth scan

4. **Ans. is a. i.e. MgSO$_4$**   *Ref. Williams 25/e, p 824*
    - Many trials have shown that if MgSO$_4$ is given to preterm neonates, it decreases the chances of cerebral palsy in them and provides neuroprotection.
    - The role of MgSO$_4$ for neuroprotection is established in preterm babies born before 28 weeks but not after 28 weeks.
    - Hence, general consensus is to give MgSO$_4$ with threatened preterm delivery from $24^{0/7}$ to $27^{6/7}$ weeks.

    Protocol: Begin I/V infusion of MgSO$_4$ loading dose, 6 g over 20–30 minutes, followed by a maintenance infusion of 2 g per hour.

    If delivery does not occur after 12 hours and is no longer considered imminent, the infusion may be discontinued. If more than 6 hours has passed since discontinuation MgSO$_4$ and delivery is again believed to be imminent, another loading dose may be given followed by maintenance dose.

5. **Ans. is c, i.e. Induce labor**

    Friends, here the question is saying best management of impending eclampsia.

    Best management in other words means definitive management. Definitive management for patient of PIH is always termination of pregnancy.

    The time at which pregnancy is terminated depends in the condition:

    In mild pre-eclampsia- TOP is done at 37 weeks.

In severe pre-eclampsia TOP is done at 34 weeks.

Immediate termination irrespective of gestational age is done in –

- Impending eclampsia
- Eclampsia
- HELLP syndrome
- Reversal of End diastolic flow.

Now this female is having impending eclampsia so we will do immediate termination of pregnancy.

6. **Ans. is a, b, c and d i.e. Oxytocin; Misoprostol; PGF$_{2\alpha}$; Dinoprostone**   *Ref. William 25/e, p 760*

Now as far as oxytocin, misoprostol, PGF$_{2\alpha}$ (carro prost) are concerned we know that these are utero tonics & are also used in prevention and treatment of PPH.

About Dinoprostone = PGE 2   *Williams 25/e, p 760 says*

"E series Prostaglandin can also prevent or treat atony. Dinoprostone PGE2 – may be used off label and given as a 20 mg suppository per rectum or per vaginum every 2 hours.

Intravenous prostaglandin E2- sulprostone is used in Europe but it is not available in the US"

Williams 25/e, p 760

'Hence' Dinoprostone is a uterotonic but is not recommended by WHO hence is used as an off label drug for this purpose.

7. **Ans. is b, i.e. Endovascular**

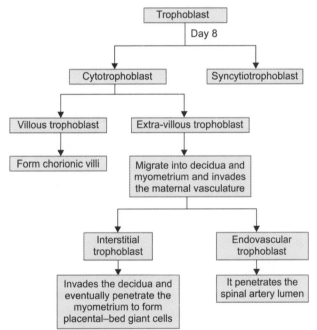

1. True statement regarding renal changes in preeclampsia:
   a. Increased GFR
   b. Glomeruloendotheliosis
   c. Increased renal blood flow
   d. Persistent after delivery

2. During delivery, the baby's head was delivered but shoulders not delivered after one minute. What's the next step?
   a. Emergency LSCS
   b. Cleidotomy
   c. Lateral traction
   d. McRoberts maneuver

3. All of the following are normal in pregnancy *except*:
   a. ALT and AST
   b. Prothrombin time
   c. ALP
   d. GGT

4. False statement regarding chorionic villous sampling:
   a. Chorionic villous sampling done at 16–21 weeks
   b. Done for chromosomal abnormality
   c. Increased nuchal translucency indication for chorionic villous sampling
   d. Trophoblastic cells are tested

5. Uteroplacental blood flow per minute:
   a. 200 mL/minute
   b. 500 mL/minute
   c. 300 mL/minute
   d. 600–700 mL/minute

6. Regarding Listeriosis in pregnancy, which of the following is false?
   a. Cause 2nd trimester loss
   b. Infection on drinking raw milk
   c. Symptoms occur after 3 days of exposure
   d. Leads to granulomatosis infantiseptica

7. Fetal blood flow through placenta:
   a. 200 mL/min
   b. 400 mL/min
   c. 900 mL/min
   d. 100 mL/min

8. A 19 years pregnant woman with mitral valve area 1.4 sq cm is admitted at 6 weeks. She is on antiarrhythmic drugs. Presently she is in NYHA2. She was diagnosed with RHD with MS at 16 years age. What is the risk of maternal mortality?
   a. < 1%
   b. 50%
   c. 15%
   d. 5%

9. Which trophoblast takes part in invasion of arteriole?
   a. Tertiary
   b. Interstitial
   c. Endovascular
   d. Extravillous

10. Drugs that have been under "FDA-X" category in pregnancy/which of the following is a category X drug?
    a. Itraconazole
    b. Isotretinoin
    c. Misoprostol
    d. Cyclophosphamide

Answers with Explanations

1. **Ans. is b, i.e. Glomeruloendotheliosis**
   Renal Changes in Preeclampsia
   - Enlarged glomerulus-**glomeruloendotheliosis**
   - Interstitial cells proliferate
   - Spasm of afferent arterioles
   - **Reduced GFR***
   - Reduced tubular absorption
   - Recovery complete after delivery
   - Bilateral renal cortical necrosis* occur in severe cases

Specific organ damage in preeclampsia	
Organ	**Damage caused due to preeclampsia**
Blood vessels	Vasospasm
Kidney	Glomerular endotheliosis
Liver	Periportal hemorrhagic necrosis, subcapsular hemorrhage
Lungs	Pulmonary edema
Heart	Subendothelial hemorrhages focal necrosis
Brain	Cerebral hemorrhage, edema
Hematology	Hemoconcentration, thrombocytopenia, disseminated intravascular coagulation

2. **Ans. is d, i.e. McRoberts maneuver**
   - If shoulder does not deliver after one minute of delivery of head, the condition is called *Shoulder dystocia*.
   - The management of shoulder dystocia is:
     - Call for help
     - Don't apply fundal pressure
     - Involve the anesthetist and pediatrician
     - Give suprapubic pressure towards the chest side of the baby which will disimpact the shoulder
     - **McRoberts maneuver**—abduct the maternal thighs and hyperflex onto the abdomen.

3. **Ans. is c, i.e. ALP**
   - With the exception of **raised ALP level**, other liver function tests like S. bilirubin, AST, ALT, CPK, LDH are unchanged in pregnancy

Changes in liver function during pregnancy
• Fall in
– Serum total protein
– Serum albumin
• Increase in
– Binding proteins
– Fibrinogen
– Transferrin
– Ceruloplasmin
– Alkaline phosphatase
• Increase in portal venous pressure

4. **Ans. is a, i.e. Chorionic villous sampling done at 16–24 weeks**
   Chorionic villous sampling (CVS)
   - Is done for prenatal diagnosis of genetic disorders
   - It is carried out between **10–13 weeks transcervically** and **transabdominally** from **10 weeks to term**
   - It is done under USG guidance with the help of the long polyethylene catherter with a metal obturator
   - Transabdominally spinal needle of 18–20 gauge is used

- Karyotype result comes in 24 hours in direct preparation and tissue culture takes 10-14 days
- **Complications** include:
  - **Fetal loss (1–2%)**—*M/C complication of chorionic villi sampling*
  - Oromandibular deformity ⎤
  - Limb deformity   ⎦ — M/C complication if CVS is done before 10 weeks
  - Chromosomal anomalies like Down's syndrome, Turner's syndrome and single gene disorders like cystic fibrosis, Tay-Sachs disease can be diagnosed using CVS.
  - If nuchal translucency is increased, it may indicate Down/Turner syndrome and hence diagnostic test karyotyping should be done. For karyotyping in 1st trimester, sample is obtained by CVS.

5. **Ans. is d, i.e. 600–700 mL/minute**   *Ref. Williams Obs 25/e, p 50*
   - Volume of blood in mature placenta —**500 mL**
   - Volume of blood in intervillous space—**150 mL**
   - Uteroplacental blood flow at term is **500-750 mL/min**. The closest answer here is 600–700 mL/min
         Williams Obs 25/e, p 50
   - Fetal blood flow through the placenta—**400 mL/min**

6. **Ans. is c, i.e. symptoms occur after 3 days of exposure**   *Ref. Williams Obs 25/e, p 1223-24*

   Listeriosis
   - Listeria monocytogenes is an **intracellular gram positive bacillus**
   - Infection is caused by consuming **infected raw food** or contact with **infected products of animals (milk).**
   - Incubation period is on an **average 30 days.**
   - Listeria infection is more common in pregnant women, immuncompromised patients and very young or old. In pregnancy incidence is 100 times more than non-pregnant.
   - **Symptoms**—Flu like illlness
   - **Amniotic fluid**—Appears meconium stained/brown in color with fetal infection.
   - **Investigations**—Blood culture during septicaemia.
   - **Complications—Late miscarriage (2nd trimester), preterm labour, still birth, meningitis, encephalitis, pneumonia, gastroenteritis and neonatal death.**
   - **Treatment**—Ampicillin plus gentamicin. In penicilin allergic women trimethaphan and sulfamethoxazole can be given
   - **Prevention**—Avoiding drinking unpasteurized milk, soft cheese, refrigerated smoked sea food.
   - Washing raw vegetable, cooking raw food.
   - Surviving neonates of fetomaternal listeriosis may suffer **granulomatosis infantiseptica**—pyogenic granulomas distributed over the whole body.

7. **Ans. is b, i.e. 400 mL/min**
   - Fetal blood flow through placenta **400 mL/min**
   - Blood flow through intervillous space 500–750 mL/min   *Ref. Dutta Obs 9/e, p 28*

8. **Ans. is a, i.e. < 1%**

Clarke's classification of risk categorization of cardiac disease in pregnancy	
Risk category	**Cardiac disease**
Low risk (maternal mortality < 1%)	• Septal defects • Mitral stenosis, NYHA class I and class II • Patent ductus arteriosus • Pulmonary/tricuspid lesions
Moderate risk (maternal mortality 5–15%)	• Mitral stenosis, NYHA class III and class IV • Marfan syndrome with normal aorta • Uncorrected TOF • Prosthetic valves • Pulmonary hypertension—Primary and secondary
High risk (maternal mortality 25–50%)	• Eisenmenger syndrome • Marfan syndrome with abdominal aorta • Dilated cardiomyopathy • Coarctation of aorta

NYHA: New York Heart Association; TOF: Tetralogy of Fallot

9. **Ans. is c, i.e. Endovascular**
    -   The **cytotrophoblast** that lines the **villous stems** are called **villous cytotrophoblast***.
    -   The cytotrophoblast which **invades the decidua** are known as **interstitial extravillous cytotrophoblast***.
    -   The cytotrophoblast that invades the **spiral arteries** are known as **intravascular/endovascular extravillous cytotrophoblast***.

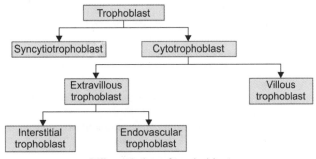

Differentiation of trophoblast

Extravillous trophoblastic invasion

• Interstitial trophoblast
  – Invades decidua basalis and myometrium
  – Forms placental bed giant cells
• Endovascular trophoblast
  – Invades spiral arteries
    - First phase (by 12 weeks): invades arteries in decidua
    - Second phase (by 16 weeks): Invades arteries in myometrium

Functions of the trophoblasts

• Syncytiotrophoblast
  – Transports nutrients and gases
  – Secretes peptide and steroid hormones
• Villous trophoblast
  – Formation of villi
  – Transports of nutrients and gases
• Interstitial trophoblast
  – Interacts with cells of maternal immune system
• Endovascular trophoblast
  – Facilitates placental blood flow

10. **Ans. is b, i.e. Isotretinoin**   *Ref. Dutta Obs 9/e, p 475*
    -   **Category X** drugs are **contraindicated** in pregnancy
    -   Proven fetal risk clearly outway any possible benefit

Drugs in this group are:
• Alcohol • ACE inhibitors • Lithium • Methotrexate • Valproic acid • Mifepristone • Danazol • Isotretinoin • Radioactive iodine

Safety rating system for drugs

Category A: Safety established
- Controlled studies in women show no risk to fetus in first trimester
- No evidence of risk in later trimesters
- Possibility of fetal harm appears remote

Category B: Safety likely
- Animal studies show to fetal risk but no controlled studies in pregnant women or
- Animal studies have shown adverse effect but not confirmed in women in first or later trimesters

Category C: Teratogenicity possible
- Studies in animals have revealed adverse effects on the fetus (teratogenic, embryoidal, or other) but no controlled studies in women *or*
- Studies in women and animals not available
- These drugs should be given only if the potential benefit justifies the potential risk to the fetus

Category D: Teratogenicity probable
- Positive evidence of human fetal risk, but the benefits from use in pregnant women may be acceptable despite the risk, if the drug is needed in:
  - A life-threatening situation *or*
  - A serious disease for which safter drugs cannot be used or are ineffective

Category X: Teratogenicity likely
- Studies in animals and humans have demonstrated fetal abnormalities and/or
- There is evidence of fetal risk based on human experience and
- The risk of the use of the drug in pregnant women clearly outweighs any possible benefit
- Contraindicated in women who are or may become pregnant

Some teratogenic prescription drugs (Category X)

- Androgens and testosterone derivatives (e.g., danazol)
- Angiotensin-converting enzyme (ACE) inhibitors (e.g., enalapril, captopril) and angiotensin II receptor blockers
- Coumadin derivatives (e.g., warfarin)
- Carbamazepine

1. Gold standard test for detection beta hCG is:
   a. β subunit Radioimmunoassay
   b. ELISA
   c. Latex agglutination test
   d. Bioassay
   e. Direct latex agglutination test

2. True about ventouse application during labor:
   a. Cup is placed 3 cm in front of posterior fontanelle
   b. Cup is placed 3 cm posterior to anterior fontanelle
   c. Useful in face presentation
   d. Contraindicated in vertex presentation
   e. Can be used in preterm fetus

3. Cardiac disease in pregnancy associated with highest mortality:
   a. Eisenmenger syndrome
   b. Ebstein's anomaly
   c. Mitral stenosis
   d. Aortic stenosis
   e. Coarctation of aorta

4. Possible complication(s) seen in an infant of diabetic mother is/are:
   a. Hypoglycemia
   b. Hypocalcemia
   c. Hyperglycemia
   d. Hyperkalemia
   e. Congenital heart defects

5. Infectious cause(s) of nonimmune hydrops fetalis is/are:
   a. Cytomegalovirus
   b. Parvovirus B19
   c. HSV 1
   d. HPV
   e. Hepatitis B virus

6. Which of the following structure(s) is/are involved 2nd degree perineal laceration:
   a. Skin, subcutaneous tissue
   b. Internal anal sphincter
   c. External anal sphincter
   d. Superficial perineal muscle
   e. Deep perineal muscles

7. Which of the following parameter(s) is/are useful in diagnosis of Choriomeningitis:
   a. Fetus heart rate > 160 bpm
   b. Purulent vaginal discharge
   c. Low glucose in amniotic fluid
   d. Mother with fever > 100.4°F
   e. WBC > 16,000/cc

8. Component(s) of active management of third stage of labor is/are:
   a. Uterine massage
   b. Controlled cord traction
   c. Immediate cord clamping
   d. Uterotonic agents
   e. Bakri-Balloon baloon

1. **Ans. is a, i.e. β subunit Radioimmunoassay**

"Since the early 1970s, the **gold standard for the measurement of hCG** has been the β subunit radioimmunoassay" — *journals.sagepub.com*

"**Bioassay with animals (*obsolete*)**: The earlier biological tests based on animals, *e.g. Aschheim-Zondek (frog) test, Friedman's test (rabbit), Galli Mainini test (frog) and Hogben test (toad) employed in the past to detect hCG in the urine of pregnant women are only of historical interest and are obsolete and no longer in use*" — *Obs by JB Sharma 1st/65*

Summary of pregnancy tests (β-hCG)

Test	Test sensitivity	Time taken	Inference	Positive on
Immunological tests (urine)				
• Agglutination inhibition test (latex test)	0.5–1 (IU/mL) (urine)	2 minutes	Absence of agglutination	2 days after missed period
• Direct latex agglutination test	0.2 (IU/mL) (urine)	2 minutes	Presence of agglutination	2-3 days after missed period
• Two-site sandwich immunoassay (membrane ELISA/card tests)	30-50 mIU/mL (urine) 1.0 mIU/mL ('67serum)	4-5 minutes	Color bands in the control as well as in test window	On the frist day of the missed period (28th day of cycle)
Various kits in card forms are available			+Pregnant (card test)	Not pregnant (card test)
Enzyme-linked immunosorbent assay	1-2 mIU/mL (serum)	2-4 hours		5 days before the first missed period
Radioimmunoassay				
Radioimmunoassay (β subunit)	0.0002 IU/mL	3-4 hours		25th day of cycle
Immunoradiometric assay (IRMA)	0.05 mIU/mL (serum)	30 minutes		8 days after conception

Hormonal tests of pregnancy

Tests	Sample	Sensitivity (mIU/mL) or IU/L	Time taken	Comments	
1. Biological tests	Urine	3500	5-6 days	45	Obsolete
• Immunological tests					
• Slide test					
• Tube test	Urine	1500	2 mins	44	Not done for low sensitivity
• Latex agglutination	Urine	500	2 mins	34	Not done for low sensitivity
inhibition test (latex test)	Urine	500-1000	2 mins	30 days (2 days after missed periods)	Absence of agglutination
• Direct latex agglutination test		200	2 mins	30 days (2 days after missed period)	Presence of agglutination
3. Home test kits	Urine	10–5	2 mins	30 days (2 days after missed period)	Commonly used in normal pregnancy
4. Enzyme-linked immunsorbent assay (ELISA)	Serum	1–2	2–4 hours		Used in medical management of ectopic pregnancy and for in vitro fertilization (IVF) pregnancies
5. Radioimmunoassay β subunit of hCG (does not cross react with LH)	Serum	2	3-4 hours	25th day (5 days before missing period)	–do–
6. Immunoradiometric assay (IRMA) (Sandwich principle)	Serum	0.05	30 mins	8 days after conception or 25th day (5 days before missing period)	–do–
7. Radio receptor assay serum (not used as it cross reacts with LH)	Serum	1	1 hour	–do–	–do–

2. **Ans. is a, i.e. Cup is placed 3 cm in front of posterior fontanelle**
   - As discussed in chapter on ventouse: The cup is placed 3 cm anterior to posterior fontanelle and 6 cm posterior to anterior fontanelle (i.e. option a is true, b is false)
   - Ventouse cannot be used in presentation other than vertex (i.e. option d is incorrect). It cannot be used in face presentation (i.e. option c is false).
   - Ventouse cannot be used in preterm fetus. (i.e. option c is false).

3. **Ans. is a, i.e. Eisenmenger syndrome**
   Repeat Question

4. **Ans. is a, b and e, i.e. Hypoglycemia; Hypocalcemia; and Congenital heart defects**

   Neonatal Complication (in diabetic mother)   *Ref. Dutta Obs 9/e, p 266; JB Sharma 1/e p 511-12*
   - Hypoglycemia (< 35 mg/dL)
   - Respiratory distress syndrome
   - Hyperbilirubinemia
   - Polycythemia
   - Hypocalcemia (≤ 7 mg/dL)
   - Hypomagnesemia (≤ 7 mg/dL)
   - Cardiomyopathy

5. **Ans. is a, b, c and e, i.e. Cytomegalovirus; Parvovirus B19; HSV 1; Hepatitis B virus**

   "Nonimmune hydrops fetalis (NIHF) has been reported in association with a number of viral, bacterial, and parasitic infectious diseases, including parvovirus, cytomegalovirus, syphilis, and toxoplasmosis. Although the associations are less clear, NIHF has also been reported to occur with Coxsackie virus, trypanosomiasis, varicella, human hypervirus 6 and 7, herpes simplex type 1, respiratory syncytial virus, congenital lymphocytic choriomeningitis virus, and leptospirosis. Parvovirus is the most commonly reported infectious cause of NIHF".–www.ajog.org

   emedicine.medscape.com

Infectious causes of hydrops fetalis
• Parvo B19V
• CMV
• Syphilis
• Herpes simplex
• Toxoplasmosis
• Hepatitis B
• Adenovirus
• Ureaplasmaurealyticum
• Coxsackievirus type B
• Listeria monocytogenes
• Enterovirus
• Lymphocytic choriomeningitis virus (LCMV)

6. **Ans. is a, d and e, i.e. Skin, subcutaneous tissue; Superficial perineal muscle and Deep perineal muscles**

   Classification of perineal tears

Degree		Classification
1		Laceration of the vaginal mucosa or perineal skin only
2		*Laceration involving the perineal muscles but not the anal sphincter*
3		Laceration involving the anal sphincter muscles, being further subdivided into 3A, 3B and 3C
	3A	Where < 50% of the external anal sphincter is torn
	3B	Where >50% of the external anal sphincter is torn
	3C	Where the external and internal anal sphincters are torn
4		Laceration extending through the anal epithelium (resulting with a communication of the vagina epithelium and anal epithelium)

7. **Ans. is a, b, c, d and e, i.e. Fetus heart rate > 160 bpm; Purulent vaginal discharge; Low glucose in amniotic fluid; Mother with fever > 100.4°F; and WBC > 16,000/cc**
   Symptoms and signs of chorioamnionitis   *Obs by JB Sharma 1/e p 468-69*
   Fever, pain abdomen, malaise, foul smelling vaginal discharge

Signs

1. **Fever > 100.4°F/37.8°C**
2. Maternal tachycardia (> 100 bpm or > 20 bpm above the base line)
3. **Fetal tachycardia (> 160 bpm)**
4. Uterine tenderness
5. Foul smelling amniotic fluid

Investigations

1. Maternal leukocytosis (> 16000/cc and shift to left)
2. Raised C reactive protein (CRP) > 2.5
3. High vaginal swab for Gram stain and culture and sensitivity
4. Ultrasound

Biophysical profile (BBP)

- Decreased fetal breathing movements
- Decreased gross fetal body movements
- Non-reactive NST
- Decreased amount of liquor (amniotic fluid volume)
- Decreased fetal tone

Diagnosis is made if there is fever along with 2 or more signs (maternal tachycardia, fetal tachycardia, uterine tenderness, foul smelling vaginal discharge) or investigations (Leukocytosis, raised CRP).

Clinical and amniotic fluid laboratory diagnosis of chorioamnionitis

Test	Result suggesting chorioamnionitis	Comments
Clinical parameters		Generally non-specific
Fever	Temperature > 100.4 twice or >101 once	95–100 sensitive
Maternal tachycardia`	> 100/min	50–80% sensitive
Fetal tachycardia	>160/min	40–70% sensitive
Fundal tenderness	Tenderness on palpation	4–25% sensitive
Vaginal discharge	Foul-smelling discharge	5–22% sensitive
Amniotic fluid parameters		
Culture	Microbial growth	Diagnostic gold-standard
Gram stain	Bacteria or white blood cells (>6/HPF)	24% sensitive, 99% specific
Glucose level	<15 mg/dL	Affected by maternal hyperglycemia 57% sensitive, 74% specific
Interleukin 6	>7.9 ng/mL	81% sensitive, 75% specific
Matrix Metalloproteinase	Positive result	90% sensitive and 80% specific
White blood cell count	> 30/cubic mm	57% sensitive, 78% specific
Leukocyte esterase	Positive (dipsticks)	85–91% sensitive, 95–100% specific

8. **Ans. is a, b and d, i.e. Uterine massage; Controlled cord traction; and Uterotonic agents**

This question has been discussed in detail throughout, I am not explaining it again.

1. **Karyotype of complete H. mole is:**
    a. XX
    b. XY
    c. XO
    d. XXY
    e. XXX

2. **Syphilis screening text in pregnancy:**
    a. RPR
    b. VDRL
    c. TPHA
    d. FTA-ABS
    e. EIA

3. **Ultrasonographic finding of intrauterine pregnancy in first trimester of antenatal period include:**
    a. True gestational sac
    b. Pseudo gestational sac
    c. Corpus luteum in ovary
    d. Fetal pole
    e. Yolk sac

4. **True regarding varicella in pregnancy is/are:**
    a. Congenital malformations are more common when the infection occurs during 12–20 weeks of gestational age
    b. Congenital malformations are more common when the infection occurs during > 20 weeks gestational age
    c. Immunoglobulin can be given to the neonates whose mother had Varicella 5 days before to 2 days after the delivery
    d. Acyclovir is unsafe in pregnancy
    e. Varicella vaccine is given in pregnancy

5. **Cephaly associated with cranio-synostosis is/are:**
    a. Dolicocephaly
    b. Scaphocephaly
    c. Anterior plagiocephaly
    d. Oxycephaly
    e. All of the above

6. **Magnesium toxicity in pregnancy:**
    a. Loss of deep tendon reflexes
    b. Decreased respiratory rate
    c. Decreased urinary output
    d. Hypertension
    e. Increased heart rate

7. **Following is true regarding immunoprophylaxis Hepatitis B in pregnancy:**
    a. A combination of hepatitis B immune globulin (HBIG) and hepatitis B vaccination should be initiated within 24 hours of delivery
    b. HBIG can be given upto 72 hours after birth
    c. In mothers with an unknown HBsAg positivity status at delivery, the birth dose of hepatitis B vaccine can be delayed upto >24 hours of birth
    d. In the case of preterm babies of HBsAg positive mothers, the birth dose is indicated only if the baby weighs more than 2 kilograms
    e. 4 doses of vaccine should be given postnatally

8. **Complication of maternal/gestational diabetes are all except:**
    a. Chromosomal abnormalities
    b. Intrauterine death
    c. Neural tube defects
    d. Macrosomia
    e. Hyperglycemia in newborn

9. **Breech presentation is predisposed by:**
    a. Nulliparity
    b. Prematurity
    c. Aneuploidy
    d. Face presentation

Answers with Explanations

1. **Ans. is a, and b, i.e. XX; and XY** *Ref. Dutta Obs 8/e, p 230; Williams 25/e p 389*
   - The genotype is typically 46,XX (diploid) due to the subsequent mitosis of the fertilizing sperm but can also be 46, XY (diploid). 46, YY (diploid) is not observed. In contrast, a partial mole occurs when a normal agg is fertilized by one or two sperm which then reduplicates itself, yielding the genotypes of 69XXX, 69XXY (triploid) or less commonly 69XYY.

2. **Ans. is a, b and e. i.e. RPR; VDRL; and EIA**
   Ref. https://www.aafp.org/afp/2010/0115/odl.html;https://www.cdc.gov/std/tg2015/syphilis-pregnancy.htm
   - Nontreponemal tests commonly used for initial screening are the Venereal Disease Research Laboratory (VDRL) test or the rapid plasma reagin (RPR) test
   - CDC also recommends treonemal test like EIA/CIA for screening
   - These are typically followed by a confirmatory fluorescent treponemal antibody absorbed test (FTA-ABS) or Treponema pallidum passive particle agglutination test (TPPA).
   - *Screening intervals*: All pregnant women should be tested at main first prenatal visit. For women in high risk groups, many organizations recommended repeated serological testing in the third trimester and delivery.

3. **Ans. is a c, d and e, i.e. True gestational sac; Corpus luteum in ovary; Fetal pole, and Yolk sac**
   Ref. Dutta Obs 7/e, p 642 and 6/e p 68
   - Intrauterine pregnancy is usually diagnosed by a positive pregnancy test and demonstration of a gestational sac in the uterus.
   - A transvaginal scan (more sensitive than a transabdominal scan) can detect an intrauterine gestational sac at 4-5 weeks, an embryo (yolk sac) at 5 weeks.
   - A fetal pole with heart sounds is typically seen by the completion of 7 menstrual weeks
   - In cases of ectopic pregnancy (extrauterine pregnancy), a pseudo sac (due to decidual reaction in the endometrium) may give a false impression of an intrauterine pregnancy.
   - In the first 8 weeks of pregnancy, the corpus luteum is often identified as a cystic mass measuring 1–3 cm in diameter.

4. **Ans. is a, and c, i.e. Congenital malformations are more common when the infection occurs during 12–20 weeks of gestational age; and Immunoglubulin can be given to the neonates whose mother had Varicella 5 days before to 2 days after the delivery**
   Ref. https://www.stanfordchildrens/org/en/topic/default?id=varicella-and-pregnancy-90-P02161
   - When a woman has a varicella infection during the first 20 weeks of pregnancy, there is a 2 percent chance for the baby to develop a group of birth defects called the "congenital varicella syndrome." This syndrome rarely occurs if the infection happens after 20 weeks of pregnancy.
   - Varicella zoster immunoglobulin should be administered to neonates whenever the onset of maternal disease is between 5 days before and 2 days after delivery.
   - If VZIG is not immediately availabe, clincans should provide prophylaxis with acyclovir (800 mg orally 5 times daily for 7 days) or valacyclovir (1000 mg orally 3 times daily for seven days).
   "*Use of acyclovir in the first trimester does not increase birth defects, and it should be the antiviral drug of choice in early pregnancy.*"
   -https://www.aafp.org/afp/2011/0801/p320a.html
   - "This drug has been safely used to treat genital herpes in women in all stages of pregnancy."

   -https://www.drugs.com/pregnancy/acyclovir.html
   - Women should not get vaccinated during pregnancy or during the 30 days before becoming pregnant.

   Varicella and Pregnancy
   - Although more than 90 percent of pregnant women are immune to chickenpox but some pregnant women will develop chickenpox during pregnancy, however, because they are not immune. Pregnant women who get chickenpox are at risk for serious complications.
   - The disease is caused by the varicella-zoster virus (VZV), which is a form of the herpes virus. Transmission occurs from person-to-person by direct contact with an infected person's rash, or through the air by a cough or sneeze. Chickenpox is contagious one to two days before the appearance of the rash until the blisters have dried and become scabs. Once exposed to the virus, chickenpox may take up to 14 to 16 days to develop.
   - *When a woman has a varicella infection during the first 20 weeks of pregnancy, there is a 2 percent chance for the baby to develop a group of birth defects called the "congenital varicella syndrome," This includes scars, defects of muscle and bone, malformed and paralyzed limbs, a small head size, blindness, seizures, and intellectual disability. This syndrome rarely occurs if the infection happens after 20 weeks of pregnancy.*

- Another time there is a concern with a varicella infection is during the newborn period, if the mother develops the rash from five days before to two days after delivery. Between 25 and 50 percent of newborns will be infected in this case, and develop a rash between 5 and 10 days after birth. Up to 30 percent of infected babies will die if not treated. If the mother develops a rash between 6 and 21 days before delivery, the baby faces some risk of mild infection.
- In 1995, the FDA approved a chickenpox vaccine. ***If the baby is treated immediately after birth with an injection of VZIG (varicella-zoster immune globulin), the infection can be prevented or the severity lessened. Varicella zoster immunoglobulin should be administered to neonates whenever the onset of maternal disease is between 5 days before and 2 days after delivery.***
- If a pregnant woman has been exposed to someone with chickenpox or shingles, VZIG can be given within 96 hours to prevent chickenpox, or lessen the severity. ***If VZIG is not immediately available, clinicians should provide prophylaxis with acyclovir (800 mg orally 5 times daily for 7 days) or valacyclovir (1000 mg orally 3 times daily for seven days). Both regimens should be comparable in effectiveness, but the former is less expensive.*** It is important for pregnant women to avoid exposure to anyone with chickenpox if they are not sure whether they are immune to this infection.
- If a patient develops acute varicella, with or without prophylaxis, she should be treated immediately with oral acyclovir or valacyclovir in above mentioned doses.
- If a patient develops evidence of pneumonia, encephalitis, severe disseminated infection, or if she is immunosuppressed, she should be hospitalized and treated with intravenous acyclovir. The appropriate dose for intravenous administration of acyclovir is 10 mg per kg every 8 hours for 10 days. In obese patients, ideal body weight should be used to calculate the dose of acyclovir.
- The best way to protect against chickenpox is to get the chickenpox vaccine. ***Women should not get vaccinated during pregnancy or during the 30 days before becoming pregnant.***

5. **Ans. is e, i.e. All of the above**   *Ref. https://www.ncbi.nlm.nih.gov/pmc/articles/PMC3056371*

- Craniosynostosis is a premature pathologic fusion of one or more cranial vault sutures that leads to abnormal shape of the skull. Dolichocephaly and scaphocephaly are cranial vault deformities that result from premature fusion of the sagittal suture, with a resultant increase in the anterior-posterior dimension as well as restriction of biparietal growth. There is a male predilection. They are the most common cephalies found in craniosynostosis.
- Brachycephaly and anterior plagiocephaly result from premature bicoronal or unicoronal fusion, respectively, with consequent restriction of anterior-posterior calvarial growth and relatively unimpeded biparietal growth. There is a female predilection.
- Oxycephaly results most commonly from a combination of severe sagittal and coronal synostoses. This condition may result in microcephaly with raised ICP and neurologic impairment.

Craniosynostosis

- Craniosynostosis is a premature pathologic fusion of one or more cranial vault sutures that leads to abnormal shape of the skull. The fused sutures lead to restricted growth in some areas and compensatory bossing in other areas. The head may assume different shapes depending upon the site and timing of the abnormally fused suture.
- Sometimes the resulting growth pattern provides the necessary space for the growing brain, but results in an abnormal head shape and abnormal facial features. In cases in which the compensation does not effectively provide enough space for the growing brain, craniosynostosis results in increased *intracranial pressure* leading possibly to visual impairment, sleeping impairment, eating difficulties, or an impairment of mental development combined with a significant reduction in IQ.
- Children born with craniosynostosis have a distinct *phenotype*, i.e., appearance—observable traits caused by the expression of a condition's genes. The features of craniosynostosis' particular phenotype are determined by which suture is closed. The fusion of this suture causes a certain change in the shape of the skull; a deformity of the skull.
- *Virchow's* law dictates that, when premature suture closure occurs, growth of the skull typically is restricted perpendicularly to the fused suture and enhanced in a plane parallel to it, thus trying to provide space for the fast-growing brain. Using this law, the pattern of skull deformity in craniosynostosis often may be predicted.

Types of craniosynostoses

Deformity	Suture (incidence, %)
Dolichocephaly	Sagittal
Scaphocephaly	Sagittal
Brachycephaly	Bicoronal
Anterior plagiocephaly	Unicoronal
Turricephaly	Bilateral lambdoid
Posterior plagiocephaly	Unilateral lambdoid
Trigonocephaly	Metopic
Oxycephaly	Sagittal + coronal
Kleeblattschädel	Sagittal + coronal + lambdoid

6. **Ans. is a, and b, i.e. Loss of deep tendon reflexes; Decreased respiratory rate**

Ref. Miller 7/e p 814; Dutta Obs 7/e p 235; Williams Obs 23/e p 737-39; www.ncbi.nlm.nih.gov)

- The first sign of magnesium toxicity is usually the loss of tendon (patella) reflexes.
- Magnesium sulphate toxicity causes diaphoresis.
- Magnesium toxicity leads to respiratory depression and decreased respiratory rate.
- Magnesium sulphate toxicity can also result in cardiac arrest.

Now as far as oliguria is concerned, it is not a sign of magnesium sulphate toxicity, we check for urine output before giving $MgSO_4$ injection because Magnesium is excreted by kidneys. So if kidneys are not functioning properly, it results in accumulation of magnesium sulphate and its toxicity.

7. **Ans. is a, b and e, i.e. A combination of hepatitis B immune gobulin (HBIG) and hepatitis B vaccination should be initiated within 24 hours of delivery; HBIG can be given upto 72 hours after birth; and 4 doses of vaccine should be given postnatally**

Ref. https://www.indianpediatrics.net/feb2013/feb-189-192.htm

- A combination of hepatitis B immune globulin (HBIG) and hepatitis B vaccination initiated within 24 hours of delivery has been shown to protect 85 to 95% of babies whose mothers were positive for both HBsAg and HBeAg
- Studies have shown that HBIG is effective when administered as late as 72 hours after birth.
- In mothers with an unknown HBsAg positivity status at delivery, the birth dose of hepatitis B vaccine is administered within 24 hours of birth, and HBIG is administered as soon as possible if the mother tests positive, ideally within 72 hours of delivery.
- In the case of preterm babies of HBsAg positive mothers, the birth dose is indicated even if the baby weighs less than 2 kilograms.
- Although the conventional schedule for hepatitis B vaccination consists of three doses including the birth dose, WHO stipulates that four doses may be given in concordance with programmatic requirements of National Schedules. A combination of HBIG and hepatitis B vaccination initiated within 24 hours of delivery, followed by a three dose immunization schedule initiated at 1-2 months of age, has been shown to protect 85 to 95% of babies whose mothers were positive for both HBsAg and HBeAg.

Hepatitis B in pregnancy

- Hepatitis is not a cause of excessive maternal mortality and morbidity in pregnancy.
- In patients of hepatitis B: A modest increase in preterm birth has been observed but no effect is seen on IUGR and pre-eclampsia.

Now copy from Williams p 1064 *-------*

Preventive Strategies

- Transplacental viral infection is uncommon, and Towers and associates (2001) reported that viral DNA is rarely found in amnionic fluid or cord blood. Interestingly, HBV DNA has been found in the ovaries of HBV-positive pregnant women, although this may not be a significant factor in perinatal transmission. The highest HBV DNA levels were found in women who transmitted the virus to their fetuses.
- In the absence of HBV immunoprophylaxis, 10 to 20 percent of women positive for HBsAg transmit viral infection to their infant. This rate increases to almost 90 percent if the mother is HBsAg and HBeAg positive. Immunoprophylaxis and hepatitis B vaccine given to newborns of HBV-infected mothers has decreased transmission dramatically and prevented approximately 90 percent of infections. But, women with high HBV viral loads---106 to 108 copies/mL—or those who are HBeAg positive still have approximately a 10-percent vertical transmission rate, regardless of immunoprophylaxis.
- The Society for Maternal-Fetal Medicine (2016) recommends antiviral therapy to decrease vertical transmission in women at highest risk because of high HBV DNA levels. Although lamivudine, a cytidine nucleoside analogue, significantly lowers the risk of fetal HBV infection in women with high HBV viral loads, recent data indicate that lamivudine may be less effective in the third trimester. Moreover, it is associated with the development of resistant mutations and is no longer recommended at a first-line agent. Newer drugs include the adenosine nucleoside analogue tenofovir and the thymidine analogue telbivudine. Both are associated with a lower risk of resistance than lamivudine. Tenofovir has been recommended as the first-line agent during pregnancy by the Society for Maternal-Fetal Medicine (2016). These antiviral medications appear safe in pregnancy and are not associated with higher rates of congenital malformations or adverse obstetrical outcomes.
- Newborns of seropositive mothers are given HBIG very soon after birth. This is accompanied by the first of a three-dose hepatitis B combinant vaccine.
- The American Academy of Pediatrics and the American College of Obstetricians and Gynecologists (2017) does not consider maternal HBV infection a contraindication to breastfeeding.
- For high-risk mothers who are seronegative, hepatitis B vaccine can be given during pregnancy. The efficacy is similar to that for nonpregnant adults, and overall seroconversion rates approach 95 percent after three doses (Stewart, 2013). The traditional vaccination schedule of 0, 1, and 6 months may be difficult to complete during pregnancy, and compliance

rates decline after delivery. Sheffeld and coworkers (2011) reported that the three-dose regimen given prenatally---initially and at 1 and 4 months---resulted in seoconversion rates of 56, 77, and 90 percent respectively. This regimen was easily completed during routine prenatal care.

A. Immunoprophylaxis

– *A combination of hepatitis B immune globulin (HBIG) and hepatitis B vaccination initiated within 24 hours of delivery has been shown to protect 85 to 95% of babies whose mothers were positive for both HBsAg and HBeAg.*

B. Birth dose of hepatitis B vaccine

– Administration of single antigen hepatitis B vaccine soon after birth is critically important for the prevention of perinatal and early postnatal transmission of HBV infection, and is much more efficacious for this purpose than doses given after the neonatal period.

– The CDC; however, recommends that the birth dose be given within 12 hours after delivery.

C. Vaccination schedule

– *Although the conventional schedule for hepatitis B vaccination consists of three doses including the birth dose, WHO stipulates that four doses may be given in concordance with programmatic requirements of National Schedules. A combination of HBIG and hepatitis B vaccination initiated within 24 hours of delivery, followed by a three dose immunization schedule initiated at 1–2 months of age, has been shown to protect 85 to 95% of babies whose mothers were positive for both HBsAg and HBeAg.*

– The widely spaced schedule with the third dose of hepatitis B vaccine administered at least 6 months after birth, is recommended by the CDC for vaccination of babies of HBsAg positive mothers. However, WHO recommends the closely spaced schedule.

D. Special situations

– *In mothers with an unknown HBsAg positivity status at delivery, the birth dose of hepatitis B vaccine is administered within 24 hours of birth, and HBIG is administered as soon as possible if the mother tests positive, ideally within 72 hours of delivery.*

– *In the case of preterm babies of HBsAg positive mothers, the birth dose is indicated even if the baby weighs less than 2 kilograms*, but should be followed by a further three doses starting at six weeks of age.

– Interruption of the vaccine series does not warrant revaccination, but rather completion of the missed dose as early as possible with a minimum interval of four weeks between two doses.

– Women who are HBsAg negative in pregnancy, but who are at high risk of acquiring hepatitis B infection, including those with a history of multiple sexual partners or of drug abuse, should receive hepatitis B vaccine.

E. Passive immunization

– HBIG is used as an adjunct to the hepatitis B vaccine to prevent vertical transmission. It provides temporary protection that lasts for 3 to 6 months. A combination of HBIG with HBV is more effective than HBV alone in prevention of transmission of hepatitis B.

– *Studies have shown that HBIG is effective when administered as late as 72 hours after birth)*

– The addition of HBIG to active immunization is particularly beneficial when the mother is both HBsAg and HBeAg positive.

8. **Ans. is e, i.e. Hyperglycemia in newborn**

   Repeat

9. **Ans. is b, and c, i.e. Prematurity; and Aneuploidy**

   Ref. Dutta Obs 8/e, p 435

   Etiology of breech presentation

   • **Prematurity**: It is the commonest cause of breech presentation.
   • **Factors preventing spontaneous version**: (a) *Breech with extended legs* (b) Twins (c) Oligohydramnions (d) Congenital malformation of the uterus such as septate or bicornuate uterus (e) short cord, relative or absolute (e) Intrauterine death of the fetus.
   • **Favourable adaptions**: (a) Hydrocephalus—big head can be well accommodated in the wide fundus (b) Placenta praevia (c) Contracted pelvis (d) Cornufundal attachment of the placenta—minimises the space of the fundus where the smaller head can be placed comfortably.
   • **Undue mobility of the fetus**: (a) Hydramnios (b) *Multiparae* with lax abdominal wall.
   • **Fetal abnormality**: Trisomies 13, 18, 21, anencephaly and myotonic dystrophy due to alteration of fetal muscular tone and mobility.